BARNES & NOBLE

Concise

Medical
Dictionary

BARNES
&NOBLE
BOOKS
NEW YORK

This edition of the *Barnes & Noble Concise Medical Dictionary* is based on the *New American Pocket Medical Dictionary, Second Edition* edited by Nancy Roper
© Churchill Livingstone 1988.

Line drawings are taken from the *Churchill's Illustrated Medical Dictionary*
© Neil O. Hardy 1989, by arrangement with Churchill Livingstone Inc. and the artist.

Additional material in this edition
© Barnes & Noble Books 1995.

ISBN 1-56619-735-X

Printed and bound in the United States of America

M 9 8 7 6 5 4 3

Contents

How to use
this dictionary

Main entries These are listed in alphabetical order and appear in **bold** type. Derivative forms of the main entry also appear in **bold** type and, along with their parts of speech, are to be found at the end of the definition.

Separate meanings of main entry Different meanings of the same word are separated by means of an arabic numeral before each meaning.

Subentries Subentries relating to the defined headword are listed in alphabetical order and appear in *italic* type, following the main definition.

Parts of speech The part of speech follows single word main entries and derivative forms of the main entry, and appears in *italic* type. For the parts of speech used in the dictionary, see the list of abbreviations on page v.

Cross-references Cross-references alert you to related words and additional information elsewhere in the dictionary. Two symbols have been used for this purpose—an arrow → and an asterisk.* At the end of a definition, the arrow indicates the word you should then look up for related subject matter. In the case of a drug trade name, it will refer you to the approved name and main definition. For anatomical terms, the arrow will indicate an illustration in Appendix 1 to show the term's position in the body.

Within a definition an asterisk placed at the end of a word means that there is a separate entry in the dictionary which may be of use in providing further information.

Abbreviations

abbr	abbreviation	*opp*	opposite
adj	adjective	*pl*	plural
e.g.	for example	*sing*	singular
esp.	especially	*syn*	synonym
i.e.	that is	™	trademark
i.m.	intramuscular	*v*	verb
i.v.	intravenous	*vi*	intransitive verb
n	noun	*vt*	transitive verb

Guide to pronunciation: consonants

ch (= tsh) as in cheese (chēz),
              stitch (stich),
              picture (pik′chėr).

j (dzh)   judge (juj),
              rigid (rij′id).

sh   dish,
              lotion (lō′-shun).

zh   vision (vizh′-'n).

ng   sing,
              think (thiŋgk).

g   Always hard as in good

th   No attempt has been made to distinguish between the
      breathed sound as in "think" and the voiced sound as
      in "them."

Accent: The accented syllable is indicated by a slanting stroke
          at its termination, e.g., fibrositis (fi-brė-sī′-tis).

Guide
to pronunciation:
vowels

a as in fat, back, tap.

ā	lame, brain (brān), vein (vān).
à	far, calf (kàf), heart (hàrt), coma (kō′mà).
e	flesh, deaf (def), said (sed).
ē	he, tea (tē), knee (nē), anemia (an-ē′-mi-à).
ė	there, air (ėr), area (ėr′-i-à).*
i	sit, busy (biz′-i).
ī	spine, my, eye, tie
o	hot, cough (kof).
ō	bone, moan (mōn), dough (dō).
u	gum, love (luv), tough (tuf), color (kul′-ėr).
ū	mute, due, new, you, rupture (rup′-tūr).
aw	saw, gall (gawl), caul (kawl), water (waw′tėr).
oy	loin, boy.
oo	foot, womb (woom), wound (woond), rude (rood).
ow	cow, sound (sownd), gout (gowt).

*When followed by "r," "e"; is often sound as in "her" or as "u" in "fur" (for example, "ferment"); in "-er" as a final unaccented syllable, the "e" is sometimes more or less elided (drawer, tower).

Prefixes which can be used as combining forms in compounded words

Prefix	Meaning	Prefix	Meaning
a-	without, not	bili-	bile
ab-	away from	bio-	life
abdo-	} abdominal	blenno-	mucus
abdomino-		bleph-	eyelid
acro-	extremity	brachio-	arm
ad-	towards	brachy-	short
adeno-	glandular	brady-	slow
aer-	air	broncho-	bronchi
amb-	} both, on both sides	calc-	chalk
ambi-		carcin-	cancer
amido-	NH₂ group united to an acid radical	cardio-	heart
		carpo-	wrist
amino-	NH₂ group united to a radical other than an acid radical	cata-	down
		cav-	hollow
		centi-	a hundredth
amphi-	on both sides, around	cephal-	head
amyl-	starch	cerebro-	brain
an-	not, without	cervic-	neck, womb
ana-	up	cheil-	lip
andro-	male	cheir-	hand
angi-	vessel (blood)	chemo-	chemical
aniso-	unequal	chlor-	green
ant-	} against, counteracting	chol-	bile
anti-		cholecysto-	gall bladder
ante-	} before, in front of	choledocho-	common bile duct
antero-		chondro-	cartilage
antro-	antrum	chrom-	color
aorto-	aorta	cine-	film, motion
app-	away, from	circum-	around
arachn-	spider	co-	
arthro-	joint	col-	} together
auto-	self	com-	
bi-	twice, two	con-	

NH_2 group united to an acid radical

NH_2 group united to a radical other than an acid radical

coli-	bowel	faci-	face
colpo-	vagina	ferri-	iron
contra-	against	ferro-	
costo-	orib	fibro-	fiber, fibrous tissue
cox-	hip	flav-	yellow
crani-	skull	feto-	fetus
cranio-		fore-	before, in front of
cryo-	cold	gala-	milk
crypt-	hidden, concealed	gastro-	stomach
cyan-	blue	genito-	genitals, reproductive
cysto-	bladder	ger-	old age
cyto-	cell	glosso-	tongue
dacryo-	tear	glyco-	sugar
dactyl-	finger	gnatho-	jaw
de-	away, from, reversing	gyne-	female
deca-	ten	hema-	blood
deci-	tenth	hemo-	
demi-	half	hemi-	half
dent-	tooth	hepa-	liver
derma-	skin	hepatico-	
dermat-		hepato-	
dextro-	to the right	hetero-	unlikeness,
dia-	through		dissimilarity
dip-	double	hexa-	six
dis-	separation, against	histo-	tissue
dorso-	at back	homeo-	like
dys-	difficult, painful,	homo-	same
	abnormal	hydro-	water
ecto-	outside, without,	hygro-	moisture
electro-	external	hyper-	above
em-	electricity	hypo-	below
	in	hypno-	sleep
en-	in, into, within	hystero-	uterus
end-		iatro-	physician
endo-		idio-	peculiar to the
ent-	within		individual
entero-	intestine	ileo-	ileum ilium
epi-	on, above, upon	ilio-	
ery-	red	immuno-	immunity
eu-	well, normal	in-	not, in, into, within
ex-	away from, out,	infra-	below
exo-	out of	inter-	between
extra-	outside	intra-	within

intro-	inward	oculo-	eye
ischio-	ischium	odonto-	tooth
iso-	equal	oligo-	deficiency, diminution
karyo-	nucleus	onc-	mass
kerato-	horn, skin, cornea	onycho-	nail
kypho-	rounded, humped	oo-	egg, ovum
lact-	milk	oophor-	ovary
laparo-	flank	ophthalmo-	eye
laryngo-	larynx	opisth-	backward
lepto-	thin, soft	orchido-	testis
leuco-	white	oro-	mouth
leuko-		ortho-	straight
lympho-	lymphatic	os-	bone, mouth
macro-	large	osteo-	bone
mal-	abnormal, poor	oto-	ear
mamm-	breast	ova-	egg
mast-		ovari-	ovary
medi-	middle	pachy-	thick
mega-	large	pan-	all
melano-	pigment, dark	para-	beside
meso-	middle	patho-	disease
meta-	between	ped-	child, foot
metro-	uterus	penta-	five
micro-	small	pento-	
milli-	a thousandth	per-	by, through
mio-	smaller	peri-	around
mono-	one, single	perineo-	perineum
muco-	mucus	pharma-	drug
multi-	many	pharyngo-	pharynx
myc-	fungus	phlebo-	vein
myelo-	spinal cord, bone marrow	phono-	voice
		photo-	light
myo-	muscle	phren-	diaphragm, mind
narco-	stupor	physio-	form, nature
naso-	nose	pleuro-	pleura
necro-	corpse	pluri-	many
neo-	new	pneumo-	lung
nephro-	kidney	podo-	foot
neuro-	nerve	polio-	grey
noct-	night	poly-	many, much
normo-	normal	post-	after
nucleo-	nucleus	pre-	before
nyct-	night	pro-	

proct-	anus	syn-	together, union, with
proto-	first	tabo-	tabes, wasting away
pseudo-	false	tachy-	fast
psycho-	mind	tarso-	foot, edge of eyelid
pyelo-	pelvis of the kidney	teno-	tendon
pyo-	pus	tetra-	four
pyr-	fever	thermo-	heat
quadri-	four	thoraco-	thorax
quint-	five	thrombo-	blood clot
radi-	ray	thyro-	thyroid gland
radio-	radiation	tibio-	tibia
re-	again, back	tox-	poison
ren-	kidney	tracheo-	trachea
retro-	backward	trans-	across, through
rhin-	nose	tri-	three
rub-	red	trich-	hair
racchar-	sugar	tropho-	nourishment
sacro-	sacrum	ultra-	beyond
salpingo-	fallopian tube	uni-	one
sapro-	dead, decaying	uretero-	ureter
sarco-	flesh	urethro-	urethra
sclero-	hard	uri-	urine
scota-	darkness	uro-	urine, urinary organs
semi-	half	utero-	uterus
sept-	seven	vaso-	vessel
sero-	serum	veno-	vein
socio-	sociology, society	ventro-	abdomen
sphygm-	pulse	vesico-	bladder
spleno-	spleen	xanth-	yellow
spondy-	vertebra	xero-	dry
steato-	fat	xiphi-	} ensiform cartilage of
sterno-	sternum	xipho-	sternum
sub-	below	zoo-	animal
supra-	above		

Suffixes which can be used as combining forms in compounded words

Suffix	Meaning	Suffix	Meaning
-able	able to, capable of	-genic	capable of causing
-agra	attack, severe pain	-gogue	increasing flow
-al	characterized by, pertaining to	-gram	a tracing
-algia	pain	-graph	description, treatise, writing
-an	belonging to, pertaining to	-iasis	condition of, state
-ase	catalyst, enzyme, ferment	-iatric	practice of healing
-asis	state of	-itis	inflammation of
-blast	cell	-kinesis	motion
-caval	pertaining to venae cavae	-kinetic	motion
-cele	tumor, swelling	-lith	calculus, stone
-centesis	to puncture	-lithiasis	presence of stones
-cide	destructive, killing	-logy	science of, study of
-clysis	infusion, injection	-lysis	breaking down, disintegration
-coccus	spherical cell	-lytic	breaking down, disintegration
-cule	little	-malacia	softening
-cyte	cell	-megaly	enlargement
-derm	skin	-meter	measure
-desis	to bind together	-morph	form
-dynia	pain	-ogen	precursor
-ectasis	dilation, extension	-odynia	pain
-ectomy	removal of	-oid	likeness, resemblance
-emia	blood	-ol	alcohol
-esthesia	sensibility, sense-perception	-ology	the study of
-facient	making	-oma	tumor
-form	having the form of	-opia	eye
-fuge	expelling	-opsy	looking
-genesis	formation, origin	-ose	sugar
-genetic	formation, origin	-osis	condition, disease, excess
		-ostomy	to form an opening or outlet

-otomy	incision of	-scope	instrument for visual examination
-ous	like, having the nature of		
-pathy	disease	-scopy	to examine visually
-penia	lack of	-somatic	pertaining to the body
-pexy	fixation		
-phage	ingesting	-somy	pertaining to chromosomes
-phagia	swallowing		
-phasia	speech	-sonic	sound
-philia	affinity for, loving	-stasis	stagnation, cessation of movement
-phobia	fear		
-phylaxis	protection	-sthenia	strength
-plasty	reconstructive surgery	-stomy	to form an opening or outlet
-plegia	paralysis	-taxis	arrangement, coordination, order
-pnea	breathing	-taxy	
-poiesis	making	-tome	cutting instrument
-ptosis	falling	-tomy	incision of
-rhage	to burst forth	-trophic	nourishing
-rhaphy	suturing	-tropic	seeking, acting on or toward
-rhea	excessive discharge		
-rhythmia	rhythm	-urea	urine
-saccharide	basic carbohydrate molecule		

A

abacterial (ā-bak-tē′-rē-ȧl) *adj* without bacteria; word used to describe a condition not caused by bacteria.

abdomen (ab′-dō-měn, ab-dō′-měn) *n* the largest body cavity, immediately below the thorax, from which it is separated by the diaphragm.* Enclosed largely by muscle and fascia, and therefore capable of change in size and shape. It is lined with a serous membrane, the peritoneum,* which is reflected as a covering over most of the organs. *acute abdomen* pathological condition within the abdomen requiring immediate surgical intervention. *pendulous abdomen* a relaxed condition of the anterior wall, allowing it to hang down over the pubis. *scaphoid abdomen* (navicular) concavity of the anterior wall.

abdominal (ab-dom′-in-al) *adj* pertaining to the abdomen. *abdominal aorta* → Figures 10, 19. *abdominal breathing* more than usual use of the diaphragm and abdominal muscles to increase the input of air to and output from the lungs. Can be done voluntarily in the form of exercises; occurring in disease it is a compensatory mechanism for inadequate oxygenation. *abdominal excision of the rectum* usually performed by two surgeons working at the same time. The rectum is mobilized through an abdominal incision. The bowel is divided well proximal to the tumor; proximal end is brought out as a permanent colostomy. Excision of distal bowel containing the tumor together with the anal canal is completed through a perineal incision.

abdominocentesis (ab-dom′-in-ō-sen-tē′-sis) *n* paracentesis* of the peritoneal cavity.

abdominoperineal (ab-dom-in-ō-per-inē′-al) *adj* pertaining to the abdomen and perineum.*

abduct *vt* to draw away from the median line of the body. → adduct *opp*—**abduction** *n*.

abductor *n* a muscle which, on contraction, draws a part away from the median line of the body. → adductor *opp*. *abductor policis longus* → Figure 3.

aberration *n* a deviation from normal. *chromosomal aberration* loss, gain or exchange of genetic material in the chromosomes of a cell resulting in deletion, duplication, inversion or translocation of genes. *mental aberration* → mental. *optical aberration* imperfect focus of light rays by a lens—**aberrant** *adj*.

abiotrophy (ab-ē-ot′-rō-fē) *n* premature loss of vitality or degeneration of certain cells or tissues, usually of genetic origin. → retinitis, chorea.

ablation (ab-lā′-shun) *n* removal. In surgery, the word means excision or amputation—**ablative** *adj*.

ABO incompatibility blood group incompatibility between maternal and fetal blood based on anti-A or anti-B agglutinins in maternal blood and presence of A or B factors in the infant's blood. May cause hemolytic disease of newborn.

abort *vt* to terminate before full development.

abortifacient (ab-ōr-ti-fā′-shent) *adj* causing abortion. Drug or agent inducing expulsion of a nonviable fetus.

abortion *n* 1 abrupt termination of a process. 2 expulsion from a uterus of the product of conception before it is viable, i.e., before 20–24 weeks gestation or before the fetus weighs 500 g. → abortus. *complete abortion* entire contents of the uterus are expelled. *criminal abortion* intentional evacuation of uterus by other than trained, licensed medical personnel, or when abortion is prohibited by law. *habitual abortion* (preferable syn: *recurrent abortion*) term used when abortion recurs in successive pregnancies. *incomplete abortion* part of the fetus or placenta is retained within the uterus. *induced abortion* (also called "artificial") intentional evacuation of uterus. *inevitable abortion* one which has advanced to a stage where termination of pregnancy cannot be prevented. *missed abortion* early signs and symptoms of pregnancy disappear and the fetus dies, but is not expelled for some time. → carneous mole. *septic abortion* one associated with uterine infection and rise in body temperature. *spontaneous abortion* one which occurs naturally without intervention. *therapeutic abortion* intentional termination of a pregnancy which is a hazard to the mother's life and health. *threatened abortion* slight blood loss per vagina while cervix remains closed. May be accompanied by abdominal pain. *tubal abortion* an ectopic* pregnancy that dies and is expelled from the fimbriated end of the Fallopian tube—**abortive** *adj*.

abortus (a-bōr′-tus) *n* an aborted fetus weighing less than 500 g. It is either dead or incapable of surviving.

abrasion (ab-rā′-zhun) *n* 1 superficial injury to skin or mucous membrane from scraping or rubbing; excoriation. 2 can be used therapeutically for removal of scar tissue (dermabrasion).

abscess (ab′-ses) *n* localized collection of pus produced by pyogenic organisms. May be acute or chronic. → quinsy. *alveolar abscess* at the root of a tooth. *amoebic abscess* one caused by *Entamoeba hystolitica;* usual site is the liver. → amoebiasis. *Brodie's abscess* chronic osteomyelitis* occurring without previous acute phase. *cold abscess* one occurring in the course of such chronic inflammation as may be due to *Mycobacterium tuberculosis. psoas abscess* → psoas.

acalculia (ā-kal-kŭl′-ē-à) *n* inability to do simple arithmetic.

acapnia (ā-kap′-nē-ȧ) *n* absence of CO_2 in the blood. Can be produced by hyperventilation—**acapnial** *adj*.

acatalasia (a-kat-al-āzh-ȧ′) *n* genetically determined absence of the enzyme catalase; predisposes to oral sepsis.

accessory nerve eleventh cranial nerve.

accommodation *n* adjustment, e.g., the power of the eye to alter the convexity of the lens according to nearness or distance of objects, so that a distinct image is always retained—**accommodative** *adj*.

accouchement (ak-koosh′-mo) *n* delivery in childbirth. Confinement.

accoucheur (ak-koo-shūr′) *n* man skilled in midwifery; an obstetrician—**accoucheuse** *fem*.

acebutolol (as-e-bū′-to-lol) *n* a β- adrenoceptor blocking agent used in cardiac dysrhythmias, angina pectoris and hypertension. (Sectral.)

acephalous (ā-sef′-a-lus) *adj* without a head.

acetabuloplasty (as-et-ab′-ūl-ō-plas-tē) *n* operation to improve the depth and shape of the hip socket (acetabulum); necessary in such conditions as congenital dislocation of the hip and osteoarthritis of the hip.

acetabulum (as-et-ab′-ūl-um) *n* a cuplike socket on the external lateral surface of the pelvis into which the head of the femur fits to form the hip joint—**acetabula** *pl*.

acetaminophen (a-sēt-a-min′-ō-fen) *n* a nonsalicylate analgesic-antipyretic. (Tylenol.)

acetazolamide (a-sē-ta-zol′-a-mīd) *n* oral diuretic of short duration. Carbonic anhydrase inhibitor. Used for treatment of glaucoma.* (Diamox.)

aceto-acetic acid (as-ē′-tō-as-ē′-tik) (*syn* diacetic acid) a monobasic keto acid. Produced at an interim stage in oxidation of fats in the human body. In some metabolic upsets, e.g., acidosis and diabetes mellitus, it is present in excess in blood and escapes in urine. (It changes to acetone if urine is left standing.) Excess acid in the blood can produce coma.

acetohexamide (as-ēt-ō-heks′-ȧ-mīd) *n* oral antidiabetic drug, one of the sulphonylureas.* (Dymelor.)

acetone (as′-e-tōn) *n* inflammable liquid with characteristic odor; valuable as a solvent. *acetone bodies* → ketone.

acetonemia (as-e-tōn-ēm′-ē-ȧ) *n* acetone bodies in the blood—**acetonemic** *adj*.

acetonuria (as-e-tō-nū′-rē-ȧ) *n* excess acetone bodies in urine, causing a characteristic sweet smell—**acetonuric** *adj*.

acetylcholine (as-et-il-kō′-lēn) *n* chemical substance released from nerve endings to activate muscle, secretory glands and other nerve cells. The nerve fibers releasing this chemical are termed cholinergic. Hydrolyzed into choline and acetic acid by the enzyme acetylcholinesterase, which is present around nerve endings and also in blood and other tissues.

acetylcysteine (as-et-il-sis′-tēn) *n* mucolytic agent, invaluable in cystic* fibrosis. Also used in treatment of paracetamol overdose. (Mucomyst.)

acetylsalicylic acid (as-et-il-sal′-is-il-ik) extensively used mild analgesic. Gastric irritant; can cause hematemesis. Aspirin is the generic name.

achalasia (ak-a-lā′-zhà) *n* failure to relax. *cardiac achalasia* → cardiac.

Achilles tendon (ak-il′-ēz) the tendinous termination of the soleus* and gastrocnemius* muscles inserted into the heel bone (os calcis).

achlorhydria (ā-klōr-hī′-drē-à) *n* absence of free hydrochloric acid in the stomach. Found in pernicious anemia and gastric cancer—**achlorhydric** *adj*.

acholia (ā-kōl′-ē-à) *n* the absence of bile*—**acholic** *adj*.

acholuria (ā-kōl-ūr′-ē-à) *n* the absence of bile* pigment from urine. → jaundice—**acholuric** *adj*.

achondroplasia (ā-kon-drō-plā′-zhà) *n* inherited condition characterized by arrested growth of the long bones resulting in short-limbed dwarfism with a big head. Intellect is not impaired. Inheritance is dominant—**achondroplastic** *adj*.

achromatopsia (ā-krō-ma-top′-zē-à) *n* complete color blindness; only monochromatic grey is visible.

Achromycin™ tetracycline.*

achylia (a-kī′-lē-à) *n* absence of chyle*—**achylic** *adj*.

acid-alcohol-fast *adj* in bacteriology, describes an organism which, when stained, is resistant to decolorization by alcohol as well as acid, e.g., *Mycobacterium tuberculosis*.

acid-base balance equilibrium between acid and base elements of the blood and body fluids.

acidemia (as-id-ē′-mē-à) *n* abnormal acidity of blood (pH* below normal). When caused by poor ventilation and increasing carbon dioxide it is termed *respiratory acidemia*. When caused by increased lactic acid production in muscles it is *metabolic acidemia*. → acidosis—**acidemic** *adj*.

acid-fast *adj* in bacteriology, describes an organism which, when stained, does not become decolorized when subjected to dilute acids.

acidosis (as-id-ō′-sis) *n* depletion of body's alkali reserve, with resulting disturbance of acid-base balance. Acidemia.* → ketosis—**acidotic** *adj*.

acid phosphatase (fos′-fa-tāz) enzyme which synthesizes phosphate esters of carbohydrates in an acid medium. *acid phosphatase test* an increase of this enzyme in blood is indicative of carcinoma of the prostate gland.

aciduria (as-id-ūr′-ē-à) *n* excretion of an acid urine. May occur as result of inborn error and associated with other manifestations.

acini (as'-in-ī) *npl* minute saccules* or alveoli,* lined or filled with secreting cells. Several acini combine to form a lobule—**acinus** *sing,* **acinous, acinar** *adj.*

acne, acne vulgaris (ak'-nē vul-gar'-is) *n* condition in which the pilosebaceous glands are overstimulated by circulating androgens, and excessive sebum* is trapped by a plug of keratin, one of the protein constituents of human hair. Skin bacteria then colonize the glands and convert trapped sebum into irritant fatty acids responsible for swelling and inflammation (pustules) which ensue. Minocycline is the drug of choice.

acneiform (ak-nē'-i-form) *adj* resembling acne.

acoustic nerve eighth cranial nerve. → Figure 13.

acquired immune deficiency syndrome (AIDS) virally caused disease of the immune system, resulting in progressively debilitating opportunistic infections* and a poor prognosis. Transmission of the virus (HIV*) is strictly by exchange of body fluids, hence infective risk is particularly high among the most sexually active and among intravenous drug users.

acriflavine (ak-ri-flā'-vin) *n* powerful antiseptic, used in a 1:1000 solution for wounds, and 1:4000 to 1:8000 for irrigation. Acriflavine emulsion is a bland, nonadherent wound dressing containing liquid paraffin. Proflavine and euflavine are similar compounds.

acrocephaly (ak-rō-sef'-a-lē) *n* (*syn* oxycephaly) congenital malformation in which the top of the head is pointed and the eyes protrude, due to premature closure of sagittal and coronal skull sutures—**acrocephalic, acrocephalous** *adj.*

acrocephalosyndactyly (ak-rō-sef'-a-lō-sin-dak'-til-ē) *n* congenital malformation with pointed head, webbed hands and feet. → Apert's syndrome.

acrocyanosis (ak-rō-sī-an-ō'-sis) *n* coldness and blueness of the extremities due to circulatory disorder—**acrocyanotic** *adj.*

acrodynia (ak-rō-dīn'-ē-à) *n* painful reddening of the extremities such as occurs in erythroedema* polyneuritis.

acromegaly (ak-rō-meg'-a-lē) *n* enlargement of hands, face and feet, occurring in an adult due to excess growth hormone. In a child this causes gigantism. → growth hormone test—**acromegalic** *adj.*

acromicria (ak-rō-mīk'-rē-à) *n* smallness of hands, face and feet, probably due to deficiency of growth hormone from the pituitary gland.

acromioclavicular (ak-rō-mi-ō-kla-vik'-ū-làr) *adj* pertaining to the acromion process (of scapula) and the clavicle.

acromion (ak-rō'-mē-on) *n* the point or summit of the shoulder; triangular process at the extreme outer end of the spine of the scapula—**acromial** *adj.*

acronyx (ak'-rō-niks) *n* ingrowing of a nail.

acroparesthesia (ak-rō-pār-es-thē'-zi-a) *n* tingling and numbness of the hands.

ACTH *abbr* adrenocorticotropic hormone. → corticotropin.

Acthar gel (ak'-thar jel) preparation of ACTH used for diagnostic testing of adrenocortical function and therapeutically for lupus erythematosus, rheumatoid arthritis and allergies.

actin (ak'-tin) *n* one of the proteins in muscle cells; it reacts with myosin to cause contraction.

actinic dermatoses skin conditions in which integument is abnormally sensitive to ultraviolet light.

Actinomyces (ak-tin-ō-mī'-sēz) *n* genus of parasitic funguslike bacteria exhibiting a radiating mycelium. Also called "ray fungus." Many antibiotic drugs are produced from this genus.

actinomycosis (ak-tin-ō-mī-kō'-sis) *n* disease caused by the bacterium *Actinomyces israeli,* the sites most affected being lung, jaw and intestine. Granulomatous tumors form which usually suppurate, discharging a thick, oily pus containing yellowish granules ("sulphur granules")—**actinomycotic** *adj.*

actinotherapy (ak-tin-ō-thė'-ra-pē) *n* treatment by infrared or ultraviolet radiation.

action *n* the activity or function of any part of the body. *antagonistic action* performed by those muscles which limit the movement of an opposing group. *reflex action* → reflex. *sexual action* coitus, cohabitation, sexual intercourse. *specific action* that brought about by certain remedial agents in a particular disease, e.g., salicylates in acute rheumatism. *specific dynamic action* the stimulating effect upon the metabolism produced by the ingestion of food, esp. proteins, causing the metabolic rate to rise above basal levels. *synergistic action* that brought about by the co-operation of two or more muscles, neither of which could bring about the action alone.

acuity (ak-ū'-it-ē) *n* sharpness, clearness, keenness, distinctness. *auditory acuity* ability to hear clearly and distinctly. Tests include use of tuning fork, whispered voice and audiometer. In infants, simple sounds, e.g., bells, rattles, cup and spoon are utilized. *visual acuity* the extent of visual perception is dependent on clarity of retinal focus, integrity of nervous elements and cerebral interpretation of the stimulus. Usually tested by Snellen's* test types at 6 meters. (20').

acupuncture (ak'-ū-punk-tūr) *n* **1** the incision or introduction of fine, hollow tubes into edematous tissue for the purpose of withdrawing fluid. **2** a technique of insertion of special needles into particular parts of the body for the treatment of disease, relief of pain or production of anesthesia.

acute *adj* short and severe; not long drawn out or chronic. *acute defibrination syndrome* (*syn* hypofibrinogenemia) excessive bleeding due to maternal absorption of thromboplastins from retained blood clot or damaged placenta within the uterus. A missed abortion, placental abruption, amniotic fluid embolus, prolonged retention in utero of a dead fetus and intravenous administration of dextran can lead to ADS. *acute dilatation of the stomach* sudden enlargement due to paralysis of the muscular wall. → paralytic ileus. *acute heart failure* cessation or impairment of heart action in previously undiagnosed heart disease or in the course of another disease. *acute yellow atrophy* acute diffuse necrosis of the liver; icterus gravis; malignant jaundice. *acute abdomen* pathological condition within the belly requiring immediate surgical intervention. *acute lymphoblastic leukemia* proliferation of circulating lymphoblasts (abnormal cells). Outlook is reasonably favorable in children and many can expect to be cured after a 2-year course of treatment. *acute myeloblastic leukemia* proliferation of circulating myeloblasts. Condition is rapidly fatal if not treated; average duration of first remission is 14 months.

acyanosis (ā-sī-an-ō′-sis) *n* without cyanosis*—**acyanotic** *adj*.

acyclovir (ā-sī′-clō-vir) *n* antiviral drug used to treat herpes simplex infections. (Zovirax.)

acyesis (ā-sī-ē′-sis) *n* absence of pregnancy—**acyetic** *adj*.

acystia (ā-sis′-tē-ȧ) *n* congenital absence of the bladder—**acystic** *adj*.

Adagen™ pegademase* bovine.

Adam's apple laryngeal prominence in front of the neck, esp. in the adult male, formed by the junction of the two wings of the thyroid cartilage.

Addison's disease (ad′-i-sonz) deficient secretion of cortisol and aldosterone by the adrenal cortex, causing electrolytic upset, diminution of blood volume, lowered blood pressure, weight loss, hypoglycemia, great muscular weakness, gastrointestinal upsets and pigmentation of skin.

adduct *vt* to draw towards the midline of the body. → abduct *opp*—**adduction** *n*.

adductor *n* any muscle which moves a part toward the median axis of the body. *adductor longus* → Figure 3. *adductor magnus* → Figure 3. → abductor *opp*.

adenectomy (ad-en-ek′-to-mē) *n* surgical removal of a gland.

adenitis (ad-en-īt′-is) *n* inflammation of a gland or lymph node. *hilar adenitis* inflammation of bronchial lymph nodes.

adenocarcinoma (ad-en-ō-kȧr-sin-ō′-mȧ) *n* a malignant growth of glandular tissue—**adenocarcinomata** *pl*, **adenocarcinomatous** *adj*.

adenofibroma (ad-en-ō-fī-brō′-mȧ) *n* → fibroadenoma.

adenoid (ad′-en-oyd) *adj* resembling a gland. → adenoids.

adenoidectomy (ad-en-oyd-ek′-to-mē) *n* surgical removal from nasopharynx of adenoid tissue.

adenoids (ad'-en-oydz) *npl* (pharyngeal tonsils) a mass of lymphoid tissue in the nasopharynx which can obstruct breathing and interfere with hearing.

adenoma (ad-en-ō'-mȧ) *n* a nonmalignant tumor of glandular tissue—**adenomata** *pl*, **adenomatous** *adj*.

adenomyoma (ad-en-ō-mī-ō'-mȧ) *n* a nonmalignant tumor composed of muscle and glandular elements, usually applied to benign growths of the uterus—**adenomyomata** *pl*, **adenomyomatous** *adj*.

adenopathy (ad-en-op'-a-thē) *n* any disease of a gland, esp. a lymphatic gland—**adenopathic** *adj*.

adenosclerosis (ad-en-ō-skle-rō'-sis) *n* hardening of a gland with or without swelling, usually due to replacement by fibrous tissue or calcification*—**adenosclerotic** *adj*.

adenosine diphosphate (ADP) (ad-en'-ō-sēn dī-fos'-fāt) important cellular metabolite involved in energy exchange within the cell. Chemical energy is replenished in the cell by phosphorylation of ADP to ATP, primarily in the mitochondrion.

adenosine triphosphate (ATP) (trī-fos'-fāt) intermediate high energy compound which on hydrolysis to ADP releases chemically useful energy. ATP is generated during catabolism and utilized during anabolism.

adenotonsillectomy (ad-en-ō-ton-sil-ek'-to-mē) *n* surgical removal of the adenoids and tonsils.

adenovirus (ad-en-ō-vī'-rus) *n* a group of DNA-containing viruses composed of 47 serologically distinct types; 31 serotypes have been found in man, and many in various animal species. Some cause upper respiratory infection, others pneumonia, others epidemic keratoconjunctivitis.

ADH *abbr* antidiuretic hormone. → vasopressin.

adhesion *n* abnormal union of two parts, occurring after inflammation; a band of fibrous tissue which joins such parts. In the abdomen such a band may cause intestinal obstruction; in joints it restricts movement; between two surfaces of pleura it prevents complete pneumothorax.

adiaphoresis (ā-dī-a-fōr-ē'-sis) *n* lack of perspiration or sweat—**adiaphoretic** *adj*.

adipose (ad'-ip-ōs) *adj* fat; of a fatty nature. Cells constituting adipose tissue contain either white or brown fat.

adiposity (ad-i-pos'-it-ē) *n* excessive accumulation of fat in the body.

aditus (ad'-i-tus) *n* in anatomy, an entrance or opening.

adjuvant (ad'-joo-vant) *n* a substance included in a prescription to aid action of other drugs. *adjuvant therapy* supportive measures in addition to main treatment.

ADL *abbr* activities of daily living.

adnexa (ad-neks′-å) *npl* structures which are in close proximity to a part. *adnexa oculi* the lacrimal apparatus. *adnexa uteri* the ovaries and Fallopian tubes—**adnexal** *adj*.

adoral (ad-ōr′-ål) *adj* near the mouth.

ADP *abbr* adenosine diphosphate.*

adrenal (ad-rē′-nal) *adj* near the kidney, by custom referring to the adrenal glands, one lying above each kidney (→ Figure 19). The *adrenal cortex* secretes mineral and glucocorticoids which control chemical constitution of body fluids, metabolism and secondary sexual characteristics. Under control of the pituitary gland via secretion of corticotropin.* The *adrenal medulla* secretes noradrenaline and adrenaline. → adrenalectomy.

adrenal function tests abnormal adrenalcortical function can be detected by measuring plasma cortisol. If hypoadrenalism is suspected, function is assessed after administration of synthetic ACTH. Increased adrenal medullary function may be detected by measuring urinary vanyl* mandelic acid (VMA) excretion.

adrenalectomy (ad-rē′-nal-ek′-to-mē) *n* removal of an adrenal gland, usually for tumor. If both adrenal glands are removed, replacement administration of cortical hormones is required.

Adrenalin™ epinephrine.*

adrenergic (ad-ren-ėr′-jik) *adj* describes nerves which liberate either noradrenaline* or adrenaline* from their terminations. Most sympathetic nerves release noradrenaline. → cholinergic *opp*.

adrenocorticotropic hormone (ad-ren′-ō-kōr- ti-kō-trōp′-ik) → corticotropin.

adrenogenital syndrome (ad-ren-ō-jen′-it-al) an endocrine disorder, usually congenital, resulting from abnormal activity of adrenal cortex. A female child will show enlarged clitoris and possibly labial fusion, perhaps being confused with a male. Male child may show pubic hair and enlarged penis. In both there is rapid growth, muscularity and advanced bone age.

adrenolytic (ad-re-nō-li′-tik) *adj* that which antagonizes the action or secretion of adrenaline and nonadrenaline.

Adriamycin™ doxorubicin.*

Adrucil™ fluorouracil.*

adsorbents *npl* solids which bind gases or dissolved substances on their surfaces. Charcoal adsorbs gases and acts as a deodorant. Kaolin adsorbs bacterial and other toxins, hence used in cases of food poisoning.

adsorption *n* property of a substance to attract and to hold to its surface a gas, liquid or solid in solution or suspension—**adsorptive** *adj*, **adsorb** *vt*.

advancement *n* operation to remedy squint. Muscle tendon opposite to the direction of the squint is detached and sutured to the sclera anteriorly.

adventitia (ad-ven-tish'-à) *n* the external coat, esp. of an artery or vein—**adventitious** *adj*.

Aerobacter *n* obsolete name for bacteria of genus *Enterobacter** and *Klebsiella*.

aerobe (ā'ėr-ōb) *n* a microorganism which requires O_2 to maintain life. *aerobic exercise* exercise which utilizes inspired O_2 for energy. anaerobe* *opp*—**aerobic** *adj*.

aerogenous (ār-oj'-en-us) *adj* gas producing.

aerophagia, aerophagy (ār-ō-fā-jà) *n* excessive air swallowing.*

Aerosporin™ polymyxin* B.

afebrile (ā-fēb'-rīl) *adj* without fever.

affect (af'-ekt) *n* emotion or mood—**affective** *adj*.

afferent (af'-ėr-ent) *adj* conducting inward to a part or organ; used to describe nerves, blood and lymphatic vessels. → efferent *opp*. *afferent degeneration* that which spreads up sensory nerves.

afibrinogenemia (ā-fī-brin'-ō-jen-ē'-mē-à) *n* inadequate fibrinogen-fibrin conversion; a serious disorder of blood coagulation—**afibrinogenemic** *adj*.

AFP *abbr* alphafetoprotein.*

afterbirth *n* the placenta, cord and membranes which are expelled from the uterus after childbirth.

afterimage *n* visual impression of an object which persists after the object has been removed. Called "positive" when image is seen in its natural colors; "negative" when bright parts become dark, while dark parts become light.

afterpains *n* pains felt after childbirth, due to contraction and retraction of uterine muscle.

agalactia (a-gal-ak'-tē-à) *n* nonsecretion or imperfect secretion of milk after childbirth—**agalactic** *adj*.

agammaglobulinemia (a-gam-a-glob'-ūl-in-ēm'-ē-à) *n* absence of gammaglobulin in blood, with consequent inability to produce immunity to infection. *Bruton's agammaglobulinemia* a congenital condition in boys, in which B-lymphocytes are absent but cellular immunity remains intact. → dysgammaglobulinemia—**agammaglobulinemic** *adj*.

aganglionosis (a-gang-li-on-ō'-sis) *n* absence of ganglia, as those of the distant bowel. → Hirschsprung's disease, megacolon.

agar (ā'gar) *n* gelatinous substance obtained from certain seaweeds; used as a bulk-increasing laxative and as a solidifying agent in bacterial culture media.

agenesis (ā-jen'-es-is) *n* incomplete and imperfect development—**agenetic** *adj*.

age-related macular degeneration (AMD) affects the elderly, cause unknown. Deteriorative changes in macula* cause loss of central vision; peripheral vision generally preserved.

agglutination (ag-gloo'-tin-ā'-shun) *n* the clumping of bacteria, red blood cells or antigen-coated particles by antibodies called "agglutinins," developed in blood serum of a previously infected or sensitized person or animal. Agglutination forms the basis of many laboratory tests—**agglutinable, agglutinative** *adj*, **agglutinate** *vt, vi*.

agglutinins (ag-gloo'-tin-inz) *npl* antibodies which agglutinate or clump organisms or particles.

agglutinogen (ag-gloo'-tin-ō-jen) *n* an antigen which stimulates formation of agglutinins,* used in the production of immunity, e.g., dead bacteria as in vaccine, particulate protein as in toxoid.

aglossia (a-glos'-ē-à) *n* absence of the tongue—**aglossic** *adj*.

aglutition (a-gloo-ti'-shun) *n* dysphagia.*

agnathia (ag-na'-thē-à) *n* absence or incomplete development of the jaw.

agnosia (ag-nō'-zhà) *n* inability to appreciate sensory impressions. *spatial agnosia* loss of spatial appreciation—**agnosic** *adj*.

agonist (ag'-on-ist) *n* a muscle which shortens to perform a movement. → antagonist *opp*.

agranulocyte (ā-gran'-ū-lō-sīt) *n* a nongranular leukocyte.

agranulocytosis (ā-gran-ū-lō-sī-tō'-sis) *n* marked reduction in or complete absence of granulocytes* (polymorphonuclear leukocytes). Usually results from bone marrow depression caused by (a) hypersensitivity to drugs, (b) cytotoxic drugs, or (c) irradiation. Characterized by fever, ulceration of the mouth and throat and quickly leads to prostration and death. → neutropenia— **agranulocytic** *adj*.

agraphia (a-graf'-ē-à) *n* loss of language facility. *motor agraphia* inability to express thoughts in writing, usually due to left precentral cerebral lesions. *sensory agraphia* inability to interpret the written word, due to lesions in the posterior part of the left parieto-occipital region—**agraphic** *adj*.

ague (ā'-gū) *n* malaria.*

AHG *abbr* antihemophilic* globulin.

AIDS *abbr* acquired* immune deficiency syndrome.

AIDS-related complex (ARC) a less severe condition than overt AIDS* which occurs in some people who have contracted the AIDS virus; may be asymptomatic or it may present as a febrile type of illness.

akathisia (ak'-a-thē'-zhà) *n* state of persistent motor restlessness; can occur as a side-effect of neuroleptic drugs.

akinetic (ā-kin-et′-ik) *adj* word applied to states or conditions where there is lack of movement—**akinesia** *n*.

Akineton™ biperiden.*

alanine transaminase (ALT) enzyme present in serum and body tissues, esp. the liver. Acute damage to hepatic cells causes increase in serum concentration.

alastrim (al-as′-trim) *n* less virulent form of smallpox.

Albers-Schönberg disease (al′-bārs–shern′-berg) → osteopetrosis.

albinism (al′-bin-izm) *n* congenital absence, either partial or complete, of normal pigmentation, so that the skin is fair, hair white and eyes pink; due to a defect in melanin synthesis.

albino (al-bī′-nō) *n* person affected with albinism—**albinotic** *adj*, **albiness** *fem*.

albumin (al-bū′-min) *n* a protein found in animal and vegetable matter; soluble in water and coagulates on heating. *serum albumin* chief protein of blood plasma and other serous fluids. → lactalbumin—**albuminous, albuminoid** *adj*.

albuminuria (al-bū-min-ūr′-ē-à) *n* presence of albumin in urine. Condition may be temporary and clear up completely, as in many febrile states. → orthostatic albuminuria. *chronic albuminuria* leads to hypoproteinemia*—**albuminuric** *adj*.

albumose (al′-bū-mōs) *n* an early product of proteolysis. Resembles albumin, but is not coagulated by heat.

albumosuria (al-bū-mōs-ū′-rē-à) *n* presence of albumose in urine—**albumosuric** *adj*.

albuterol (al-bū′-tèr-ol) *n* bronchodilator derived from isoprenaline.* Does not produce cardiovascular side-effects when inhaled in recommended dosage. (Ventolin.)

alcohol (al′-ko-hol) *n* (*syn* ethanol) a constituent of wines and spirits. Absolute alcohol is occasionally used by injection for relief of trigeminal neuralgia and other intractable pain; rectified spirit (90% alcohol) is widely used in preparation of tinctures; methylated spirit contains 95% alcohol with wood naphtha and is for external application only. Enhances action of hypnotics and tranquilizers. *alcohol psychosis* Korsakoff's syndrome.*

alcohol-fast *adj* in bacteriology, describes an organism which, when stained is resistant to decolorization by alcohol.

alcoholuria (al-ko-hol-ū′-rē-à) *n* alcohol in the urine; the basis of one test for fitness to drive after drinking alcohol.

Aldactone™ spironolactone.*

Aldoclor™ drug containing methyldopa* and chlorothiazide.*

aldolase test an enzyme test; the serum enzyme aldolase is increased in diseases affecting muscle.

Aldomet™ methyldopa.*

aldosterone (al-dos'-tėr-ōn) *n* adrenocortical steroid which, by its action on renal tubules, regulates electrolyte metabolism; hence described as a "mineralocorticoid." Secretion is regulated by the renin*- angiotensin system. It increases excretion of potassium and conserves sodium and chloride.

aldosteronism (al-dos'-tėr-ōn-izm) *n* condition resulting from tumors of the adrenal cortex in which electrolyte imbalance is marked and alkalosis and tetany may ensue.

alexia (a-leks'-ē-à) *n* word blindness; inability to interpret significance of the printed or written word, but without loss of visual power. Can be due to a brain lesion or insufficient/inappropriate sensory experience during "ab initio" stage of learning—**alexic** *adj*.

ALG *abbr* antilymphocyte* globulin.

algesia (al-jē'-zi-à) *n* excessive sensitiveness to pain; hyperesthesia. → analgesia *opp*—**algesic** *adj*.

algesimeter (al-jēz-im'-et-er) *n* instrument which registers degree of sensitivity to pain.

algid (al'-jid) *adj* used to describe severe attack of fever, esp. malaria, with collapse, extreme coldness of the body, suggesting a fatal termination. During this stage rectal temperature may be high.

alginates (al'-jin-ātz) *npl* seaweed derivatives which, when applied locally, encourage the clotting of blood. Available in solution and in specially impregnated gauze.

alimentary (al-i-ment'-à-rē) *adj* pertaining to food.

alimentation (al-i-men-tā'-shun) *n* the act of nourishing with food; feeding.

aliquot (al'-i-kwot) *n* part contained by the whole an integral number of times.

alkalemia (al-kal-ēm'-ē-à) *n* → alkalosis—**alkalemic** *adj*.

alkali (al'-ka-lī) *n* soluble corrosive bases, including soda, potash and ammonia, which neutralize acids forming salts and combine with fats to form soaps. Alkaline solutions turn red litmus blue. *alkaline reserve* a biochemical term denoting amount of buffered alkali (normally bicarbonate) available in blood for neutralization of acids (normally dissolved CO_2) formed in or introduced into the body.

alkaline (al'-ka-līn) *adj* 1 possessing the properties of or pertaining to an alkali. 2 containing an excess of hydroxyl over hydrogen ions. *alkaline phosphatase test* an increase in the enzyme alkaline phosphatase in the blood is indicative of such conditions as obstructive jaundice and various forms of bone disease.

alkalinuria (al-ka-lin-ūr'-ē-à) *n* alkalinity of urine—**alkalinuric** *adj*.

alkaloid (al'-ka-loyd) *n* resembling an alkali. Name often applied to a large group of organic bases found in plants and which possess important physiological actions. Morphine, quinine, caffeine, atropine and strychnine are well-known examples of alkaloids—**alkaloidal** *adj*.

alkalosis (al-ka-lō'-sis) *n* (*syn* alkalemia) excess of alkali or reduction of acid in the body. Develops from a variety of causes such as overdosage with alkali, excessive vomiting or diarrhea and hyperventilation. Results in neuromuscular excitability expressed clinically as tetany.*

alkaptonuria (al-kap-tōn-ūr'-ē-à) *n* presence of alkaptone (homogentisic acid) in urine, resulting from only partial oxidation of phenylalanine and tyrosine. Condition usually noticed because urine goes black in the diapers, or when left to stand. Apart from this, and a tendency to arthritis in later life, there are no ill-effects from alkaptonuria.

Alkeran™ melphalan.*

alkylating agents (al'-kil-ā-ting) disrupt the process of cell division affecting DNA in the nucleus, probably by adding to it alkyl groups. Some are useful against malignant cell growth.

allelomorphs (a-lē'-lō-mōrfs) *npl* originally used to denote inherited characteristics that are alternative and contrasting, such as normal color vision contrasting with color blindness, or the ability to taste or not to taste certain substances, or different blood groups. The basis of Mendelian inheritance of dominants and recessives. In modern usage allelomorph(s) is equivalent to allele(s), namely, alternative forms of a gene at the same chromosomal location (locus)—**allelomorphic** *adj*, **allelomorphism** *n*.

allergen (al'-ėr-jen) *n* any antigen* capable of producing manifestation of an immune response—**allergenic** *adj*, **allergenicity** *n*.

allergy (al'-ėr-jē) *n* an altered or exaggerated susceptibility to various foreign substances or physical agents. Sometimes caused by interaction of an antigen with IgE antibody on the surface of mast cells. Scientifically, describes diseases due to altered immune response, a state of altered reactivity. Some drug reactions, hay fever, insect bite reactions, urticarial reactions and asthma are classed as allergic diseases. → anaphylaxis, sensitization—**allergic** *adj*.

allocheiria (al-ō-chīr'-ē-à) *n* an abnormality of tactile sensibility under test, wherein patient refers a given stimulus to the other side of the body.

allograft (al'-lō-graft) *n* grafting or transplanting an organ or tissue from one person to another who does not share the same transplantation antigens.

allopurinal (al-lō-pū′-rin-ol) *n* substance which prevents formation of deposits of crystals from insoluble uric acid. Diminishes tophus* in gout and substantially reduces frequency and severity of further attacks. Can cause skin rash. (Zyloprim.)

alopecia (al-ō-pē′-shē-à) *n* baldness, which can be congenital, premature or senile. *alopecia areata* a patchy baldness, usually of a temporary nature. Cause unknown, probably autoimmune, but shock and anxiety are common precipitating factors. Exclamation mark hairs are diagnostic. *cicatrical alopecia* progressive alopecia of the scalp in which tufts of normal hair occur between many bald patches. Folliculitis decalvans is an alopecia of the scalp characterized by pustulation and scars.

Alophen™ drug containing phenolphthalin.*

alphachymotrypsin (al-fa-kī-mō-trip′-sin) *n* pancreatic enzyme used in ophthalmic surgery to dissolve the capsular ligament and allow the lens to be extracted through the pupil and out of the wound without undue physical manipulation. An anti-inflammatory agent when taken orally.

alphafetoprotein (al-fa-fē′-tō-prō′-tēn) *n* present in maternal serum and amniotic fluid in cases of fetal abnormality.

alphatocopherol (al-fa-tō-kof′-er-ol) *n* vitamin* E.

alprazolam (al-pra′-zō-lam) *n* anti-anxiety drug; benzodiazepine compound acting on the central nervous system. (Xanax.)

ALS *abbr* antilymphocyte* serum. Also advanced life support. Also amyotrophic* lateral sclerosis.

ALT *abbr* alanine* transaminase.

alternative medicine term in use for such diverse techniques as acupuncture, biofeedback, chiropractic, homeopathy, relaxation and yoga.

alum (al′-um) *n* potassium or ammonium aluminum sulfate. Used for its astringent properties as a mouthwash (1%) and as a douche (0.5%). Also used for precipitating toxoid. → APT.

aluminum hydroxide (hī-droks′-īd) antacid with a prolonged action in treatment of peptic ulcer; usually given as a thin cream or gel. No risk of alkalosis with long treatment, as the drug is not absorbed.

aluminum paste mixture of aluminum powder, zinc oxide and liquid paraffin, used as a skin protective in ileostomy; sometimes known as "Baltimore paste."

Alupent™ metaproterenol sulfate.*

alveolar abscess (al-vē′-o-lar) → abscess.

alveolar-capillary block syndrome rare syndrome of unknown etiology characterized by breathlessness, cyanosis* and right heart failure, due to thickening of alveolar cells of the lungs, thus impairing diffusion of oxygen.

alveolitis (al-vē-ōl-ī'-tis) *n* inflammation of alveoli, by custom usually referring to those in the lung; when caused by inhalation of an allergen such as pollen, termed *extrinsic allergic alveolitis*.

alveolus (al-vē'-ol-us) *n* **1** an air vesicle of the lung. **2** bone of the tooth socket, providing support for the tooth, partially absorbed when the teeth are lost. **3** a gland follicle or acinus—**alveoli** *pl*, **alveolar** *adj*.

Alzheimer's disease (alts'-hī-mėrz) a dementing disease also referred to as pre-senile dementia*; there are specific brain abnormalities.

Bronchiole
Pulmonary arteriole
Pulmonary venule
Smooth muscle
Alveolar duct
Alveolar sac
Capillary bed on alveolar sac

alveoli

amalgam (à-mal'-gam) *n* any of a group of alloys containing mercury. *dental amalgam* an amalgam which is used for filling teeth; contains mercury, silver and tin.

amantadine (am-an'-ta-dēn) *n* antiviral agent which reduces length of illness in virus A_2 influenza (Hong Kong flu) and frequency of respiratory complications. Evokes a response similar to but less powerful than that of dopa in relieving tremor and rigidity in Parkinson's disease. (Symmetrel.)

amastia (a-maś-tē-à) *n* congenital absence of the breasts.

amaurosis (am-aw-rō'-sis) *n* partial or total blindness—**amaurotic** *adj*.

amblyopia (am-blē-ōp'-ē-à) *n* defective vision approaching blindness. → smoker's blindness—**amblyopic** *adj*.

ambulant (am'-bū-lant) *adj* able to walk.

ambulatory (am'-bū-là-tor-ē) *adj* mobile, walking about. *ambulatory treatment* term for monitoring a patient at intermittent visits to the outpatients' department of a hospital. Also known as outpatient treatment.

AMD *abbr* age-related* macular degeneration.

ameba (àm-ē'-bà) *n* → *amoeba*.

amelia (à-mē'-lē-à) *n* congenital absence of a limb or limbs. *complete amelia* absence of both arms and legs.

amenorrhea (ā-men-ō-rē'-à) *n* absence of the menses. When menstruation has not been established at the time when it should have been, it is *primary amenorrhea;* absence of the menses after they have once commenced is referred to as *secondary amenorrhea*—**amenorrheal** *adj.*

amentia (a-men'-shà) *n* mental subnormality from birth; to be distinguished from dementia which is acquired mental impairment.

ametria (ā-mēt'-rē-à) *n* congenital absence of the uterus.

ametropia (ā-mēt-rō'-pē-à) *n* defective sight due to imperfect retractive power of the eye—**ametropic** *adj,* **ametrope** *n.*

Amicar™ aminocaproic* acid.

amikacin (a-mi-kā'-sin) *n* antibiotic for especial use in serious Gram-negative gentamicin-resistant infections; a semisynthetic derivative of kanamycin,* altered structurally to resist degradation by bacterial enzymes. (Amikin.)

Amikin™ amikacin.*

amiloride (am-il-ōr'-īd) *n* fairly mild diuretic, but has unusual potassium-conserving properties. When used, potassium supplements are rarely required, but continued use may lead to increased potassium in the blood. (Midamor.)

aminacrine (a-min'-à-krin) *n* nonstaining antiseptic similar to acriflavine, and used for similar purposes in the same strength.

aminoacidopathy (àm-ēn'-ō-as-id-op'-ath-ē) *n* disease caused by imbalance of amino acids.

amino acids (am-ēn'-ō) organic acids in which one or more hydrogen atoms are replaced by the amino group, NH_2. They are the end product of protein hydrolysis and from them the body resynthesizes its own proteins. Ten cannot be elaborated in the body and are therefore essential in the diet—arginine, histidine, isoleucine, leucine, lysine, methionine, phenylalanine, threonine, tryptophan and valine. Remainder are designated nonessential amino acids.

aminoaciduria (am-ēn'-ō-às-id-ūr'-ē-à) *n* abnormal presence of amino acids in urine; usually indicates an inborn error of metabolism as in cystinosis* and Fanconi's syndrome*—**aminoaciduric** *adj.*

aminocaproic acid (am-ēn'-ō-kap-rō'-ik) *n* inhibits plasminogen activators and has a direct hemostatic action by preventing breakdown of fibrin. An antifibrinolytic agent. (Amicar.)

aminoglutethimide (am-ēn-ō-gloo-teth'-i-mīd) *n* drug used to produce adrenal suppression in hormone-dependent cancers. (Cytadren.)

aminophylline (am-in-of'-il-in) *n* theophylline with ethylenediamine. A soluble derivative of theophylline,* widely used in treatment of asthma, congestive heart failure and cardiac edema. (Somophyllin.)

Aminoplex™ synthetic preparation suitable for intravenous infusion. Contains those amino acids normally ingested as protein; has been used to irrigate wounds with good results.

aminosalicylic acid (am-ēn-ō-sal-is-il′-ik) antibacterial drug, used orally as a tuberculostatic.

Aminosyn™ solution of amino acids administered orally or intravenously.

amitosis (a-mi-tō′-sis) *n* division of a cell by direct fission—**amitotic** *adj*.

amitriptyline (am-i-trip′-til-in) *n* a tricyclic antidepressant similar to imipramine* but possessing a pronounced sedative effect which is of particular value in the agitated depressive. (Elavil, Endep.)

ammonia (am-ō′-ni-à) *n* naturally occurring compound of nitrogen and hydrogen. In humans, several inborn errors of ammonia metabolism can cause mental retardation, neurological signs and seizures. *ammonia solution* colorless liquid with a characteristic pungent odor. Used in urine testing—**ammoniated, ammoniacal** *adj*.

ammonium bicarbonate (am-ō′-ni-um bī-kar′-bo-nāt) widely used in cough mixtures as a mild expectorant, and occasionally as a carminative in flatulent dyspepsia.

ammonium chloride (klōr′-īd) used to increase acidity of urine in urinary infections. Occasionally given as a mild expectorant.

amnesia (am-nē′-zhà) *n* complete loss of memory; can occur after concussion, in dementia, hysteria and following ECT. The term *anterograde amnesia** is used for impairment of memory for recent events after an accident, etc., and *retrograde amnesia* when impairment is for past events—**amnesic** *adj*.

amniocentesis (am-nē-o-sen-tē′-sis) *n* piercing the amniotic cavity through the abdominal wall to withdraw a sample of fluid for examination to establish prenatal diagnosis of chromosomal abnormalities, spina bifida, metabolic errors, fetal hemolytic disease, and so on.

amniography (am-nē-og′-ra-fē) *n* X-ray of the amniotic sac after injection of opaque medium; outlines umbilical cord and placenta—**amniographical** *adj*.

amnion (am′-nē-on) *n* innermost membrane enclosing the fetus and containing the amniotic* fluid. It ensheaths the umbilical cord and is connected with the fetus at the umbilicus—**amnionic, amniotic** *adj*.

amnionitis (am-nē-on-īt′-is) *n* inflammation of the amnion.*

amnioscopy (am-nē-os′-ko-pē) *n* amnioscope passed through the abdominal wall enables viewing of the fetus and amniotic fluid. Clear, colorless fluid is normal; yellow or green staining is due to meconium and occurs in cases of fetal hypoxia. *cervical amnioscopy* can be performed late in pregnancy. A different instrument is inserted via the vagina and cervix for the same reasons—**amnioscopic** *adj*.

amniotic cavity (am-nē-ot'-ik) the fluid-filled cavity between the embryo and the amnion.

amniotic fluid liquid produced by the fetal membranes and the fetus, which surrounds the fetus throughout pregnancy. As well as providing the fetus with physical protection, amniotic fluid is a medium of active chemical exchange, secreted and reabsorbed by cells lining the amniotic cavity and swallowed, metabolized and excreted as fetal urine. → amnioscopy. *amniotic fluid embolism* formation of an embolus in the amniotic sac and its transference in the blood circulation of mother to lung or brain. A rare complication of pregnancy. May occur at any time after rupture of the membranes. *amniotic fluid infusion* escape of amniotic fluid into the maternal circulation.

amniotome (am'-nē-o-tōm) *n* instrument for rupturing the fetal membranes. Also called amnihook.

amniotomy (am-nē-ot'-o-mē) *n* artificial rupture of the fetal membranes to induce or expedite labor.

amlodipine besylate (am-lōd'-i-pēn be'-sil-āt) calcium channel blocker. (Norvasc.)

amoeba (am-ē'-bȧ) *n* a protozoon. An elementary, unicellular form of life. The single cell is capable of ingestion and absorption, respiration, excretion, movement and reproduction by amitotic fission. One strain, *Entamoeba histolytica*, is the parasitic pathogen which produces amoebic dysentery* in man. → protozoon—**amoebae** *pl*, **amoebic** *adj*. Also spelled ameba.

amoebiasis (am-ē-bī'-ȧ-sis) *n* infestation of large intestine by the protozoon *Entamoeba histolytica*, causing ulceration and passage per rectum of necrotic mucous membrane and blood (hence "amoebic dysentery"). If amoebae enter the portal circulation they may cause liver necrosis (hepatic abscess). Diagnosis is by isolating the amoeba in the stools.

amoebicide (am-ē'-bi-sīd) *n* agent which kills amoebae—**amoebicidal** *adj*.

amoeboid (am-ē'-boyd) *adj* resembling an amoeba in shape or in mode of movement, e. g., white blood cells.

amoeboma (am-ē-bō'-mȧ) *n* a tumor in the cecum or rectum caused by *Entamoeba hystolytica*. Fibrosis may occur and obstruct the bowel.

Amoxil™ amoxicillin.*

amoxicillin (a-moks-i-sil'-lin) *n* antibiotic; penetrates bronchial secretions more readily than ampicillin,* therefore preferable in chronic lower respiratory tract infections. In acute infections the sole advantage is its greater absorption and high blood levels for equivalent dose. (Amoxil.)

amphetamine (am-fet'-à-mēn) *n* sympathomimetic agent (structurally related to adrenaline*) which is a potent CNS stimulant; formerly used as an appetite suppressant and in the treatment of depression but, because of its addictive potential and frequent abuse, its use is now restricted.

amphotericin B (am-fō-tèr'-i-sin) anti-fungal agent given by i.v. infusion to treat serious systemic infections, e.g., histoplasmosis, candidiasis. It is taken as lozenges to eradicate *Candida* from the mouth; as cream or pessaries for the vagina and orally for treatment of bowel infections. (Fungizone.)

ampicillin (am-pi-sil'-lin) *n* antibiotic active against many, but certainly not all, strains of *Esch. coli, Proteus, Salmonella* and *Shigella;* these are bacteria against which penicillin G* is far less active. Has a wide range of activity and is a broad-spectrum antibiotic. Given orally and by injection. (Omnipen, Polycillin.)

ampule (am'-pūl) *n* hermetically sealed glass or plastic phial containing a single sterile dose of a drug.

ampulla (am-pool'-à) *n* any flasklike dilatation (Figure 17). *ampulla of Vater* the enlargement formed by the union of the common bile duct with the pancreatic duct where they enter the duodenum—**ampullae** *pl*, **ampullar, ampullary, ampullate** *adj*.

amputation *n* removal of an appending part, e.g., breast, limb.

amylase (am'-i-lāz) *n* any enzyme which converts starches into sugars. *pancreatic amylase* amylopsin.* *salivary amylase* ptyalin.* *amylase test* urine is tested for starch to assess kidney function.

amyl nitrite (am'il nīt'-rīt) volatile rapid-acting vasodilator, used by inhalation from crushed ampules. Its action is brief; main use is in treatment of angina.

amyloid (am'-i-loyd) *adj, n* resembling starch. An abnormal complex material which accumulates in certain disorders known as amyloidosis.*

amyloidosis (am-i-loyd-ō'-sis) *n* formation and deposit of amyloid* in any organ, notably the liver and kidney. *primary amyloidosis* has no apparent cause. *secondary amyloidosis* can occur in any prolonged toxic condition such as Hodgkin's disease, tuberculosis and leprosy. Common in the genetic disease familial Mediterranean* fever.

amylolysis (am-il-ol'-is-is) *n* the digestion of starch—**amylolytic** *adj*.

amylopsin (am-il-op'-sin) *n* a pancreatic enzyme, which in an alkaline medium converts insoluble starch into soluble maltose.

amylum (am'-il-um) *n* starch.*

amyotonia congenita (ā-mī-ō-tō'-nē-à con-jen'-it-à) (*syn* floppy baby syndrome) benign congenital hypotonia present at birth in the absence of demonstrable musculoneural pathology. Improvement occurs and the child's progress becomes normal.

amyotrophic lateral sclerosis (ALS) (ā-mī-ō-trō′-fik) (*syn* Lou Gehrig's disease) syndrome of progressive muscular weakness and atrophy with poor prognosis.

anabolic compound (an-ab-ol′-ik) chemical substance which causes a synthesis of body protein. Useful in convalescence. Many of the androgens* are in this category.

anabolism (an-ab′-ol-izm) *n* the series of chemical reactions in the living body requiring energy to change simple substances into complex ones. → adenosine diphosphate, adenosine triphosphate, metabolism.

anacidity (an-as-id′-it-ē) *n* lack of normal acidity, esp. in the gastric juice. → achlorhydria.

anacrotism (an-ak′-rot-izm) *n* an oscillation in the ascending curve of a sphygmographic pulse tracing, occurring in aortic stenosis—**anacrotic** *adj*.

Anadrol™ oxymetholone.*

anaerobe (an′-er-ōb) *n* microorganism which will not grow in the presence of molecular oxygen. When this is strictly so, it is termed an *obligatory anaerobe*. The majority of pathogens are indifferent to atmospheric conditions and will grow in the presence or absence of oxygen and are therefore termed *facultative anaerobes*. aerobe* *opp*—**anaerobic** *adj*.

anaerobic respiration (an-er-ōb′-ik) occurs when oxygen available to the fetus is limited, with the consequent production of lactic and pyruvic acids and a fall in the pH value of fetal blood. This can be measured in labor once the cervix has dilated—by taking a microsample of blood from the fetal scalp.

Anafranil™ clomipramine.*

analeptic (an-à-lep′-tik) *adj*, *n* restorative. Analeptics in current use include caffeine, amphetamines, monoamine oxidase inhibitors and tricyclic antidepressants.

analgesia (an-al-jē′-zhȧ) *n* loss of painful impressions without loss of tactile sense. → algesia *opp*—**analgesic** *adj*.

anaphia (an-af′-ē-ȧ) *n* loss of or reduction in sense of touch.

anaphylactic reaction (an-a-fil-ak′-tik) adverse reaction due to release of the constituents of acute inflammatory cells, generally as a result of antigens binding to IgE on mast cells and basophils. In hayfever* the reaction occurs mainly in the nose; in asthma* it occurs in the lower respiratory tract. In anaphylaxis* it occurs in many tissues throughout the body.

anaphylactoid (an-a-fil-ak′-toyd) *adj* pertaining to or resembling anaphylaxis.

anaphylaxis (an-a-fil-aks'-is) *n* (*syn* serum sickness) a hypersensitive state of the body to a foreign protein (e.g., horse serum) so that injection of a second dose after ten days brings about an acute reaction which may be fatal; in lesser degree it produces bronchospasm, pallor and collapse. → allergy, sensitization—**anaphylactic** *adj*.

anaplasia (an-a-plā'-zhà) *n* loss of the distinctive characteristics of a cell, associated with proliferative activity as in cancer—**anaplastic** *adj*.

anarthria (an-àr'-thrē-à) *n* loss of physical ability to form speech.

anasarca (an-a-sar'-kà) *n* serous infiltration of cellular tissues and serous cavities; generalized edema—**anasarcous** *adj*.

anastomosis (an-as-to-mō'-sis) *n* **1** the intercommunication of the branches of two or more arteries or veins. **2** in surgery, establishment of an intercommunication between two hollow organs, vessels or nerves—**anastomoses** *pl*, **anastomotic** *adj*, **anastomose** *vt*.

anatomical position anterior view of the upright body facing forward, hands by the sides with palms facing forwards. Posterior view is of the back of the upright body in that position.

anatomy (an-at'-o-mē) *n* science which deals with the structure of the body by means of dissection—**anatomical** *adj*.

ancillary (an'-sil-ār-ē) *n* something that aids an action but is not necessary for performance of the action.

Ancobon™ flucytosine.*

Ancylostoma (angk-sil-os'-to-mà) *n* (*syn* human hookworm). *Ancylostoma duodenale* is predominantly found in southern Europe and the Middle and Far East. *Necator americanus* is found in the Americas and tropical Africa. Mixed infections are not uncommon. Only clinically significant when infestation is moderate or heavy. Worm inhabits duodenum and upper jejunum; eggs are passed in stools, hatch in moist soil and produce larvae which can penetrate bare feet and reinfect people. Prevention is by wearing shoes and using latrines.

ancylostomiasis (angk-sil-os-to-mī'-a-sis) *n* (*syn* hookworm disease) infestation of intestine with Ancylostoma, giving rise to malnutrition and severe anemia.

androblastoma (an-drō-blas-tō'-mà) *n* (*syn* arrhenoblastoma) a tumor of the ovary; can produce male or female hormones and can cause masculinization in women or precocious puberty in girls.

androgens (an'-drō-jenz) *npl* hormones secreted by the testes and adrenal cortex, or synthetic substances, which control the building up of protein and the male secondary sex characteristics, e.g., distribution of hair and deepening of voice. When given to females they have a masculinizing effect. → testosterone—**androgenic, androgenous** *adj*.

anemia (an-ē'-mē-à) *n* deficiency of hemoglobin in blood due to lack of red blood cells and/or their hemoglobin content. Produces clinical manifestations arising from hypoxemia,* such as lassitude and breathlessness on exertion. Treatment is according to cause and there are many. *aplastic anemia* is the result of complete bone marrow failure. *pernicious anemia* results from the inability of bone marrow to produce normal red cells through lack of a protein released by gastric glands, the intrinsic factor, which is necessary for absorption of vitamin B_{12} from food. An autoimmune mechanism may be responsible. *sickle-cell anemia* familial, hereditary hemolytic anemia peculiar to blacks. The red cells are crescent-shaped. *splenic anemia* (*syn* Banti's disease) leukopenia, thrombocytopenia, alimentary bleeding, and splenomegaly which in turn is caused by portal hypertension. → Addison's disease, hemolytic disease of the newborn, spherocytosis, thalassemia—**anemic** *adj*.

anencephaly (an-en-sef'-a-lē) *n* congenital absence of the brain; the condition is incompatible with life. Detected by raised levels of alphafetoprotein in amniotic fluid—**anencephalous, anencephalic** *adj*.

anesthesia (an-es-thē'-zhà) *n* loss of sensation. *general anesthesia* loss of sensation with loss of consciousness. In *local anesthesia* nerve conduction is blocked directly and painful impulses fail to reach the brain. *spinal anesthesia* may be caused by (a) injection of a local anesthetic into the spinal subarachnoid space, (b) a lesion of the spinal cord.

anesthesiology (an-es-thēz-ē-ol'-o-jē) *n* science dealing with anesthetics, their administration and effect.

anesthetic (an-es-thet'-ik) *n, adj* 1 a drug which produces anesthesia. 2 causing anesthesia. 3 insensible to stimuli. *general anesthetic* drug which produces general anesthesia by inhalation or injection. *local anesthetic* a drug which injected into issues or applied topically causes local insensibility to pain. *spinal anesthetic* → spinal—**anesthetize** *vt*.

aneurine (a-nū'-rin) *n* thiamine or vitamin B_1.

aneurysm (an'-ūr-izm) *n* dilation of a blood vessel, usually an artery, due to local fault in the wall through defect, disease or injury, producing a pulsating swelling over which a murmur may be heard. True aneurysms may be saccular, fusiform, or dissecting where the blood flows between the layers of the arterial wall—**aneurysmal** *adj*.

angiectasis (an-jē-ek'-tà-sis) *n* abnormal dilatation of blood vessels. → telangiectasis—**angiectatic** *adj*.

angiitis (an-jē-ī'-tis) *n* inflammation of a blood or lymph vessel. → vasculitis—**angiitic** *adj*.

angina (an-jī′-ná) *n* sense of suffocation or constriction. *angina pectoris* severe but temporary attack of cardiac pain which may radiate to the arms. Results from myocardial ischemia. Often the attack is induced by exercise (angina of effort)—**anginal** *adj*.

angiocardiography (an-jē-ō-kár-dē-og′-raf-ē) *n* demonstration of the chambers of the heart and great vessels after injection of an opaque medium—**angiocardiographic** *adj*, **angiocardiogram** *n*, **angiocardiograph** *n*.

angioedema (an-jē-ō-e-dē′-má) *n (syn* angioneurotic edema) severe form of urticaria* which may involve skin of the face, hands or genitals and the mucous membrane of mouth and throat; edema of the glottis may be fatal. Immediately there is an abrupt local increase in vascular permeability, as a result of which fluid escapes from blood vessels into surrounding tissues. Swelling may be due to an allergic hypersensitivity reaction to drugs, pollens or other known allergens, but in many cases no cause can be found.

angiography (an-jē-og′-ra-fē) *n* demonstration of the arterial system after injection of an opaque medium—**angiographic** *adj*, **angiogram** *n*, **angiograph** *n*.

angiology (an-jē-ol′-o-jē) *n* science dealing with blood and lymphatic vessels—**angiological** *adj*.

angioma (an-jē-ō′-má) *n* nonmalignant tumor of blood vessels, usually capillaries. *spider angioma* appears as central lesion with radiating tendrils; develops in liver cirrhosis and in pregnancy.

angioplasty (an′-jē-ō-plas-tē) *n* plastic surgery of blood vessels. *percutaneous transluminal coronary angioplasty* a balloon is passed into a stenosed coronary artery and inflated with contrast medium; it presses the atheroma against the vessel wall, thereby increasing the lumen—**angioplastic** *adj*.

angiosarcoma (an-jē-ō-sár-kō′-má) *n* malignant tumor arising from blood vessels—**angiosarcomata** *pl*, **angiosarcomatous** *adj*.

angiospasm (an′-jē-ō-spazm) *n* constricting spasm of blood vessels—**angiospastic** *adj*.

angiotensin (an-jē-ō-ten′-sin) *n* inactive substance formed by action of renin* on a protein in blood plasma. In the lungs angiotensin I is converted into angiotensin II, a highly active substance which constricts blood vessels and causes release of aldosterone* from the adrenal cortex. (Hypertensin.)

angular stomatitis → stomatitis.

anhidrosis (an-hī-drō′-sis) *n* deficient sweat secretion—**anhidrotic** *adj*.

anhidrotics (an-hī-dro′-tiks) *n* any agent which reduces perspiration.

anhydremia (an-hīd-rēm′-ē-á) *n* deficient fluid content of blood—**anhydremic** *adj*.

anhydrous (an-hīd′-rus) *adj* entirely without water, dry.

anicteric (an-ik'-tėr-ik) *n* without jaundice.

aniridia (an-i-rid'-ē-à) *n* lack or defect of the iris*; usually congenital.

anisocoria (an-i-sō-kō'-rē-à) *n* inequality in diameter of the pupils.

anisocytosis (an-i-sō-sī-tō'-sis) *n* inequality in size of red blood cells.

anisomelia (an-i-sō-mē'-lē-à) *n* unequal length of limbs—**anisomelous** *adj*.

anisometropia (an-i-sō-me-trō'-pē-à) *n* a difference in the refraction* of the two eyes—**anisometropic** *adj*.

ankle clonus *n* series of rapid muscular contractions of the calf muscle when the foot is dorsiflexed by pressure upon the sole.

ankyloblepharon (ang-ki-lō-blef'-à-ron) *n* adhesion of the ciliary edges of the eyelids.

ankylosing spondylitis (ang-ki-lō'-sing spon-dil-ī'-tis) → spondylitis.

ankylosis (ang-ki-lō'-sis) *n* stiffness or fixation of a joint as a result of disease. → spondylitis—**ankylosed** *adj*, **ankylose** *vt, vi*.

Ankylostoma (ang-kil-os'-to-mà) *n* Ancylostoma.*

annular (an'-ū-làr) *n* ring-shaped. *annular ligaments* hold in proximity two long bones, as in the wrist and ankle joints.

anodyne (an'-ō-dīn) *n* remedy which relieves pain. → analgesic.

anogenital (ā-nō-jen'-it-al) *adj* pertaining to the anus and genital region.

anomia (an-ōm'-ē-à) *n* inability to name objects or persons.

anonychia (an-o-nik'-ē-à) *n* absence of nails.

anoperineal (ān'-ō-pėr-in-ē'-al) *adj* pertaining to the anus and perineum.

anoplasty (ān'-ō-plas-tē) *n* plastic surgery of the anus—**anoplastic** *adj*.

anorchism (an-ōr'-kizm) *n* congenital absence of one or both testes—**anorchic** *adj*.

anorectal (ān-ō-rek'-tal) *adj* pertaining to the anus and rectum.

anorectic (an-or-ek'-tik) *n* 1 appetite depressant. 2 one who suffers from anorexia nervosa.

anorexia (an-or-eks'-ē-à) *n* loss of or impaired appetite for food. *anorexia nervosa* a psychological illness, most common in female adolescents. There is minimal food intake leading to loss of weight and sometimes death from starvation—**anorexic, anorectic** *adj*.

anosmia (an-oz'-mē-à) *n* absence of the sense of smell—**anosmic** *adj*.

anovular (an-ov'-ū-làr) *adj* absence of ovulation. *anovular menstruation* is the result of taking contraceptive pills. *anovular bleeding* occurs in metropathia* hemorrhagica. An endometrial biopsy following an *anovular cycle* shows no progestational changes.

anoxemia (an-oks-ēm'-ē-à) *n* literally, no oxygen in the blood, but used to mean hypoxemia*—**anoxemic** *adj*.

anoxia (an-oks'-ē-à) *n* literally, no oxygen in the tissues, but used to signify hypoxia*—**anoxic** *adj*.

Antabuse™ disulfiram.*

antacid (ant-as'-id) *n* substance which neutralizes or counteracts acidity. Commonly used in alkaline stomach powders and mixtures.

antagonist *n* a muscle that relaxes to allow the agonist to perform a movement. When applied to a drug it is one which blocks, nullifies or reverses the effects of another drug—**antagonistic** *adj*, **antagonism** *n*.

antaphrodisiac (ant-af-rō-dēz'-ē-ak) *n* an agent that diminishes sexual desire; absence of sexual impulse. Also anaphrodisiac.

anteflexion (an'-tē-flek'-shun) *n* the bending forward of an organ, commonly applied to the position of the uterus. → retroflexion *opp*.

antemortem (an-tē-mor'-tem) *adj* before death. → postmortem *opp*.

antenatal (an-tē-nā'-tal) *adj* prenatal.* → postnatal *opp*—**antenatally** *adj*.

Antepar™ elixir or tablets containing piperazine.

antepartum (an'-tē-pàr'-tum) *adj* before birth. → postpartum *opp*. *antepartum hemorrhage* → placental abruption.

anterior (an-tē'-rē-ėr) *adj* in front of; the front surface of; ventral. → posterior *opp*. *anterior chamber of the eye* space between posterior surface of the cornea and anterior surface of the iris. → aqueous. *anterior tibial syndrome* severe pain and inflammation over anterior tibial muscle group, with inability to dorsiflex the foot.

anterograde (an'-tėr-ō-grād) *adj* proceeding forward. → retrograde *opp*. → amnesia.

anteversion (an'-tē-vėr'-shun) *n* normal forward tilting, or displacement forward, of an organ or part. → retroversion *opp*—**anteverted** *adj*, **antevert** *vt*.

anthelmintic (ant-hel-min'-tik) *adj* describes any remedy for the destruction or elimination of intestinal worms.

anthracemia (an-thra-sēm'-ē-à) *n* anthrax septicemia—**anthracemic** *adj*.

anthracosis (an-thra-kō'-sis) *n* accumulation of carbon in the lungs due to inhalation of coal dust; may cause fibrotic reaction. A form of pneumoconiosis*—**anthracotic** *adj*.

Anthra-Derm™ anthralin.*

anthralin (an'-thra-lin) *n* ointment applied to the skin for treatment of psoriasis. (Anthra-Derm.)

anthrax (an'-thraks) *n* a contagious disease of cattle, which may be transmitted to man by inoculation, inhalation and ingestion, causing malignant pustule, woolsorter's disease and gastrointestinal anthrax respectively. Causative organism is *Bacillus* anthracis*. Preventive measures include prophylactic immunization of cattle and man.

anthropoid (an'-thrō-poyd) *adj* resembling man. Also used to describe a pelvis that is narrow from side to side, a form of contracted pelvis.*

anthropometry (an-thrō-pom'-et-rē) *n* measurement of the human body and its parts for comparison and establishing norms for sex, age, weight, race and so on—**anthropometric** *adj*.

antianemic (an-tē-an-ēm'-ik) *adj* used to prevent hemorrhage, e.g., vitamin* K.

antiarrhythmic (an-tē-ā-rith'-mik) *adj* describes drugs and treatments used in a variety of cardiac rhythm disorders.

antibiosis (an-tē-bī-ōs'-is) *n* an association between organisms which is harmful to one of them. → symbiosis *opp*—**antibiotic** *adj*.

antibiotics (an-tē-bī-ot'-iks) *npl* antibacterial substances derived from fungi and bacteria, exemplified by penicillin.* Later antibiotics such as tetracycline* are active against a wider range of pathogenic organisms, and are also effective orally. Others, such as neomycin* and bacitracin,* are rarely used internally owing to high toxicity, but are effective when applied topically, and skin sensitization is uncommon.

antibodies *npl* → immunoglobulins. *monoclonal antibodies* laboratory-grown copies of a single antibody isolated from patient sample and multiplied in vitro through several stages and techniques. Uses are experimental, in demonstrating immune mechanisms and in cancer treatment.

anticholinergic (an-tē-kōl-in-ėrj'-ik) *adj* inhibitory to the action of a cholinergic nerve* by interfering with the action of acetylcholine,* a chemical by which such a nerve transmits its impulses at neural or myoneural junctions.

anticholinesterase (an-tē-kōl-in-es'-tėr-ās) *n* drug that blocks or inactivates the enzyme cholinesterase* at nerve endings. Used for reversing the effects of muscle relaxant drugs.

anticoagulant (an-tē-kō-ag'-ūl-ant) *n* agent which prevents or retards clotting of blood; a small amount is made in the human body. Uses: (a) to obtain specimens suitable for pathological investigaton and chemical analyses where whole blood or plasma is required instead of serum; the anticoagulant is usually oxalate; (b) to obtain blood suitable for transfusion, the anticoagulant usually being sodium citrate; (c) as a therapeutic agent in treatment of coronary thrombosis, phlebothrombosis (thrombophlebitis), etc., when aspirin should not be given.

anti-D *n* anti-Rh_0, an immunoglobulin,* Rho Gam.

antidepressants (an-tē-dē-pres'-ants) *npl* drugs which relieve depression. Those in the tricyclic group are the most often prescribed; useful for endogenous depression. Monoamine* oxidase inhibitors, another group, are not so widely used, as strict dietary controls are needed to prevent toxic side-effects.

antidiabetic (an-tē-dī-ab-et'-ik) *adj* literally "against diabetes." Used to describe therapeutic measures in diabetes mellitus; the hormone insulin,* oral diabetic agents, e.g., tolbutamide.*

antidiuretic (an-tē-dī-ūr-et'-ik) *adj* reducing the volume of urine. *antidiuretic hormone (ADH)* vasopressin.*

antidote *n* remedy which counteracts or neutralizes action of a poison.

antiembolic (an-tē-em'-bol-ik) *adj* against embolism.* Antiembolic stockings are worn to decrease risk of deep vein thrombosis.

antiemetic (an-tē-ē-met'-ik) *adj* against emesis.* Any agent which prevents nausea and vomiting.

antienzyme (an-tē-en'-zīm) *n* a substance which exerts a specific inhibiting action on an enzyme. Found in digestive tract to prevent digestion of its lining, and in blood, where they act as immunoglobulins.*

antifebrile (an-tē-fēb'-ril) *adj* describes any agent which reduces or allays fever.

antifibrinolytic (an-tē-fī-brin-ō-lit'-ik) *adj* describes any agent which prevents fibrinolysis.*

antifungal (an-tē-fun'-gal) *adj* describes any agent which destroys fungi.

antigen (an'-tē-jen) *n* any substance which, under favorable conditions, can stimulate production of antibodies* (specific immune* response)—**antigenic** *adj*.

antihemophilic globulin (AHG) factor VIII involved in blood* clotting, present in plasma; absent from serum; deficient in hemophilia.*

antihemorrhagic (an-tē-hem-or-aj'-ik) *adj* describes any agent which prevents hemorrhage; used to describe vitamin* K.

antihistamines (an-tē-hist'-à-mēnz) *npl* drugs which suppress some effects of released histamine.* Widely used in palliative treatment of hay fever, urticaria, angioneurotic edema and some forms of pruritis. Also have antiemetic* properties, and are effective in motion and radiation sickness. Side-effects include drowsiness.

antihypertensive (an-tē-hī-pér-ten'-siv) *adj* describes any agent which reduces high blood pressure.

antileprotic (an-tē-lep-rot'-ik) *adj* describes any agent which prevents or cures leprosy.

antiluetic (an-tē-loo-et'-ik) *adj* describes any agent which prevents or cures syphilis (lues).

antilymphocyte globulin immunoglobulin* containing antibodies to lymphocyte membrane antigens, causing their inactivation or lysis and thus diminishing immune response.

antilymphocyte serum (ALS) serum containing antibodies which bind to lymphocytes inhibiting their function. Used to induce immunosuppression in a patient undergoing kidney transplant.

antimetabolite (an-tē-met-ab'-ō-līt) *n* a compound which is sufficiently similar to the chemicals needed by a cell to be incorporated into nucleoproteins of that cell, thereby preventing its development. Examples are methotrexate,* a folic acid antagonist, and mercaptopurine,* a purine antagonist. Antimetabolites are used in treatment of cancer.

Antiminth™ pyrantel* pamoate.

antimitotic (an-tē-mī-tot'-ik) *adj* preventing reproduction of a cell by mitosis. Describes many of the drugs used to treat cancer.

antimutagen (an-tē-mū'-ta-jen) *n* substance which nullifies the action of a mutagen*—**antimutagenic** *adj*.

antimycotic (an-tē-mī-kot'-ik) *adj* describes any agent which destroys fungi.

antineoplastic (an-tē-nē-ō-plas'-tik) *adj* describes any substance or procedure which works against neoplasms.* → alkylating agents, cytotoxic, radiotherapy.

antineuritic (an-tē-nū-rit'-ik) *adj* describes any agent which prevents neuritis. Specially applied to vitamin* B complex.

antioxidants (an-tē-oks'-id-ants) *npl* describes any substances which delay the process of oxidation.

antiparkinson(ism) drugs (an-tī-pàr'-kin-son-izm) term for major tranquilizing drugs, such as the phenothiazines. They counter side-effects of neuroleptic or antipsychotic drugs.

antipellagra (an-tē-pel-ā'-grà) *adj* against pellagra; a function of the nicotinic acid portion of vitamin* B complex.

antiperiodic (an-tē-pēr-ē-od'-ik) *n* agent which prevents periodic return of a disease, e.g., use of quinine in malaria.

antiperistalsis (an-tē-per-i-stal'-sis) *n* reversal of normal peristaltic action—**antiperistaltic** *adj*.

antiphlogistic (an-tē-flō-jis'-tik) *adj* agent that helps relieve inflammation, e.g., kaolin.

antiprothrombin (an-tē-prō-throm'-bin) *n* arrests blood clotting by preventing conversion of prothrombin into thrombin. Anticoagulant.

antipruritic (an-tē-proo-rit'-ik) *adj* describes any agent which relieves or prevents itching.

antipyretic (an-tē-pī-ret'-ik) *adj* describes any agent which allays or reduces fever.

antirachitic (an-tē-rak-it'-ik) *adj* describes any agent which prevents or cures rickets, a function of vitamin D.*

antireflux (an-tē-rē'-fluks) *adj* against backward flow. Usually refers to reimplantation of ureters into bladder in cases of chronic pyelonephritis* with associated vesicoureteric reflux.

antiRhesus (Rh) serum (an-tē-rē'-sus) given to Rh-negative women who have an Rh-positive baby to prevent development of Rhesus antibodies which might cause erythroblastosis* fetalis in a subsequent pregnancy. Rho Gam.

antischistosomal (an-tē-skis-tō-sō'-mal) *adj* describes any agent which works against *Schistosoma*.

antiscorbutic (an-tē-skor-bū'-tik) *adj* describes any agent which prevents or cures scurvy, a function of vitamin* C.

antisecretory (an-tē-sē'-kret-or-ē) *adj* describes any agent which inhibits secretion.

antisepsis (an-tē-sep'-sis) *n* prevention of sepsis (tissue infection); introduced into surgery in 1880 by Lord Lister, who used carbolic acid—**antiseptic** *adj*.

antiseptics (an-tē-sep'-tiks) *npl* chemical substances which destroy or inhibit growth of microorganisms. Can be applied to living tissues.

antiserotonin (an-tē-sē'-rō-tōn'-in) *n* substance which neutralizes or lessens effect of serotonin.*

antiserum (an-tē-sēr'-um) *n* substance prepared from the blood of an animal which has been immunized by the requisite antigen; contains a high concentration of antibodies.

antisialagogue (an-tē-sī-al'-à-gog) *n* substance which inhibits salivation.

antistreptolysin (an-tē-strep-tō-lī'-sin) *adj* against streptolysins.* Raised antistreptolysin titer in blood is indicative of recent streptococcal infection.

antithrombins (an-tē-throm'-binz) *npl* interactions and blood substances which inhibit thrombin* activity. → heparin.

antithrombotic (an-tē-throm-bot'-ik) *adj* describes measures that prevent or cure thrombosis.*

antithymocyte globulin (ATG) (an-tē-thī'-mō-sīt) immunoglobulin* which binds to antigens on thymic lymphocytes and inhibits lymphocyte-dependent immune responses.

antithyroid (an-tē-thī'-royd) *n* any agent used to decrease activity of the thyroid gland.

antitoxin (an-tē-toks'-in) *n* antibody which neutralizes a given toxin. Made in response to invasion by toxin-producing bacteria, or injection of toxoids—**antitoxic** *adj*.

antitreponemal (an-tē-trep-ō-nēm'-ål) *adj* describes measures against infections caused by *Treponema*.

antitussive (an-tē-tus'-iv) *adj* describes measures which suppress cough.

antivenin (an-tē-ven'-in) *n* serum prepared from animals injected with snake venom; used as antidote in cases of poisoning by snakebite.

antivitamin (an-tē-vīt'-å-min) *n* substance interfering with absorption or utilization of a vitamin.

antrectomy (an-trek'-tō-mē) *n* in treatment of duodenal ulcer, excision of pyloric antrum* of stomach, thus removing source of the hormone gastrin.

antrooral (an-trō-ōr'-ål) *adj* pertaining to the maxillary antrum and the mouth. *antrooral fistula* can occur after extraction of an upper molar tooth, the root of which has protruded into the floor of the antrum.

antrostomy (an-tros'-tom-ē) *n* an artificial opening from nasal cavity to antrum* of Highmore (maxillary sinus) for drainage.

antrum (ant'-rum) *n* a cavity, esp. in bone. *antrum of Highmore* in the superior maxillary bone—**antral** *adj*.

Antuitrin™ extract of the anterior pituitary gland.

Anturane™ sulfinpyrazone.*

anuria (an-ū'-rē-å) *n* absence of secretion of urine by the kidneys. → suppression—**anuric** *adj*.

anus (ā'-nus) *n* the end of the alimentary canal, at the extreme termination of the rectum. Formed of a sphincter muscle which relaxes to allow fecal matter to pass through. *artificial anus* → colostomy. *imperforate anus* → imperforate—**anal** *adj*.

anvil *n* the incus, the middle of the three small bones of the middle ear. Shaped like an anvil.

anxiolytics (ank-si-ō-lit'-iks) *npl* agents which reduce anxiety.

aorta (ā-ōr'-tà) *n* main artery arising out of the left ventricle of the heart. → Figure 9.

aortic (ā-ōr′-tik) *adj* pertaining to the aorta. *aortic incompetence* regurgitation of blood from aorta back into the left ventricle. *aortic murmur* abnormal heart sound heard over aortic area; a systolic murmur alone is the murmur of aortic stenosis, a diastolic murmur denotes aortic incompetence. The combination of both systolic and diastolic murmurs causes the so-called "to and fro" aortic murmur. *aortic stenosis* narrowing of aortic valve; usually due to rheumatic heart disease or a congenital bicuspid valve defect predisposing to deposit of calcium.

aortitis (ā-ōr-tī′-tis) *n* inflammation of the aorta.

aortography (ā-ōr-tog′-raf-ē) *n* demonstration of the aorta after introduction of an opaque medium, either via a catheter passed along the femoral or brachial artery or by direct translumbar injection—**aortographic** *adj*, **aortogram** *n*, **aortograph** *n*.

APC *n* tablets containing aspirin, phenacetin, and caffeine.

aperients (a-pėr′-ē-ents) *npl* → laxatives.

aperistalsis (ā-pėr-is-tal′-sis) *n* absence of peristaltic movement in the bowel. Characterizes the condition of paralytic ileus—**aperistaltic** *adj*.

Apert's syndrome (ā′-pėrts) congenital craniosynostosis accompanied by deformities of the hands. → syndactyly, acrocephalosyndactyly.

apex *n* the summit or top of anything which is cone-shaped, e.g., the tip of the root of a tooth. → Figure 7. In a heart of normal size the *apical beat* (systolic impulse) can be seen or felt in the 5th left intercostal space in the mid-clavicular line—**apices** *pl*, **apical** *adj*.

Apgar score (ap′gàr) measure used to evaluate general condition of a newborn baby, developed by an American anesthetist, Dr. Virginia Apgar. A score of 0, 1, or 2 is given using criteria of heart rate, respiratory effort, skin color, muscle tone and reflex response to a nasal catheter. A score of between 8 and 10 would indicate a baby in excellent condition, whereas a score below 7 would cause concern.

aphagia (a-fā′-jà) *n* inability to swallow—**aphagic** *adj*.

aphakia (a-fā′-kē-à) *n* absence of the crystalline lens. Describes the eye after removal of a cataract—**aphakic** *adj*.

aphasia (a-fā′-zhà) *n* often used interchangeably with dysphasia.* Disorder of the complex language function, in spite of normal hearing over the whole frequency range, which is thought to be due to brain lesion. Several classifications but the most commonly used terms are *expressive* (*motor*) aphasia and *receptive* (*sensory*) *aphasia*, although many patients exhibit deficiencies in both types—**aphasic** *adj*.

aphonia (a-fō′-nē-à) *n* loss of voice from a cause other than a cerebral lesion—**aphonic** *adj*.

aphrodisiac (af-rō-dēz'-ē-ak) *n* an agent which stimulates sexual excitement.

aphthae (af'-thē) *npl* small ulcers of oral mucosa surrounded by a ring of erythema—**aphtha** *sing*, **aphthous** *adj*.

aphthous stomatitis (af'-thus stō-má-tī'-tis) → stomatitis.

apicectomy (āp-is-ek'-to-mē) *n* excision of the apex of the root of a tooth.

aplasia (a-plā'-zhá) *n* incomplete development of tissue; absence of growth.

aplastic (ā-plas'tik) *adj* 1 without structure or form. 2 incapable of forming new tissue. *aplastic anemia* → anemia.

apnea (ap-nē'-á) *n* transitory cessation of breathing as seen in Cheyne-Stokes respiration.* Due to lack of necessary CO_2 tension in the blood for stimulation of the respiratory center. *apnea of the newborn* → periodic breathing. *sleep apnea* failure of autonomic control of respiration which becomes more pronounced during sleep—**apneic** *adj*.

apocrine glands (ap'-ō-krin) modified sweat glands, esp. in axilary, genital and perineal regions. Responsible after puberty for body odor.

apodia (ā-pō'-dē-á) *n* congenital absence of the feet.

apomorphine (a-pō-mor'-fēn) *n* powerful emetic* when injected.

aponeurosis (ap-ō-nū-rō'-sis) *n* a broad glistening sheet of tendonlike tissue which serves to invest and attach muscles to each other, and also to the parts which they move—**aponeuroses** *pl*, **aponeurotic** *adj*.

aponeurositis (ap-ō-nū-rō-sī'-tis) *n* inflammation of an aponeurosis.

apophysis (ap-of'-is-is) *n* a projection, protuberance or outgrowth, usually in context with bone.

apoplexy (ap'-ō-plek-sē) *n* condition more commonly referred to as cerebrovascular* accident (stroke)—**apoplectic, apoplectiform** *adj*.

appendectomy (ap-pen-dek'-to-mē) *n* excision of the appendix* vermiformis.

appendicitis (ap-pen-di-sī'-tis) *n* inflammation of the appendix* vermiformis.

appendix (ap-pen'-diks) *n* an appendage. *appendix vermiformis* a wormlike appendage of the cecum about the thickness of a pencil and usually measuring from 50.8 to 152.4 mm in length (→ Figure 18). Its position is variable, and it is apparently functionless—**appendices** *pl*, **appendicular** *adj*.

apposition (ap-o-zish'-un) *n* the approximation or bringing together of two surfaces or edges.

apraxia (a-praks'-ē-á) *n* inability to deal effectively with or manipulate objects as a result of a brain lesion. *constructional apraxia* inability to arrange objects to a plan—**apraxic, apractic** *adj*.

Apresoline™ hydralazine.*

APT *abbr* alum precipitated diphtheria toxoid. A diphtheria prophylactic used mainly for children.

apyrexia (ā-pī-reks'-ē-à) *n* absence of fever—**apyrexial** *adj*.

apyrogenic (ā-pī-rō-jen'-ik) *adj* not fever producing.

aqua (ak'-wà) *n* water. *aqua fortis* nitric acid. *aqua menthae piperitae* peppermint water.

aqueduct *n* a canal. *aqueduct of Sylvius* canal connecting the 3rd and 4th ventricles of the brain; aqueductus cerebri.

aqueous (ā'-kwi-us) *adj* watery. *aqueous humor* fluid contained in the anterior and posterior chambers of the eye. → Figure 15.

arachidonic acid (ar-ak'-id-on-ik) one of the essential fatty acids. Found in small amounts in human and animal liver and organ fats. A growth factor.

arachnodactyly (ar-ak-nō-dak'-til-ē) *n* congenital abnormality resulting in spider fingers.

arachnoid (ar-ak'-noyd) *adj* resembling a spider's web. *arachnoid membrane* a delicate membrane enveloping the brain and spinal cord, lying between the pia mater internally and the dura mater externally; the middle serous membrane of the meninges—**arachnoidal** *adj*.

Aralen™ chloroquine.*

Aramine™ metaraminol.*

arborization (àr-bor-ī-zā'-shun) *n* an arrangement resembling the branching of a tree. Characterizes both ends of a neuron, i.e., the dendrons and the axon as it supplies each muscle fiber.

arboviruses (àr-bō-vī'-rus-es) *npl* RNA viruses transmitted by arthropods. Members of the mosquito-borne group include those causing yellow fever, dengue and viruses causing infections of the CNS. Sandflies transmit the virus causing sandfly fever. The tickborne viruses can cause hemorrhagic fevers.

ARC *abbr* AIDS*-related complex.

arcus senilis (àr'-kus sen-il'-is) opaque ring round the edge of the cornea, seen in old people.

areola (ar-ē'-o-là) *n* pigmented area round the nipple of the breast. A *secondary areola* surrounds the primary areola in pregnancy—**areolar** *adj*.

ARF *abbr* 1 acute renal* failure. 2 acute respiratory* failure.

Arfonad™ trimetaphan.*

arginase (àr'-jin-āz) *n* enzyme found in the liver, kidney and spleen. It splits arginine into ornithine and urea.

arginine (àr'-jin-ēn) *n* an essential amino acid. Used in treatment of acute liver failure to counter acute ammonia intoxication.

argininosuccinuria (àr-jin-ēn'-ō-suks-in-ū'-rē-à) *n* presence of arginine and succinic acid in urine; associated with mental subnormality.

Argyll Robertson pupil (àr-gil') one which reacts to accommodation, but not to light. Diagnostic sign in neurosyphilis,* but not all examples are syphilitic. Other important causes include disseminated sclerosis and diabetes mellitus. In the nonsyphilitic group the pupil is not small, but often dilated and unequal and is called atypical.

ariboflavinosis (ā-rī-bō-flāv-in-ōs'-is) *n* deficiency state caused by lack of riboflavin* and other members of the vitamin B complex. Characterized by cheilosis, seborrhea, angular stomatitis, glossitis and photophobia.

Aristocort™ triamcinalone.*

Arnold-Chiari malformation (àr'-nōlt kē'-a-rē) a group of disorders affecting the base of the brain. Commonly occurs in hydrocephalus associated with meningocele and myelomeningocele. There are degrees of severity but usually there is some "kinking" or "buckling" of the brain stem with cerebellar tissue herniating through the foramen magnum at the base of the skull.

AROM *abbr* active range of motion; artificial rupture of membranes.

arrectores pilorum (àr-ek-tōr'-ēz pi-lōr'-um) internal, plain, involuntary muscles (→ Figure 12) attached to hair follicles, which, by contraction, erect the follicles, causing "gooseflesh"—**arrector pili** *sing*.

arrhenoblastoma (a-rēn-ō-blas-tō'-mà) *n* → androblastoma.

arrhythmia (a-rith'-mē-à) *n* any deviation from the normal rhythm, usually referring to the heart beat. → sinus extrasystole, fibrillation, heart, Stokes-Adams syndrome, tachycardia.

Artane™ trihexyphenidyl.*

artefact (àr'-te-fakt) *n* → artifact.

arteralgia (àr'-ter-al'-jē-à) *n* pain in an artery.

arterectomy (àr-tèr-ek'-to-mē) *n* excision of an artery or part of an artery.

arteriography (àr-tēr-ē-og'-ra-fē) *n* demonstration of the arterial system after injection of an opaque medium—**arteriographic** *adj*, **arteriogram, arteriograph** *n*.

arteriole (àr-tēr'-ē-ōl) *n* a small artery, joining an artery to a capillary.

arteriopathy (àr-tēr-ē-op'-à-thē) *n* disease of any artery—**arteriopathic** *adj*.

arterioplasty (àr-tēr'-ē-ō-plas-tē) *n* plastic surgery to an artery—**arterioplastic** *adj*.

arteriorrhaphy (àr-tē-rē-ōr'-raf-ē) *n* a plastic procedure or suturing of an artery, as in obliteration of an aneurysm.

arteriosclerosis (ȧr-tēr-ē-ō-sklér-ō′-sis) *n* degenerative arterial change associated with advancing age. Primarily a thickening of the media and usually associated with some degree of atheroma.* *cerebral arteriosclerosis* syndrome characterized by progressive memory loss, confusion and childlike behavior—**arteriosclerotic** *adj*.

arteriotomy (ȧr-tēr-ē-ot′-ō-mē) *n* incision or needle puncture of an artery.

arteriovenous (ȧr-tēr-ē-ō-vēn′-us) *adj* pertaining to an artery and a vein, e.g., an arteriovenous aneurysm, fistula, or shunt for hemodialysis. *arteriovenous filtration* hemofiltration.*

arteritis (ȧr-tēr-ī′-tis) *n* inflammatory disease affecting the middle walls of arteries. May be due to an infection such as syphilis or it may be part of a collagen disease. Arteries may become swollen and tender and blood may clot in them. *giant cell arteritis, temporal arteritis* occurs in the elderly and mainly in scalp arteries. Blindness can ensue if there is thrombosis of the ophthalmic vessels. Treatment with cortisone is effective—**arteritic** *adj*.

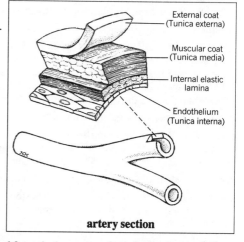

External coat (Tunica externa)

Muscular coat (Tunica media)

Internal elastic lamina

Endothelium (Tunica interna)

artery section

artery *n* a vessel carrying blood from the heart to various tissues. Internal endothelial lining provides a smooth surface to prevent clotting of blood. A middle layer of plain muscle and elastic fibers allows for distension as blood is pumped from the heart. The outer, mainly connective tissue layer prevents overdistension. Lumen is largest nearest to the heart; it gradually decreases in size. *artery forceps* forceps used to produce hemostasis*—**arterial** *adj*.

arthralgia (ȧrth-ral′-jȧ) *n* (*syn* articular neuralgia, arthrodynia) pain in a joint, used especially when there is no inflammation—**arthralgic** *adj*.

arthrectomy (ȧrth-rek′-to-mē) *n* excision of a joint.

arthritis (ȧrth-rī′-tis) *n* inflammation of one or more joints which swell, become warm to touch, are painful and are restricted in movement. There are many causes and treatment varies according to the cause. → arthropathy. *arthritis deformans juvenilis* → Still's disease. *arthritis nodosa* gout*—**arthritic** *adj*.

arthroclasis (àrth-rō-klā'sis) *n* breaking down of adhesions within the joint cavity to produce a wider range of movement.

arthrodesis (àrth-rō-dē'-sis) *n* stiffening of a joint by operative means.

arthrodynia (àrth-rō-dī'-nē-à) *n* → arthralgia—**arthrodynic** *adj*.

arthroendoscopy (àrth-rō-en-dos'-kop-ē) *n* visualization of the interior of a joint using an endoscope*—**arthroendoscopic** *adj*.

arthrography (àrth-rog'-raf-ē) *n* radiographic examination to determine internal structure of a joint, outlined by contrast media—either a gas or opaque medium or both—**arthrographic** *adj*, **arthrogram** *n*, **arthrograph** *n*.

arthrology (àrth-rol'-oj-ē) *n* study of structure and function of joints, their diseases and treatment.

arthropathy (àrth-rop'-ath-ē) *n* any joint disease. Condition is currently classified as: *enteropathic arthropathies* resulting from chronic diarrheal diseases; *psoriatic arthropathies* psoriasis; *seronegative arthropathies* include all other instances of inflammatory arthritis other than rheumatoid arthritis; *seropositive arthropathies* include all instances of rheumatoid arthritis—**arthropathies** *pl*, **arthropathic** *adj*.

arthroplasty (àrth'-rō-plas-tē) *n* surgical remodelling of a joint. *cup arthroplasty* articular surface is reconstructed and covered with a vitallium cup. *excision arthroplasty* gap is filled with fibrous tissue. *Girdlestone arthroplasty* excision arthroplasty of the hip. *replacement arthroplasty* insertion of an inert prosthesis of similar shape. *total replacement arthroplasty* replacement of the head of femur and the acetabulum, both being cemented into the bone—**arthroplastic** *adj*.

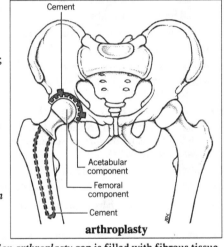

Cement

Acetabular component

Femoral component

Cement

arthroplasty

arthroscope (àrth'-rō-skōp) *n* instrument used for visualization of interior of a joint cavity. → endoscope—**arthroscopy** *n*, **arthroscopic** *adj*.

arthrosis (àr-thrō'-sis) *n* degeneration in a joint.

arthrotomy (àrth-rot'-o-mē) *n* incision into a joint.

articular (àr-tik'-ū-làr) *adj* pertaining to a joint or articulation. Applied to cartilage, surface, capsule, etc., *articular neuralgia* → arthralgia.

articulation (ár-tik-ū-lā′-shun) *n* **1** junction of two or more bones; a joint. **2** enunciation of speech—**articular** *adj*.

artifact (árt′-i-fakt) *n* any artificial product; an unnatural change in a structure or tissue. Also spelled artefact.

artificial anus → colostomy.

artificial blood a fluid able to transport O_2; used successfully in the USA and Japan. Jehovah's Witnesses acted as subjects for clinical trials.

artificial feeding → enteral.

artificial insemination → insemination.

artificial kidney → dialyser.

artificial limb → prosthesis, orthosis.

artificial lung → respirator.

artificial pneumothorax → pneumothorax.

artificial respiration → resuscitation.

ascariasis (as-kár-ī′-a-sis) *n* infestation by ascarides.* The bowel is most commonly affected but, in the case of roundworm, infestation may spread to the stomach, liver and lungs.

ascaricide (as-kar′-is-īd) *n* substance lethal to ascarides*—**ascaricidal** *adj*.

ascarides (as-kar′-i-dēz) *npl* nematode worms of the family *Ascaridae*, to which belong the roundworm (*Ascaris lumbricoides*) and the threadworm (*Oxyuris vermicularis*).

ascending colon → Figure 18.

Aschoff's nodules (ash′-hofs) nodules in the myocardium in rheumatism.

ascites (a-sī′-tēz) *n* (*syn* hydroperitoneum) free fluid in the peritoneal cavity—**ascitic** *adj*.

ascorbic acid (a-skor′-bik) vitamin* C. A water-soluble vitamin necessary for healthy connective tissue, particularly collagen fibers and cell walls. Present in fresh fruits and vegetables. It is destroyed by cooking in the presence of air and by plant enzymes released when cutting and grating food; it is also lost by storage. Deficiency causes scurvy. Used as nutritional supplement in anemia and to promote wound healing.

asepsis (ā-sep′-sis) *n* the state of being free from living pathogenic microorganisms—**aseptic** *adj*.

aseptic technique precautionary method used in any procedure where possibility exists of introducing organisms into the patient's body. Every article used must be sterilized.

ASLO *abbr* antistreptolysin* O.

asparaginase (as-par'-a-jin-āz) *n* enzyme derived from microorganisms. Rarely useful in treatment of asparagine-requiring acute lymphoblastic leukemias.

aspartate transaminase enzyme present in serum and body tissues, esp. heart and liver. Released into serum following tissue damage such as myocardial infarction or acute damage to liver cells.

aspergillosis (as-pėr-ji-lō'-sis) *n* opportunistic infection,* mainly of lungs, caused by any species of *Aspergillus*. → bronchomycosis.

Aspergillus (as-pėr-jil'-us) *n* genus of fungi, found in soil, manure and on various grains. Some species are pathogenic.

aspermia (ā-sperm'-ē-à) *n* lack of secretion or expulsion of semen—**aspermic** *adj*.

asphyxia (as-fiks'-ē-à) *n* suffocation; cessation of breathing. O_2 content of air in the lungs falls while CO_2 rises and similar changes follow rapidly in the arterial blood. *blue asphyxia, asphyxia livida* deep blue appearance of a newborn baby; good muscle tone, responsive to stimuli. *white (pale) asphyxia, asphyxia pallida* more severe condition of newborn; pale, flaccid, unresponsive to stimuli. → respiratory distress syndrome.

aspiration *n* (*syn* paracentesis, tapping) withdrawal of fluids from a body cavity by means of a suction or siphonage apparatus. *aspiration pneumonia* inflammation of lung from inhalation of foreign body, usually fluid or food particles—**aspirate** *vt*.

aspirator *n* a negative pressure apparatus for withdrawing fluids from cavities.

aspirin *n* acetylsalicylic* acid.

assimilation *n* process whereby already digested foodstuffs are absorbed and utilized by tissues—**assimilable** *adj*, **assimilate** *vt, vi*.

assisted ventilation mechanical assistance with breathing. Babies requiring extended periods of assisted ventilation are at great risk of developing bronchopulmonary dysplasia, which can result in repeated chest infections.

AST *abbr* aspartate* transaminase.

astereognosis (as-stėr-ē-og-nō'-sis) *n* loss of power to recognize shape and consistency of objects.

asthenia (as-thē'-nē-à) *n* lack of strength; weakness, debility—**asthenic** *adj*.

asthenopia (as-thē-nō'-pē-à) *n* poor vision—**asthenopic** *adj*, **asthenope** *n*.

asthma (az'-mà) *n* paroxysmal dyspnea* characterized by wheezing and difficulty in expiration because of muscular spasm in the bronchi. Recent advances in immunology reveal that mast cells in bronchial walls produce immunoglobulin on encountering pollen grains; when more are inhaled, alveolar mast cells burst, causing an asthmatic attack. New anti-asthmatic drugs can prevent this. → bronchial asthma, renal asthma—**asthmatic** *adj*.

astigmatism (as-tig'-màt-izm) *n* defective vision caused by inequality of one or more refractive surfaces, usually the corneal, so that light rays do not converge to a point on the retina. May be congenital or acquired—**astigmatic, astigmic** *adj*.

astringent (as-trin'-jent) *adj* describes an agent which contracts organic tissue, thus lessening secretion—**astringency, astringent** *n*.

astrocytoma (as-trō-sī-tō'-mà) *n* slowly growing tumor of the glial tissue of brain and spinal cord.

AST test aspartate transferase is an enzyme normally present in liver, heart, muscles and kidneys. Values greater than 400 units per ml of serum are abnormal and are the commonest indication of liver disease.

Astrup test (as'-trup) estimates degree of acidosis by measuring pressures of oxygen and carbon dioxide in arterial blood.

asymptomatic (ā-simp-tom-at'-ik) *adj* symptomless.

asynclitism (ā-sin'-klit-izm) *n* anterior or posterior deflection of the saggital suture in presentation of the fetal head.

Atabrine™ quinacrine.*

ataractic (at-a-rak'-tik) *adj* describes drugs that, without drowsiness, relieve anxiety. → tranquilizers.

Atarax™ hydroxyzine.*

atavism (at'-à-vizm) *n* reappearance of a hereditary trait which has skipped one or more generations—**atavic, atavistic** *adj*.

ataxia, ataxy (a-taks'-ē-à, a-taks'-ē) *n* defective muscular control resulting in irregular and jerky movements; staggering. *ataxic gait* → gait. → *Friedreich's ataxia*—**ataxic** *adj*.

atelectasis (at-el-ek'-ta-sis) *n* numbers of pulmonary alveoli do not contain air due to failure of expansion (congenital atelectasis) or resorption of air from the alveoli (collapse*)—**atelectatic** *adj*.

atenolol (at-en'-ol-ol) *n* cardioselective beta adrenoceptor antagonist; an effective hypotensive. (Tenormin.)

ATG *abbr* antithymocyte* globulin.

atherogenic (ath-er-ō-jen'-ik) *adj* capable of producing atheroma*—**atherogenesis** *n*.

atheroma (ath-er-ō'-mà) *n* deposition of hard yellow plaques of lipoid material in the intimal layer of arteries. May be related to high level of cholesterol in blood. Of significance in coronary arteries in predisposing to coronary thrombosis—**atheromatous** *adj*.

atherosclerosis (ath-er-ō-skle-rō'-sis) *n* co-existing atheroma and arteriosclerosis—**atherosclerotic** *adj*.

athetosis (ath-e-tō'-sis) *n* condition marked by purposeless movements of hands and feet and generally due to a brain lesion—**athetoid, athetotic** *adj.*

athlete's foot tinea pedis. → tinea.

Ativan™ lorazepam.*

atonic (ā-ton'-ik) *adj* without tone; weak—**atonia, atony, atonicity** *n.*

atopic syndrome (ā-top'-ik) constitutional tendency to develop infantile eczema, asthma, hay fever or all three, when there is a positive family history.

ATP *abbr* adenosine* triphosphate.

atracurium (at-rà-cū'-rē-um) *n* nondepolarizing relaxant drug which is destroyed spontaneously in the body by the Hofmann* reaction. (Tracrium.)

atresia (ā'-trē'-zhà) *n* imperforation or closure of a normal body opening, duct or canal—**atresic, atretic** *adj.*

atrial fibrillation (ā'-trē-al fib-ril-ā'-shun) chaotic irregularity of atrial rhythm without any semblance of order. The ventricular rhythm, depending on conduction through the atrioventricular node, is irregular. Commonly associated with mitral stenosis or thyrotoxicosis.

atrial flutter rapid regular cardiac rhythm caused by irritable focus in atrial muscle and usually associated with organic heart disease. Speed of atrial beats between 260 and 340 per minute. Ventricles usually respond to every second beat, but may be slowed by carotid sinus pressure.

atrial septal defect nonclosure of foramen ovale at birth resulting in congenital heart defect.

atrioventricular *adj* pertaining to the atria and the ventricles of the heart. Applied to a node, tract and valves.

atrium (ā'-trē-um) *n* cavity, entrance or passage. One of the two upper cavities of the heart (→ Figure 9)—**atria** *pl,* **atrial** *adj.*

Atromid-S™ clofibrate.*

atrophic rhinitis (ā-trō'-fik rīn-ī'-tis) (*syn* ozena) an atrophic condition of the nasal mucous membrane with associated crusting and fetor.

atrophy (at'-rō-fē) *n* wasting, emaciation, diminution in size and function. *acute yellow atrophy* massive necrosis of liver associated with severe infection, toxemia of pregnancy or ingested poisons. *progressive muscular atrophy* (*syn* motor neuron disease) disease of the motor neurons of unknown cause, characterized by loss of power and wasting in the upper limbs. May also have upper motor neuron involvement (spasticity) in lower limbs—**atrophied, atrophic** *adj.*

atropine (at'-rō-pēn) *n* principal alkaloid of belladonna. Has spasmolytic, mydriatic and central nervous system depressant properties. Given before anesthetic to decrease secretion in bronchial and salivary systems and to prevent cardiac depression. *atropine methonitrate* is used in pylorospasm and in spray preparations for asthma and bronchospasm.

attenuation (at-ten-ū-ā'-shun) *n* process by which pathogenic microorganisms are induced to develop or show less virulent characteristics. They can then be used in the preparation of vaccines—**attenuant, attenuated** *adj*, **attenuate** *vt*, *vi*.

attrition *n* wear of the occlusal* surfaces of teeth by use.

audiogram *n* visual record of the acuity of hearing tested with an audiometer.

audiology (aw-dē-ol'-o-jē) *n* scientific study of hearing—**audiological** *adj*.

audiometer (aw-dē-om'-et-ėr) *n* apparatus for clinical testing of hearing. It generates pure tones over a wide range of pitch and intensity—**audiometric** *adj*, **audiometry** *n*.

auditory (aw'-di-tor-ē) *adj* pertaining to the sense of hearing. *auditory acuity* → acuity. *auditory area* that portion of the temporal lobe of the cerebral cortex which interprets sound. *auditory canal* → Figure 13. *auditory meatus* canal between the pinna and eardrum. *auditory nerves* the eighth pair of cranial nerves. *auditory ossicles* the three small bones—malleus, incus and stapes—stretching across the cavity of the middle ear.

aura (aw'-rȧ) *n* a premonition; a peculiar sensation or warning of an impending attack, such as occurs in epilepsy.*

aural (awr'-ȧl) *adj* pertaining to the ear.

Aureomycin™ chlortetracycline.* → tetracycline.

auricle (aw'-rik-l) *n* **1** the pinna of the external ear. → Figure 13. **2** an appendage to the cardiac atrium.* **3** obsolete term for atrium*—**auricular** *adj*.

auriscope (aw'-ris-kōp) *n* instrument for examining the ear, usually incorporating both magnification and illumination.

aurothiomalate (aw-rō-thī'-ō-mȧl-āt) *n* gold injection useful in chronic discoid lupus erythematosus and rheumatoid arthritis. Urine should be tested for albumen before each injection. (Myochrysine.)

auscultation (aws-kul-tā'-shun) *n* a method of listening to body sounds, particularly the heart, lungs and fetal circulation for diagnostic purposes. It may be: (a) immediate, by placing the ear directly against the body, (b) mediate, by the use of a stethoscope—**auscultatory** *adj*, **auscult, auscultate** *v*.

Australian antigen an antigen* associated with hepatitis* B virus. Found in blood of 0.1 percent of Americans without manifestations of disease. Rates are higher in tropical areas. This blood may induce hepatitis in other people, so must not be used for transfusion.

Australian lift better described as shoulder lift. Method of lifting a heavy patient, whereby weight is taken by the upper shoulder muscles of two lifters, who then rise by straightening flexed hips and knees.

autism (aw'-tizm) *n* a condition of self-absorption with retreat from reality into a private world of thought, fantasies and in extreme cases hallucinations.

autoagglutination (aw-tō-a-glōō-ti-nā'-shun) *n* clumping together of the body's own red blood cells caused by autoantibodies; occurs in acquired hemolytic anemia, an autoimmune disease.

autoantibody (aw-tō-an'-ti-bod-ē) *n* an antibody which can bind to normal constituents of the body, such as DNA, smooth muscle and parietal cells.

autoantigen (aw-tō-an'-ti-jen) *n* antigens in normal tissues which can bind to autoantibodies.

autoclave (aw'-tō-klāv) **1** *n* apparatus for high-pressure steam sterilization. **2** *vt* sterilize in an autoclave.

autodigestion *n* self-digestion of tissues within the living body. → autolysis.

autoeroticism (aw-tō-e-rot'-is-izm) *n* self-gratification of the sex instinct. → masturbation—**autoerotic** *adj*.

autograft *n* tissue grafted from one part of the body to another.

autoimmune disease (aw-tō-im-mūn') illness caused by, or associated with, the development of an immune response to normal body tissues. Hashimoto's disease, myxedema, Graves' disease and pernicious anemia are examples.

autoimmunization (aw-to-im'-mūn-īz-ā'-shun) *n* process which leads to an autoimmune disease.

autoinfection *n* → infection.

autointoxication *n* poisoning from faulty or excessive metabolic products elaborated within the body. Such products may be derived from infected or dead tissue.

autolysis (aw-tol'-is-is) *n* autodigestion* which occurs if digestive enzymes escape into surrounding tissues—**autolytic** *adj*.

automatism (aw-tom'-at-izm) *n* organized behavior which occurs without subsequent awareness of it; somnambulism, hysterical and epileptic states.

autonomic (aw-tō-nom'-ik) *adj* independent, self-governing. *autonomic nervous system* (*ANS*) is divided into parasympathetic and sympathetic portions. They are made up of nerve cells and fibers which cannot be controlled at will and carry on reflex control of bodily functions.

autoplasty (aw'-tō-plas-tē) *n* replacement of tissue by a graft of tissue from the same body—**autoplastic** *adj*, **autoplast** *n*.

autopsy (aw'-top-sē) *n* examination of a dead body (cadaver) for diagnostic purposes.

autosome (aw'-tō-sōm) *n* a chromosome other than a sex chromosome (gonosome).

autosuggestion *n* self-suggestion; uncritical acceptance of ideas arising in the individual's own mind. Occurs in hysteria.*

autotransfusion *n* infusion into a patient of the actual blood lost by hemorrhage, esp. when hemorrhage occurs into the abdominal cavity.

avascular (ā-vas'-kū-lar) *adj* bloodless; not vascular, i.e., without blood supply. *avascular necrosis* death of bone from deficient blood supply following injury or possibly through disease, often a precursor of osteoarthritis—**avascularity** *n*, **avascularize** *vt, vi*.

Avazyme™ chymotrypsin.*

Aventyl™ nortriptyline.*

avidin (av'-i-din) *n* high molecular weight protein with high affinity for biotin* and which can interfere with absorption of biotin. Found in raw egg white.

avirulent (ā-vir'-ū-lent) *adj* without virulence.*

avitaminosis (ā-vīt-a-min-ōs'-is) *n* any disease resulting from a deficiency of vitamins.

Avlosulfan™ dapsone.*

avulsion (a-vul'-shun) *n* a forcible wrenching away, as of a limb, nerve or polypus.

axilla (aks-il'-à) *n* the armpit.

axillary (aks'-il-ār-ē) *adj* applied to nerves, blood and lymphatic vessels, of the armpit. *axillary artery* → Figure 10. *axillary vein* → Figure 11.

axis *n* **1** the second cervical vertebra. **2** an imaginary line passing through the center; the median line of the body—**axial** *adj*.

axon (aks'on) *n* that process of a nerve cell conveying impulses away from the cell; the essential part of the nerve fiber and a direct prolongation of the nerve cell—**axonal** *adj*.

axonotmesis (aks-on-ot-mēs'-is) *n* (*syn* neurotmesis) peripheral degeneration as a result of damage to axons of a nerve. Internal architecture is preserved and recovery depends upon regeneration of the axons, and may take many months (about 25.4 mm a month is usual speed of regeneration). Such a lesion may result from pinching, crushing or prolonged pressure.

azacytidine (az-à-sī'-ti-dēn) *n* antimetabolite used in treatment of leukemia.

azathioprine (az-à-thī'-ō-prēn) *n* immunosuppressive drug. Works by competing against purine, an essential metabolite for cell division. (Imuran.)

azlocillin (az-lō-sil'-in) *n* pencillin antibiotic particularly active against *Pseudomonas* infections. (Azlin.)

Azolid™ phenylbutazone.*

azoospermia (ā-zō-ō-spérm'-ē-à) *n* sterility of the male through nonproduction of spermatozoa.

azotemia (az-ōt-ēm'-ē-à) *n* uremia.

azoturia (az-ōt-ūr'-ē-à) *n* pathological excretion of urea in urine—**azoturic** *adj.*

AZT *abbr* azidothymidine; drug acting on the immune system used for AIDS.* (Retrovir.)

Azulfidine™ sulfasalazine.*

azygos (az'-i-gos) *adj* occurring singly, not paired. *azygos veins* three unpaired veins of the abdomen and thorax which empty into the inferior vena cava— **azygous** *adj.*

B

B cells major constituent of the immune system; lymphocytes that produce immunoglobulins (antibodies). They can be activated either by T-cell released cytokines* or by presence of antigen.

Babinski's reflex (bab-in'-skēz) or sign. Movement of great toe upwards (dorsiflexion) instead of downwards (plantar flexion) on stroking sole of the foot. Indicative of disease or injury to upper motor neurons and present in organic but not hysterical hemiplegia. Babies exhibit dorsiflexion, but after learning to walk show normal plantar flexion response.

bacillemia (bas-il-ēm'-ē-à) *n* presence of bacilli in blood—**bacillemic** *adj*.

Bacille-Calmette-Gueria (ba-sēl'-kal-met'-gār'-ē-à) → BCG.

bacilluria (bas-il-ū'-rē-à) *n* presence of bacilli in urine—**bacilluric** *adj*.

Bacillus (bas-il'-us) *n* genus of bacteria consisting of aerobic, Gram-positive, rod-shaped cells which produce endospores. Majority are motile by means of peritrichate flagella. These organisms are saprophytes and their spores are common in soil and dust of the air. *B. anthracis* causes anthrax in man and in animals.

bacitracin (bas-i-trā'-sin) *n* antibiotic used mainly for external application in conditions resistant to other forms of treatment. Does not cause sensitivity reactions.

baclofen (bak'-lō-fen) *n* drug which reduces spasticity of voluntary muscle; mode uncertain. Side-effects include nausea, vomiting, diarrhea, gastric discomfort, muscular incoordination, hypotonia, mental confusion, vertigo and drowsiness. Particularly useful for multiple sclerosis. (Lioresal.)

bacteremia (bak-te-rēm'-ē-à) *n* presence of bacteria in blood—**bacteremic** *adj*.

bacteria (bak-tē'-rē-à) *n* a group of microorganisms, also called the "schizomycetes." Typically small cells of about 1 micron in transverse diameter. Structurally there is a protoplast, containing cytoplasmic and nuclear material (not seen by ordinary methods of microscopy) within a limiting cytoplasmic membrane, and a supporting cell wall. Other structures such as flagella, fimbriae and capsules may also be present. Individual cells may be spherical, straight or curved rods or spirals; they may form chains or masses and some show branching with mycelium formation. May produce various pigments including chlorophyll. Some form endospores. Reproduction is chiefly by simple binary fission. They may be free living, saprophytic or parasitic; some are pathogenic to man, animals and plants—**bacterium** *sing,* **bacterial** *adj.*

bactericide (bak-tēr′-i-sīd) *n* any agent which destroys bacteria—**bactericidal** *adj.*

bactericidin (bak-tēr-i-sīd′-in) *n* antibody which kills bacteria.

bacteriology (bak-tēr-ē-ol′-oj-ē) *n* scientific study of bacteria—**bacteriological** *adj.*

bacteriolysin (bak-tē-rē-ō-lī′-sin) *n* a specific antibody formed in the blood which causes dissolution of bacteria.

bacteriolysis (bak-tēr-ē-ol′-is-is) *n* the disintegration and dissolution of bacteria—**bacteriolytic** *adj.*

bacteriophage (bak-tēr′-ē-ō-fāj) *n* a virus parasitic on bacteria.

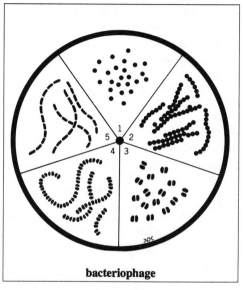

bacteriophage

bacteriostasis (bak-tēr-ē-ō-stā′-sis) *n* arrest or hindrance of bacterial growth—**bacteriostatic** *adj.*

bacteriuria (bak-tē-rē-ū′-rē-à) *n* presence of bacteria in urine (100,000 or more pathogenic microorganisms per ml). Acute urinary tract infection may be preceded by, and active pyelonephritis may be associated with, asymptomatic bacteriuria.

Bactocill™ oxacillin.*

Bactrim™ cotrimoxazole.*

BAL *abbr* British antilewisite. → dimercaprol.

balanitis (bal-an-ī′-tis) *n* inflammation of the glans penis.

balanoposthitis (bal-an-ō-pos-thī′-tis) *n* inflammation of the glans penis and prepuce.

balanus (bal′-an-us) *n* the glans of the penis or clitoris.

baldness *n* → alopecia.

ballottement (bal-lot'-ment) *n* testing for a floating object, esp. used to diagnose pregnancy. A finger is inserted into the vagina and the uterus is pushed forward; if a fetus is present it will fall back again, bouncing in its bath of fluid—**ballottable** *adj*.

balsam of Peru viscous aromatic liquid from the trunks of South American trees. Mild antiseptic used with zinc ointment for sores.

balsam of Tolu brown aromatic resin. Used as syrup of Tolu in cough syrups.

Baltimore paste → aluminum paste.

bandage *n* traditionally a piece of cloth, calico, cotton, flannel, etc., of varying size and shape applied to some part of the body: (a) to retain a dressing or a splint; (b) to support, compress, immobilize; (c) to prevent or correct deformity.

Banthine™ methantheline.*

Banti's disease (ban'-tēz) → anemia.

barbiturates (bár-bit'-ū-rātz) *npl* widely used group of sedative drugs derived from barbituric acid (a combination of malonic acid and urea). Small changes in basic structure result in formation of rapid-acting, medium or long-acting barbiturates. Continual use may result in addiction. Action potentiated in presence of alcohol. As barbiturates produce tolerance and psychological and physical dependence, have serious toxic side-effects and can be fatal following large overdose, they have been replaced in clinical use by safer drugs, e.g., benzodiazepines.

barbiturism (bár-bit'-ū-rizm) *n* addiction to barbiturates. Characterized by confusion, slurring of speech, yawning, sleepiness, depressed respiration, cyanosis and even coma.

barbotage (bár'-bot-ázh) *n* method of extending spread of spinal anesthesia: local anesthetic is directly mixed with aspirated cerebrospinal fluid and reinjected into the subarachnoid space.

barium enema retrograde introduction of barium sulfate suspension, plus a quantity of air, into the large bowel via a rectal catheter, during fluoroscopy.

barium sulfate heavy insoluble powder used, in an aqueous suspension, as a contrast agent in X-ray visualization of alimentary tract.

barium sulfide chief constituent of depilatory creams. → depilatories.

Barlow's disease (bár'-lōz) infantile scurvy.*

barotrauma (bār-ō-traw'-mà) *n* injury due to a change in atmospheric or water pressure, e.g., ruptured eardrum.

bartholinitis (bár-tol-in-ī'-tis) *n* inflammation of Bartholin's* glands.

Bartholin's glands (bár'-to-linz) two small glands situated at each side of external orifice of the vagina. Their ducts open just outside the hymen.

bartonellosis (bår-to-nel-ō'-sis) *n* nonprotozoal hemolytic anemia. *syn* Oroya fever.

basal cell cell type of the lowest layer of the epidermis. *basal cell carcinoma* also "rodent ulcer," slow-growing but nonmetastisizing neoplasm of the skin, usually with defined border and a confusion of blood vessels at the surface. Particularly seen in the elderly, esp. occurring on the face.

basal ganglia (bā'-sal gang'-glē-à) grey cells at the cerebral base concerned with modifying and coordinating voluntary muscle movement. Site of degeneration in Parkinson's disease.

basal metabolic rate (BMR) oxygen consumption as measured when energy output has been reduced to a basal minimum, that is, when patient is fasting and is physically and mentally at rest. Result is expressed in kilocalories as a percentage of the norm for a subject of same age, sex and surface area.

basal narcosis (når-kō'-sis) pre-anesthetic administration of narcotic drugs which reduce fear and anxiety, induce sleep and thereby minimize postoperative shock.

basic life support (BLS) maintenance of a clear airway and cardiopulmonary function.

basilarvertebral insufficiency (bā'-si-lar vér'-te-bral) vertebrobasilar* insufficiency.

basilic (bas-il'-ik) *adj* prominent. *basilic vein* on the inner side of the arm (→ Figure 10). *median basilic* a vein at the bend of the elbow which is generally chosen for venepuncture.

basophil (bā'-sō-fil) *n* **1** a cell which has an affinity for basic dyes. **2** a basophilic granulocyte (white blood cell) which takes up a particular dye; function appears to be phagocytic and it contains heparin and histamine.

basophilia (bā-sō-fil'-ē-à) *n* **1** increase of basophils in the blood. **2** basophilic staining of red blood corpuscles.

Bazin's disease (ba-zaz') (*syn* erythema induratum) chronic recurrent disorder, involving skin of the legs in women; with deep-seated nodules which later ulcerate.

BCG *abbr* Bacille-Calmette-Guerin. An attenuated form of tubercle bacilli; without power to cause tuberculosis, but retaining antigenic function; used in vaccine for immunization against tuberculosis.

bearing down **1** term for the expulsive pains in second stage of labor. **2** feeling of weight and descent in the pelvis associated with uterine prolapse or pelvic tumors.

beat *n* pulsation of the blood in the heart and blood vessels. *apical beat* → apex. *dropped beat* loss of an occasional ventricular beat as occurs in extrasystoles.* *premature beat* an extrasystole.*

beclomethasone (bek-lō-meth'-à-sōn) *n* anti-asthmatic corticosteroid drug prepared in inhaler (Beclovent, Vanceril).

Beclovent™ beclomethasone.*

bedsore *n* → pressure sore.

bedwetting *n* → enuresis.

Behçet syndrome (bā'-set) described by Behçet in 1937. Starts with ulceration of mouth and/or genitalia with eye changes such as conjunctivitis, keratitis or hypopyon iritis. One site may be affected months or years before others. There may also be skin nodules, thrombophlebitis and arthritis of one or more of the large joints. Pulmonary, gastrointestinal and neurological complications are being increasingly reported. Cause unknown; some favor virus, others an allergic vasculitis. No effective treatment apart from attempts to suppress worst phases with steroids. Blindness may result from ocular complications.

bejel (bej'-el) *n* long-lasting, nonvenereal form of syphilis* mainly affecting children in the Middle East and Africa. Usually starts in the mouth and then affects the skin, so that it is easily transmitted. Rarely fatal and is treated with penicillin.

belching *n* noisy oral emission of gas, mainly swallowed air, from the gullet and stomach.

belladonna (bel-à-don'-à) *n* deadly nightshade (*Atropa belladonna*). Powerful antispasmodic. The alkaloid from deadly nightshade is poisonous, but from it atropine* and scopolamine* are extracted.

Bellergal™ combination of phenobarbital,* belladonna* alkaloids and ergotamine.* Useful for menopausal syndrome, premenstrual tension and migraine.

Bellocq's sound or cannula (bel-oks') a curved tube used for plugging the posterior nares.

Bell's palsy facial hemiparesis* from edema of the seventh (facial) cranial nerve. Cause unknown.

bemegride (bem'-i-grīd) *n* respiratory stimulant; can be given intravenously.

benactyzine (ben-ak'-ti-zēn) *n* tranquilizing drug with selective action, producing sense of detachment from environment. Used in anxiety and tension neuroses. (Deprol.)

Benadryl™ diphenhydramine.*

Bence-Jones protein (bens-jōnz') protein bodies appearing in the urine of some patients with myclomatosis.* On heating the urine they are precipitated out of solution at 50°–60° C; they redissolve on further heating to boiling point and reprecipitate on cooling.

bendroflumethiazide (bend-rō-flōō-meth-ī'-à-zīd) *n* oral diuretic of the thiazide group: it decreases reabsorption of sodium and chloride in the kidney tubules; duration of action is about 20–24 hours. Used with caution in renal or hepatic failure. → diuretics, thiazides. (Corzide, Naturetin, Rauzide.)

bends *n* → caisson disease.

Benedict's solution (ben'-e-dikts) solution of copper sulfate which is easily reduced, producing color changes. Used to detect the presence of glucose.

Benemid™ probenecid.*

benign (bē-nīn') *adj* 1 noninvasive, noncancerous (of a growth). 2 describes a condition or illness which is not serious and does not usually have harmful consequences. *benign myalgic encephalomyelitis* (*BME*) flulike illness with symptoms including dizziness, muscle fatigue and spasm, headaches and other neurological pain. A high percentage of BME sufferers have a higher level of Coxsackie B antibodies in blood than the rest of the population.

Bennett's fracture (ben'-ets) fracture of proximal end of first metacarpal involving the articular surface.

Bentyl™ dicyclomine.*

benzalkonium (ben-zal-kō'-nē-um) *n* antiseptic with detergent action. Used as 1% solution for skin preparation, 1:20,000–1:40,000 for irrigation of wounds. Incompatible with soap, with loss of activity.

benzocaine (ben'-zō-kān) *n* relatively nontoxic surface anesthetic for skin and mucous membranes. Used as dusting powder (10%), ointment (10%), suppositories (5 g), and lozenges. Occasionally given orally in gastric carcinoma.

benzodiazepines (ben-zō-dī-az'-e-pēns) *npl* group of minor tranquilizers which have similar pharmacological activities, such as sedation, reducing anxiety, relaxing muscles. Includes Ativan, Librium, Valium, Xanax.

benzoic acid (ben-zō'-ik) antiseptic* and antifungal* agent used as a food preservative and in pharmaceutical preparations; also in keratolytic* ointments. Rarely given orally owing to irritant effects. Saccharin* is a derivative of this acid.

benzoin (ben'-zō-in) *n* a resin of balsam used as a topical protective and as an expectorant.

benzphetamine (benz-fet'-à-mēn) *n* drug similar to amphetamine*; used orally in treatment of obesity. (Didrex.)

benzthiazide (benz-thī'-à-zīd) *n* thiazide diuretic. (Exna.) → diuretics.

benztropine (benz-trō'-pēn) *n* drug similar to atropine* but also has antihistaminic, local anesthetic and sedative effects; reduces muscle rigidity and cramp of parkinsonism. (Cogentin.)

benzyl benzoate (ben'-zil ben'-zō-āt) aromatic liquid; has ascaricidal properties and is used mainly in treatment of scabies.*

bephenium hydroxynaphthoate (be-fen'-ē-um hī-droks-ē-naf'-thō-āt) anthelmintic effective against hookworm and roundworm; given on an empty stomach at least 1 hour before food.

beriberi (ber'-ē-ber'-ē) *n* deficiency disease caused by lack of vitamin B_1. Occurs mainly in those countries where staple diet is polished rice. Symptoms are pain from neuritis, paralysis, muscular wasting, progressive edema, mental deterioration and, finally, heart failure.

berylliosis (ber-il-ē-ō'-sis) *n* industrial disease; impaired lung function because of interstitial fibrosis from inhalation of beryllium. Steroids are used in treatment.

Besnier's prurigo (bez'-nē-āz prōō-rī'gō) an inherited flexural neurodermatitis with impaired peripheral circulation giving rise to dry thickened epidermis and outbreaks of eczema in childhood. Old term for atopic* syndrome. → eczema.

beta blocker (bā'-tȧ) drug which prevents stimulation of beta adrenergic receptors, thus decreasing heart activity.

Betadine™ povidone* iodine, available as aerosol spray, surgical scrub, scalp lotion and ointment.

betamethasone (bā-ta-meth'-ȧ-sōn) *n* synthetic corticosteroid drug effective on low dosage; similar to prednisolone.* (Betnelan, Celestone.)

bethanechol (beth-an'-e-kol) *n* compound resembling carbachol* in activity, but relatively nontoxic. Used in urinary retention, abdominal distension and myasthenia gravis. (Duvoid, Urecholine.)

Betnelan™ betamethasone.*

Betnovate™ cream or ointment containing betamethasone.* More effective than those containing hydrocortisone, but can be absorbed through skin and can produce local or systemic side-effects.

bicarbonate (bī-kȧr'-bon-āt) *n* a salt of carbonic acid. *blood bicarbonate* that in the blood, indicating alkali reserve. Also called "plasma bicarbonate."

bicellular (bī-sel'-ū-lȧr) *adj* composed of two cells.

biceps (bī'-seps) *n* a muscle possessing two heads or points of origin. → Figure 4. *biceps femoris* → Figure 5.

Bicillin™ penicillin* G.

biconcave (bī-kon'-kāv) *adj* concave or hollow on both surfaces.

biconvex (bī-kon'-veks) *adj* convex on both surfaces.

bicornuate (bī-kōrn'-ū-āt) *adj* having two horns, generally applied to a double uterus or a single uterus possessing two horns.

bicuspid (bī-kus'-pid) *adj* having two cusps or points. *biscuspid teeth* the pre-molars. *biscuspid valve* the mitral valve between the left atrium and ventricle of the heart.

bifid (bī'-fid) *n* divided into two parts. Cleft or forked.

bifurcation (bī-fur-kā'-shun) *n* division into two branches—**bifurcate** *adj, vt, vi.*

biguanides (bī'-gwan-īdz) *npl* (*syn* diguanides) oral antidiabetic agents. They do not act on the islets of Langerhans but appear to stimulate uptake of glucose by muscle tissue in diabetic subjects. Unwanted side-effects include lactic acidosis.

bilateral (bī-lat'-ėr-al) *adj* pertaining to both sides.

bile (bīl) *n* a bitter, alkaline, viscid, greenish-yellow fluid secreted by the liver and stored in the gallbladder. Contains water, mucin, lecithin, cholesterol, bile salts and the pigments bilirubin and biliverdin. *bile ducts* the hepatic and cys-tic, which join to form the common bile duct (→ Figure 18). *bile salts* emulsi-fying agents, sodium glycocholate and taurocholate—**bilious, bilary** *adj.*

Bilharzia (bil-hår'-zē-á) *n* → *Schistosoma.*

bilharziasis (bil-hår-zī'-á-sis) *n* → schistosomiasis.

biliary (bil'-ē-ār-ē) *adj* pertaining to bile. *biliary colic* pain in right upper quad-rant of the abdomen, due to obstruction of the gallbladder or common bile duct, usually by a stone; it is severe and often occurs about an hour after a meal; it may last several hours and is usually steady, which differentiates it from other forms of colic. Vomiting may occur. *biliary fistula* an abnormal track convey-ing bile to the surface or to some other organ.

bilirubin (bil-ē-roo'-bin) *n* pigment largely derived from breakdown of hemo-globin from red blood cells destroyed in the spleen. When released it is fat sol-uble, gives an indirect reaction with Van* den Bergh's test and is potentially harmful to metabolically active tissues in the body, particularly basal nuclei of the immature brain. *indirect bilirubin* is transported to the blood attached to albumen to make it less likely to enter and damage brain cells. In the liver the enzyme glucuronyl transferase conjugates indirect fat-soluble bilirubin with glucuronic acid to make it water soluble, in which state it is relatively nontoxic, reacts directly with Van den Bergh's test *(direct bilirubin)* and can be excreted in stools and urine. → phototherapy.

biliuria (bil-ē-ū'-rē-á) *n* (choluria) the presence of bile pigments in urine—**bili-uric** *adj.*

biliverdin (bil-ē-vėr'-din) *n* green pigment of bile formed by oxidation of bilirubin.

bilobate (bī-lō'-bāt) *adj* having two lobes.

bilobular (bī-lob'-ū-lár) *adj* having two little lobes or lobules.

bimanual (bī-man'-ū-ȧl) *adj* performed with both hands. A method of examination used in gynecology: internal genital organs are examined between one hand on the abdomen and the other or a finger within the vagina.

binaural (bīn-aw'-rȧl) *adj* pertaining to, or having two ears. Applied to a type of stethoscope.*

binder *n* type of many-tailed bandage which can be applied to the abdomen to provide external pressure while internal pressure is decreasing, e.g., in childbirth, paracentesis of the abdomen.

Binet's test (be-nāz') properly Binet-Simon scale. First used in 1905. Series of graded intelligence tests in which an individual's intelligence level (mental age) is compared with chronological age. A forerunner of IQ tests.

binge-purge syndrome → bulimia.

binocular vision focusing of both eyes on one object at the same time in such a way that only one image is seen. Not an inborn ability but acquired in the first few months of life.

binovular (bīn-ov'-ū-lȧr) *adj* derived from two separate ova. Binovular twins may be of different sexes. → uniovular *opp.*

biofeedback *n* presentation of immediate visual or auditory information about usually unconscious body functions such as blood pressure, heart rate and muscle tension. Either by trial and error or by operant conditioning, a person can learn to repeat behavior which results in a satisfactory level of body functions.

biohazard *n* anything which presents a hazard to life. Some specimens for the pathological laboratory are so labelled.

biopsy (bī'-op-sē) *n* excision of tissue from a living body for microscopic examination to establish diagnosis.

biorhythm (bī-ō-rith'-um) *n* any of the recurring cycles of physical, emotional and intellectual activity which affect people's lives—**biorhythmic** *adj.*

biosensors (bī-ō-sens'-ors) *npl* noninvasive instruments which measure the result of biological processes, for example, local skin temperature and humidity; or biological response to, for example, external pressure.

biotin (bī'-o-tin) *n* member of vitamin B complex; also known as vitamin H and as coenzyme R. Probably synthesized by intestinal flora. Lack of it may cause dermatitis in humans.

biparous (bip'-ār-us) *adj* producing two offspring at one birth.

biperiden (bī-pėr'-i-den) *n* drug which acts on the autonomic nervous system: useful for drug-induced parkinsonism. (Akineton.)

bipolar (bī-pō'-lȧr) *adj* having two poles.

birth *n* act of expelling the young from the mother's body; delivery; being born. *birth canal* cavity or canal of the pelvis through which baby passes during labor. *birth control* prevention or regulation of conception by any means; contraception. *birth injury* any injury occurring during parturition, e.g., fracture of a bone, subluxation of a joint, injury to peripheral nerve, intracranial hemorrhage. *birth mark* nevus.* *premature birth* one occurring after the infant is viable, but before term. *birth rate* number of live births per 1000 people in a given year.

bisacodyl (bis-à-kō'-dil) *n* synthetic laxative; not absorbed when taken orally but has a contact stimulant action on the bowel lining. Also available as suppositories. (Dulcolax.)

bisexual (bī-seks'-ū-ál) *adj* **1** having some of the physical genital characteristics of both sexes; a hermaphrodite. True hermaphrodite possesses gonadal tissue of both sexes. **2** describes a person who is sexually attracted to both men and women.

bismuth (biz'-muth) *n* a greyish metal. *bismuth carbonate* mild antacid used with other alkalis in dyspepsia and peptic ulcer. *bismuth salicylate* gastric sedative used in gastroenteritis. *bismuth sodium tartrate* soluble compound used occasionally by intramuscular injection in infective arthritis. *bismuth subgallate* yellow, insoluble powder. Used as dusting powder in eczema and in suppositories for hemorrhoids. Occasionally given orally as an astringent.

Bitot's spots (bē'-tōz) (*syn* xerosis conjunctivae) collections of dried epithelium, flaky masses and microorganisms at the sides of the cornea. A manifestation of vitamin A deficiency.

blackhead *n* → comedo.

black lung disease a form of pneumoconiosis arising from exposure to coal dust; an industrial disease of coal miners.

blackwater fever a malignant form of malaria* occurring in the tropics, esp. Africa; with great destruction of red blood cells, causing a very dark colored urine.

bladder *n* membranous sac containing fluid or gas.

blastocyst (blas'-tō-sist) *n* stage in mammalian embryo development consisting of the inner cell mass and a trophoblast layer enclosing the blastocele. Also called blastodermic vesicle.

Blastomyces (blas-tō-mī'-sēz) *n* genus of pathogenic yeastlike organisms—**blastomycetic** *adj*.

blastomycosis (blas-tō-mī-kō'-sis) *n* granulomatous condition caused by budding, yeastlike organisms called *Blastomyces*. May affect skin, viscera and bones—**blastomycotic** *adj*.

blastula (blas′-tū-là) *n* early stage in development of the fertilized ovum when the morula* becomes cystic and infolds to become the gastrula.

bleb (bleb) *n* a large blister.* → bulla, vesicle.

bleeder *n* one who is subject to frequent loss of blood, as one suffering from hemophilia.*

"bleeding time" time required for spontaneous arrest of bleeding from a skin puncture; under controlled conditions this forms a clinical test.

blennorrhagia (blen-or-āj′-ē-à) *n* **1** copious mucous discharge particularly from the vagina or male urethra. **2** Gonorrhea.

blennorrhea (blen-ōr-ē′-à) *n* blennorrhagia.*

bleomycin (blē-ō-mī′-sin) *n* antibiotic. (Blenoxane.)

blepharitis (blef-àr-īt′-is) *n* inflammation of the eyelids, particularly the edges —**blepharitic** *adj*.

blepharon (blef′-àr-on) *n* the eyelid; palpebra—**blephara** *pl*.

blepharoplasty (blef-àr-ō-plast′-ē) *n* tarsoplasty*—**blepharoplastic** *adj*.

blepharoptosis (blef-àr-op′-to-sis) *n* → ptosis—**blepharoptotic** *adj*.

blepharospasm (blef′-àr-ō-spazm) *n* spasm of muscles in the eyelid. Excessive winking—**blepharospastic** *adj*.

blind loop syndrome resulting from intestinal obstruction of surgical anastomosis; stasis in the small intestine which encourages bacterial growth thus producing diarrhea and malabsorption.

blind sight following damage to visual cortex, some patients have been diagnosed blind after traditional testing. However, they may be trained to use functional residual vision.

blind spot spot at which the optic nerve leaves the retina. It is insensitive to light.

blister *n* separation of the epidermis from the dermis by collection of fluid, usually serum or blood.

blistering fluid liquor* epispasticus, a counterirritant.

Blocadren™ timolol* maleate.

blood *n* red viscid fluid filling the heart and blood vessels. Consists of a colorless fluid, plasma, in which are suspended red blood corpuscles (erthrocytes), white corpuscles (leukocytes), and platelets (thrombocytes). Plasma contains a great many substances in solution, including factors which enable blood to clot. *defibrinated blood* fibrin removed by agitation. *laked blood* red cells hemolysed. *occult blood* blood which is not visible to the naked eye but whose presence can be detected by chemical tests.

blood bank special refrigerator in which blood is kept after withdrawal from donors until required for transfusion.

blood-brain barrier membranes between circulating blood and the brain. Some drugs can pass from blood through this barrier to the cerebrospinal fluid, others cannot.

blood casts casts of coagulated red blood corpuscles, formed in renal tubules and found in urine.

blood clotting primary phase: vessel closes itself off from circulation and a plug of tiny particles (platelets) collects to fill the gap, attracted by collagen present in blood vessel walls. Collagen is normally separated from flowing blood by a thin layer of cells which line the vessel wall: blood only comes into contact with collagen when a break occurs in this lining and the first platelets stick to it. These first two steps—contraction, plug—are normal in hemophilia A and B. Secondary phase: involves coagulation over and through the platelet mass. Plasma coagulation factors are as follows:

Factor No.	Synonyms
I	fibrinogen
II	prothrombin
III	tissue thromboplastin
IV	calcium ions
V	proaccelerin
VII	factor VII
VIII	antihemophilic factor (AHF)
IX	Christmas factor
X	Stuart factor (Prower factor)
XI	plasma thromboplastin antecedent (PTA)
XII	Hageman factor
XIII	fibrin-stabilizing factor

Factor VIII is affected in hemophilia A; factor IX is affected in hemophilia B (Christmas disease). In von Willebrand's disease there is a deficiency in both factor VIII and in platelet function.

blood count calculation of the number of red or white cells per cubic millimeter of blood, using a hemocytometer. *complete blood count* largely automated determination of blood content, including amounts of hematocrit and hemoglobin, and numbers of red and white cells per unit volume. Additionally, figure for MCV (mean corpuscular volume), MCH (mean corpuscular hemoglobin) and MCHC (mean corpuscular hemoglobin concentration). → Appendix. *differential blood count* estimation of relative proportions of different leukocyte cells in blood. Normal differential count is: polymorphs 65%–70%, lymphocytes 20%–25%, monocytes 5%, eosinophils 0%–3%, basophils 0%–0.5%. In childhood the proportion of lymphocytes is higher.

blood cross-matching method of mixing a sample of donor's red blood cells with recipient's serum (major cross-matching), and mixing a sample of recipient's cells with donor's serum (minor cross-matching). Done before a blood transfusion to determine blood compatibility.

blood culture incubation of blood sample in suitable medium at an optimum temperature, so that any contained organisms can multiply and so be isolated and identified under a microscope. → septicemia.

blood formation hemopoiesis.*

blood gas tension → tension.

blood glucose profiles used to make adjustments to treatment of individual diabetic patients; show peaks and troughs and duration of action of a given insulin preparation, which can vary from patient to patient. Blood samples are taken on fasting, 2 h after breakfast, before lunch, 2 h after lunch, before evening meal, at bedtime and possibly during the night. Patients may perform these tests at home.

blood groups ABO system. Four groups: A, B, AB and O. Cells of these groups contain the corresponding antigens, A, B, A and B, except group O cells, which contain neither antigen A nor B. For this reason group O blood can be given to any of the other groups and is known as the "universal donor." In plasma there are agglutinins* which will cause agglutination of any cell carrying the corresponding antigen, e.g., group A plasma contains anti-B agglutinins; group AB plasma contains no agglutinins. Group AB is therefore known as the "universal recipient" and can receive A, B and O blood. This grouping is determined by (a) testing a suspension of red cells with anti-A and anti-B serum or (b) testing serum with known cells. Transfusion with an incompatible ABO group will cause a severe hemolytic reaction and death may occur unless transfusion is promptly stopped. High titer agglutinins: in some persons anti-A or anti-B content of plasma is unusually high and their agglutinating and hemolytic effect cannot be neutralized by dilution in a recipient's blood stream. Such blood can be transfused only to a recipient of the same ABO group as the donor. Blood containers are usually labelled to show presence of high titer agglutinins. *Rhesus blood group* red cells contain four pairs of antigens which are known by the letters Cc, Dd, Ee and Ff. The letters denote allelomorphic genes which are present in all cells except the sex cells, where a chromosome can carry C or c, but not both. In this way the Rhesus genes and blood groups are derived equally from each parent. When cells contain only the cde groups, then the blood is said to be Rhesus negative (Rh–); when they contain C, D or E singly or in combination with cde, then the blood is Rhesus positive (RH +). These groups are antigenic and can, under suitable conditions, produce the corresponding antibody in serum. These antibodies are then used to detect presence of Rh groups in cells. Antibodies to the Rh group are produced by (a) transfusion with Rh incompatible blood, (b) immunization during pregnancy by fetal cells containing antigen entering the mother's circulation. This can cause erythroblastosis* fetalis. → rhesus incompatibility.

blood-letting venesection.*

blood plasma → plasma.

blood pressure pressure exerted by blood on blood vessel walls. Usually refers to pressure within arteries, which may be measured in mm of mercury using a sphygmomanometer. Arterial blood pressure fluctuates with each heart beat, having a maximum value (the systolic pressure) which is related to the ejection of blood from the heart into the arteries and a minimum value (diastolic pressure) when aortic and pulmonary valves are closed and the heart is relaxed. Usually values for both systolic and diastolic pressures are recorded (e.g., 120/70). → hypertension, hypotension.

blood serum fluid which exudes when blood clots; it is plasma minus clotting agents.

blood sugar amount of glucose in circulating blood; varies within normal limits. Level is controlled by various enzymes and hormones, most important single factor being insulin.* → hyperglycemia, hypoglycemia.

blood transfusion → transfusion.

blood urea amount of urea* (the end product of protein metabolism) in blood; varies within normal range. Virtually unaffected by amount of protein in diet when the kidneys, which are the main organs of urea excretion, are normal. When diseased, blood urea quickly rises. → uremia.

BLS *abbr* basic* life support.

"blue baby" appearance produced by some congenital heart defects. The appearance, by contrast, of a newborn child suffering from temporary anoxia is described as "blue asphyxia."

blue pus bluish discharge from a wound infected with *Pseudomonas aeruginosa* (*pyocyanea*).

BME *abbr* benign* myalgic encephalomyelitis.

BMR *abbr* basal* metabolic rate.

BM stix chemically impregnated "stick" for estimating capillary blood sugar by color change.

BMT *abbr* bone marrow transplant/transplantation. → transplantation.

body image image in an individual's mind of one's own body. Distortions occur in anorexia* nervosa, parietal lobe tumors and trauma.

Boeck's disease (beks) form of sarcoidosis.*

Bohn's nodules (bōns) tiny white nodules on the palate of the newly born.

boil *n* (*syn* furuncle) acute inflammatory condition surrounding a hair follicle; caused by *Staphylococcus aureus*. Usually attended by suppuration; it has one opening for drainage in contrast to a carbuncle.*

bolus (bō'-lus) *n* **1** a soft, pulpy mass of masticated food. **2** a large dose of a drug given at beginning of a treatment program to raise blood concentration rapidly to a therapeutic level.

bone *n* connective tissue in which salts, such as calcium carbonate and calcium phosphate, are deposited to make it hard and dense. The separate bones make up the skeleton.*

bone graft transplantation of a piece of bone from one part of the body to another, or from one person to another. Used to repair bone defects or to supply osteogenic tissue.

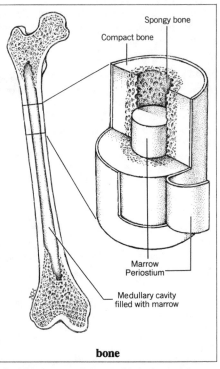

Spongy bone
Compact bone
Marrow
Periosteum
Medullary cavity filled with marrow

bone

bone marrow substance contained within bone cavities. At birth the cavities are filled with blood-forming *red marrow,* but in later life deposition of fat in long bones converts the red into *yellow bone marrow. bone marrow puncture* investigatory procedure whereby a sample of marrow is obtained by aspiration after piercing the sternum or iliac crest. *bone marrow transplant* → transplantation.

Bonnevie-Ullrich syndrome (bun-vē' ul'-rik) → Noonan syndrome.

borborygmi (bor-bor-ig'-mē) *n* rumbling noises caused by the movement of gas in the intestines.

Bordetella (bor-de-tel'-à) *n* genus of bacteria. *B. pertussis* causes whooping cough.

boric acid (bōr'-ik) (*syn* boracic acid) mild antiseptic used mainly as eye lotions and ear drops. Dusting powders and lotions should not be applied to large raw areas, as there is danger of boric poisoning.

Bornholm disease (bōrn'-hŏm) (*syn* epidemic pleurodynia) viral disease due to B group of coxsackieviruses; named after Danish island where it was described by Sylvest in 1934. 2–14 days incubation. Symptoms include sudden onset of severe pain in lower chest or abdominal or lumbar muscles. Breathing may be difficult, because of pain, and fever is common. May last up to one week. No specific treatment.

botulism (bot'-ū-lizm) *n* poisoning with the preformed exotoxin of *Clostridium botulinum*. Vomiting, constipation, ocular and pharyngeal paralysis and sometimes aphonia manifest within 24–72 h of eating food contaminated with spores, which require anaerobic conditions to produce toxin. Hence the danger of home-canned vegetables and meat.

bougie (boo'-zhē) *n* cylindrical instrument made of gum elastic, metal or other material. Used in varying sizes for dilating strictures, e.g., esophageal or urethral.

bowel (bow'-el) *n* the large intestine. → intestine.

bowleg *n* varum genu.*

Boyle's anesthetic machine (boilz) apparatus by which chloroform, ether, nitrous oxide gas and oxygen may be administered. Adapted for use with cyclopropane.*

brachial (brā'-kē-al) *adj* pertaining to the arm. Applied to vessels in this region and a nerve plexus at the root of the neck. *brachial artery* → Figure 9. *brachial vein* → Figure 10.

brachialis (brā-kē-al'-is) *n* → Figure 4.

brachiocephalic artery (brā-kē-ō-sef-al'-ik) → Figure 9.

brachiocephalic vein → Figure 10.

brachioadialis (brā'-kē-ō-rā-dē-al'-is) → Figure 4.

brachium (brā'-kē-um) *n* the arm (esp. from shoulder to elbow), or any armlike appendage—**brachia** *pl*, **brachial** *adj*.

bradycardia (brā-di-kár'-dē-à) *n* slow rate of heart contraction, resulting in a slow pulse rate. In febrile states, for each degree rise in body temperature the expected increase in pulse rate is ten beats per minute. When the latter does not occur, the term "relative bradycardia" is used.

brain *n* the encephalon; the largest part of the central nervous system: contained in the cranial cavity and surrounded by three membranes called meninges. Fluid inside the brain contained in the ventricles, and outside in the subarachnoid space, acts as a shock absorber to the delicate nerve tissue. → Figure 1.

branchial (brang'-kē-al) *adj* pertaining to the fissures or clefts which occur on each side of the neck of the human embryo and which enter into the development of nose, ears and mouth. *branchial cyst* a cyst* in the neck arising from abnormal development of the branchial* cleft/s.

Braxton Hicks sign (braks'-ton hiks) intermittent painless contractions of the uterus observed throughout pregnancy.

break-bone fever → dengue.

breast *n* 1 anterior upper part of the thorax. 2 the mammary gland. *breast bone* the sternum.

breath-H$_2$ (hydrogen) test for disaccharide intolerance. An indirect method for detecting lactase deficiency.

breech *n* the buttocks. → buttock.

breech/birth presentation refers to position of a baby in the womb such that the buttocks would be born first: normal position is head first.

bregma (breg'-mà) *n* the anterior fontanel. → fontanel.

bretylium tosylate (bre-til'-ē-um to'-sil-āt) antihypertensive drug. (Bretylol.)

Bretylol™ bretylium* tosylate.

Brevital™ methohexital.*

Bricanyl™ terbutaline.*

Bright's disease (brīts) inflammation of the kidneys. → nephritis.

Broadbent's sign (brod'-bents) visible retraction of the left side and back, in the region of the 11th and 12th ribs, synchronous with each heart beat and due to adhesions between the pericardium and diaphragm. → pericarditis.

broad ligaments lateral ligaments; double fold of parietal peritoneum which hangs over the uterus and outstretched Fallopian tubes, forming a lateral partition across the pelvic cavity.

broad thumb syndrome Rubenstein-Taybi* syndrome.

Broca's area (brōk'-às) often described as the motor center for speech; situated at the commencement of the sylvian fissure in the left hemisphere of the cerebrum. Injury to this center can result in language deficiency, including inability to speak.

Brodie's abscess (brō'-dēz) chronic abscess* in bone.

bromides (brō'-mīdz) *npl* a small group of drugs, exemplified by potassium bromide, which have a mild depressant action on the central nervous system. Used extensively in epilepsy before phenobarbital was introduced; now rarely used in nervous insomnia and restlessness, sometimes in association with chloral* hydrate.

bromidrosis (brom-i-drō'-sis) *n* profuse, fetid perspiration, esp. associated with the feet—**bromidrotic** *adj*.

bromism (brō'-mizm) *n* chronic poisoning due to continued or excessive use of bromides.*

bromocriptine (brō-mō-krip'-tēn) *n* dopamine receptor agonist useful in parkinsonism and hyperprolactinemia. (Parlodel.)

bromosulphthalein test (brō-mō-sulf'-tha-lēn) used to assess liver function; 5 mg per kg of body weight of the blue dye are injected intravenously. If more than 5% of dye is circulating in blood 45 min after injection, there is impaired hepatic function.

brompheniramine maleate (brom-fen-ir'-à-mēn mal'-ē-āt) antihistamine used for rhinitis and allergy symptoms. (Dimetane.)

Brompton cocktail (bromp'-ton) mixture containing alcohol, morphine and cocaine for relieving pain in terminally-ill patients. Name is applied to different mixtures.

bronchi (brong'-kī) *npl* the two tubes into which the trachea* divides at its lower end. → Figures 6, 7—**bronchus** *sing,* **bronchial** *adj.*

bronchial asthma (brong'-kē-àl az'-mà) reversible airflow obstruction precipitated in different patients by intake of allergens, infection, vigorous exercise or emotional stress. Often with family history of asthma* and/or other allergic conditions.

bronchial tubes *npl* subdivisions of the bronchi* after they enter the lungs.

bronchiectasis (brong-kē-ek'-ta-sis) *n* dilatation of the bronchial tubes which, when localized, is usually result of pneumonia or lobar collapse in childhood, but when more generalized is due to some inherent disorder of bronchial mucous membrane as in cystic fibrosis. Associated with profuse, fetid, purulent expectoration. Characterized by recurrent respiratory infections and digital clubbing. Leads to eventual respiratory failure—**bronchiectatic** *adj.*

bronchiole (brong'-kē-ōl) *n* one of the minute subdivisions of the bronchi,* which terminate in the alveoli or air sacs of the lungs—**bronchiolar** *adj.*

bronchiolectasis (brong-kē-ō-lek'-ta-sis) *n* dilatation of the bronchioles.

bronchiolitis (brong-kē-ōl-īt'-is) *n* inflammation of the bronchioles,* usually in children in first year of life—**bronchiolitic** *adj.*

bronchitis (brong-kī'-tis) *n* inflammation of the bronchi. *acute bronchitis* as an isolated incident is usually a primary viral infection occurring in children as a complication of the common cold, influenza, whooping cough, measles or rubella. Secondary infection occurs with bacteria, commonly *Streptococcus pneumoniae* or *Haemophilus influenzae.* Acute bronchitis in adults is usually an acute exacerbation of chronic bronchitis precipitated by a viral infection but sometimes by a sudden increase in atmospheric pollution. In *simple chronic bronchitis* bronchial mucous glands are hypertrophied and patient's only complaint is of cough productive of mucoid sputum. In *chronic obstructive bronchitis* bronchial mucous membrane has so hypertrophied that bronchial lumen is narrowed, causing airflow obstruction resulting in wheezing and leading to respiratory insufficiency and sometimes eventual respiratory failure—**bronchitic** *adj.*

bronchoconstrictor (brong-kō-con-strik'-tor) *n* any agent which constricts the bronchi.

bronchodilator (brong-kō-dī'-lā-tor) *n* any agent which dilates the bronchi.

bronchogenic (brong-kō-jen'-ik) *adj* arising from one of the bronchi.

bronchography (brong-kog'-raf-ē) *n* radiological demonstration of the bronchial tree after introduction of a small amount of a liquid contrast medium—**bronchographic** *adj*, **bronchogram** *n*, **bronchograph** *n*.

bronchomycosis (brong-kō-mī-kō'-sis) *n* general term used to cover a variety of fungal infections of the bronchi and lungs, e.g., pulmonary candidiasis,* aspergillosis*—**bronchomycotic** *adj.*

bronchophony (brong-kof'-ō-nē) *n* abnormal transmission of voice sounds heard over consolidated lung or over a thin layer of pleural fluid.

bronchopleural fistula (brong-kō-ploo'-ràl fis'-tūl-à) pathological communication between the pleural cavity and one of the bronchi.

bronchopneumonia (brong'-kō-nū-mō'nē-à) *n* term describing a form of pneumonia in which areas of consolidation are distributed widely around bronchi and not in a lobar pattern—**bronchopneumonic** *adj.*

bronchopulmonary (brong'-kō-pul'-mon-ār-ē) *adj* pertaining to the bronchi and the lungs—**bronchopulmonic** *adj.*

bronchorrhea (brong-kō-rē'-à) *n* excessive discharge of mucus from bronchial mucous membrane—**bronchorrheal** *adj.*

bronchoscope (brong'-kō-skōp) *n* endoscope* used for examining and taking biopsies from interior of the bronchi. Also used for removal of inhaled foreign bodies. Traditional bronchoscopes are rigid tubes; modern bronchoscopes are flexible fiberoptic instruments—**bronchoscopic** *adj*, **bronchoscopy** *n.*

bronchospasm (brong'-kō-spazm) *n* sudden constriction of the bronchial tubes due to contraction of involuntary plain muscle in their walls—**bronchospastic** *adj.*

bronchospirometer (bron'-kō-spī-rom'-et-ér) *n* instrument for measuring capacity of one lung—**bronchospirometric** *adj*, **bronchospirometry** *n.*

bronchostaxis (brong'-kō-stak'-sis) *n* hemorrhage from a bronchial wall.

bronchostenosis (brong'-kō-sten-ōs'-is) *n* narrowing of one of the bronchi—**bronchostenotic** *adj.*

bronchus (brong'-kus) → bronchi.

Bronkaid Mist™ epinephrine.*

Bronkephrine™ ethylnorepinephrine.*

Bronkosol™ isoetharine.*

Brucella (broo-sel′-là) *n* genus of bacteria causing brucellosis* (undulant fever in man; contagious abortion in cattle). *Brucella abortus* is the bovine strain. *Brucella melitensis* the goat strain, both transmissible to man via infected milk.

brucellosis (broo-sel-lō′-sis) *n* (*syn* melitensis) an infective reticulosis. Generalized infection in man resulting from one of the species of *Brucella;* with recurrent attacks of fever and mental depression, which may last for months. An industrial disease in occupations involving contact with bovine animals infected by *Brucella abortus,* their carcasses or untreated products; or with laboratory specimens containing *Brucella abortus.* Also called "Malta fever," "abortus fever," "Mediterranean fever" and "undulant fever."

Brudzinski's sign (brood-zin′-skēz) immediate flexion of knees and hips on raising head from pillow. Seen in meningitis.

bruise *n* (*syn* contusion) a discoloration of skin due to an extravasation of blood into underlying tissues; there is no abrasion of the skin. → ecchymosis.

bruit (broo′-ē) *n* → murmur.

bruxism (bruks′-izm) *n* teeth clenching; can cause headache from muscle fatigue and excessive wear of teeth.

BSE *abbr* breast self-examination.

bubo (bū′-bō) *n* enlargement of lymphatic glands, esp. in the groin. A feature of soft sore (chancroid), lymphogranuloma inguinale and plague—**bubonic** *adj*.

buccal (buk′-àl) *adj* pertaining to the cheek or mouth.

Buerger's disease (bėr′-gėrz) (*syn* thromboangiitis obliterans) chronic obliterative vascular disease of peripheral vessels which results in intermittent claudication.* In an investigation, incidence of HLA-A9 and HLA-B5 was significantly greater in those with Buerger's disease than in the controls. *Buerger's exercises* were designed to treat this condition; legs are placed alternately in elevation and dependence to assist perfusion of the extremities with blood.

buffer *n* **1** generally, a mixture of substances in solution with ability to bind both hydrogen and hydroxyl ions and the property of resistance to pH change when acids or alkalis are added. **2** anything used to reduce shock or jarring due to contact.

bulbar (bul′-bàr) *adj* pertaining to the medulla* oblongata. *bulbar palsy or paralysis* paralysis* which involves the labioglossopharyngeal (lips, tongue and pharynx) region and results from degeneration of motor nuclei in the medulla oblongata. Patient is deprived of safety reflexes and is in danger of choking and aspiration pneumonia. Associated with feeding difficulties in profoundly handicapped children.

bulbourethral (bul-bō-ūr-ēth′-ràl) *adj* applied to two racemose* glands (Cowper's) which open into the bulb of the male urethra. Their secretion is part of seminal fluid.

bulimarexia (bū-lēm-à-reks′-ē-à) *n* bulimia.*

bulimia (bū-lēm′-ē-à) *n* eating disorder involving repeated episodes of uncontrolled consumption of large quantities of food in a short time. Many anorectics have a history of such episodes. *bulimia nervosa* (*syn* binge-purge syndrome) self-induced vomiting after meals.

bulla (bool′-là) *n* a large watery blister. In dermatology, bulla formation is characteristic of the pemphigus group of dermatoses, but occurs sometimes in other diseases of the skin, e.g., in impetigo, in dermatitis herpetiformis, etc.— **bullae** *pl,* **bullate, bullous** *adj.*

bumetanide (bū-met′-an-īd) *n* potent loop diuretic. → diuretics. (Bumex.)

Bumex™ bumetanide.*

BUN *abbr* blood urea nitrogen.*

bundle *n* a group of fibers. *bundle of His* atrioventricular bundle; a bundle of fibers in the heart for conducting impulses.

bunion (bun′-yun) *n* (*syn* hallux valgus) deformity on the head of the metatarsal bone at its junction with the great toe. Friction and pressure of shoes at this point cause a bursa to develop. The prominent bone, with its bursa, is known as a bunion.

buphthalmos (buf-thal′-mos) *n* (*syn* oxeye) congenital glaucoma.

bupivacaine (bū-piv′-à-kān) *n* one of the longer acting local anesthetics suitable for regional nerve block. Synthetic; less toxic than cocaine.* (Marcaine.)

buprenorphine (bū-pre′-nōr-fēn) *n* analgesic with a longer action than morphine and of low dependence. (Buprenex.)

Burkitt's lymphoma (bur′-kits lim-fō′-mà) a malignant lymphoma frequently of the jaw but other sites as well. Affects principally children. Occurs almost exclusively in areas of Africa and New Guinea where malaria is endemic.

Burow's solution (bur′-ōwz) aluminum acetate, an antiseptic solution.

burr *n* attachment for a surgical drill, used for cutting into tooth or bone.

bursa (bur′-sà) *n* fibrous sac lined with synovial membrane and containing a small quantity of synovial fluid. Bursae are found between (a) tendon and bone, (b) skin and bone, (c) muscle and muscle. Function is to facilitate movement without friction between these surfaces—**bursae** *pl.*

bursitis (bur-sī′-tis) *n* inflammation of a bursa. *olecranon bursitis* inflammation of bursa over the point of the elbow. *prepatellar bursitis* (*syn* housemaid's knee) a fluid-filled swelling of the bursa in front of the knee cap (patella); frequently associated with excessive kneeling. A blow can result in bleeding into the bursa, with infection by pyogenic pathogens.

Buscopan™ derivative of hyoscine (hyoscine-N-butyl bromide), antispasmodic which relaxes smooth muscle in peptic ulcer, colic and related conditions; most effective by injection.

busulfan (bū-sul'-fan) *n* cytotoxic, alkylating drug used in chronic myeloid leukemia and polycythemia. Regular blood counts are essential, as the compound is a powerful depressant of bone marrow. (Myleran.)

butacaine (bū'-tà-kān) *n* synthetic local anesthetic similar to cocaine.* Used in ophthalmology as 2% solution which, unlike cocaine, does not dilate the pupil. (Butyn.)

Butazolidin™ phenylbutazone.*

buttock (but'-ok) *n* one of the two projections posterior to the hip joints. Formed mainly of the gluteal* muscles.

butylaminobenzoate (bū-til-am-ēn-ō-ben'-zō-āt) *n* local anesthetic used as ointment (1%), suppositories (1 g), or dusting powder.

Butyn™ butacaine.*

butyrophenones (bū'-ti-rō-fē'-nonz) *npl* substances which are dopamine blockers; they produce extrapyramidal side-effects.

bypass surgery → cardiac* bypass operation.

byssinosis (bis-in-ō'-sis) *n* form of pneumoconiosis* caused by inhalation of cotton or linen dust.

C

cachet (kash-ā′) *n* flat capsule formed of rice paper, enclosing any bitter powdered drug to be taken orally.

cachexia (ka-keks′-ē-à) *n* state of constitutional disorder, malnutrition and general ill-health. Chief signs are bodily emaciation, sallow unhealthy skin and heavy lusterless eyes—**cachectic** *adj*.

CaEDTA *abbr* calcium disodium edetate, a chelating agent. Used in lead poisoning and as eyedrops in treatment of lime burns.

caisson disease (kā′-son) (*syn* the bends; decompression sickness) results from sudden reduction in atmospheric pressure, as experienced by divers on return to surface, airmen ascending to great heights. Caused by bubbles of nitrogen which are released from solution in blood; symptoms include pain in limbs, joints, and chest. Largely preventable by proper and gradual decompression technique.

Caladryl™ lotion and cream containing calamine* and diphenhydramine.*

calamine (kal′-à-mīn) *n* zinc carbonate tinted pink with ferric oxide. Widely employed in lotions and creams for its mild astringent action on the skin. *calamine lotion* calamine dissolved in a weak solution of carbolic acid (phenol) for its anesthetic effect in relieving itch.

Calan™ verapamil.*

calcaneus (kal-kā′-nē-us) *n* the heel bone; the os calcis, largest of the tarsal bones.

calcareous (kal-kā′-rē-us) *adj* pertaining to or containing lime or calcium; of a chalky nature.

calciferol (kal-sif′-e-rol) *n* one of a group of fat-soluble compounds which have antirachitic properties and can be produced artificially. This, or natural vitamin D, is essential for the uptake and utilization of calcium. Given in rickets and to prevent hypocalcemia in celiac disease, in parathyroid deficiency and lupus vulgaris. (Sterogyl 15.)

calcification (kal-sif-i-kā′-shun) *n* hardening of an organic substance by deposit of calcium salts within it. May be normal, as in bone, or pathological, as in arteries.

calcitonin (kal-si-tōn′-in) *n* (*syn* thyrocalcitonin) hormone produced in the thyroid parafollicular or "C" cells. May play a role in regulating blood calcium level. In therapeutic doses it lowers serum calcium and inhibits resorption of bone. May be of benefit in Paget's* disease.

calcium gluconate (glū′-kon-āt) well tolerated and widely used salt of calcium. Indicated in all calcium deficiency states, in allergic conditions and in lead poisoning.

calcium lactate (lak′-tāt) a soluble salt of calcium, less irritating than calcium chloride. Used orally like calcium gluconate in all calcium deficiency states.

calcium oxalate (oks′-à-lāt) salt which, if it occurs in high concentrations in urine, may lead to formation of urinary calculi.

calculus (kal′-kū-lus) *n* abnormal concretion composed chiefly of mineral substances and formed in the passages which transmit secretions, or in cavities which act as reservoirs for them. *dental calculus* mineralized dental plaque deposited on the tooth surface—**calculi** *pl,* **calculous** *adj.*

callosity (kal-os′-it-ē) *n* (*syn* keratoma) a local hardening of skin caused by pressure or friction. The epidermis becomes hypertrophied. Most commonly seen on feet and palms of the hands.

callus (kal′-us) *n* **1** a callosity. **2** partly calcified tissue which forms about the ends of a broken bone and ultimately accomplishes repair of a fracture. When complete the bony thickening is known as *permanent callus*—**callous** *adj.*

calor (kal′-or) *n* heat; one of the four classic local signs of inflammation—others are dolor,* rubor,* tumor.*

calorie *n* unit of heat. In practice the calorie is too small a unit to be useful and the kilocalorie is the preferred unit in metabolic studies. A kilocalorie (kcal, Cal) is the amount of heat required to raise the temperature of 1 kg of water by 1° C. In science generally, the calorie has been replaced by the joule as a unit of energy, work and heat; a joule is approximately 1/4 calorie—**calorific** *adj.*

calvarium (kal-vār′-ē-um) *n* the vault of the skull; the skull cap.

camphor (kam′-for) *n* carminative and expectorant internally, and used as a camphorated tincture of opium in cough mixtures. Applied externally in the form of camphorated oil as an analgesic and as a rubefacient—**camphorated** *adj.*

Campylobacter (kam′-pil-ō-bak′-ter) *n* a Gram-negative motile rod bacterium; causes an acute diarrheal illness lasting several days.

canal *n* a duct or channel. *canal of Schlemm* → Figure 15.

canaliculotomy (kan-a-lik′-ūl-ot′-o-mē) *n* excision of the posterior wall of the ophthalmic canaliculus* and conversion of drainage "tube" into a bony channel.

canaliculus (kan-a-lik′-ū-lus) *n* a minute capillary passage. Any small canal, such as the passage leading from the edge of the eyelid to the lacrimal sac or one of the numerous small canals leading from the haversian canals—**canaliculi** *pl*, **canalicular** *adj*, **canaliculization** *n*.

cancellous (kan'-sel-lus) *n* resembling latticework; light and spongy; like a honeycomb.

cancer *n* general term for any malignant growth in any part of the body. The growth is purposeless, parasitic, and flourishes at the expense of the human host. Characteristics are tendency to cause local destruction, to invade adjacent tissues and to spread by metastasis. Frequently recurs after removal. Carcinoma refers to malignant tumors of epithelial tissue, sarcoma to malignant tumors of connective tissue—**cancerous** *adj*.

cancericidal (kan-sėr-i-sīd'-ål) *adj* lethal to cancer.

cancrum oris (kan'-krum ōr'-is) gangrenous stomatitis of cheek in debilitated children. Often called "noma." Associated with measles in malnourished African children.

Candida (kan'-di-då) *n* (*syn* Monilia) genus of dimorphic fungi. Yeastlike cells which form some filaments; widespread in nature. *Candida (Monilia) albicans* a commensal of the gastrointestinal tract. Causes infections such as thrush, vulvovaginitis, balanoprosthitis and systemic disease in some physiological and pathological states. Disease can result from disturbed flora due to use of wide-spectrum antibiotics, steroids, immunosuppressive and/or cytotoxic drugs. Infection can also occur during pregnancy or secondary to debilitating general disease such as diabetes mellitus or Cushing's syndrome. Oral infection can be due to poor oral hygiene, including carious teeth and ill-fitting dentures.

candidiasis (kan-di-dī'-å-sis) *n* (*syn* candidosis, moniliasis, thrush) disease caused by infection with a species of *Candida*.

canine *adj* of or resembling a dog. *canine teeth* four in all, two in each jaw, situated between the incisors and the premolars. Those in the upper jaw are popularly known as the "eye teeth."

canker (kang'-kėr) *n* white spots on mucous membrane of the mouth.

cannula (kan'-ū-là) *n* hollow tube for introduction or withdrawal of fluid from the body—**cannulae** *pl*, **cannulation** *n*.

cantharides (kan-thar'-i-dēz) *n* blistering agent prepared from the dried Spanish beetle *Cantharides*.

canthus (kan'-thus) *n* angle formed by the junction of the eyelids. Inner one is known as the *nasal canthus* and outer as the *temporal canthus*—**canthi** *pl*, **canthal** *adj*.

Capastat™ capreomycin.*

CAPD *abbr* continuous* ambulatory peritoneal dialysis.

capillary *n* (literally, hairlike) any tiny thin-walled vessel forming part of a network which facilitates rapid exchange of substances between the contained fluid and the surrounding tissues. *bile capillary* begins in a space in the liver and joins others, eventually forming a bile duct. *blood capillary* unites an arteriole and a venule. *capillary fragility* relative ease with which blood capillaries may rupture. *lymph capillary* begins in tissue spaces throughout the body and joins others, eventually forming a lymphatic vessel.

Capoten™ captopril.

capreomycin (kap-rē-ō-mī′-sin) *n* peptide antibiotic derived from *Streptomyces capreolus;* mainly a secondary drug in treating drug-resistant tuberculosis. (Capastat.)

capsule *n* 1 ligaments which surround a joint. 2 a gelatinous or rice paper container for noxious drugs. 3 the outer membranous covering of certain organs, such as the kidney, liver, spleen, adrenals—**capsular** *adj*.

capsulectomy (kap-sūl-ek′-to-mē) *n* surgical excision of a capsule. Refers to a joint or lens; less often to the kidney.

capsulitis (kap-sūl-ī′-tis) *n* inflammation of a capsule. Sometimes used as a synonym for frozen* shoulder.

capsulotomy (kap-sūl-ot′-om-ē) *n* incision of a capsule, usually referring to that surrounding the crystalline lens of the eye.

captopril (kap′-tō-pril) *n* drug which inhibits angiotensin-converting enzyme (ACE), thus preventing formation of active angiotensin II. → angiotensin. (Capoten.)

caput succedaneum (kap′-ut suk-sē-dā′-nē-um) edematous swelling of the baby's soft scalp tissue, apparent at or shortly after birth. Swelling is diffuse, not delineated by scalp suture lines and usually disappears rapidly.

Carbacel™ carbachol.*

carbachol (kår′-ba-kol) *n* parasympathetic nervous system stimulant similar to acetylcholine* but active orally and has a sustained action by injection. Given in postoperative retention of urine and intestinal atony, and as eye drops for glaucoma. (Carbacel, Miostat.)

carbamazepine (kår-bam-az′-e-pēn) *n* anticonvulsant which also relieves pain; esp. useful in trigeminal neuralgia. (Tegretol.)

carbaminohemoglobin (kår-bam-ēn′-ō-hē-mo-glō′-bin) *n* compound formed between CO_2 and hemoglobin. Part of the CO_2 in the blood is carried in this form.

carbenicillin (kår-ben-i-sil′-in) *n* the only semisynthetic penicillin to show any reasonable activity against the antibiotic-resistant *Pseudomonas aeruginosa*. High concentrations can be achieved in urine to destroy *Pseudomonas* there, but much larger doses, of the order of 30–40 g a day, are needed to achieve sufficient concentration in tissues. Such large doses can only be given by intravenous infusion. (Geopen, Pyopen.)

carbidopa (kår-bi-dō'-på) *n* when added to levodopa* allows reduction of dose, decreases frequency of adverse reactions and improves control of symptoms.

carbinoxamine maleate (kår-bin-oks'-å-mēn mal'-ē-āt) antihistamine; used for rhinitis and symptoms of allergy. (Clistin.)

Carbocaine™ mepivacaine.*

carbohydrate (kår-bō-hī'-drāt) *n* organic compound containing carbon, hydrogen and oxygen. Formed in nature by photosynthesis in plants. Carbohydrates are heat producing; they include starches, sugars and cellulose, and are classified in three groups: monosaccharides, disaccharides and polysaccharides. *carbohydrate intolerance* widespread and of highly variable degree, lack of one or more enzymes necessary to split disaccharides into monosaccharides. Ingestion of most sugars causes bloating, nausea, diarrhea, cramps.

carbolic acid (kår-bol'-ik) → phenol.

carboluria (kår-bol-ū'-rē-å) *n* green or dark-colored urine due to excretion of carbolic acid, as occurs in carbolic acid poisoning—**carboluric** *adj*.

carbon dioxide a gas; waste product of many forms of combustion and metabolism, excreted via the lungs. Accumulates in respiratory insufficiency or respiratory failure and carbon dioxide tension* in arterial blood (P_2CO_2) increases above the reference range of 36–44 mmHg (c 5.0 kPa).

carbon monoxide a poisonous gas which forms a stable compound with hemoglobin, thus blocking its normal reversible oxygen-carrying function and causing signs and symptoms of hypoxia to ensue.

carbonic anhydrase (kår-bon'-ik an-hī'-drāz) a zinc-containing enzyme which facilitates transfer of CO_2 from tissues to blood and to alveolar air by catalyzing the decomposition of carbonic acid into CO_2 and water.

carboxyhemoglobin (kår-boks'-ē-hēm-ō-glō'-bin) *n* stable compound formed by union of carbon monoxide and hemoglobin; deprives red blood cells of respiratory function.

carboxyhemoglobinemia (kår-boks'-ē-hēm-ō-glō'-bin-ē'-mē-å) *n* carboxyhemoglobin* in the blood—**carboxyhemoglobinemic** *adj*.

carboxyhemoglobinuria (kår-boks'-ē-hēm-ō-glō'-bin-ūr'-ē-å) *n* carboxyhemoglobin* in urine—**carboxyhemoglobinuric** *adj*.

carbuncle (kår'-bung-kl) *n* acute inflammation (usually caused by *Staphylococcus*) involving several hair follicles and surrounding subcutaneous tissue, forming an extensive slough with several discharging sinuses.

carcinogen (kår-sin'-ō-jen) *n* any cancer-producing substance or agent—**carcinogenic** *adj*, **carcinogenicity** *n*.

carcinogenesis (kår-sin-ō-jen'-e-sis) *n* the production of cancer—**carcino-** genetic *adj*.

carcinoid syndrome (kàr′-sin-oyd) a histologically malignant but clinically mostly benign tumor of the appendix that may secrete serotonin,* which stimulates smooth muscle causing diarrhea, asthmatic spasm, flushing and other miserable symptoms. Methysergide may give prompt relief of diarrhea.

carcinoma (kàr-sin-ō′-mà) *n* a cancerous growth of epithelial tissue (e.g., mucous membrane) and derivatives such as glands. *carcinoma-in-situ* asymptomatic condition with cells closely resembling cancer cells. A very early cancer; previously called pre-invasive carcinoma—**carcinomata** *pl*, **carcinomatous** *adj*.

carcinomatosis (kàr-sin-ō-mà-tō′-sis) *n* condition in which cancer is widespread throughout the body.

cardia (kàr′-dē-à) *n* the esophageal opening into the stomach.

cardiac (kàr′-dē-ak) *adj*
1 pertaining to the heart; **2** pertaining to the cardia. *cardiac achalasia* food fails to pass normally into the stomach, though there is no obvious obstruction. The esophagus does not demonstrate normal waves of contraction after swallowing; this prevents normal relaxation of the cardiac sphincter. Associated with loss of ganglion cells within muscle layers of at least some areas of the affected esophagus. *cardiac arrest* complete cessation of the heart's activity. Failure of heart action to maintain an adequate cerebral circulation in the absence of a causative and irreversible disease. The clinical picture of cessation of circulation in a patient who

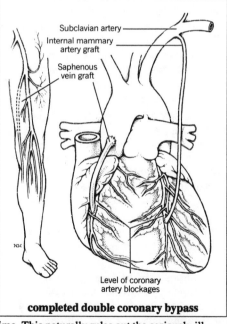

Subclavian artery

Internal mammary artery graft

Saphenous vein graft

Level of coronary artery blockages

completed double coronary bypass

was not expected to die at the time. This naturally rules out the seriously ill patient who is dying slowly with an incurable disease. *cardiac asthma* nocturnal paroxysmal dyspnea precipitated by pulmonary congestion resulting from left-sided heart failure. → asthma. *cardiac bed* one which can be manipulated so that patient is supported in a sitting position. *cardiac bypass operation* bypassing of sclerosed vessels supplying heart muscle by grafting a vein from the leg. *cardiac catheterization* → catheterization. *cardiac cycle* series of movements through which the heart passes in performing one heart beat; corresponds to one pulse beat and takes about one second. → diastole, systolic. *cardiac edema* gravitational edema. Such patients excrete excessive aldosterone which increases excretion of potassium and conserves sodium and chloride. Anti-aldosterone drugs useful, e.g., spironalactone, triamterine. Both act as diuretics. → edema. *cardiac pacemaker* electrical apparatus for maintaining myocardial contraction by stimulating heart muscle. A pacemaker may be permanent, emitting the stimulus at a constant rate, or it may fire only on demand when the heart does not spontaneously contract at a minimum rate. *cardiac tamponade* compression of heart. Can occur in surgery and penetrating wounds or rupture of the heart—from hemopericardium.

cardialgia (kȧr-dē-al′-jē-ȧ) *n* literally, pain in the heart. Often used to mean heartburn (pyrosis*).

cardiogenic (kȧr-dē-ō-jen′-ik) *adj* of cardiac origin, such as shock in coronary thrombosis.

cardiograph (kȧr′-dē-ō-graf) *n* instrument for recording graphically the force and form of the heart beat—**cardiographic** *adj,* **cardiogram** *n.*

cardiology (kȧr′-dē-ol′-o-jē) *n* study of structure, function and diseases of the heart—**cardiologist** *n.*

cardiomegaly (kȧr′-dē-ō-meg′-a-lē) *n* enlargement of the heart.

cardiomyopathy (kȧr′-dē-ō-mī-op′-ath-ē) *n* an acute, subacute, or chronic disorder of heart muscle, of unknown etiology or association, often with endocardial or sometimes with pericardial involvement (WHO definition)—**cardiomyopathic** *adj.*

cardiopathy (kȧr-dē-op′-ath-ē) *n* heart disease—**cardiopathic** *adj.*

cardiophone (kȧr′-dē-ō-fōn) *n* a microphone strapped to patient which allows audible and visual signal of heart sounds. By channelling pulse through an electrocardiograph, a graphic record can be made. Can be used for the fetus.

cardioplasty (kȧr′-dē-ō-plas′-tē) *n* plastic operation to cardiac sphincter of the stomach.

cardioplegia (kȧr′-dē-ō-plē′-jȧ) *n* induction of electromechanical cardiac arrest. *cold cardioplegia* cardioplegia combined with hypothermia to reduce oxygen consumption of the myocardium during open heart surgery.

cardiopulmonary (kȧr′-dē-ō-pul′-mon-ā-rē) *adj* pertaining to heart and lungs. *cardiopulmonary bypass* used in open heart surgery. Heart and lungs are excluded from the circulation and replaced by a pump oxygenator. *cardiopulmonary resuscitation (CPR)* → resuscitation—**cardiopulmonic** *adj.*

Cardioquin™ quinidine.

cardiorator (kår'-dē-ō-rā'-tor) *n* apparatus for visual recording of the heart beat.

cardiorenal (kår'-dē-ō-rēn'-al) *adj* pertaining to the heart and kidney.

cardiorespiratory (kår'-dē-ō-resp'-ir-atōr-ē) *adj* pertaining to the heart and respiratory system.

cardiorraphy (kår-dē-ōr'-af-ē) *n* stitching of the heart wall; usually reserved for traumatic surgery.

cardioscope (kår'-dē-ō-skōp) *n* instrument fitted with a lens and illumination, for examining interior of the heart—**cardioscopic** *adj*.

cardiospasm (kår'-dē-ō-spazm) *n* spasm of the cardiac sphincter between the esophagus and the stomach, causing retention within the esophagus. Usually no local pathological change is found.

cardiothoracic (kår'-dē-ō-thōr-as'-ik) *adj* pertaining to the heart and thoracic cavity. A specialized branch of surgery.

cardiotocography (kår'-dē-ō-to-kog'-raf-ē) *n* procedure in which fetal heart rate is measured either by external microphone or by application of an electrode to the fetal scalp, recording fetal ECG and from it the fetal heart rate. Using either an internal catheter which is passed into the amniotic cavity, or an external transducer placed on the mother's abdomen, maternal contractions can also be measured. Both measurements are fed through a monitor in such a way that extraneous sounds are excluded, and both measurements are recorded on heat-sensitive paper—**cardiotocograph** *n*.

cardiotomy syndrome (kår-dē-ot'-o-mē) pyrexia, pericarditis and pleural effusion following heart surgery; may develop weeks or months after operation and is thought to be an autoimmune reaction.

cardiotoxic (kår-dē-ō-toks'-ik) *adj* describes any agent which has injurious effect on the heart.

cardiovascular (kår'-dē-ō-vas'-kū-lår) *adj* pertaining to the heart and blood vessels.

cardioversion (kår'-dē-ō-ver'-shun) *n* use of electrical countershock for restoring heart rhythm to normal.

carditis (kår-dī'-tis) *n* inflammation of the heart. A word seldom used without the appropriate prefix, e.g., endo-, myo-, pan-, peri-.

caries (kår'-ēz) *n* **1** inflammatory decay of bone, usually associated with pus formation. **2** a microbial disease of the calcified tissue of the teeth characterized by demineralization of inorganic portion and destruction of organic substance of the tooth—**carious** *adj*.

carina (kå-rē'-nà) *n* keellike structure exemplified by the keel-shaped cartilage at the bifurcation of the trachea into two bronchi—**carinal** *adj*.

cariogenic (kā-rē-ō-jen′-ik) *adj* any agent causing caries,* by custom referring to dental caries.

carminative (kår-min′-a-tiv) *adj, n* having the power to relieve flatulence and associated colic. Chief carminatives administered orally are aromatics: cinnamon, cloves, ginger, nutmeg and peppermint.

carmustine (kår-mus′-tēn) *n* an alkylating cytotoxic agent.

carneous mole (kår′-nē-us) fleshy mass in the uterus comprising blood clot and a dead fetus or parts thereof which have not been expelled with abortion.

carotenes (kär′-ō-tēns) *npl* group of naturally occurring pigments within the larger group of carotenoids.* Carotene occurs in three forms—alpha (α), beta (β) and gamma (γ). The β form is converted in the body to vitamin A; it is therefore a provitamin.

carotenoids (ka-rot′-e-noyds) *npl* group of about 100 naturally occurring yellow to red pigments found mostly in plants, some of which are carotenes.*

carotid (kår-ot′-id) *n* principal artery on each side of the neck. At the bifurcation of the common carotid into the internal and external carotids there are: (a) the *carotid bodies,* a collection of chemoreceptors which, being sensitive to chemical changes in the blood, protect the body against lack of O_2, (b) the *carotid sinus,* a collection of receptors sensitive to pressure changes; increased pressure causes slowing of the heart beat and lowering of blood pressure.

carpal tunnel syndrome nocturnal pain, numbness and tingling in the distribution of the median nerve in the hand. Due to compression as the nerve passes under the fascial band. Most common in middle-aged women.

carphology (kår-fol′-o-jē) *n* involuntary picking at the bedclothes, as seen in exhaustive or febrile delirium. *syn* floccillation.

carpometacarpal (kår′-pō-met-å-kår′-pal) *adj* pertaining to the carpal and metacarpal bones, joints between them and ligaments joining them.

carpopedal (kår′-pō-pē′-dal) *adj* pertaining to hands and feet. *carpopedal spasm* (*syn* Trousseau's sign) spasm of hands and feet in tetany,* provoked by constriction of the limb.

carpus (kår′-pus) *n* the wrist, consisting of eight small bones arranged in two rows. → Figure 3—**carpal** *adj*.

cartilage (kår′-til-aj) *n* dense connective tissue capable of withstanding pressure; several types according to function. There is relatively more cartilage in a child's skeleton but much of it has been converted into bone by adulthood—**cartilaginous** *adj*.

caruncle (ka-rung′-kl) *n* a red fleshy projection. Hymenal caruncles surround the entrance to the vagina after rupture of the hymen. The lacrimal caruncle is the fleshy prominence at the inner angle of the eye.

caseation (kā-sē-ā'-shun) *n* formation of a soft, cheeselike mass, as occurs in tuberculosis—**caseous** *adj*.

casein (kā'-sēn) *n* protein produced when milk enters the stomach; result of precipitation of caseinogen. Coagulation occurs and is due to action of rennin* upon the caseinogen* in milk, splitting it into two proteins, one being casein, which combines with calcium forming a clot. *casein hydrolysate* predigested protein food derived from casein, easily added to other foods to increase protein content. *syn* paracasein.

caseinogen (kā-sēn'-o-jen) *n* principal protein in milk; insoluble in water but kept in solution in milk by inorganic salts. Proportion to lactalbumin* is much higher in cows' milk than in human milk. Converted into insoluble casein in the presence of chymosin.

caseous degeneration (kā'-sē-us) cheeselike tissue resulting from atrophy in a tuberculoma or gumma.

Casoni test (ka-sō'-nē) intradermal injection of fresh, sterile hydatid fluid. A white papule indicates a hydatid* cyst.

cast *n* **1** fibrous material and exudate which has been molded to the form of a cavity or tube in which it has collected. **2** a rigid casing made with plaster of Paris and applied to immobilize a part of the body.

castor oil a vegetable oil with purgative action when taken orally. Also used with zinc ointment for diaper rash and pressure sores.

castration (kas-trā'-shun) *n* surgical removal of testicles in the male, or of ovaries in the female. May be part of treatment for a hormone-dependent cancer—**castrated** *adj*, **castrate** *n*, *vt*.

CAT *abbr* computed* axial tomography.

catabolism (kat-ab'-ol-izm) *n* series of chemical reactions in the living body in which complex substances, taken in as food, are broken down into simpler ones accompanied by release of energy, needed for anabolism and the other activities of the body. → adenosine triphosphate, metabolism—**catabolic** *adj*.

catalase (kat'-a-lāz) *n* enzyme present in most human cells to catalyze breakdown of hydrogen peroxide.

catalysis (kat-al'-i-sis) *n* increase in the rate at which a chemical action proceeds to equilibrium through the medium of a catalyst or catalyser. If there is retardation it is negative catalysis—**catalytic** *adj*.

catalyst (kat'-a-list) *n* (*syn* catalyser, enzyme, ferment) agent which produces catalysis.* It does not undergo any change during the process.

cataplexy (kat'-a-pleks-ē) *n* condition of muscular rigidity induced by severe mental shock or fear; patient remains conscious—**cataplectic** *adj*.

Catapres™ clonidine.*

cataract (kat'-à-rakt) *n* an opacity of the crystalline lens or its capsule; congenital, senile, traumatic or due to metabolic defects, in particular, diabetes mellitus. *hard cataract* contains a hard nucleus, tends to be dark in color and occurs in older people. *soft cataract* one without a hard nucleus, occurs at any age, but particularly in the young. Cataract usually develops slowly and when mature is called a *ripe cataract*—**cataractous** *adj*.

catarrh (ka-tàr') *n* chronic inflammation of a mucous membrane with constant flow of a thick sticky mucus—**catarrhal** *adj*.

catatonic schizophrenia (kat-a-ton'-ik skitz-ō-frēn'-ē-à) → schizophrenia.

cat-cry syndrome produced by partial loss of one of the number 5 chromosomes, leading to mental subnormality with certain physical abnormalities and a curious, flat, toneless catlike cry in infancy.

catecholamines (kat-e-kōl'-a-mēns) *npl* any of a group of amines secreted in the body to act as neurotransmitters; epinephrine, norepinephrine and dopamine are examples. Some have been synthesized and can be prescribed as treatment.

catgut *n* form of ligature and suture of varying thickness, strength and absorbability, prepared from sheep's intestines. The "plain" variety is usually absorbed in 5–10 days. "Chromicized" catgut and "iodized" catgut will hold for 20–40 days.

catheter (kath'-e-tèr) *n* hollow tube of variable length and bore, usually having one fluted end and a tip of varying size and shape according to function; made of many substances including soft and hard rubber, gum elastic, glass, silver, other metals and plastic materials, some of which are now radioopaque. They have many uses, from insufflation of hollow tubes to introduction and withdrawal of fluid from body cavities. A recent innovation is the fiberoptic cardiac catheter which, when in situ, picks up pulses of light from which the oxygen saturation of the blood can be determined.

catheterization (kath-e-ter-īz-ā'-shun) *n* insertion of a catheter, most usually into urinary bladder. *cardiac catheterization* long plastic catheter or tubing inserted into an arm vein and passed along to right atrium, ventricle and pulmonary artery for (a) recording pressure in these areas, (b) introducing contrast medium prior to X-ray and high speed photography. Esp. useful in the diagnosis of congenital heart defects—**catheterize** *vt*.

cat scratch fever bacterial infection resulting from a scratch or bite by a cat; fever and glandular swelling about a week after the incident. Recovery is usually complete, although there may be some abscesses.

cauda (kaw'-dà) *n* a tail or taillike appendage—**caudal, caudate** *adj*.

caudal anesthetic (kaw'-dal) anesthetic administered by means of an approach to the epidural space through the caudal canal in the sacrum.

caul (kawl) *n* the amnion, instead of rupturing as is usual to allow the baby through, persists and covers the baby's head at birth.

cauliflower growth proliferative free-growing type of cancer which forms an excrescence on the affected surface.

causalgia (kaws-al′-jē-à) *n* excruciating neuralgic pain, resulting from physical trauma to a cutaneous nerve. Also known as reflex sympathetic dystrophy.

cauterize (kaw′-tėr-īz) *vt* to cause destruction of tissue by applying a heated instrument, a cautery—**cauterization** *n*.

cavernous (kav′-ėr-nus) *adj* having hollow spaces, *cavernous sinus* a channel for venous blood, on either side of the sphenoid bone; drains blood from lips, nose and orbits. Sepsis in these areas can cause cavernous sinus thrombosis.

cavitation (kav-it-ā′-shun) *n* formation of a cavity, as in pulmonary tuberculosis.

cavity *n* a hollow; an enclosed area. *abdominal cavity* that below the diaphragm; the abdomen. *buccal cavity* the mouth. *cerebral cavity* the ventricles of the brain. *cranial cavity* the brain box formed by the bones of the cranium. *medullary cavity* hollow center of a long bone, containing yellow bone marrow or medulla. *nasal cavity* that in the nose, separated into right and left halves by the nasal septum. *oral cavity* buccal cavity. *pelvic cavity* that formed by the pelvic bones, more particularly the part below the iliopectineal line. *peritoneal cavity* potential space between parietal and visceral layers of the peritoneum. Similarly, the *pleural cavity* is the potential space between pulmonary and parietal pleurae which in health are in contact in all phases of respiration. *synovial cavity* potential space in a synovial joint. *uterine cavity* that of the uterus, the base extending between the orifices of the uterine tubes.

CCU *abbr* coronary care unit. → intensive care/therapy unit.

cecostomy (sē-kos′-to-mē) *n* surgically established fistula between the cecum* and anterior abdominal wall, usually to achieve drainage and/or decompression of the cecum; usually created by inserting a widebore tube into the cecum.

cecum (sē′-kum) *n* blind, pouchlike commencement of the colon* in the right iliac fossa. To it is attached the vermiform appendix; it is separated from the ileum by the ileocecal valve—**cecal** *adj*.

Cedilanid-D™ deslanoside.*

ceftriaxone (sef-tri-aks′-ōn) *n* semisynthetic cephalosporin with a half life of 8 h, a single i.m. dose of which is claimed to be extremely effective against gonorrhea. (Rocephin.)

cefuroxime (sef-ūr-oks′-ēm) *n* useful drug for penicillin-resistant strains of microorganisms. (Ceftin, Zinacef.)

Celestone™ betamethasone.*

celiac (sē′-lē-ak) *adj* relating to the abdominal cavity; applied to arteries, veins, nerves and a plexus. *celiac disease* (*syn* gluten enteropathy, celiac sprue, non-tropical sprue) due to intolerance of the protein gluten* in wheat and rye. Sensitivity occurs in villi of the small intestine, producing malabsorption syndrome. Symptoms become apparent at 3–6 months, soon after a child is weaned on to cereals, as up to this time the digestion is not interfered with. On weaning, absorption of fats is impaired, and large amounts of split fats may be excreted in the stools (steatorrhea*).

celioscopy (sē-lē-os'-ko-pē) *n* laparoscopy.*

cell *n* a minute mass of protoplasm containing a nucleus. Some cells, e.g., erythrocytes, are non-nucleated and others may be multinucleated—**cellular** *adj*.

cell mediated immunity → immunity.

cellulitis (sel-ū-lī'-tis) *n* diffuse inflammation of connective tissue, esp. the loose subcutaneous tissue. When it involves pelvic tissues in the female, it is called parametritis; in the floor of the mouth, Ludwig's angina.

cellulose (sel'-ū-lōs) *n* a carbohydrate forming the outer walls of plant and vegetable cells. A polysaccharide which cannot be digested by man but supplies fiber for stimulation of peristalsis.

Celontin™ methsuximide.*

cementum (se-men'-tum) *n* layer of calcified tissue covering the surface of the root of a tooth.

central cyanosis → cyanosis.

central nervous system (CNS) the brain and spinal cord and their nerves and end organs. Controls voluntary acts.

central venous pressure pressure of blood within the right atrium; measured by an indwelling catheter and a pressure manometer.

centrifugal (sen-trif'-ū-gál) *adj* efferent. Having a tendency to move outwards from the center, as the rash in smallpox.

centripetal (sen-trip'-et-al) *adj* afferent. Having a tendency to move towards the center, as the rash in chickenpox.

centrosome (sen'-trō-sōm) *n* minute spot in the cytoplasm of a fertilized ovum, influencing division of the nucleus.

cephalalgia (sef-al-al'-jà) *n* pain in the head; headache.

cephalexin (sef-al-eks'-in) *n* cephalosporin*; antibiotic which, unlike cephaloridine,* is well absorbed when given orally. Useful for urinary infections. (Keflex.)

cephalhematoma (sef-al-hēm-a-tō'-mà) *n* a collection of blood in subperiosteal tissues of the scalp.

cephalic (sef-al'-ik) *adj* pertaining to the head; near the head. *cephalic vein* → Figure 10. *cephalic version* → version.

cephalocele (sef-al'-ō-sēl) *n* hernia of the brain; protrusion of part of the brain through the skull.

cephalohematoma (sef-al-ō-hēm-a-tō'-ma) *n* cephalhematoma.*

cephalometry (sef-al-om'-et-rē) *n* measurement of the living human head.

cephalopelvic disproportion (CPD) inability of fetus to pass safely through pelvis in labor, due to contraction of the pelvis, unfavorable attitude, position or presentation of the fetus, or large size of fetus in relation to pelvic size. May be associated with inefficient uterine contractions, lack of moldability of fetal head, or rigidity of perineum.

cephalosporin (sef-al-ō-spōr'-in) *n* large group of antibiotics produced by a mold obtained from sewage in Sardinia in 1948.

cephalothin (sef'-al-ō-thin) *n* semisynthetic broad spectrum cephalosporin antibiotic. (Keflin.)

cephradine (sef'-ra-dīn) *n* a mixed antibiotic used mainly for urinary tract infections; usually given orally but injectable form also available. (Velosef.)

Cephulac™ preparation of lactulose.*

cerebellar gait → gait.

cerebellum (sėr-i-bel'-um) *n* that part of the brain which lies behind and below the cerebrum (→ Figures 1, 11). Its chief functions are co-ordination of fine voluntary movements and control of posture—**cerebellar** *adj.*

cerebral (sėr'-e-bral; sėr-ē'-bral) *adj* pertaining to the cerebrum. *cerebral compression* arises from any space-occupying intracranial lesion. *cerebral palsy* nonprogressive brain damage before completion of brain development, resulting in mainly motor conditions ranging from clumsiness to severe spasticity.

cerebration (sėr-e-brā'-shun) *n* mental activity.

cerebrospinal (sėr-i-brō-spī'-nal) *adj* pertaining to brain and spinal cord. *cerebrospinal fluid, CSF* clear fluid filling ventricles of the brain and central canal of the spinal cord. Also found beneath cranial and spinal meninges in the pia-arachnoid space.

cerebrovascular (sėr-i-brō-vas'-kū-lar) *adj* pertaining to blood vessels of the brain. *cerebrovascular accident (CVA)* interference with cerebral blood flow due to embolism, hemorrhage or thrombosis. Signs and symptoms vary according to duration, extent and site of tissue damage: a passing, even momentary inability to move a hand or foot; weakness or tingling in a limb; stertorous breathing; incontinence of urine and feces; coma; paralysis of a limb or limbs and speech deficiency (aphasia). *syn* stroke.

cerebrum (sėr'-e-brum; sėr-ē'-brum) *n* largest and uppermost part of the brain (→ Figure 11); it does not include the cerebellum, pons and medulla. The longitudinal fissure divides it into two hemispheres, each containing a lateral ventricle. Internal substance is white, outer convoluted cortex is grey—**cerebral** *adj.*

Cerubidine™ daunorubicin.*

cerumen (se-roo'-men) *n* waxlike, brown secretion from special glands in the external auditory canal—**ceruminous** *adj.*

cervical (sėr'-vi-kal) *adj* 1 pertaining to the neck; 2 pertaining to the cervix (neck) of an organ. *cervical amnioscopy* → amnioscopy. *cervical canal* lumen of the cervix uteri, from internal to external os. *cervical nerve roots* → Figure 11. *cervical rib* (*syn* thoracic inlet syndrome) a supernumerary rib in the cervical region, which may present no symptoms or may press on nerves of the brachial plexus. *cervical smear* → Pap test. *cervical vertebrae* → Figure 3.

cervicectomy (sėr-vi-sek'-to-mē) *n* amputation of the uterine cervix.

cervicitis (sėr-vis-ī'-tis) *n* inflammation of the uterine cervix.

cervix (sėr'-viks) *n* a neck. *cervix uteri, uterine cervix* neck of the uterus (→ Figure 17)—**cervical** *adj.*

cesarean section (ses-ār'-ē-an) delivery of fetus through an abdominal incision. Said to be named after Caesar, who may have been born in this way. When delivery is accomplished extraperitoneally, a "low cervical cesarian section."

cestode (ses'-tōd) *n* tapeworm. → Taenia.

Cetamide™ sulfacetamide.*

CFT *abbr* complement* fixation test.

Chadwick's sign (chad'-wiks) dark blue or purple coloration of vaginal mucous membrane; a presumptive sign of pregnancy.

chalazion (ka-lā'-zē-on) *n* cyst on the edge of the eyelid from retained secretion of the meibomian* glands.

chalone (kā'-lōn) *n* substance which inhibits rather than stimulates, e.g., enterogastrone inhibits gastric secretions and motility.

chancre (shang'-kėr) *n* the primary syphilitic ulcer, associated with swelling of local lymph glands. The picture of chancre plus regional adenitis constitutes "primary syphilis." Chancre is painless, indurated, solitary and highly infectious.

chancroid (shang'-kroyd) *n* (*syn* soft sore) type of venereal disease prevalent in warmer climates. Causes multiple, painful, ragged ulcers on penis or vulva; often associated with bubo* formation. Infection is by *Haemophilus ducreyi.*

Charcot's joint (shàr'-kōs) complete disorganization of a joint associated with syringomyelia or advanced cases of tabes dorsalis (locomotor ataxia). The condition is painless. *Charcot's triad* manifestation of disseminated sclerosis—nystagmus, intention tremor and staccato speech.

cheilitis (kī-lī'-tis) *n* inflammation of the lip.

cheiloplasty (kī'-lō-plas-tē) *n* any plastic operation on the lip.

cheilosis (kī-lō'-sis) *n* maceration at the angles of the mouth, fissures occur later. May be due to riboflavin* deficiency.

cheiropompholyx (kī-rō-pom'-fo-liks) *n* symmetrical eruption of skin of hands (esp. fingers) characterized by formation of tiny vesicles and associated with itching or burning. On the feet the condition is called "podopompholyx."

chelating agents (kē'-lā-ting) soluble organic compounds that can fix certain metallic ions into their molecular structure. When given in cases of poisoning the new complex so formed is excreted in urine.

chemonucleolysis (kē-mō-nū-klē-ol'-is-is) *n* injection of an enzyme, usually into an invertebral disk, for dissolution of same—**chemonucleolytic** *adj.*

chemopallidectomy (kē-mō-pal-id-ek'-to-mē) *n* destruction of a predetermined section of globus pallidus in the nucleus of the brain by chemicals.

chemoprophylaxis (kē-mō-prō-fil-aks'-is) *n* prevention of disease (or recurrent attack) by administration of chemicals—**chemoprophylactic** *adj.*

chemoreceptor *n* 1 cellular area having a chemical affinity for, and capable of combining with, specific substances. 2 a sensory end-organ capable of reacting to a chemical stimulus.

chemosis (kē-mō'-sis) *n* edema or swelling of the bulbar conjunctiva*— **chemotic** *adj.*

chemotaxis (kēm-ō-taks'-is) *n* movements of a cell (e.g., leukocyte) or an organism in response to chemical stimuli; attraction is *positive chemotaxis,* repulsion is *negative chemotaxis*—**chemotactic** *adj.*

chemotherapy (kēm-ō-ther'-à-pē) *n* use of a specific chemical agent to arrest progress of, or eradicate, disease in the body without causing irreversible injury to healthy tissues. Chemotherapeutic agents are administered mainly by oral, intramuscular and intravenous routes, and are distributed usually by the blood stream.

chenodeoxycholic acid (ken'-ō-dē-oks-ē-kōl'-ik) a detergentlike molecule normally present in bile; may be taken orally to dissolve gallstones.

Cheyne-Stokes respiration (chān'-stōks) cyclical waxing and waning of breathing, characterized at one extreme by deep fast breaths and at the other by apnea; generally with ominous prognosis.

CHF *abbr* congestive* heart failure.

chiasma, chiasm (kī-az'-mà) *n* an X-shaped crossing or decussation. *optic chiasma* the meeting of the optic nerves, where fibers from medial or nasal half of each retina cross the middle line to join optic tract of the opposite side (→ Figure 1)—**chiasmata** *pl.*

chickenpox *n* (*syn* varicella) mild, specific infection with varicella zoster virus. Successive crops of vesicles appear first on the trunk; they scab and heal.

chilblain (chil'-blān) *n* (*syn* crythema pernio) congestion and swelling attended with severe itching and burning sensation in reaction to cold.

Chinese restaurant syndrome *n* postprandial disturbance due to eating monosodium* glutamate.

chiniofon (kin'-i-ō-fen) *n* amebicide used in prophylaxis and treatment of acute and chronic amebiasis, often in association with emetine.*

chiropody (kī-rop'-o-dē) *n* podiatry.*

chiropractic (kī-rō-prak'-tik) *n* manipulation of vertebrae to relieve impingement of subluxated transverse processes on the nerve roots.

chiropractor (kī'-rō-prak-tor) *n* person who believes many diseases arise from interference with nerve flow and is skilled in vertebral manipulation.

Chlamydia (kla-mid'-ē-å) *n* genus of bacterialike microorganisms causing disease in man and birds. Some *Chlamydia* infections of birds can be transmitted to man. *C. trachomatis* causes trachoma.* Sexual transmission occurs. → ornithosis, psittacosis.

chloasma (klō-az'-må) *n* patchy brown discoloration of the skin, esp. the face. Can appear during pregnancy.

chloral hydrate (klōr'-al hī'-drāt) rapid-acting sedative and hypnotic of value in nervous insomnia.

chlorambucil (klōr-am'-bū-sil) *n* oral alkylating agent used in lymphoproliferative disorders. (Leukeran.)

chloramphenicol (klōr-am-fen'-ik-ol) *n* orally effective wide-range antibiotic. Drug of choice in typhoid and paratyphoid fevers, valuable in many infections resistant to other drugs. Used locally in eye and ear infections. Can cause aplastic anemia.* (Chloromycetin.)

chlorcyclizine (klōr-sīk'-li-zēn) *n* long-acting antihistamine with few sideeffects. Also used in travel sickness.

chlordiazepoxide (klōr-dī-az-e-poks'-īd) *n* drug which relieves anxiety and tension and has a muscle relaxant function; administered by mouth or by injection. (Librium.)

chlorhexidine (klōr-heks'-i-dēn) *n* bactericidal solutions effective against a wide range of bacteria. Used in 1:2000 solution as general antiseptic, 1:5000 for douches and irrigation. Hand cream (1%) effective in reducing cross infection. (Hibiclens, Hibistat.)

chlorocresol (klōr'-ō-krē'-sol) *n* bactericidal phenolic cresol* particularly useful as preservative for injections in multiple dose vials.

chloroform (klōr'-ō-form) *n* a heavy liquid, once used extensively as a general anesthetic. Much used in the form of chloroform water as a flavoring and preservative in aqueous mixtures.

chloroma (klōr-ō'-mà) *n* condition producing multiple greenish-yellow growths on periosteum of facial and cranial bones, and on vertebrae, in association with acute* myeloid leukemia.

Chloromycetin™ chloramphenicol.*

chlorophyll (klōr'-ō-fil) *n* green coloring matter which enables photosynthesis in plants. Prepared medicinally for external use as a deodorant.

chloroquine (klōr'-ō-kwin) *n* potent antimalarial effective in treatment and suppression of the disease. Added to table salt in some endemic areas. Also used in amebic hepatitis and collagen diseases. Can cause ocular complications. Has a mild anti-inflammatory effect and in the long term lowers titer of the rheumatoid factor in serum. (Aralen.)

chlorothiazide (klōr-ō-thī'-à-zīd) *n* diuretic with a mild blood pressure lowering action; rarely gives rise to symptoms of hypotension. (Diuril.)

chlorotrianisene (klōr-ō-trī-an'-i-sēn) *n* alternative to stilbestrol.* Prescribed for some menopausal symptoms, because of its prolonged estrogenic action by slow release, but this is not an advantage if side-effects occur, as the effect of the hormone cannot be immediately discontinued. (TACE.)

chloroxylenol (klōr-oks'-i-len'-ol) *n* a phenolic cresol* used as a germicide.

chlorpheniramine (klōr-fen-ēr'-à-mēn) *n* antihistamine of high potency and of value in allergic conditions and also in treatment of transfusion reactions. Given orally or by injection.

chlorpromazine (klōr-prō'-mà-zēn) *n* drug of exceptional pharmacological action: sedative, antiemetic, antispasmodic and hypotensive. Increases effectiveness of hypnotics, anesthetics, alcohol and analgesics. Valuable in psychiatric conditions and management of senile patients. May cause skin sensitization, leukopenia, parkinsonism, jaundice and hypothermia. (Thorazine.)

chlorpropamide (klōr-prō'-pa-mīd) *n* antidiabetic agent; one of the sulfonylureas.* (Diabinese.)

chlorprothixene (klōr-prō-thicks'-ēn) *n* tranquilizer useful in acute schizophrenic conditions, but less effective when treatment is prolonged. (Taractan.)

chlortetracycline (klōr-tet-rà-sī'-klin) *n* a preparation of tetracyline.* (Aureomycin.)

chlorthalidone (klōr-thal'-i-dōn) *n* oral diuretic given on alternate days; action lasts up to 48 h. (Hygroton.)

choanae (kō-ān'-ē) *npl* funnel-shaped openings. → nares—**choana** *sing*, **choanal** *adj*.

chocolate cyst endometrial cyst* containing altered blood. Ovaries are the most usual site.

choked disk → papilledema.

cholagogue (kōl'-a-gog) *n* a drug which causes an increased flow of bile into the intestine.

cholangiography (kōl-an-jē-og'-raf-ē) *n* radiographic examination of hepatic, cystic and bile ducts. Can be performed: (a) after oral or intravenous administration of radioopaque substance, (b) by direct injection at operation to detect any further stones in the ducts, (c) during or after operation by way of a T-tube in the common bile duct, (d) by means of injection via skin on the anterior abdominal wall to the liver, called percutaneous transhepatic cholangiography. → endoscopic* retrograde cholangiopancreatography—**cholangiographic** *adj*, **cholangiograph** *n*.

cholangiohepatitis (kōl-an'-jē-ō-hep-à-tī'-tis) *n* inflammation of the liver and bile ducts.

cholangitis (kōl-an-jī'-tis) *n* inflammation of the bile ducts.

cholecystangiography (kōl-e-sist-anj-ē-og'-raf-ē) *n* radiographic examination of gallbladder, cystic and common bile ducts.

cholecystectomy (kōl-ē-sist-ek'-to-mē) *n* surgical removal of the gallbladder. Usually advised for stones, inflammation and occasionally for new growths.

cholecystenterostomy (kōl-ē-sist-en-tėr-os'-to-mē) *n* establishment of an artificial opening (anastomosis*) between gallbladder and small intestine.

cholecystitis (kōl-ē-sist-ī'-tis) *n* inflammation of the gallbladder.

cholecystoduodenal (kōl-ē-sist-ō-dū-ō-dēn'-àl) *adj* pertaining to gallbladder and duodenum, as an anastomosis* between them.

cholecystoduodenostomy (kōl-ē-sist-ō-dū-ō-dēn-os'-to-mē) *n* establishment of an anastomosis* between gallbladder and duodenum. Usually necessary in stricture of common bile duct, which may be congenital or due to previous inflammation or operation.

cholecystography (kōl-ē-sis-tog'-rà-fē) *n* radiographic examination of the gallbladder after administration of opaque medium—**cholecystographic** *adj*, **cholecystogram** *n*.

cholecystojejunostomy (kōl-ē-sis-tō-je-jūn-os'-to-mē) *n* anastomosis* between gallbladder and jejunum. Performed for obstructive jaundice due to growth in head of pancreas.

cholecystokinin (kōl-ē-sis-to-kin'-in) *n* hormone which contracts the gallbladder. Secreted by upper intestinal mucosa.

cholecystolithiasis (kōl-ē-sis-tō-lith-ī'-à-sis) *n* presence of stone or stones in the gallbladder.

cholecystostomy (kōl-ē-sis-tos'-to-mē) *n* surgically established fistula between gallbladder and the abdominal surface; used to provide drainage, in empyema of the gallbladder or after removal of stones.

cholecystotomy (kōl-ē-sis-tot'-o-mē) *n* incision into the gallbladder.

choledochography (kōl-ē-dok-og'-ra-fē) cholangiography.*

choledocholithiasis (kōl-ē-dok-ō-lith-ī'-à-sis) *n* presence of a stone or stones in the bile ducts.

choledocholithotomy (kōl-ē-dok-ō-lith-ot'-o-mē) *n* surgical removal of a stone from the common bile duct.

choledochostomy (kōl-ē-dok-os'-to-mē) *n* drainage of the common bile duct using a T tube, usually after exploration for a stone.

choledochotomy (kōl-ē-dok-ot'-o-mē) *n* incision into the common bile duct.

Choledyl™ oxtriphylline.*

cholelithiasis (kōl-ē-lith-ī'-à-sis) *n* presence of stones in gallbladder or bile ducts.

cholemia (kōl-ēm'-ē-à) *n* presence of bile* in blood—**cholemic** *adj*.

cholera (kol'-e-rà) *n* acute epidemic disease, caused by *Vibrio comma,* occurring in the East. Main symptoms are evacuation of copious "rice-water" stools accompanied by agonizing cramp and collapse. Spread mainly by contaminated water, overcrowding and insanitary conditions. High mortality.

cholestasis (kōl-ē-stā'-sis) *n* diminution or arrest of the flow of bile. *intrahepatic cholestasis* syndrome comprising jaundice of an obstructive type, itching, pale stools and dark urine, but in which the main bile ducts outside the liver are patent—**cholestatic** *adj*.

cholesteatoma (kol-es-tē-à-tō'-mà) *n* benign encysted tumor containing cholesterol. Mainly occurs in the middle ear—**cholesteatomatous** *adj*.

cholesterol (kol-es'-tėr-ol) *n* crystalline substance of a fatty nature found in the brain, nerves, liver, blood and bile. Not easily soluble and may crystallize in gallbladder and along arterial walls. When irradiated it forms vitamin D.

cholesterosis (kol-es-tėr-os'-is) *n* abnormal deposition of cholesterol.*

cholestyramine (kol-es-tī'-rà-mēn) *n* a basic ion-exchange resin which combines with bile acids in the intestine to form a product which is not absorbed, hence lowering blood levels of cholesterol.* (Questran.)

choline (kōl'-ēn) *n* chemical found in animal tissues as a constituent of lecithin* and acetylcholine.* Thought to be part of the vitamin* B complex, and known to be a growth factor. Necessary for fat transportation in the body. Useful in preventing fat deposition in the liver in cirrhosis. Richest sources are dairy products.

choline magnesium trisalicylate (trī-sal-is´-il-āt) derivative of salicylic* acid; has a nonsteroidal anti-inflammatory action.

cholinergic (kōl-in-ėr´-jik) *adj* applied to nerves which liberate acetylcholine* at their termination. Includes nerves that cause voluntary muscle to contract and all parasympathetic nerves. → adrenergic *opp. cholinergic crisis* respiratory failure resulting from overtreatment with anticholinesterase* drugs; distinguished from myasthenic* crisis by giving 10 mg edrophonium chloride intravenously: with no improvement cholinergic crisis is confirmed, and 1 mg atropine sulfate is given intravenously together with immediate mechanical respiration. → edrophonium test.

cholinesterase (kōl-in-es´-tėr-āz) *n* enzyme that hydrolyzes acetylcholine into choline and acetic acid at nerve endings.

choluria (kō-lū´-rē-à) *n* biluria*—**choluric** *adj*.

chondritis (kon-drī´-tis) *n* inflammation of cartilage.

chondrocostal (kon-drō-kos´-tàl) *adj* pertaining to costal cartilages and ribs.

chondrodynia (kon-drō-dī´-nē-à) *n* pain in a cartilage.

chondrolysis (kon-drol´-is-is) *n* dissolution of cartilage—**chondrolytic** *adj*.

chondroma (kon-drō´-mà) *n* benign tumor of cartilage. Tends to recur after removal.

chondromalacia (kon-drō-mā-lā´-sē-à) *n* softening of cartilage.

chondrosarcoma (kon-drō-sàr-kō´-mà) *n* malignant neoplasm of cartilage—**chondrosarcomata** *pl*, **chondrosarcomatous** *adj*.

chondrosternal (kon-drō-stėr´-nàl) *adj* pertaining to rib cartilages and sternum.

chordee (kōr´-dē) *n* painful erection of the penis lately associated with urethritis.

chorditis (kōr-dī´-tis) *n* inflammation of spermatic or vocal cords.

chordotomy (kōr-do´-to-mē) *n* → cordotomy.

chorea (kōr-ē´-à) *n* disease manifested by irregular and spasmodic movements, beyond the patient's control. Even voluntary movements are rendered jerky and ungainly. Childhood disease often called rheumatic chorea or "St. Vitus Dance"; adult form is part of a cerebral degenerative process called Huntington's* chorea—**choreal, choreic** *adj*.

choreiform (kōr-ē´-i-form) *n* resembling chorea.*

choriocarcinoma (kōr-ē-ō-kàr-sin-o´-mà) chorionepithelioma.*

chorion (kōr´-ē-on) *n* outer membrane forming the embryonic sac. *chorion biopsy* → chorionic villus biopsy—**chorial, chorionic** *adj*.

chorionepithelioma (kōr-ē-on-ep-i-thē-lē-ō´-mà) *n* a highly malignant tumor arising from chorionic cells, usually after a hydatidiform* mole, although it may follow abortion or even normal pregnancy, quickly metastasizing especially to the lungs. Cytotoxic drugs have improved the prognosis.

chorionic villi (kōr-ē-on'-ik vil'-lī) projections from the chorion* from which the fetal part of the placenta is formed. Through the chorionic villi diffuse gases, nutrient and waste products from maternal to fetal blood and vice versa.

chorionic villus biopsy (kōr-ē-on'-ik vil'-us) biopsy of a chorionic villus for prenatal diagnosis of many disorders.

chorioretinitis (kōr-ē-ō-ret-in-īt'-is) *n* (*syn* choroidoretinitis) inflammation of the choroid and retina.

choroid (kōr'-oyd) *n* the middle pigmented, vascular coat of the posterior five-sixths of the eyeball, continuous with the iris in front (→ Figure 15). It lies between the sclera* externally and the retina* internally, and prevents the passage of light rays—**choroidal** *adj*.

choroiditis (kōr-oyd-īt'-is) *n* inflammation of the choroid. *Tay's choroiditis* degenerative change affecting the retina around the macula* lutea.

choroidocyclitis (kōr-oyd-ō-sīk-lī'-tis) *n* inflammation of the choroid and ciliary body.

Christmas disease → hemophilias.

chromatography (krō-ma-tog'-raf-ē) *n* method of separating and identifying substances in a complex mixture based on their differential movement through a two-phase system; effected by a flow of liquid or gas (mobile phase) which percolates through an absorbent (stationary phase). Stationary phase may be solid (e.g., paper), liquid or a mixture of both. Mobile phase may be liquid or gaseous and fills the spaces of the stationary phase through which it flows. Stationary and mobile phases are so selected that the compounds which are to be separated have different distribution coefficients between the phases due to differences in their physicochemical properties—**chromatogram** *n*.

chromic acid (krō'-mik) in 5% solution an astringent, used in preparation of chromicized catgut; stronger solutions are caustic and can be painted on warts.

chromosome (krō'-mō-sōm) *n* one of the staining bodies seen within a cell nucleus as it prepares to divide and during division. Chromosomes split longitudinally in the process. They carry hereditary factors (genes). Chromosomes are made essentially of DNA,* of which the genes are made, and the chromosome number is constant for each species. In man, there are 46 in each cell, except in mature ovum and sperm, in which the number is halved as a result of reduction division (meiosis). A set of 23 chromosomes is inherited from each parent. The human male produces two types of sperm: with Y chromosomes to generate males and with X chromosomes for females—**chromosomal** *adj*.

chronic *adj* lingering, lasting; implies nothing as to severity of a condition. *chronic lymphocytic leukemia* proliferation of lymphocytes in blood, which occurs mainly in the elderly. Little active treatment is necessary and patients may live comfortably for many years. *chronic myelocytic leukemia* proliferation of myelocytes in blood; may run a static course over several years but eventually an acute phase supervenes (blast crisis). *chronic obstructive pulmonary disease* range of deteriorative changes causing chronic limitation of air intake— **chronicity** *n*.

chronic fatigue syndrome characterized by various symptoms but usually including lymphadenopathy, low-grade fever, muscular or bone pain, impaired mental concentration, and recurrent fatigue. May continue for years; cause unknown.

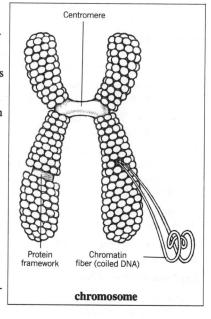

chromosome

Chronulac™ preparation of lactulose.*

Chvostek's sign (shvos′-teks) excessive twitching of the face on tapping the facial nerve; a sign of tetany.*

chyle (kīl) *n* digested fats which, as an alkaline, milky fluid, pass from the small intestine via the lymphatics to the blood stream—**chylous** *adj*.

chylothorax (kīl-ō-thōr′-aks) *n* leakage of chyle from thoracic duct into pleural cavity.

chyluria (kīl-ūr′-ē-à) *n* chyle* in the urine, which can occur in some nematode infestations, either when a fistulous communication is established between a lymphatic vessel and the urinary tract or when distension of the urinary lymphatics causes them to rupture—**chyluric** *adj*.

chyme (kīm) *n* partially digested food which as an acidic, creamy-yellow, thick fluid passes from the stomach to the duodenum. Its acidity controls the pylorus so that chyme is ejected at frequent intervals—**chymous** *adj*.

chymopapain (kī-mō-pap′-ān) *n* proteolytic enzyme obtained from latex of the pawpaw tree.

Chymoral™ mixture of enzymes trypsin* and chymotrypsin.*

chymotrypsin (kī-mō-trip'-sin) *n* protein-digesting enzyme secreted by the pancreas; activated by trypsin. A pharmaceutical preparation is useful in debridment of necrotic tissue and for loosening secretions, e.g., in respiratory tract. Also facilitates lens extraction. (Avazyme.)

cicatrix (sik'-à-triks) *n* → scar.

cilia (sil'-ē-à) *npl* 1 the eyelashes. 2 microscopic hairlike projections from certain epithelial cells. Membranes containing such cells, e.g., those lining the trachea and Fallopian tubes, are known as ciliated membranes—**cilium** *sing*, **ciliary, ciliated, cilial** *adj*.

ciliary (sil'-ē-ār-ē) *adj* hairlike. *ciliary body* specialized structure in the eye connecting anterior part of the choroid to circumference of the iris (→ Figure 15); composed of the ciliary muscles and processes. *ciliary muscles* fine hairlike muscle fibers arranged circularly to form a greyish-white ring immediately behind the corneoscleral junction. *ciliary processes* about 70 in number, are projections on the undersurface of the choroid, attached to the ciliary muscles.

cimetidine (sī-met'-i-dēn) *n* a histamine H_2-receptor antagonist which inhibits both resting and stimulated gastric acid secretion. Useful for active peptic ulcers; should be taken after evening meal; single daily dose at night gives better control of nocturnal gastric acid output and lowers mean 24 h acidity as effectively as divided doses. Antacids interfere with its absorption. (Tagamet.)

cinchonism (sin'-kon-ism) *n* quininism.*

cineangiocardiography (sin-ē-an-jē-ō-kàr-dē-og'-raf-ē) *n* motion picture technique of recording passage of contrast medium through heart and blood vessels.

cineangiography (sin-ē-an-jē-og'-raf-ē) *n* motion picture technique of recording images during angiography.*

circadian rhythm (sir-kā'-dē-an) cycle with periodicity of 24 h.

circinata (sir-sin-a'-tà) *n* → tinea.

circinate (sir'-sin-āt) *adj* in the form of a circle or segment of a circle, e.g., skin eruptions of late syphilis, ringworm, etc.

circulation *n* passage in a circuit; usually of the blood. *circulation of bile* passage of bile from liver cells, where it is formed, via gallbladder and bile ducts to the small intestine, where its constituents are partly reabsorbed into the blood and thus return to the liver. *circulation of blood* passage of blood from heart to arteries to capillaries to veins and back to heart. *circulation of cerebrospinal fluid* takes place from the ventricles of the brain to the cisterna magna, bathing the surface of the brain and the spinal cord, including its central canal; absorbed into the blood in the cerebral venous sinuses. *circulation of lymph* lymph is collected from tissue spaces and passed in the lymphatic capillaries, vessels, glands and ducts to reenter blood stream. *collateral circulation* alternative route provided for blood by secondary blood vessels when a primary vessel is blocked. *greater circulation* circulation of blood from left ventricle to aorta, to tissue, and back to right atrium of heart. *lesser circulation* circulation of blood from right ventricle to pulmonary artery, to lungs, and back to left atrium of heart—**circulatory** *adj,* **circulate** *vi, vt.*

circumcision (sir-kum-sizh'-un) *n* excision of the prepuce of the penis, usually for religious or ethnic reasons. The operation is sometimes required for phimosis* or paraphimosis.* *female circumcision* excision of parts of external genitalia.

circumcorneal (sir-kum-kōr'-nē-ȧl) *adj* around the cornea.

circumoral (sir-kum-ōr'-ȧl) *adj* surrounding the mouth. *circumoral pallor* a pale appearance of the skin around the mouth. A characteristic of scarlatina.*

circumvallate (sir-kum-val'-āt) *adj* surrounded by a raised ring, as the large circumvallate papillae at the base of the tongue.

cirrhosis (sir-ō'-sis) *n* hardening of an organ; result of degenerative changes in tissues with resulting fibrosis. *biliary cirrhosis* inflammation of the bile ducts leading to lesions, scarring and finally fibrous obstruction; cause unknown. *cirrhosis of liver* as a result of damage from virus, microorganisms, toxic substances or dietary deficiencies interfering with nutrition of liver cells—often a result of alcoholism. Associated developments include ascites,* obstruction of portal vein circulation, with hematemesis,* jaundice and enlargement of the spleen—**cirrhotic** *adj.*

cirsoid (sir'-soyd) *adj* resembling a tortuous, dilated vein (varix*). *cirsoid aneurysm* a tangled mass of pulsating blood vessels appearing as a subcutaneous tumor, usually on the scalp.

cisplatin (sis'-pla-tin) *n* platinum compound used in treatment of malignancy.

cisterna (sis-tėr'-nȧ) *n* any closed space serving as a reservoir for a body fluid. *cisterna magna* subarachnoid space in the cleft between cerebellum and medulla oblongata—**cisternal** *adj.*

cisternal puncture → puncture.

Citanest™ prilocaine.*

citric acid (sit'-rik) acid present in lemons. Widely used as potassium* citrate, a diuretic. *citric acid cycle* → Kreb's cycle.

claudication (klaw-di-kā'-shun) *n* limping caused by impaired blood supply to the legs. Cause may be spasm or disease of the vessels themselves. In *intermittent claudication* patient experiences severe pain in the calves while walking; abated by rest.

clavicle (klav'-ik-l) *n* collarbone (→ Figures 2, 3)—**clavicular** *adj.*

clavulanic acid (klav-ū-lan'-ik) used in combination with amoxycillin* to inhibit the enzyme penicillinase produced by penicillin-resistant bacteria.

clavus (klā'-vus) *n* a corn.*

claw-foot *adj, n* (*syn* pes cavus) deformity in which longitudinal arch of the foot is increased in height and associated with clawing of the toes; acquired or congenital in origin.

claw-hand *n* hand contracted to clawlike appearance; may be due to injury or disease.

Cleocin™ clindamycin.*

climacteric (kli-mak'-te-rik) *n* in the female, the menopause.* A corresponding period occurs in men, called the *male climacteric*.

clindamycin (klin-dȧ-mī'-sin) *n* derivative of lincomycin*; more active than parent compound.

clinical *adj* pertaining to a clinic. Describes the practical observation and treatment of sick persons as opposed to theoretical study.

Clistin™ carbinoxamine* maleate.

clitoridectomy (klit-or-i-dek'-to-mē) *n* surgical removal of the clitoris.

clitoriditis (klit-or-id-ī'-tis) *n* inflammation of the clitoris.

clitoris (klit'-or-is) *n* small erectile organ of the female genitalia situated just below the mons veneris at the junction anteriorly of the labia minora.

cloaca (klō-ā'-kȧ) *n* in osteomyelitis,* opening through the involucrum* which discharges pus—**cloacal** *adj*.

clobetasol propionate (klō-bet'-a-sol prō'-pē-on-āt) soothing steroid application for such skin conditions as eczema. (Temovate.)

clofazimine (klō-faz'-i-mēn) *n* a red dye, given orally. Controls symptoms of erythema nodosum leprosum reaction in lepromatous leprosy better than prednisolone.*

clofibrate (klō-fī'-brāt) *n* lowers blood cholesterol and is used to prevent fat embolism, particularly in patients with bone injury. (Atromid-S.)

Clomid™ clomiphene.*

clomiphene (klō'-mi-phēn) *n* synthetic nonsteroidal compound that induces ovulation and subsequent menstruation in some otherwise anovulatory women, thereby enhancing fertility. (Clomid.)

clomipramine (klom-ip'-ra-mēn) *n* antidepressive drug of the tricyclic group with unique ability to counteract obsessional symptoms. (Anafranil.)

clonic (klon'-ik) *adj* → clonus.

clonidine (klōn'-i-dēn) *n* similar to methyldopa,* but causes less postural hypotension though it gives some patients a very dry mouth. In small doses, of value in preventing migraine. (Catapres, Dixarit.)

clonus (klō'-nus) *n* a series of intermittent muscular contractions and relaxations. → tonic *opp;* ankle clonus—**clonic** *adj,* **clonicity** *n*.

Clostridium (klos-trid'-ē-um) *n* bacterial genus. *Clostridia* are large Grampositive anaerobic bacilli found as commensals of the gut in animals and man and as saprophytes in the soil. Endospores* are produced which are widely distributed. Pathogenic species produce exotoxins, e.g., *C. tetani* (tetanus), *C. botulinum* (botulism), *C. perfringens (welchii)* (gas gangrene), *C. difficile* (pseudomembranous colitis).

clot *v* to coagulate. *n* a thrombus or coagulation.

clotting time time taken by shed blood to coagulate.

clove oil oil extracted from cloves, which has antiseptic, carminative and anodyne properties. Used to relieve toothache.

cloxacillin (kloks-à-sil'-lin) *n* semisynthetic penicillin* which is active against penicillin-resistant staphylococci; acid-stable and given orally or parenterally. (Tegopen.)

clozapine (kloz'-a-pēn) *n* antipsychotic drug; binds to dopamine receptors, preferring limbic to striatal sites. (Clozaril.)

Clozaril™ clozapine.*

clubbed fingers thickening and broadening of the bulbous fleshy portion of the fingers under the nails. Cause unknown; occurs in people who have heart and/or lung disease.

clubfoot *n* a congenital malformation, either unilateral or bilateral. → talipes.

clumping *n* agglutination.*

Clutton's joints (klut'-ons) joints which show symmetrical swelling, usually painless, the knees often being involved. Associated with congenital syphilis.

clysis (klī'-sis) *n* **1** cleansing or washing out of a cavity. **2** term used when administering fluids by other than oral route: subcutaneously (hypodermoclysis); intravenously (venoclysis); and rectally (proctoclysis).

CMV *abbr* cytomegalovirus.*

CNS *abbr* central nervous* system.

coagulase (kō-ag'-ū-lāz) *n* enzyme produced by some bacteria of the genus *Staphylococcus:* it coagulates plasma and is used to classify staphylococci as coagulase-negative or coagulase-positive.

coagulate (kō-ag'-ū-lāt) *v* to form a clot or solidify—**coagulation** *n*.

coagulum (kō-ag'-ū-lum) *n* any coagulated mass; a scab.

coalesce (kō-à-les') *vt* to grow together; to unite into a mass. Often used to describe development of a skin eruption, when discrete areas of affected skin merge to form sheets of a similar appearance—**coalescence** *n,* **coalescent** *adj*.

coal tar black substance obtained by distillation of coal; used in ointment for psoriasis and eczema.

coarctation (kō-ark-tā′-shun) *n* contraction, stricture, narrowing; applied to a vessel or canal.

coarse tremor violent trembling.

cobalamin (kō-bal′-à-min) *n* generic term for the vitamin B_{12} group. → cyanocobalamin.

cocaine (kō-kān′) *n* powerful local anesthetic obtained from leaves of the coca plant. Toxic, esp. to the brain; may cause agitation, disorientation, convulsions and can induce addiction. It has vasoconstrictor properties, hence the blanching which occurs when applied to mucous membranes. Now largely replaced by less toxic compounds such as procaine* and xylocaine,* but still used in eye drops, often with homatropine.*

cocainism (kō-kān′-izm) *n* mental and physical degeneracy caused by morbid craving for, and excessive use of, cocaine.*

coccidioidomycosis (kok-sid-ē-oy′-dō-mī-kō′-sis) *n* disease acquired by inhaling dust containing spores of the fungus *Coccidioides immitis*. Symptoms vary, including bronchitis, fever, chest pain, chills, hemoptysis.* Occurs in southwestern U.S. Usually self limiting, but progressive form is often fatal. Also called Valley fever.

coccus (kok′-us) *n* a spherical or nearly spherical bacterium—**cocci** *pl*, **coccal, coccoid** *adj*.

coccydynia (kok-si-din′-ē-à) *n* pain in the region of the coccyx.

coccygectomy (kok-si-jek′-to-mē) *n* surgical removal of the coccyx.

coccyx (kok′-siks) *n* the last bone of the vertebral column (→ Figure 3). It is triangular in shape and curved slightly forward; composed of four rudimentary vertebrae, cartilaginous at birth, ossification being completed at about the 30th year—coccygeal *adj*.

cochlea (kōk′-lē-à) *n* spiral canal resembling the interior of a snail shell, in the anterior part of the bony labyrinth of the ear (→ Figure 13)—**cochlear** *adj*.

codeine (kō′-dēn) *n* an alkaloid of opium* with mild analgesic properties; often combined with aspirin.* Valuable as a cough sedative in dry, unproductive cough.

cod liver oil contains vitamins A and D; used on that account as a dietary supplement in mild deficiency. It can be applied as a dressing to promote healing.

co-enzyme (kō-en′-zīm) *n* an enzyme activator.

coffee ground vomit vomit containing blood, which in its partially digested state resembles coffee grounds. Indicative of slow upper gastrointestinal bleeding. → hematemesis.

Cogentin™ benztropine.*

coitus (kō'-it-us) *n* insertion of the erect penis into the vagina: the act of sexual intercourse or copulation. *coitus interruptus* removal from the vagina of the penis before ejaculation of semen as a means of contraception. The method is unreliable—**coital** *adj*.

Colace™ docusate* sodium.

colchicine (kōl'-chi-sēn) *n* drug used to treat gout.

cold abscess → abscess.

cold sore oral herpes.*

colectomy (kō-lek'-to-mē) *n* excision of part or all of the colon.

colic (kol'-ik) *n* severe pain

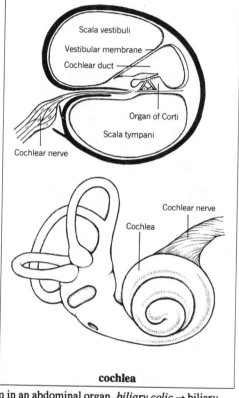

cochlea

resulting from periodic spasm in an abdominal organ. *biliary colic* → biliary. *intestinal colic* abnormal peristalic movement of an irritated gut. *painter's (lead) colic* spasm of intestine and constriction of mesenteric vessels, resulting from lead poisoning. *renal colic* spasm of ureter due to a stone. *uterine colic* dysmenorrhea*—**colicky** *adj*.

coliform (kol'-i-form) *adj* describes any bacterium of fecal origin which is morphologically similar to *Escherichia coli*.

colistin (kol'-is-tin) *n* antibiotic active against many Gram-negative organisms. Useful in *Pseudomonas aeruginosa* infections. Less toxic than polymyxin* B. (Coly-Mycin S.)

colitis (kō-lī'-tis) *n* inflammation of the colon. May be acute or chronic, and may be accompanied by ulcerative lesions. *ulcerative colitis* inflammatory and ulcerative condition of the colon. Evidence has accumulated for an immunological basis for the condition rather than a psychosomatic one, as was previously thought. Usually affects young and early middle-aged adults, producing periodic bouts of diarrheal stools containing mucus and blood; varies in severity from a mild form with little constitutional upset to a severe, dangerous and prostrating illness.

collagen (kol'-à-jen) *n* main protein constituent of white fibrous tissue (skin, tendon, bone, cartilage and all connective tissue); composed of bundles of tropocollagen molecules, which contain three intertwined polypeptide chains. The *collagen diseases* are characterized by an inflammatory lesion of unknown etiology affecting collagen and small blood vessels (possibly due to a hypersensitivity state); they include dermatomyositis, lupus erythematosus, polyarteritis (periarteritis) nodosa, purpura, rheumatic fever, rheumatoid arthritis and scleroderma. *collagen proline hydroxylase* an enzyme necessary for wound healing; vitamin* C is necessary for this enzyme's maintenance and function. Research indicates that tissues which are rapidly synthesizing collagen (e.g., healing wounds) have high levels of this enzyme—**collagenic, collagenous** *adj*.

collapsing pulse water-hammer pulse of aortic incompetence, with high initial upthrust which quickly falls away.

collarbone *n* clavicle (→ Figures 2, 3).

Colles' fracture (kol'-ēz) break at lower end of the radius following a fall on the outstretched hand. Backward displacement of the hand produces a "dinner fork" deformity.

colliquative (kol-lik'-wà-tiv) *adj* profuse, excessive.

collodion (kol-lō'-dē-on) *n* solution of pyroxylin* with ether and alcohol. It forms a flexible film on the skin, a protective dressing.

colloid (kol'-oyd) *n* a gluelike noncrystalline substance, diffusible but not soluble in water; unable to pass through an animal membrane. Some drugs can be prepared in colloidal form. *colloid degeneration* mucoid degeneration of tumors. *colloid goiter* abnormal enlargement of thyroid gland, due to accumulation of viscid, iodine-containing colloid.

colloidal gold test carried out on cerebrospinal fluid to assist diagnosis of neurosyphilis.

coloboma (kol-ō-bō'-mà) *n* congenital fissure or gap in the eyeball or one of its parts, particularly the uvea—**colobomata** *pl*.

colocystoplasty (kol-ō-sis'-to-plas-tē) *n* operation to increase capacity of the urinary bladder, using part of the colon—**colocystoplastic** *adj*.

Cologel™ methylcellulose.*

colon (kō'-lon) *n* the large bowel extending from the cecum* to the rectum* (→ Figure 18). In its various parts it has appropriate names—ascending, transverse, descending and sigmoid colon. → flexure. *spasmodic colon* megacolon*—**colonic** *adj*.

colonize *vt* of commensals,* to establish a presence on or in the human body. Soon after birth commensals form a natural flora and do not usually cause infection.* Tissue can therefore be "colonized" but not infected. Infection results from imbalance between commensals and defense mechanisms.

colonoscopy (kol-on-os-kop'-ē) *n* use of a fiberoptic colonoscope to view inner membrane of the colon—**colonoscopic** *adj*.

colony *n* a mass of bacteria of one or more types. May grow to macroscopic* size, presenting species-characteristic features.

colorectal (kō-lō-rek'-tǎl) *adj* pertaining to colon and rectum.

colostomy (kol-os'-to-mē) *n* surgically established fistula between the colon and surface of the abdomen; acts as an artificial anus.

colostrum (kol-os'-trum) *n* relatively clear fluid secreted in the breasts during first 3 days after parturition, before formation of true milk. Also may be secreted during pregnancy.

colotomy (kol-ot'-o-mē) *n* incision into the colon.

color blindness applies to various conditions in which certain colors are confused with one another. Inability to distinguish between reds and greens is called daltonism. → achromatopsia.

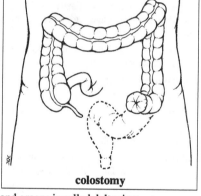

colostomy

colpitis (kol-pī'-tis) *n* inflammation of the vagina. Also vaginitis.

colpocele (kol'-pō-sēl) *n* protrusion or prolapse of either the bladder or rectum so that it presses on the vaginal wall.

colpocentesis (kol-pō-sen-tē'-sis) *n* withdrawal of fluid from the vagina, as in hematocolpos.*

colpohysterectomy (kol-pō-his-tėr-ek'-to-mē) *n* removal of the uterus through the vagina.

colpoperineorrhaphy (kol-pō-pėr-in-ē-ōr'-af-ē) *n* surgical repair of injured vagina and deficient perineum.

colpophotography (kol-pō-fō-tog'-raf-ē) *n* filming the cervix with camera and colposcope.

colporrhaphy (kol-pōr'-af-ē) *n* surgical repair of the vagina. An anterior colporrhaphy repairs a cystocele* and a posterior colporrhaphy repairs a rectosele.*

colposcope (kol'-pō-skōp) *n* instrument which, when inserted into the vagina, holds the walls apart, permitting inspection of cervix and upper vagina—**colposcopy** *n*.

colpotomy (kol-pot'-om-ē) *n* incision of the vaginal wall. A posterior colpotomy drains an abscess in the pouch* of Douglas through the vagina.

Coly-Mycin-S™ colistin.*

coma (kō'-mà) *n* state of unrousable unconsciousness, the severity of which can be assessed by corneal and pupillary reflexes and withdrawal responses to painful stimuli.

comatose (kōm'-à-tōs) *adj* in a state of coma.*

combined oral contraceptive commonly referred to as "the pill." Many brands available; all contain varying concentrations of two hormones, estrogen and progestogen. → contraceptive.

comedo (kom'-ē-dō) *n* wormlike cast formed of sebum* which occupies the outlet of a hair follicle; a feature of acne* vulgaris—**comedones** *pl*.

commensals (kom-en'-sàls) *npl* parasitic microorganisms adapted to grow on skin and mucous surfaces of the host, forming part of the normal flora. Some commensals are potentially pathogenic.

communicable *adj* transmissible directly or indirectly from one person to another.

Compazine™ prochlorperazine.*

complement *n* a normal constituent of plasma of great importance in immunity mechanisms, as it combines with antigen-antibody complex (complement fixation), completing reactions such as bacteriolysis in the killing of bacteria. *complement fixation test* measures amount of complement fixed by any given antigen-antibody complex; may confirm infection with a specific microorganism.

complemental air the extra air that can be drawn into the lungs by deep inspiration.

compos mentis (kom'-pōs men'-tis) of sound mind.

compress (kom'-press) *n* usually refers to a wet dressing of several layers of lint. A cold compress on the forehead relieves headache.

computed axial tomography (CAT) computed* tomography.

computed tomography (CT) (tom-og'-ra-fē) computer-constructed imaging technique of a thin slice through the body, derived from X-ray absorption data collected during a circular scanning motion.

conception *n* creation of a state of pregnancy; impregnation of the ovum by the spermatozoon—**conceptive** *adj*.

concha *n* → Figure 14.

concretion (kon-krē'-shun) *n* a deposit of hard material; a calculus.*

concussion *n* condition resulting from a violent jar or shock. *cerebral concussion* characterized by loss of consciousness, pallor, coldness and usually an increase in pulse rate. There may be incontinence of urine and feces.

conditioned reflex reflex in which response occurs, not to the sensory stimulus which caused it originally, but to another stimulus which the subject has learned to associate with the original stimulus; it can be acquired by training and repetition. In Pavlov's classic experiments, dogs learned to associate the sound of a bell with the sight and smell of food; even when food was not presented, salivation occurred at the sound of a bell.

conditioning *n* encouragement of new (desirable) behavior by modifying stimulus/response associations. *operant conditioning* a program to reward (or punish) a response each time it occurs, so that given time, it occurs more (or less) frequently.

condom (kon'-dom) *n* latex sheath used as a male contraceptive.* Helps protect both partners against sexually transmitted disease.

condyloma (kon-dil-ō'-må) *n* papilloma.* *Condylomata acuminato* are acuminate (pointed) dry warts found under prepuce (male), on the vulva and vestibule (female) or on skin of the perianal region (both sexes). *Condylomata lata* are highly infectious, moist, warty excrescences found in moist areas of the body (vulva, anus, axilla, etc.) as a manifestation of late secondary syphilis*—**condylomata** *pl*, **condylomatous** *adj*.

confabulation (kon-fab-ū-lā'-shun) *n* symptom common in confusional states when there is impairment of memory for recent events. Gaps in memory are filled in with fabrications, which patient nevertheless appears to accept as fact. Occurs in senile and toxic confusional states, cerebral trauma and Korsakoff* syndrome.

confluence (kon'-floo-ens) *n* becoming merged; flowing together; a uniting, as of neighboring pustules—**confluent** *adj*.

congenital (kon-jen'-it-al) *adj* of abnormal conditions, present at birth, often genetically determined. → genetic. *congenital dislocation of the hip* is due to laxity of the hip capsule. Recognized in the neonate by limitation of hip abduction. *congenital heart disease* developmental abnormalities in anatomy of the heart, resulting postnatally in imperfect circulation of blood and often manifested by murmurs, cyanosis, breathlessness and sweating. Later there may be clubbing of the fingers. → "blue baby." *congenital syphilis* → syphilis.

congestion *n* hyperemia.* Passive congestion results from obstruction or slowing down of venous return, as in lower limbs or the lungs—**congestive** *adj*, **congest** *vi*, *vt*.

congestive heart failure chronic inability of the heart to maintain an adequate output of blood from one or both ventricles, resulting in manifest congestion and overdistension of certain veins and organs with blood, and inadequate blood supply to body tissues.

conization (kōn-īz-ā′-shun) *n* removal of a cone-shaped part of the cervix by the knife or cautery.

conjugate *n* measurement of the bony pelvis. *diagonal conjugate* clinical measurement taken in pelvic assessment, from lower border of the symphysis pubis to the sacral promontory = 12.5 cm. It is 1.5–2 cm greater than *obstetrical conjugate,* the available space for the fetal head, i.e., distance from sacral promontory to the posterior surface of the top of the symphysis pubis = 10.6 cm. *true conjugate* distance from sacral promontory to summit of the symphysis pubis = 11 cm.

conjunctiva (kon-jungk-tī′-và) *n* delicate transparent membrane that lines the inner surface of the eyelids (palpebral conjunctiva) and reflects over the front of the eyeball (bulbar or ocular conjunctiva)—**conjunctival** *adj*.

conjunctivitis (kon-jungk-ti-vī′-tis) *n* inflammation of the conjunctiva. → pinkeye. *inclusion conjunctivitis* (*syn* inclusion blennorrhea) occurs in countries with low standards of hygiene; reservoir of infection is urogenital tract. → TRIC.

Conn's syndrome (konz) hyperplasia or adenoma of the adrenal cortex producing increased aldosterone.* Results in hypertension, hypokalemia and muscular weakness.

Conradi-Hünermann syndrome (kon-rad′-ē hun′-ėr-man) skeletal dysplasia genetically transmitted as an autosomal dominant trait. Skeletal abnormalities are variable; present at birth. After the first few weeks, life expectancy is normal. Mental development is not retarded.

conservative treatment aims at preventing a condition from becoming worse without using radical measures.

consolidation *n* becoming solid as, for instance, the lung due to exudation and organization in lobar pneumonia.

constipation *n* condition of infrequent and often difficult evacuation of feces due to insufficient food or fluid intake, or to sluggish or disordered action of the bowel musculature or nerve supply, or to habitual failure to empty the rectum. *acute constipation* signifies obstruction or paralysis of the gut; of sudden onset.

consumption *n* **1** act of consuming or using up. **2** once-popular term for pulmonary tuberculosis*—**consumptive** *adj*.

contact *n* **1** direct or indirect exposure to infection. **2** person who has been so exposed. *contact lens* of glass or plastic, worn under the eyelids in direct contact with conjunctiva (in place of eyeglasses) for therapeutic or cosmetic purposes.

contagious *adj* capable of transmitting infection or of being transmitted.

continuous ambulatory peritoneal dialysis (CAPD) patient remains ambulant while on peritoneal* dialysis.

continuous positive airways pressure (CPAP) treatment for babies with a tendency to alveolar collapse from hyaline membrane disease. → respiratory distress syndrome.

contraceptive *n, adj* describes an agent used to prevent conception, e.g., condom, spermicidal vaginal pessary or cream, rubber cervical cap, intrauterine device. → intrauterine device, combined oral contraceptive—**contraception** *n*.

contractile (kon-trak'-tīl) *adj* possessing the ability to shorten, usually when stimulated; special property of muscle tissue—**contractility** *n*.

contracture (kon-trak'-tūr) *n* shortening of muscle or scar tissue, producing deformity. → Dupuytren's contracture, Volkmann's ischemic contracture.

contraindication (kon-trà-in-dik-ā'-shun) *n* a sign or symptom suggesting that a certain line of treatment (in use for that disease) should be discontinued or avoided.

contralateral (kon-trà-lat'-ėr-ål) *adj* on the opposite side.

contre-coup (kon'-tre–koo) *n* injury or damage at a point opposite impact, resulting from transmitted force; can occur in an organ or part containing fluid, as the skull.

controlled-dose transdermal absorption of drugs application of a drug patch to the skin; gradual absorption gives a constant level in the blood.

contusion (kon-tū'-zhun) *n* → bruise—**contuse** *vt*.

conversion *n* a psychological conflict* manifesting as a physical symptom.

convolutions *npl* folds, twists or coils as found in the intestine, renal tubules and surface of the brain—**convoluted** *adj*.

convulsions *npl* involuntary contractions of muscles resulting from abnormal cerebral stimulation; there are many causes. They occur with or without loss of consciousness. *clonic convulsions* show alternating contraction and relaxation of muscle groups. *tonic convulsions* exhibit sustained rigidity—**convulsive** *adj*.

convulsive therapy electroconvulsive* therapy.

Cooley's anemia (koo'-lēz) thalassemia.*

Coombs' test (koomz) highly sensitive test to detect antibodies to red blood cells; "direct" method detects those bound to red cells; "indirect" method detects those circulating unbound in serum. The "direct" method is especially useful in diagnosis of hemolytic syndromes.

COPD *abbr* chronic* obstructive pulmonary disease. → bronchitis.

coprolalia (kop-rō-lā'-lē-à) *n* filthy or obscene speech. Occurs as a symptom most commonly in cerebral deterioration or trauma affecting frontal lobes of the brain. → Tourette's syndrome.

coprolith (kop'-rō'-lith) *n* fecalith.*

coproporphyrin (kop-rō-pōr-fī'-rin) *n* naturally occurring porphyrin* in the feces, formed in the intestine from bilirubin.

coracobrachialis muscle (kōr-à-kō-brā-kē-al'-is) → Figure 14.

cord *n* a threadlike structure. *spermatic cord* that which suspends the testicles in the scrotum. *spinal cord* cordlike structure in the spinal column, reaching from the foramen magnum to the first or second lumbar vertebra. It is a direct continuation of the medulla oblongata; about 45 cm long in the adult. *umbilical cord* the navel-string, attaching fetus to the placenta. *vocal cord* membranous bands in the larynx, vibrations of which produce the voice.

cordectomy (kōr-dek'-to-mē) *n* surgical excision of a cord (usually vocal cord).

cordotomy (kōr-dot'-o-mē) *n* (*syn* chordotomy) division of the anterolateral nerves in the spinal cord to relieve intractable pain in the pelvis or lower limbs.

corn *n* painful, cone-shaped overgrowth and hardening of the epidermis, produced by friction or pressure. A *hard corn* usually occurs over a toe joint; a *soft corn* occurs between the toes.

cornea (kōr'-nē-à) *n* outwardly convex transparent membrane forming part of the anterior outer coat of the eye; situated in front of the iris and pupil and merges backwards into the sclera. → Figure 15—**corneal** *adj*.

corneal graft (kōr'-nē-al) (*syn* corneoplasty, keratoplasty) a corneal opacity is excised and replaced by healthy, transparent, human cornea from a donor.

corneoplasty (kōr-nē-ō-plas'-tē) *n* corneal* graft.

corneoscleral (kōr'-nē-ō-sklir'-àl) *adj* pertaining to the cornea and sclera, as the circular junction of these structures.

coronal suture (kōr'-ō-nàl) transverse line of union between parietal and frontal bones in the skull.

coronary (kōr'-on-ār-ē) *adj* crownlike; encircling, as of a vessel or nerve. *coronary arteries* those supplying the heart; the first pair off the aorta as it leaves the left ventricle. Spasm or narrowing of these vessels produces angina pectoris. *coronary sinus* channel receiving most cardiac veins and opening into right atrium. *coronary thrombosis* occlusion of a coronary vessel by a clot of blood. The area deprived of blood becomes necrotic and is called an infarct.* → ischemic heart disease, myocardial infarction.

coronaviruses (kōr-ōn-à-vī'-rus-es) *npl* group of viruses that can cause the common cold.

cor pulmonale (kōr pul-mon-al'-ē) heart disease following on disease of lung (emphysema,* silicosis,* etc.) which strains the right ventricle.

corpus (kōr'-pus) *n* any mass of tissue which is easily distinguishable from its surroundings. *corpus callosum* → Figure 1. *corpus cavernosa* → Figure 16. *corpus luteum* → luteum. *corpus quadrigemina* → Figure 1. *corpus spongiosum* → Figure 16—**corpora** *pl.*

corpuscle (kōr'-pus-l) *n* a microscopic mass of protoplasm. Many varieties, but generally refers to red and white blood cells. → erythrocytes, leukocytes— **corpuscular** *adj.*

Corrigan's pulse (kōr'-i-gans) collapsing pulse.*

cortex (kōr'-teks) *n* **1** outer bark or covering of a plant. **2** outer layer of an organ beneath its capsule or membrane. *cortex of the cerebellum* → Figure 1. *cortex of the kidney* → Figure 20—**cortices** *pl*, **cortical** *adj.*

corticoids (kōr'-ti-koyds) *npl* a name for the several groups of natural hormones produced by the adrenal cortex and for synthetic compounds with similar actions.

corticosteroids (kōr-tik-ō-ster'-oyds) *npl* hormones produced by the adrenal cortex. The word is also used for synthetic steroids such as prednisolone* and dexamethasone.*

corticotropin (kōr-ti-kō-trōp'-in) *n* hormone of the anterior pituitary gland which specifically stimulates the adrenal cortex to produce corticosteroids. Synthetic 1–34 corticotropin is available as tetracosactrin,* given by injection, usually for test purposes.

cortisol (kōr'-ti-zol) *n* hydrocortisone, a principal adrenal cortical steroid. Increased in Cushing's disease and syndrome, and decreased in Addison's disease; essential to life. Given as physiological replacement treatment in Addison's disease and hypopituarism. Synthetic steroids such as prednisolone* and dexamethasone* are usually used when larger doses are required for antiinflammatory or immunosuppressive purposes, e.g., in asthma, some skin conditions or following transplant surgery.

cortisone (kōr'-ti-zōn) *n* a hormone of the adrenal gland; converted into cortisol* before use by the body. *cortisone suppression test* differentiates primary from secondary hypercalcemia.* Sarcoidosis causes secondary hypercalcemia; primary hyperparathyroidism causes primary hypercalcemia.

Cortisporin™ antibacterial preparation containing polymixin B, neomycin, bacitracin and hydrocortisone; cream, ointment or eye drops.

Corynebacterium (kōr-nē-bak-tēr'-ē-um) *n* bacterial genus of Gram-positive, rod-shaped bacteria averaging 3 μm in length, showing irregular staining in segments (metachromatic granules). Many strains are parasitic and some are pathogenic, e.g., *C. diphtheriae,* producing a powerful exotoxin.

coryza (kōr-ī'-zà) *n* acute upper respiratory infection of short duration; highly contagious; causative viruses include rhinoviruses, coronaviruses and adenoviruses.

Corzide™ bendroflumethazide.

Cosmegen™ dactinomycin.

cosmetic *adj, n* that which is done to improve appearance or prevent disfigurement.

costal (kos'-tal) *adj* pertaining to the ribs. *costal cartilages* those which attach ribs to the sternum.

costochondral (kos-tō-kon'-dràl) *adj* pertaining to a rib and its cartilage.

costochondritis (kos-tō-kon-drī'-tis) *n* inflammation of costochondral cartilage. → Tietze syndrome.

costoclavicular (kos-tō-klav-ik'-ū-làr) *adj* pertaining to ribs and the clavicle. *costoclavicular syndrome* synonym for cervical rib syndrome → cervical.

Cotazym™ pancreatic enzyme preparation.

cotrimoxazole (kō-trī-moks'-à-zōl) *n* antibacterial agent comprising sulfamethoxazole,* an early folic acid blocking agent, and trimethoprim,* a late folic acid blocking agent; particularly useful for urinary infections. (Bactrim, Septra.)

cotyledon (kot-il-ē'-don) *n* one of the subdivisions of the uterine surface of the placenta.*

Coumadin™ warfarin.*

counterirritant *n* an agent which, when applied to the skin, produces a mild inflammatory reaction (hyperemia) and relief of pain and congestion associated with a more deep-seated inflammatory process—**counterirritation** *n.*

couvade (kōō-vahd') *n* a custom in some cultures whereby a father exhibits the symptoms of his partner's pregnancy and childbirth.

Cowper's glands (kow'-perz) bulbourethral* glands.

cowpox (kow'-poks) *n* vaccinia; virus disease of cows. Lymph is used in vaccination of humans against smallpox (variola).

coxa (koks'-à) *n* the hip joint. *coxa valga* increase in the normal angle between neck and shaft of femur. *coxa vara* decrease in the normal angle plus torsion of the neck, e.g., slipped femoral epiphysis—**coxae** *pl.*

coxalgia (koks-al′-jà) *n* pain in the hip joint.

Coxiella (koks-ē-el′-là) *n* genus closely related to *Rickettsia* including *C. burnetii* which causes Q fever.

coxitis (koks-īt′-is) *n* inflammation of the hip joint.

coxsackie virus (koks′-ak-ē) first isolated at Coxsackie, NY. Divided into groups A and B. Many in group A appear to be nonpathogenic, some cause aseptic meningitis and herpangina. Those in group B also cause aseptic meningitis, Bornholm* disease and myocarditis.

CPAP *abbr* continuous* positive airways pressure.

CPK *abbr* creatinephosphokinase. → creatine kinase.

CPR *abbr* cardiopulmonary resuscitation. → resuscitation.

crab louse pediculus* pubis.

cradle cap scaling of the scalp of infants, often due to atopic dermatitis* or seborrheic dermatitis.

cramp *n* spasmodic contraction of a muscle or group of muscles; involuntary and painful; may result from fatigue. Occurs in tetany, food poisoning and cholera. *occupational cramp* is such as occurs amongst miners and other workers who use the same muscles continuously.

cranial (krā′-nē-àl) *adj* pertaining to the cranium.*

craniometry (krā-nē-om′-et-rē) *n* the science which deals with the measurement of skulls.

craniopharyngioma (krā-nē-ō-fār-in-jē-ōm′-à) *n* tumor which develops between the brain and the pituitary gland.

cranioplasty (krā-nē-ō-plas′-tē) *n* operative repair of a skull defect— **cranioplastic** *adj*.

craniosacral (krā-nē-ō-sāk′-ràl) *adj* pertaining to the skull and sacrum. Applied to the parasympathetic nervous system.

craniostenosis (krā-nē-ō-sten-ōs′-is) *n* condition in which the skull sutures fuse too early and the fontanels close; may cause increased intracranial pressure requiring surgery.

craniosynostosis (krā-nē-ō-sin-os-tō′-sis) *n* premature ossification of skull bones with closure of suture lines, giving rise to facial deformities. → Apert's syndrome.

craniotabes (krā-nē-ō-tā′-bēz) *n* thinning or wasting of the cranial bones, occurring in infancy and usually due to rickets*—**craniotabetic** *adj*.

craniotomy (krā-nē-ot′-o-mē) *n* surgical opening of the skull to remove a growth, relieve pressure, evacuate blood clot or arrest hemorrhage.

cranium (krā'-nē-um) *n* the part of the skull enclosing the brain. It is composed of eight bones: occipital, two parietals, frontal, two temporals, sphenoid and ethmoid—**cranial** *adj*.

c-reactive protein test a normal constituent of plasma; raised in bacterial meningitis.

creatinase (krē-at'-in-āz) *n* → creatine kinase.

creatine (krē'-at-en) *n* a nitrogenous compound synthesized in vitro. *phosphonylated creatine* is an important storage form of high-energy phosphate. *creatine kinase* (creatine phosphotransferase) occurs as three isoenzymes each having two components labelled M and B; the form in brain tissue is BB, in skeletal muscle and serum MM and in myocardial tissue both MM and MB. *creatine kinase test* the MB isoenzyme is raised in serum only in acute myocardial infarction and not in other cardiopathies. *creatine test* estimation of amount of creatine in blood. Serum creatine is raised in hyperthyroidism, and values above 0.6 mg per 100 ml of blood (40 μmol/l) suggest hyperthyroidism; also higher in muscle-wasting disorders and in renal failure.

creatinine (krē-at'-in-ēn) *n* an anhydride of creatine,* a waste product of protein (endogenous) metabolism found in muscle and blood and excreted in normal urine.

creatinuria (krē-at-in-ūr'-rē-à) *n* excess of the nitrogenous compound creatine* in urine. Occurs in conditions in which muscle is rapidly broken down, e.g., acute fevers, starvation.

creatorrhea (krē-at-ōr-ē'-à) *n* presence of excessive nitrogen in the feces; occurs particularly in pancreatic dysfunction.

Crede's method (krē-dāz') method of delivering the placenta by gently rubbing the fundus uteri until it contracts and then, by squeezing the fundus, expressing the placenta into the vagina whence it is expelled.

crepitation (krep-i-tā'-shun) *n* **1** (crepitus) grating of bone ends in fracture. **2** crackling sound in joints, e.g., in osteoarthritis. **3** crackling sound heard via stethoscope. **4** crackling sound elicited by pressure on tissue containing air (surgical emphysema).

cresol (krē'-sol) *n* chemically related to phenol* but a more powerful germicide. Cresol and/or related phenols are present in many general disinfectants.

cretinism (krē'-tin-izm) *n* due to congenital thyroid deficiency; results in a dull-looking child, underdeveloped mentally and physically, dwarfed, large head, thick legs, pug nose, dry skin, scanty hair, swollen eyelids, short neck, short thick limbs, clumsy uncoordinated gait—**cretin** *n*.

Creutzfeldt-Jakob disease (krutz'-feld–Jā'-kob) a presenile dementia and psychosis; cause is now thought to be a transmissible agent known as a "slow virus."

CRF *abbr* chronic renal failure. → renal.

crib death (*syn* sudden infant death syndrome) the unexpected sudden death of an infant, usually occurring overnight while sleeping in a crib. The commonest mode of death in infants between the ages of 1 month and 1 year; neither clinical nor postmortem findings account for phenomenon. Commoner in late winter, among low-birth-weight male infants around the age of 2 months.

cribriform (krib'-ri-form) *adj* perforated, like a sieve. *cribriform plate* that portion of the ethmoid bone allowing passage of fibers of olfactory nerve.

cricoid (krī'-koyd) *adj* ring-shaped. Applied to cartilage forming the inferior posterior part of larynx.

"cri du chat" syndrome cat-cry* syndrome.

crisis *n* **1** turning point of a disease—as the point of defervescence in fever, the arrest of an anemia. **2** muscular spasm in tabes dorsalis referred to as visceral crisis (gastric, vesical, rectal, etc.)—**crises** *pl.*

Crohn's disease (krōnz) → regional ileitis.

cromolyn sodium (krōm'-ō-lin) antihypersensitivity agent useful in prevention of asthma in some individuals with allergic responses. (Intal.)

Crosby capsule (kroz'-bē) special tube passed through the mouth to the small intestine; maneuver of the tube selects tissue for biopsy.

crotamiton (krō-tà-mī'-ton) *n* agent effective for scabies, esp. in infants, as it kills the mite and prevents itching. (Eurax.)

croup (kro͞op) *n* laryngeal obstruction. Croupy breathing in a child is often called "stridulous," meaning noisy or harsh-sounding. Narrowing of the airway which gives rise to typical attack with crowing inspiration; may be the result of edema or spasm, or both.

CRP *abbr* → c-reaction protein test.

cruciate (kroo'-shē-āt) *adj* shaped like a cross.

crus (kroos) *n* leglike or rootlike structure; applied to various body parts, e.g., crus of the diaphragm—**crura** *pl,* **crural** *adj.*

"crush" syndrome traumatic uremia. Following extensive trauma to muscle, there is a period of delay before effects of renal damage manifest themselves: increase of nonprotein nitrogen in blood, with oliguria, proteinuria and urinary excretion of myohemoglobin. Loss of blood plasma to damaged area is marked. Where hypotension has occurred, renal failure will be exacerbated by tubular* necrosis.

crutch palsy paralysis* of extensor muscles of wrist, fingers and thumb from repeated pressure of a crutch upon the radial nerve in the axilla.

cryesthesia (krī-es-thē'-zhà) *n* **1** sensation of coldness. **2** exceptional sensitivity to low temperature.

cryoanalgesia (krī-ō-an-al-jē'-zhȧ) *n* relief of pain by use of a cryosurgical probe to block peripheral nerve function.

cryoextractor (krī-ō-eks-trak'-tor) *n* type of cryoprobe* used for removal of a cataractous lens.

cryogenic (krī-ō-jen'-ik) *adj, n* anything produced by low temperature. Also describes any means or apparatus involved in production of low temperature.

cryoglobulins (krī-ō-glob'-ū-lins) *npl* abnormal proteins—immunoglobulins—which may be present in the blood in some diseases. They are characteristically insoluble at low temperatures, which can lead to obstruction of small blood vessels, as in the fingers and toes.

cryopexy (krī'-ō-peks-ē) *n* surgical fixation by freezing, as replacement of a detached retina.

cryophake (krī'-ō-fāk) *n* cataract extraction using freezing.

cryoprecipitate therapy (krī-ō-prē-sip'-i-tāt) use of Factor VIII to prevent or treat bleeding in hemophilia. Refers to preparation of Factor VIII for injection. Subarctic temperatures separate it from plasma. → blood clotting.

cryoprobe (krī'-ō-prōb) *n* freezing probe. Can be used for biopsy. A flexible metal tube attached to liquid nitrogen equipment. Cryoprobe has tips of various sizes, which can be cooled to −180°C. Causes less tissue trauma and "seeding" of malignant cells.

cryosurgery (krī-ō-sur'-je-rē) *n* use of intense, controlled cold to remove or destroy diseased tissue. Instead of a knife, a cryoprobe* is used.

cryothalamectomy (krī-ō-thal-a-mek'-to-mē) *n* freezing applied to destroy groups of neurons within the thalamus in treatment of Parkinson's disease and other hyperkinetic conditions.

cryotherapy (krī-ō-ther'-ȧ-pē) *n* use of cold for treatment of disease.

cryptococcosis (krip-tō-kok-kō'-sis) *n* disease resulting from infection of a human with the yeast *Cryptococcus neoformans*. Has a marked predilection for the central nervous system, causing subacute or chronic disease.

Cryptococcus (krip-tō-kok'-kus) *n* genus of fungi. *C. neoformans* is pathogenic to man.

cryptogenic (krip-tō-jen'-ik) *adj* of unknown or obscure cause.

cryptomenorrhea (krip-tō-men-or-ē'-ȧ) *n* retention of the menses due to congenital obstruction, such as imperforate hymen or atresia of the vagina. → hematocolpos.

cryptorchism (krip-tor'-kizm) *n* developmental defect whereby the testes do not descend into the scrotum; they are retained within the abdomen or inguinal canal—**cryptorchid, cryptorchis** *n*.

crystal violet (*syn* gentian violet) brilliant violet-colored, antiseptic aniline dye, used as 0.5% solution for ulcers and skin infections, and as a stain.

crystallin (kris′-tȧ-lin) *n* a globulin,* principal constituent of the lens of the eye.

crystalluria (kris-tȧ-lū′-rē-ȧ) *n* excretion of crystals in urine—**crystalluric** *adj*.

Crystodigin™ digitoxin.*

CSF *abbr* cerebrospinal* fluid.

CT *abbr* computed* tomography.

cubital tunnel external compression syndrome ulnar paralysis* resulting from compression of the ulnar nerve within the cubital tunnel situated on the inner and posterior aspect of the elbow—sometimes referred to as the "funny bone."

cubital vein (kū′-bi-tal) → Figure 9.

cubitus (kū′-bi-tus) *n* the forearm; elbow—**cubital** *adj*.

cuirass (kwir-as′) *n* mechanical apparatus fitted to the chest for artificial respiration.

cul de sac (kul-de-sak′) a blind cavity or pouch. *cul de sac of Douglas* an extension of the peritoneal cavity which lies behind the uterus between the posterior uterine wall and the rectum.

culdocentesis *n* aspiration of the cul de sac of Douglas via posterior vaginal wall.

culdoscope (kul′-do-skōp) *n* endoscope* used via the vaginal route—**culdoscope** *n*, **culdoscopic** *adj*.

cumulative action if the dose of a slowly excreted drug is repeated too frequently, an increasing action is obtained. This can be dangerous if, as the drug accumulates, toxic symptoms occur, sometimes quite suddenly. Long acting barbiturates, strychnine, mercurial salts and digitalis are examples of drugs with a cumulative action.

cupping *n* method of counterirritation. A small bell-shaped glass (in which the air is expanded by heating, or exhausted by compression of an attached rubber bulb) is applied to the skin, resultant suction producing hyperemia (*dry cupping*). If skin is scarified before application of cup, the term is *wet cupping*.

Cuprimine™ penicillamine.*

curare (kū-rȧr′-ē) *n* crude extract from which tubocurarine* is obtained.

curettage (kūr-et-tazh′) *n* scraping of unhealthy or exuberant tissue from a cavity; may be as treatment or to establish a diagnosis after laboratory analysis of the scrapings.

curette (kūr-et′) *n* spoon-shaped instrument or a metal loop which may have sharp, and/or blunt edges for scraping out (curetting) cavities.

curettings *npl* material obtained by scraping or curetting and usually sent for examination to the pathology department.

Curling's ulcer (kur'-lingz) ulcer* which occurs either in the stomach or duodenum as a complication of extensive burns or scalds.

cushingoid (kush'-ing-oyd) *adj* describes the moon face and central obesity common in people with elevated levels of plasma corticosteroid from whatever cause.

Cushing's disease (kush'-ingz) rare disorder, mainly of females, characterized principally by functional obesity, hyperglycemia, glycosuria, hypertension and hirsutism. Due to excessive cortisol production by hyperplastic adrenal glands as a result of increased corticotropin secretion by a tumor or hyperplasia of anterior pituitary gland.

Cushing's reflex (kush'-ingz) rise in blood pressure and a fall in pulse rate; occurs in cerebral space-occupying lesions.

Cushing's syndrome (kush'-ingz) disorder clinically similar to Cushing's* disease and also due to elevated levels of plasma corticosteroid, but primary pathology is not in the pituitary gland. It can be due to adenoma or carcinoma of the adrenal cortex and to the secretion of ACTH* by nonendocrine tumors such as bronchial carcinoma; may also be iatrogenic, due to excessive administration of corticosteroids.

cutaneous (kū-tān'-ē-us) *adj* relating to the skin. *cutaneous nerve* → Figure 12. *cutaneous ureterostomy* ureters transplanted so that they open on to skin of the abdominal wall.

cuticle (kū'-tik-l) *n* the epidermis* or dead epidermis, as that which surrounds a nail—**cuticular** *adj*.

CVA *abbr* cerebrovascular* accident.

CVP *abbr* central* venous pressure.

cyanocobalamin (sī-an-ō-kō-bal'-a-mēn) *n* vitamin* B_{12}, found in liver, fish, meat and eggs. Needed for maturation of erythrocytes. Only absorbed in the presence of intrinsic* factor secreted in the gastric juice. → cobalamin.

cyanosis (sī-an-ō'-sis) *n* bluish tinge manifested by hypoxic tissue, observed most frequently under nails, lips and skin. Always due to lack of oxygen, the causes of which are legion. *central cyanosis* blueness seen on warm surfaces such as the oral mucosa and tongue. It increases with exertion. *peripheral cyanosis* blueness of limb extremities, nose and ear lobes—**cyanosed, cyanotic** *adj*.

cyclamates (sī'-kla-māts) *npl* salts of cyclamic acid, which are 30 times as sweet as sugar and stable to heat. Banned as food additives when suspected of causing cancer.

cyclandelate (sī-klan′-del-āt) *n* vasodilator used particularly for cerebral vascular disorders. (Cyclospasmol.)

cyclical vomiting periodic attacks of vomiting in children, usually associated with ketosis and usually with no demonstrable pathological cause. Occurs mainly in highly-strung children.

cyclitis (sī-klī′-tis) *n* inflammation of the ciliary body of the eye, shown by deposition of small collections of white cells on the posterior cornea called "keratitic precipitates" (KP). Often coexistent with inflammation of the iris. → iridocyclitis.

cyclizine (sī′-kli-zēn) *n* antihistamine. (Marezine.)

cyclobenzaprine (sī-klō-benz′-á-prēn) *n* muscle relaxant. (Flexeril.)

cyclodialysis (sī-klō-dī-al′-is-is) *n* establishment of communication between anterior chamber and perichoroidal or suprachoroidal space to relieve intraocular pressure in glaucoma.

cyclodiathermy (sī-klō-dī-á-ther′-mē) *n* destruction of the ciliary body by diathermy.*

Cyclogyl™ cyclopentolate.*

cyclopentolate (sī-klō-pen′-tō-lāt) *n* synthetic, spasmolytic drug. Causes cycloplegia and mydriasis. (Cyclogyl.)

cyclophosphamide (sī-klō-fos′-fá-mīd) *n* cytotoxic agent, a nitrogen mustard. Alkylating agent that interferes with synthesis of nucleic acid in cell chromosomes, particularly in rapidly dividing cells such as those which occur in bone marrow, skin, gastrointestinal tract and fetal tissues. The main side-effects therefore occur in these tissues, causing anorexia, nausea, vomiting, diarrhea, depression of bone marrow and alopecia. Main indications are malignancy of lymphoid tissue. (Cytoxan.)

cycloplegia (sī-klō-plē′-já) *n* paralysis of the ciliary muscle of the eye—**cycloplegic** *adj*.

cycloplegics (sī-klō-plē′-jiks) *npl* drugs which cause paralysis of the ciliary muscle, e.g., atropine, homatropine, and scopolamine.

cycloserine (sī-klō-sēr′-ēn) *n* antibiotic active against many microorganisms; main use is for severe pulmonary tuberculosis caused by microorganisms resistant to other antitubercular drugs. Must be used together with other antitubercular compounds.

Cyclospasmol™ cyclandelate.*

cyclosporine (sī-klō-spōr′-in) *n* selective immunosuppressive agent which does not suppress production of antibodies. (Sandimmune.)

cyclothymia (sī-klō-thī′-mē-á) *n* tendency to alternating but relatively mild mood swings between elation and depression—**cyclothymic** *adj*.

cyclotomy (sī-klot'-o-mē) *n* drainage operation for relief of glaucoma, with incision through the ciliary body.

cyesis (sī-ē'-sis) *n* pregnancy. When there are signs and symptoms of pregnancy in a woman who believes she is pregnant, and this is not so, it is called pseudocyesis. → phantom pregnancy.

cylindroma (sil-in-drō'-mȧ) *n* tumor of the endothelial element of apocrine tissue such as a sweat gland or a salivary gland. The supporting stroma is hyalinized.

cyllosis (sil-ō'-sis) *n* clubfoot.

cyproheptadine (sī-prō-hep'-tȧ-dēn) *n* antihistamine* with antiserotonin* action. (Periactin.)

cyst (sist) *n* a sac with membranous wall, enclosing fluid or semisolid matter—**cystic** *adj*.

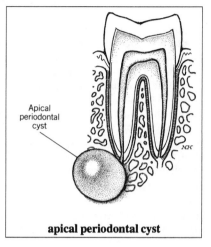

Apical periodontal cyst

apical periodontal cyst

cystadenoma (sist-ad-en-ō'-mȧ) *n* an innocent cystic new growth of glandular tissue. Liable to occur in the female breast.

cystalgia (sis-tal'-jȧ) *n* pain in the urinary bladder.

cystathioninuria (sis-tȧ-thī-on-in-ū'-rē-ȧ) *n* inherited disorder of cystathionine metabolism marked by excessive excretion, in urine, of cystathionine, an intermediate product in conversion of methionine to cysteine. Sometimes associated with mental subnormality.

cystectomy (sis-tek'-to-mē) *n* usually refers to removal of part or all of urinary bladder, which necessitates urinary diversion. The ureters may then be implanted into an isolated ileal segment (ileal conduit) or into sigmoid colon.

cysteine (sis'-tēn) *n* sulfur-containing amino acid produced by breakdown of proteins during the digestive process. Easily oxidized to cystine.*

cysticercosis (sis-ti-sėr-kō'-sis) *n* infection of man with cysticercus.*

cysticercus (sis-ti-sėr'-kus) *n* larval form of taenia.* After ingestion, ova do not develop beyond this stage in man, but form "cysts" in subcutaneous tissues, skeletal muscles and the brain, where they provoke epilepsy.

cystic fibrosis (sis'-tik fī-brō'-sis) (*syn* fibrocystic disease of the pancreas, mucoviscidosis) commonest genetically-determined disease in Caucasian populations; an abnormality of secretion of the exocrine glands. Thick mucus can block the intestinal glands and cause meconium ileus in a baby; later may cause steatorrhea, creatorrhea and malabsorption. Thick mucus in respiratory glands predisposes to repeated infections and bronchiectasis. Abnormality of sweat glands increases chloride content of sweat, which is a diagnostic aid. → sweat test.

cystine (sis′-tēn) *n* sulfur-containing amino acid, produced by breakdown of proteins during the digestive process; readily reduced to two molecules of cysteine.*

cystinosis (sis-tin-ō′-sis) *n* recessively inherited metabolic disorder in which crystalline cystine* is deposited in the body. Cystine and other amino acids are excreted in urine.

cystinuria (sis-tin-ū′-rē-à) *n* metabolic disorder in which cystine* and other amino acids appear in urine. A cause of renal stones—**cystinuric** *adj*.

cystitis (sis-tī′-tis) *n* inflammation of urinary bladder; cause is usually bacterial. May be acute or chronic, primary or secondary to stones, etc. More frequent in females, as the urethra is short.

cystitome (sis′-ti-tōm) *n* delicate ophthalmic instrument for incision of the lens capsule.

cystocele (sis′-tō-sēl) *n* prolapse of the posterior wall of the urinary bladder into the anterior vaginal wall. → colporrhaphy.

cystodiathermy (sis′-tō-dī-ath-ėr′-mē) *n* application of a cauterizing electrical current to the walls of the urinary bladder through a cystoscope, or by open operation.

cystography (sis-tog′-ra-fē) *n* radiographic examination of the urinary bladder, after it has been filled with a contrast medium—**cystographic** *adj*, **cystograph** *n*, **cystogram** *n*.

cystolithiasis (sis-tō-lith-ī′-à-sis) *n* presence of a stone or stones in the urinary bladder.

cystometer (sis-tom′-e-tėr) *n* apparatus for measuring pressure under various conditions in the urinary bladder—**cystometry** *n*.

cystometrogram (sis-tō-met′-rō-gram) *n* record of cystometer* measurements; used in study of voiding disorders.

cystopexy (sis′-tō-peks-ē) *n* a "sling" operation for stress incontinence whereby the bladder neck is supported from the back of the symphysis pubis.

cystoplasty (sis′-tō-plas-tē) *n* surgical repair of the urinary bladder—**cystoplastic** *adj*.

cystoscope (sis′-tō-skōp) *n* endoscope* used in diagnosis and treatment of bladder, ureter and kidney conditions—**cystoscopic** *adj*, **cystoscopy** *n*.

cystostomy (sis-tos′-to-mē) *n* (*syn* vesicostomy) fistulous opening is made into the urinary bladder via the abdominal wall. Usually the fistula can be allowed to heal when its purpose has been achieved.

cystotomy (sis-tot'-o-mē) *n* incision into the urinary bladder via the abdominal wall, often done to remove a large stone or tumor or to gain access to the prostate gland in the operation of transvesical prostatectomy.*

cystourethritis (sis-tō-ū-rē-thrī'-tis) *n* inflammation of urinary bladder and urethra.

cystourethrography (sis-tō-ū-rē-throg'-rá-fē) *n* radiographic examination of urinary bladder and urethra, after they have been rendered radioopaque—**cystourethrographic** *adj*, **cystourethrogram** *n*, **cystourethrograph** *n*.

cystourethropexy (sis-tō-ū-rē'-thrō-peks-ē) *n* forward fixation of urinary bladder and upper urethra in an attempt to combat incontinence of urine.

Cytadren™ aminoglutethimide.*

cytarabine (sī-tār'-a-bēn) *n* antimetabolite which interferes with DNA synthesis; used for treating acute leukemias. (Cytosar-U.)

cytodiagnosis (sī-tō-dī-ag-nō'-sis) *n* diagnosis by microscopic study of cells—**cytodiagnostic** *adj*.

cytogenetics (sī-tō-jen-et'-iks) *n* the study of normal and abnormal chromosomes, and of their behavior.

cytokines (sī'-tō-kīnz) *npl* substances secreted by lymphocytes to control magnitude of overall immune response; these include interleukin (IL), interferon (IFN), tumor necrosis factor (TNF), colony-stimulating factor (CSF) and transforming growth factor (TGF), all of which are further subdivided into specific types.

cytology (sī-tol'-o-jē) *n* microscopic study of cells. The term *exfoliative cytology* is used when the cells studied have been shed, or exfoliated, from the surface of an organ or lesion—**cytological** *adj*.

cytolysis (sī-tol'-is-is) *n* the degeneration, destruction, disintegration or dissolution of cells—**cytolytic** *adj*.

cytomegalovirus (sī-tō-meg'-á-lō-vī'-rus) *n* belongs to the same group of viruses as herpes simplex. Can cause latent and symptomless infection. Virus excreted in urine and saliva. Congenital infection is the most severe form of *cytomegalovirus infection,* can infect the fetus in utero, sometimes causing microcephaly, intracranial calcification and mental defect, or an illness at birth characterized by hepatosplenomegaly and thrombocytopenia. Infection also transmitted by blood transfusion, esp. in patients with impaired immunity, in whom it causes a glandular fever-like illness and pneumonia.

Cytomel™ preparation of liothyranine* with a standardized activity.

cytopathic (sī-tō-path'-ik) *adj* pertaining to abnormality of the living cell.

cytoplasm (sī'-tō-plazm) *n* (*syn* protoplasm) the complex chemical compound constituting the main part of the living substance of the cell, other than the contents of the nucleus—**cytoplasmic** *adj*.

Cytosar-U™ cytarabine.*

cytostasis (sī-tō-stā′-sis) *n* arrest or hindrance of cell development—**cytostatic** *adj*.

cytotoxic (sī-tō-toks′-ik) *adj* any substance which is toxic to cells. Applied to drugs used for treatment of carcinomas and the reticuloses. Two main groups: (a) antimetabolites which block action of an enzyme system, e.g., methotrexate, fluorouracil mercaptopurine; (b) alkylating agents which poison cell directly, e.g., cyclophosphamide, mustine. There are known and potential dangers while handling cytotoxic drugs—dermatitis, nasal sores, pigmentation of the skin, blisters and excessive lacrimation have been reported.

cytotoxins (sī-tō-toks′-ins) *npl* antibodies which are toxic to cells.

Cytoxan™ cyclophosphamide.*

D

D and C *abbr* dilatation* and curettage.

Da Costa syndrome (dà-kos'-tà) cardiac neurosis. Anxiety* state in which palpitations and left-sided chest pain are the most prominent symptoms.

dacryoadenitis (dak-rē-ō-ad-en-ī'-tis) *n* inflammation of a lacrimal gland; a rare condition which may be acute or chronic. May occur in mumps.*

dacryocyst (dak'-rē-ō-sist) *n* dated term for lacrimal sac (tear sac), but still used in compound forms (see below).

dacryocystectomy (dak-rē-ō-sis-tek'-to-mē) *n* excision of any part of the lacrimal sac.

dacryocystitis (dak-rē-ō-sis-tī'-tis) *n* inflammation of the lacrimal sac; usually results in abscess formation and obliteration of the tear duct, giving rise to epiphora.*

dacryocystography (dak-rē-ō-sis-tog'raf-ē) *n* radiographic examination of the tear drainage apparatus after it has been rendered radio-opaque— **dacryocystographic** *adj,* **dacryocystogram** *n.*

dacryocystorhinostomy (dak-rē-ō-sis'tō-rīn-os'-to-mē) *n* (*syn* Toti's operation) operation to establish drainage from lacrimal sac into the nose when there is obstruction of the nasolacrimal duct.

dacryolith (dak'-rē-ō-lith) *n* a concretion in the lacrimal passages.

dactinomycin (dak-tin-ō-mī'-sin) *n* intravenous cytostatic antibiotic useful in Wilm's tumor, Burkitt's lymphoma, soft tissue sarcomas and teratomas; a potent radiosensitizer. (Cosmegen.)

dactyl (dak'-tl) *n* a digit, finger or toe—**dactylar, dactylate** *adj.*

dactylitis (dak-til-ī'-tis) *n* inflammation of finger or toe. Digit becomes swollen due to periostitis. Met with in congenital syphilis, tuberculosis, sarcoid, etc.

Dakin's solution (dā'-kinz) aqueous solution of sodium hypochlorite used to irrigate wounds and as a wet dressing.

Dalmane™ flurazepam.*

dandruff *n* (*syn* scurf) common scaly condition of the scalp. May be forerunner of skin diseases of the seborrheic type, such as flexural dermatitis.

Dantrium™ dantrolene.*

dantrolene (dan'-trō-lēn) *n* antispasmodic useful in severe spasticity, multiple sclerosis, spinal cord injury and stroke. (Dantrium.)

dapsone (dap'-sōn) *n* sulfone derivative used mainly in leprosy. Prolonged treatment may produce hemolytic anemia with Heinz body formation, clinical signs of which are cyanosis of the lips; the patient is generally off-color. (Avlosulfan.)

Daranide™ dichlorphenamide.*

Daraprim™ pyrimethamine.*

Darbid™ isopropamide.*

Darvon™ dextropropoxyphene.

daunorubicin (daw-nō-rōō'-bi-sin) *n* similar to doxorubicin*; antibiotic used in acute leukemia. Believed to act by inhibiting DNA synthesis. Can cause severe bone marrow depression and toxicity of heart muscle. (Cerubidine.)

DDST *abbr* Denver Developmental Screening Test.*

deafness (def'-nes) *n* partial or complete loss of hearing. *conductive deafness* due to an obstruction which prevents conduction of sound waves from the atmosphere to the inner ear. *perceptive* or *nerve deafness* due to a lesion in the inner ear, auditory nerve or the auditory centers in the brain. *congenital deafness* can be caused by mother contracting german measles in early pregnancy.

deamination (dē-am-in-ā'-shun) *n* removal of the amino group from organic compounds such as amino acids.

death *n* cessation of the body's vital functions, usually assessed by absence of pulse and breathing. Mechanical ventilation may maintain vital functions despite the fact that the brain stem is fatally and irreversibly damaged *(brain death)*. Consequently stringent tests are necessary to diagnose death. In different countries, different criteria are used to diagnose brain death.

debility *n* condition of weakness with lack of muscle tone.

débridement (dā-brēd'-mo) *n* removal of foreign matter and injured or infected tissue from a wound. *chemical medical debridement* accomplished by external application of a substance to the wound. *surgical debridement* accomplished by using surgical instruments and aseptic technique.

Decadron™ dexamethasone.*

decalcification (dē-kal-si-fi-kā'-shun) *n* removal of mineral salts, as from teeth in dental caries, bone in disorders of calcium metabolism.

decapsulation (dē-kap-sū-lā'-shun) *n* surgical removal of a capsule.

decerebrate (dē-sėr'-e-brāt) *adj* without cerebral function: a state of deep unconsciousness. *decerebrate posture* a condition of the unconscious patient in which all four limbs are spastic and which indicates severe damage to the cerebrum.

Decholin™ dehydrocholic acid*; cholagogue.*

decidua (dē-sid′-ū-à) *n* the endometrial lining of the uterus thickened and altered for reception of the fertilized ovum. Shed when pregnancy terminates. *decidua basalis* that part which lies under the embedded ovum and forms the maternal part of the placenta; *decidua capsularis* that part which lies over the developing ovum. *decidua vera* the decidua lining the rest of the uterus— **decidual** *adj*.

deciduous (dē-sid′-ū-us) *adj* by custom refers to the primary teeth, which on shedding are normally replaced by permanent teeth.

Declomycin™ demeclocyline.*

decompensation *n* failure of compensation, usually referring to heart disease.

decompression *n* removal of pressure or a compressing force. *decompression of brain* achieved by trephining the skull. *decompression of bladder* in cases of chronic urinary retention, by continuous or intermittent drainage via catheter inserted per urethra. *decompression chamber* used when returning deep-sea divers to the surface. → caisson disease.

decongestants *npl* agents which reduce or eliminate congestion, usually referring to nasal congestion. Can be taken by mouth or applied locally as drops or sprays.

decortication (dē-kört-ik-ā′-shun) *n* surgical removal of cortex or outer covering of an organ. *decortication of lung* carried out when thickening of visceral pleura prevents re-expansion of lung, as may occur in chronic emphysema. The visceral pleura is peeled off the lung, which is then re-expanded by positive pressure through an anesthetic apparatus.

decubitus (dē-kū′-bit-us) *n* the recumbent position; lying down. *decubitus ulcer* → pressure sore—**decubiti** *pl*, **decubital** *adj*.

decussation (dē-kus-ā′-shun) *n* intersection; crossing of nerve fibers at a point beyond their origin, as in the optic and pyramidal tracts.

deep muscles → Figures 4, 5.

defecation (de-fe-kā′-shun) *n* voiding of feces per anus—**defecate** *vi*.

deferent duct → Figure 16.

deferoxamine (de-fėr-oks′-à-mēn) *n* iron chelating agent which can be used in iron poisoning. (Desferal.)

defervescence (def-er-ves′ens) *n* time during which a fever is declining. If body temperature falls rapidly it is termed "crisis"; if slowly, "lysis" is used.

defibrillation (dē-fib-ril-lā′-shun) *n* the arrest of fibrillation* of the cardiac muscle (atrial or ventricular), and restoration of normal cycle—**defibrillate** *vt*.

defibrillator (dē-fib′-ril-ā-tor) *n* any agent, e.g., an electric shock, which arrests ventricular fibrillation* and restores normal rhythm.

defibrinated (dē-fī'-brin-ā-ted) *adj* rendered free from fibrin.* Necessary process in preparation of serum from whole blood. → blood—**defibrinate** *v*.

deficiency disease disease resulting from dietary deficiency of any substance essential for good health, esp. vitamins.

degeneration *n* deterioration in quality or function. Regression from more specialized to less specialized type of tissue—**degenerative** *adj*, **degenerate** *vi*.

deglutition (dē-glōō-tish'-un) *n* process of swallowing, partly voluntary, partly involuntary.

dehiscence (dē-his'-ens) *n* process of splitting or bursting open, as of a wound.

dehydration *n* loss or removal of fluid. Arises in the body when fluid intake fails to replace fluid loss; liable to occur when there is bleeding, diarrhea, excessive exudation from a raw area, excessive sweating, polyuria or vomiting, and usually upsets the body's electrolyte balance. If suitable fluid replacement cannot be achieved orally then parenteral administration must be instituted—**dehydrate** *vt, vi*.

dehydrocholic acid (de-hīd-rō-kōl'-ik) a cholagogue.*

deja vu phenomenon (dā'-zhà vōō) occurs in epilepsy involving temporal lobes of the brain and in certain epileptic dream states. An intense feeling of familiarity, as if everything had happened before.

Delalutin™ hydroxyprogesterone* caproate.

deliquescent (del-i-kwes'-ent) *adj* capable of absorption, thus becoming fluid.

delirium *n* abnormal mental condition based on hallucinations or illusion. May occur in high fever, in mental disease, or be toxic in origin. *delirium tremens* results from alcoholic intoxication; with confusion, terror, restlessness and hallucinations—**delirious** *adj*.

Delta-Cortef™ prednisolone.*

Deltasone™ prednisone.*

deltoid (del'-toyd) *adj* triangular. *deltoid muscle* → Figures 4, 5.

demarcation (dē-már-kā'-shun) *n* an outlining of the junction of diseased and healthy tissue, often used when referring to gangrene.

dementia (dē-men'-shà) *n* (*syn* organic brain syndrome—OBS) irreversible organic brain disease causing memory and personality disorders, deterioration in personal care, impaired cognitive ability and disorientation. → Jakob-Creutzfeldt disease. *dementia praecox* early but obsolete description of what is now called schizophrenia.* *presenile dementia* signs and symptoms of dementia* occurring in people between 50 and 60 years of age; due to early hyaline degeneration of both medium and small cerebral blood vessels. → Alzheimer's disease. Pick's disease.

Demerol™ meperidine.*

demeclocycline (dē-mek-lō-sī'-klin) *n* a tetracycline.* (Declomycin.)

Demser™ metyrosine.*

demulcent (dē-mul'-sent) *n* a slippery, mucilaginous fluid which allays irritation and soothes inflammation, esp. of mucous membranes.

demyelinization (dē-mī-el-in-īz-ā'-shun) *n* destruction of the myelin* sheaths surrounding nerve fibers; occurs in multiple sclerosis.

dendrite (den'-drīt) *n* (*syn* dendron) one of the branched filaments from the body of a nerve cell; that part of a neuron which transmits an impulse to the nerve cell—**dendritic** *adj*.

dendritic ulcer (den-drit'-ik) a linear corneal ulcer that sends out treelike branches. Caused by herpes simplex. Treated with idoxuridine.

dendron (den'-dron) *n* → dendrite.

denervation (dē-nėr-vā'-shun) *n* means by which a nerve supply is cut off. Usually refers to incision, excision or blocking of a nerve.

dengue (deng'-gē) *n* (*syn* "break-bone fever") one of the mosquito*-transmitted hemorrhagic fevers, a disease of the tropics. Causative agent is an arbovirus conveyed by a mosquito. Characterized by rheumatic pains, fever and a skin eruption. The hemorrhagic form has a high mortality.

dental plaque *n* noncalcified deposit on the surface of a tooth composed of a soft mass of bacteria and cellular debris which accumulates rapidly in the absence of oral hygiene.

dentate (den'-tāt) *adj* having teeth present.

dentine (den'-tēn) *n* calcified tissue forming the body of the tooth beneath the enamel and cementum enclosing the pulp chamber and root canals.

dentition (den-ti'-shun) *n* refers to teeth. In man the primary or deciduous* teeth are called *primary dentition* and are normally 20 in number. The adult, permanent teeth are called the *secondary dentition,* and are normally 32 in number.

Denver Developmental Screening Test (DDST) developmental test for young children.

deodorant *n, adj* any substance that destroys or masks an (unpleasant) odor. Potassium permanganate and hydrogen peroxide are deodorants by their powerful oxidizing action; chlorophyll has some reputation as a deodorant for foul-smelling wounds, but its value in masking other odors is doubtful—**deodorize** *vt*.

deoxygenation (dē-oks-i-jen-ā'-shun) *n* the removal of oxygen—**deoxygenated** *adj*.

deoxyribonucleic acid (DNA) (dē-oks-i-rī-bō-nū-klē'-ik) polymers of deoxyribonucleotides which occur in complex molecules called chromosomes* found in cell nuclei and viruses. DNA carries, in coded form, instructions for passing on hereditary characteristics.

depilate (dep'-il-āt) *vt* to remove hair from—**depilatory** *adj, n,* **depilation** *n.*

depilatory (dē-pil'-åt-ōr-ē) *n* substance usually made in pastes (e.g., barium sulfide) which removes excess hair only temporarily; does not act on the papillae, consequently hair grows again. → epilation. *preoperative depilation* lessens risk of wound infection because it is nonabrasive.

DepoProvera™ medroxyprogesterone* acetate.

depression *n* **1** a hollow place or indentation. **2** diminution of power or activity. **3** emotional disorder characterized by feelings of profound sadness. Most clinicians recognize two distinct types, neurotic and psychotic. Neurotic type is called *reactive depression;* it occurs as a reaction to stress. Psychotic type is called *endogenous depression;* it arises spontaneously in the mind. Symptoms vary from mild to fatal and are: insomnia, headaches, exhaustion, anorexia, irritability, emotionalism or loss of affect, loss of interest, impaired concentration, feelings that life is not worth living and suicidal thoughts. Symptoms of endogenous depression are more severe, but paradoxically respond better to treatment. When the condition occurs in middle life it is sometimes referred to as climacteric depression or involutional melancholia.

derangement (dē-rānj'-ment) *n* insanity, mental disorder.

dereistic (dē-rē-is'-tik) *adj* of thinking, not adapted to reality. Describes autistic thinking.

dermabrasion (dėr-må-brā'-zhun) *n* → *abrasion.*

dermatitis (dėr-må-tī'-tis) *n* inflammation of the skin (by custom limited to an eczematous reaction). → eczema. *atopic dermatitis* that variety of infantile eczema which may be associated with asthma or hay fever. *contact dermatitis* inflammation caused by contact with chemically irritant or allergenic substances. *dermatitis herpetiformis* (*syn* hydroa) intensely itchy skin eruption of unknown cause, most commonly with vesicles, bullae and pustules on urticarial plaques, which remit and relapse. Associated with gluten-sensitive enteropathy. *juvenile dermatitis herpetiformis* recurrent bullous eruption on genitalia, lower abdomen, buttocks and face, mainly in children under 5, boys being affected more than girls. *nummular dermatitis* coin-shaped, crusted lesions; cause unknown but associated with dry skin, esp. in cold weather. *stasis dermatitis* chronic condition involving lower legs, often with brown pigmentation; associated with poor venous circulation.

dermatoglyphics (dėr-må-tō-glif'-iks) *n* study of ridge patterns of the skin of the fingertips, palms and soles to discover developmental anomalies.

dermatographia (dėr-må-tō-graf'-ē-å) *n* → dermographia.

dermatology (dėr-mȧ-tol′-ō-jē) *n* science that deals with the skin, its structure, functions, diseases and treatment—**dermatological** *adj,* **dermatologist** *n.*

dermatome (dėr′-mat-ōm) *n* instrument for cutting slices of skin of varying thickness, usually for grafting.

dermatomycosis (dėr-mat-ō-mī-kō′-sis) *n* fungal infection of the skin— **dermatomycotic** *adj.*

dermatomyositis (dėr′-mat-ō-mī-ōs-īt′-is) *n* an acute inflammation of skin and muscles which presents with edema and muscle weakness. May result in the atrophic changes of scleroderma.* → collagen.

dermatophytes (dėr′-ma-tō-fīts) *npl* a group of fungi which invade the superficial skin.

dermatophytosis (dėr-ma-tō-fī-tō′-sis) *n* infection of skin with dermatophyte species.

dermatosis (dėr-ma-tō′-sis) *n* generic term for skin disease—**dermatoses** *pl.*

dermis (dėr′-mis) *n* the true skin; the cutis vera; the layer below the epidermis (→ Figure 12)—**dermal** *adj.*

dermographia (dėr-mog-raf′-ē-ä) *n* (*syn* dermatographia, factitial urticaria) condition in which weals occur on skin after a blunt instrument or fingernail has been lightly drawn over it. Seen in vasomotor instability and urticaria— **dermographic** *adj.*

dermoid (dėr′-moyd) *adj* pertaining to or resembling skin. *dermoid cyst* a cyst* which is congenital in origin and usually occurs in the ovary; contains elements of hair, nails, skin, teeth, etc.

Dermoplast™ preparation of benzocaine* for use as a topical anesthetic and antipruritic.

DES *abbr* diethylstilbestrol.*

descending colon → Figure 18.

desensitization (dē-sen-sit-īz-ā′-shun) *n* **1** injection of antigens* to diminish hypersensitivity to insect venoms, drugs, pollen and other causes of acute hypersensitivity reactions. **2** of phobic patients, using intravenous methohexital sodium to achieve psychological relaxation, so that phobic situation is imagined without discomfort and patient may "unlearn" irrational fear—**desensitize** *vt.*

deserpidine (dē-sėr′-pi-dīn) *n* drug related to reserpine*; has an antihypertensive function.

Desferol™ deferoxamine.*

desiccation (de-sik-ā′-shun) *n* drying out, as desiccation of the nucleus pulposus, diminishing the "water cushion" effect of a healthy intervertebral disk.

desipramine (dez-ip'-ra-mēn) *n* antidepressant. (Norpramin.)

deslanoside (des-lan'-ō-sīd) *n* a natural glycoside; cardiac therapeutic agent. (Cedilanid-D.)

desloughing (dē-sluf'-ing) *n* process of removing slough* from a wound.

desmopressin (dez-mō-pres'-in) *n* antidiuretic → vasopressin.

desoxycorticosterone (DOCA) (dez-oks'-ē-kort-i-kō-ster'-ōn) *n* important hormone of the adrenal cortex, controlling metabolism of sodium and potassium.

desquamation (des-kwá-mā'-shun) *n* shedding; flaking off, casting off—
desquamate *vi, vt.*

detached retina separation of neuroretina from the pigment epithelium, usually accompanied by retinal tears or holes (thegmatogenous retinal detachment). *Exudative* retinal separation of the combined neuroretina and pigment epithelium from the choroid. Treatment aims to produce scar tissue between all layers of the retina and choroid.

detoxication *n* process of removing the poisonous property of a substance—
detoxicant *adj, n,* **detoxicate** *vt.*

detritus (dē-trī'-tus) *n* matter produced by detrition; waste matter from disintegration.

detrusor (dē-trōō'-sėr) *n* muscle of the urinary bladder.

detumescence (dē-tū-mes'-ens) *n* subsidence of a swelling.

dexamethasone (deks-à-meth'-à-sōn) *n* 30 times as active as cortisone* in suppressing inflammation. Less likely to precipitate diabetes than the other steroids. Sometimes used to prevent cerebral edema. (Decadron.)

Dexedrine™ dextroamphetamine.*

dextran (deks'-tran) *n* a blood plasma substitute, obtained by the action of a specific bacterium on sugar solutions. Used as a 6% or 10% solution in hemorrhage, shock, etc.

dextranase (deks'-tran-āz) *n* an enzyme that reduces the formation of dextran* from sucrose; has been used to prevent formation of dental plaque.

dextrin (deks'-trin) *n* soluble polysaccharide formed during hydrolysis of starch.

dextroamphetamine (deks-trō-am-fet'-à-mēn) *n* central nervous system stimulant similar to amphetamine* and used for similar purposes. Sometimes used as an appetite suppressant in obesity. (Dexedrine.)

dextrocardia (deks-trō-kàr'-dē-à) *n* transposition of the heart to the right side of the thorax—**dextrocardial** *adj.*

dextromethorphan (deks-trō-meth-ōr'-fàn) *n* cough suppressant; available as lozenges, syrup and a linctus.

dextropropoxyphene (deks-trō-prō-poks'-i-fēn) *n* milder type of analgesic used as morphine substitute. (Darvon.)

dextrose (deks'-trōs) *n* (*syn* glucose) a soluble carbohydrate (monosaccharide) widely used by intravenous infusion in dehydration, shock and postoperatively. Also given orally as a readily absorbed sugar in acidosis and other nutritional disturbances.

dextroxylase test (deks-troks'-i-lāz) xylose* test.

DFP *abbr* dyflos.*

D.H.E. 45™ dihydroergotamine.*

diabetes (dī-à-bē'-tēz) *n* a disease characterized by polyuria. Used without qualification it means diabetes mellitus. *diabetes insipidus* polyuria and polydipsia caused by deficiency of ADH. Usually due to trauma or tumor involving posterior pituitary but may be idiopathic. Treated with desmopressin. *nephrogenic diabetes insipidus* polyuria resulting from abnormality or disease rendering renal tubules insensitive to ADH. *diabetes mellitus* condition characterized by hyperglycemia due to deficiency or diminished effectiveness of insulin. The hyperglycemia leads to glycosuria, which in turn causes polyuria and polydipsia. Severe dehydration, sometimes sufficient to cause unconsciousness may occur (hyperosmolar nonketotic coma). Impaired utilization of carbohydrate is associated with increased secretion of antistorage hormones such as glucagon and growth hormone in an attempt to provide alternative metabolic substrate. Glycogenolysis, gluconeogenesis and lipolysis are all increased. The latter results in excessive formation of ketone bodies which in turn leads to acidosis. If untreated this will eventually cause coma (ketoacidotic diabetic coma) and death. Diabetic patients are either *insulin dependent* or *noninsulin dependent,* irrespective of patient's age at onset of the condition. *potential diabetics* have a normal glucose tolerance test but are at increased risk of developing diabetes for genetic reasons. *latent diabetics* have a normal glucose tolerance test but are known to have had an abnormal test under conditions imposing a burden on the pancreatic beta cells, e.g., during infection or pregnancy. In the latter instance the term *gestational diabetes* is commonly used. → hyperosmolar diabetic coma, insulin dependent diabetes mellitus—**diabetic** *adj, n.*

diabetogenic (dī-à-bēt-ō-jen'-ik) *adj* 1 causing diabetes.* 2 applied to an anterior pituitary hormone.

Diapid™ lypressin.*

Diabinese™ chlorpropamide.*

diacetic acid (dī-à-sē'-tik) → acetoacetic acid.

diagnosis *n* art or act of distinguishing one disease from another. *differential diagnosis* making a correct decision between diseases presenting a similar clinical picture—**diagnoses** *pl,* **diagnose** *vt.*

diagnostic *adj* 1 pertaining to diagnosis. 2 serving as evidence in diagnosis— **diagnostician** *n*.

diaguanides (dī'-à-gwan-īds) *npl* → biguanides.

dialysate (dī-al'-i-sāt) *n* type of fluid used in dialysis.*

dialyser (dī'-à-lī-zėr) *n* (*syn* artificial kidney) contains two compartments, one for blood and one for dialysate; these are separated by a semipermeable membrane. → hemodialysis.

dialysis (dī-ål'-is-īs) *n* separation of substances in solution by taking advantage of their differing diffusability through a porous membrane as in the artificial kidney. → hemodialysis. *peritoneal dialysis* the peritoneum is used as the porous membrane in performing dialysis for removal of urea and other waste products into the irrigation fluid, which is then withdrawn from the abdominal cavity. Peritoneal dialysis can be used intermittently or continuously—**dialyses** *pl*, **dialyse** *vt*.

Diamox™ acetazolamide.*

diapedesis (dī-à-pe-dē'-sis) *n* passage of cells from within blood vessels through vessel walls into the tissues—**diapedetic** *adj*.

diaper rash an erythema of the diaper area. Usual causes are ammoniacal decomposition of urine, thrush, infantile psoriasis, allergy to detergents, or excoriation from diarrhea.

diaphoresis (dī-à-fōr-ē'-sis) *n* perspiration.

diaphoretic (dī-à-fōr-et'-ik) *adj, n* agent which induces diaphoresis (sweating). → sudorific.

diaphragm (dī'-à-fram) *n* 1 domeshaped muscular partition between the thorax above and the abdomen below. 2 any partitioning membrane or septum. 3 a rubber cap which encircles the cervix to act as a contraceptive. It should be used with a spermicidal jelly or cream—**diaphragmatic** *adj*.

diaphysis (dī-åf'-i-sis) *n* shaft of a long bone—**diaphyses** *pl*, **diaphyseal** *adj*.

diaplacental (dī-à-plà-sen'-tal) *adj* through the placenta.*

diarrhea (dī-à-rē'-à) *n* deviation from established bowel rhythm, with increase in frequency and fluidity of the stools. Epidemic diarrhea of the newborn is a highly contagious infection of maternity hospitals. → arthropathy spurious diarrhea.

diarthrosis (dī-àr-thrō'-sis) *n* a synovial, freely movable joint—**diarthroses** *pl*, **diarthrodial** *adj*.

diastase (dī'-as-tāz) *n* an amylase* produced by animal, plant and bacterial cells. *pancreatic diatase* excreted in urine (and saliva), thus estimation of urinary diastase may be used as test of pancreatic function.

diastasis (dī-as′-tas-is) *n* separation of bones without fracture; dislocation. *diastasis recti* separation of the rectus abdominus muscle, seen in pregnancy and the postpartum period.

diastole (dī-as′-to-lē) *n* relaxation period of the cardiac cycle, as opposed to systole*—**diastolic** *adj*.

diathermy (dī′-à-thér-mē) *n* passage of a high frequency electric current through tissues, so that heat is produced. When both electrodes are large, heat is diffused over a wide area, according to electrical resistance of the tissues. Widely used in treatment of inflammation, esp. when deeply seated (e.g., sinusitis, pelvic cellulitis). When one electrode is very small, heat is concentrated in this area and becomes great enough to destroy tissue (surgical diathermy); used to stop bleeding at operation by coagulation of blood, or to cut through tissue in operation for malignant disease.

diazepam (dī-az′-e-pam) *n* tranquilosedative with muscle-relaxant properties. Useful in intravenous infusion for status epilepticus and tetanus and as a premedicant. (Valium.)

diazoxide (dī-az-oks′-īd) *n* suppresses activity of insulin-producing beta cells, thus useful in hypoglycemia from pancreatic tumor. Main use as hypotensive agent by rapid intravenous injection in hypertensive emergencies. (Hyperstat.)

Dibenzyline™ phenoxybenzamine.*

dibucaine (dī′-bū-kān) *n* powerful local anesthetic used for surface anesthesia, infiltration and spinal anesthesia. Available as cream, ointment and suppositories. (Nupercainal.)

DIC *abbr* disseminated* intravascular coagulation.

dicephalous (dī-sef′-à-lus) *adj* two-headed.

dichloralphenazone (dī-klōr-al-fen′-à-zōn) *n* causes less gastric irritation than chloral* hydrate. Hypnotic of the chloral group. Particularly suitable for children. (Midrin.)

dichlorphenamide (dī-klōr-fen′-à-mīd) *n* oral diuretic of short duration. Carbonic anhydrase inhibitor. Used for systemic treatment of glaucoma. (Daranide.)

dicloxacillin (dī-cloks-à-sil′-lin) *n* a penicillin active against infections caused by penicillinase-producing staphylococci. (Dynapen.)

dicrotic (dī-krot′-ik) *adj, n* pertaining to, or having a double beat, as indicated by a second expansion of the artery during diastole. *dicrotic wave* second rise in the tracing of a dicrotic pulse.

dicyclomine (dī-sī′-klō-mēn) *n* antispasmodic resembling atropine,* but less potent. Used in pylorospasm and gastric hypermotility. (Bentyl.)

didanosine (di-dan'-ō-sin) *n* antiviral agent; inhibits viral replication by competing for sites in mechanism of reverse transcription. Used in treatment for HIV* infection. (Videx.)

Didrex™ benzphetamine.*

dienestrol (dī-en-es'-trol) *n* synthetic estrogen similar to stilbestrol,* but less active. (OrthoDienestrol.)

dietary fiber coarse food containing much indigestible vegetable fiber, composed mainly of cellulose. Its bulk helps to stimulate peristalsis and eliminate feces. Now thought to be useful in preventing diseases such as constipation, obesity, diabetes mellitus and bowel cancer. → bran.

dietetics (dī-e-tet'-iks) *n* interpretation and application of the scientific principles of nutrition to feeding in health and disease—**dietician** *n*.

diethylpropion (dī-eth-yl-prō'-pē-on) central nervous system stimulant used as appetite suppressant. (Tenuate.)

diethylstilbestrol (DES) (dī-eth-yl-stil-bes'-trol) *n* hormone preparation used to treat symptoms of the menopause, menstrual disorders, inflammation of female reproductive organs and cancer of breast and prostate. Was previously used to prevent miscarriage in pregnancy but no longer, as is thought to cause cancer of reproductive organs in the children born of these pregnancies.

Dietl's crisis (dēt'-lz) rare complication of "floating" kidney. Kinking of the ureter is thought to be responsible for the severe colic produced in the lumbar region.

diflunisal (dif-lūn'-is-al) *n* nonsteroidal, anti-inflammatory analgesic drug derived from salicylic* acid. (Dolobid.)

digestion *n* process by which food is rendered absorbable—**digestible, digestive** *adj*, **digestibility** *n*, **digest** *vt*.

digestive system → Figure 18.

digit *n* a finger or toe—**digital** *adj*.

digital compression pressure applied by the fingers, usually to an artery to stop bleeding.

digitalis (dij-it-al'-is) *n* leaf of the common foxglove. Powerful cardiac tonic, used in congestive heart failure and atrial fibrillation. Active principle of Australian foxglove, digoxin,* is now preferred, as action is more consistent and reliable.

digitalization (dij-it-al-īz-ā'-shun) *n* physiological saturation with digitalis* to obtain optimum therapeutic effect.

digitoxin (dij-it-oks'-in) *n* glycoside of digitalis.* (Purodigin.)

digoxin (dij-oks'-in) *n* glycoside of digitalis.* (Lanoxin.)

diguanides (dī'-gwan-īds) *npl* → biguanides.

dihydrocodeine (dī-hī-drō-kō′-dēn) *n* nonhabit-forming analgesic, useful for suppression of cough, respiratory infections and painful wounds. Can be given orally or by injection.

dihydroergotamine (dī-hī-drō-ér-got′-à-mēn) *n* derived from ergotamine,* used in migraine. (D.H.E. 45.)

dihydromorphinone (dī-hī-drō-mōr′-fin-ōn) *n* morphinelike analgesic of high potency but short action; little hypnotic effect. Occasionally used as a depressant in severe cough. Considered less habit-forming than morphine. (Dilaudid.)

dihydrotachysterol (dī-hī-drō-tak-is′-tér-ol) *n* prepared in oil; used to raise blood calcium, esp. in parathyroid tetany.

diiodotyrosine (dī-ī-ō-dō-tī′-rō-sēn) *n* organic iodine-containing precursor of thyroxine.*

Dilantin™ phenytoin* sodium.

dilatation (dī-là-tā′-shun) *n* stretching or enlargement. May occur physiologically, pathologically or be induced artificially. *dilatation and curettage* by custom refers to artificial stretching of the cervical os to procure scrapings of the uterine epithelium.

Dilaudid™ dihydromorphinone.*

dimenhydrinate (dī-men-hīd′-rin-āt) *n* powerful antiemetic for travel sickness and vertigo. (Dramamine.)

dimercaprol (BAL) (dī-mér-kap′-rol) *n* organic compound used as antidote for poisoning by arsenic and gold. Also useful in mercury poisoning if treatment is prompt, but is not suitable for lead poisoning. Forms soluble compounds with metals, which are then rapidly excreted.

Dimetane™ brompheniramine* maleate.

diodone (dī′-o-dōn) *n* organic iodine compound used as X-ray contrast agent in intravenous pyelography.

Diogenes syndrome (dī-oj′-en-ēz) gross self-neglect.

diopter (dī-op′-tér) *n* unit of measurement in refraction. A lens of one diopter has focal length of 1 meter.

diphenhydramine (dī-fen-hīd′-rà-mēn) *n* one of the first antihistamines.* Widely used in allergic conditions and travel sickness. Also has sedative action. (Benadryl.)

diphenoxylate (dī-fen-oks′-il-āt) *n* prescribed for acute and chronic diarrhea, and gastrointestinal upsets; has some morphinelike actions: (a) depresses the respiratory center, (b) acts as a cortical depressant, (c) reduces intestinal mobility. Atropine* is included (Lomotil) to provide dryness of mouth should patient take an overdose.

diphtheria (dif-thē′-rē-à) *n* acute, specific, infectious notifiable disease caused by *Corynebacterium diptheriae;* with a grey, adherent, false membrane growing on a mucous surface, usually that of the upper respiratory tract. Locally there is pain and swelling which may be suffocating. Systemically, toxins attack heart muscle and nerves—**diphtheritic** *adj*.

diphtheroid (dif'-thėr-oyd) *adj* any bacterium morphologically and culturally resembling *Corynebacterium diphtheriae.*

diplegia (dī-plē'-jä) *n* symmetrical paralysis of legs, usually associated with cerebral damage—**diplegic** *adj*.

diplococcus (dip-lō-kok'-us) *n* coccal bacterium characteristically occurring in pairs.

diploid (dip'-loyd) *adj* refers to chromosome complement of organisms, like man, in which each chromosome exists in duplicate form, one member of each pair being derived from mother, and one from the father. The two sets are united at fertilization. Humans have a diploid number of 46 chromosomes; 23 pairs.

diplopia (dip-lō'-pē-à) *n* seeing two objects where only one exists (double vision).

dipsomania (dip-sō-mā'-nē-à) *n* alcoholism* in which drinking occurs in bouts, often with long periods of sobriety between—**dipsomaniac** *adj, n*.

dipyridamole (dī-pī-rid'-à-mōl) *n* drug with antianginal and antihypertensive properties; also reduces blood platelet aggregation. (Persantine.)

Diquinol™ iodoquinol.*

disaccharide (dī-sak'-à-rīd) *n* a sugar (as lactose, maltose, sucrose) which yields two molecules of monosaccharide on hydrolysis.

Disalcid™ salsalate.*

disarticulation (dis-àr-tik-ū-lā'-shun) *n* amputation at a joint.

discission (di-sish'-un) *n* (*syn* needling) rupturing of lens capsule to allow absorption of lens substance in the condition of cataract.

disclosing tablet contains erythrosine*; used to identify dental* plaque.

discogenic (dis-kō-jen'-ik) *adj* arising in or produced by a disk, usually an intervertebral disk.

disease *n* deviation from or interruption of normal structure and function of any part of the body. Manifested by a characteristic set of signs and symptoms, and in most instances the etiology, pathology and prognosis is known.

disimpaction (dis-im-pak'-shun) *n* separation of broken ends of a bone that have been driven into each other during the impact which caused fracture. Traction may then be applied to maintain bone ends in good alignment and separate.

disinfectants *npl* term usually reserved for germicides which are too corrosive or toxic to be applied to tissues, but which are suitable for application to inanimate objects.

disinfection *n* removal or destruction of harmful microbes but not usually bacterial spores; commonly achieved with heat or chemicals.

Disipal™ orphenadrine.*

disk *n* intervertebral disk; one of the cartilaginous spacers between vertebrae,* uniting the spinal column and holding vertebrae in position. *slipped disk* → prolapse.

diskectomy (disk-ek'-to-mē) *n* surgical removal of a disk, usually an intervertebral disk.

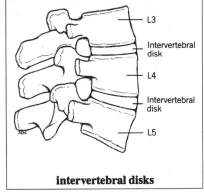

intervertebral disks

Labels: L3, Intervertebral disk, L4, Intervertebral disk, L5

diskography (dis-kog'-rȧ-fē) *n* x-ray of an intervertebral disk, after rendering radio-opaque.

dislocation *n* displacement of organs or articular surfaces, so that all apposition between them is lost. May be congenital, spontaneous, traumatic, or recurrent—**dislocated** *adj*, **dislocate** *vt*.

disobliteration *n* rebore. Removal of that which blocks a vessel, most often intimal plaques in an artery (called endarterectomy*).

disopyramide (dis-ō-pī'-rȧ-mīd) *n* drug with antiarrhythmic action similar to that of quinidine.*

dissection (dī-sek'-shun) *n* separation of tissues by cutting. *block dissection of glands* total excision of a group of lymph nodes; usually part of treatment for carcinoma.

disseminated (dis-em'-in-āt-ed) *adj* widely spread or scattered. *disseminated intravascular coagulation (DIC)* condition with overstimulation of body's clotting and anticlotting process in response to disease or injury. *disseminated sclerosis* → multiple sclerosis.

dissociation (dis-sō-shē-ā'-shun) *n* in psychiatry, abnormal mental process by which the mind achieves nonrecognition and isolation of certain unpalatable facts; involves actual splitting off from consciousness of all the unpalatable ideas so that the individual is no longer aware of them. Dissociation is a common symptom in hysteria but is seen in most exaggerated form in delusional psychoses.

distal (dis'-tȧl) *adj* farthest from the head or source.

distichiasis (dis-tik-ī′-as-is) *n* extra row of eyelashes at the inner lid border, which is turned inward against the eye.

disulfiram (dī-sulf′-ir-am) *n* sulfur compound that in the presence of alcohol causes nausea and vomiting. Hence used in treatment of alcoholism. (Antabuse.)

Diucardin™ hydroflumethiazide.*

Diulo™ metolazone.*

diuresis (dī-ū-rē′-sis) *n* increased secretion of urine; sometimes part of intensive therapy, esp. in poisoning (forced diuresis).

diuretics (dī-ū-ret′-iks) *npl* drugs which increase flow of urine. Those which enhance excretion of sodium and other ions, thereby increasing urinary output, are called *saluretic diuretics* and comprise the thiazide group of drugs. Those which act on the loop of Henle are called *loop diuretics;* they produce a rapid diuresis, onset of action being 5–10 min when given parenterally or 20–30 min if given orally; duration of action is 4–6 h.

Diuril™ chlorothiazide.*

divers' paralysis caisson* disease.

diverticulitis (dī-ver-tik-ū-lī′-tis) *n* inflammation of a diverticulum.*

diverticulosis (dī-vėr-tik-ū-lō′-sis) *n* condition with many diverticula, esp. in the intestines.

diverticulum (dī-vėr-tik′-ū-lum) *n* a pouch or sac protruding from the wall of a tube or hollow organ. May be congenital or acquired. *Meckel's diverticulum* occurs in distal ileum, causing cramps and vomiting; corrected by surgery. *Zenker's diverticulum* pouching of the esophagus through cricopharyngeal muscle; patient may regurgitate food on bending or lying down—**diverticula** *pl*.

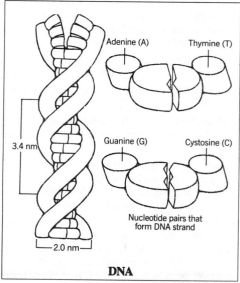

Adenine (A) Thymine (T)

Guanine (G) Cystosine (C)

3.4 nm

Nucleotide pairs that form DNA strand

2.0 nm

DNA

DNA *abbr* deoxyribonucleic* acid. *DNA probe* blood from a finger prick is applied to a radioactively labelled probe; malarial DNA combines with human DNA causing a dark spot to appear on X-ray film, diagnostic of malaria.

DOA *abbr* dead on arrival.

dobutamine (dō-bū'-tȧ-mēn) *n* directly acting stimulant of heart muscle which augments myocardial contractility in severe cardiac failure and shock syndrome, e.g., after myocardial infarction. (Dobutrex.)

Dobutrex™ dobutamine.*

DOCA *abbr* → deoxycorticosterone acetate.

docusate (dok'-ū-sāt) *n* stool softener helpful in prevention of fecal impaction.

Döderlein's bacillus (dod'-er-līnz) nonpathogenic Gram-positive rod which normally lives in the vagina and by its action provides an acid medium.

Dolobid™ diflunisal.*

Dolophine™ methadone.*

dolor (dō'-lor) *n* pain; esp. in the context of the four classical signs of inflammation—the others being calor,* rubor,* tumor.*

dominant *adj* describes a character possessed by one parent which, in the offspring, overrides the corresponding alternative character derived from the other parent. The words, and concepts, of dominance and recessivity are now often extended to the genes themselves that control the respective characters; → recessive *opp.*

dominant hemisphere on opposite side of the brain to that of the preferred hand. Dominant hemisphere for language is the left in 90% of right-handed and 30% of left-handed people.

Donnatal™ phenobarbital.*

Donovan bodies (don'-ō-van) Leishman-Donovan* bodies.

dopa (dō-pȧ) *n* dihydroxyphenylalanine, an important compound formed in the intermediate stage in synthesis of catecholamines* from tyrosine.*

dopamine (dōp'-ȧ-mēn) *n* a catecholamine neurotransmitter, closely related to adrenalin* and noradrenalin.* Increases cardiac output and renal blood flow but does not produce peripheral vasoconstriction. Most valuable in hypotension and shock of cardiac origin. Normally present in high concentration in those regions of the brain which are selectively damaged in parkinsonism.

Dopram™ doxapram.*

Doriglute™ glutethimide.*

dorsal (dōr'-sȧl) *adj* pertaining to the back, or to posterior part of an organ. *dorsal position* lying on the back with head supported on a pillow.

dorsiflexion (dōr-si-flek'-shun) *n* bending backwards. In the case of the great toe, upwards (Babinski's* reflex).

dorsocentral (dōr-sō-sen'-tråi) *adj* at the back and in the center.

dorsolumbar (dōr-sō-lum'-bår) *adj* pertaining to lumbar region of the back.

dosimeter (dō-sim'-e-tėr) *n* instrument worn by personnel or placed within equipment to measure incident X-rays or gamma rays. Commonly a small photographic film in a special filter holder.

double vision → diplopia.

douche (doosh) *n* stream of fluid directed against the body externally or into a body cavity.

Down syndrome (*syn* mongolism) congenital condition, with generally severe mental subnormality and facial features vaguely resembling the Mongoloid races; stigma include oval tilted eyes, squint and a flattened occiput. Chromosome abnormality is of two types: (a) primary trisomy, caused by abnormal division of chromosome 21 (atmeiosis). resulting in an extra chromosome instead of the normal pair. The infant has 47 chromosomes and is often born of an elderly mother. (b) Structural abnormality involving chromosome 21, with a total of 46 chromosomes, one of which has an abnormal structure as result of a specific translocation. Such infants are usually born of younger mothers; higher risk of recurrence in subsequent pregnancies.

doxapram (doks'-å-pram) *n* stimulant of the vital medullary centers, useful in barbiturate poisoning.

doxepin (doks'-e-pin) *n* a tricyclic antidepressant.* Effective after 3–15 days medication. (Sinequan.)

doxorubicin (doks-ō-roo'-bi-sin) *n* cytotoxic antibiotic particularly effective in childhood malignancies. Similar to daunorubicin* but less cardiotoxic. (Adriamycin.)

doxycycline (doks-i-sī'-klin) *n* rapidly absorbed, slowly excreted tetracycline.* (Vibramycin.)

doxylamine (doks-il'-å-mēn) *n* antihistamine useful in treatment of allergies.

DP *abbr* Depo-Provera → medroxyprogesterone acetate.

DPT *abbr* combination immunization providing immunity against diphtheria, pertussis, and tetanus.

dracontiasis (drak-on-tī'-å-sis) *n* infestation with *Dracunculus* * *medinensis* common in India and Africa.

Dracunculus medinensis (drak-un'-kū-lus med-in-en'-sis) (*syn* Guinea worm), nematode parasite which infests man from contaminated drinking water. From the intestine the adult female migrates to skin surface to deposit larvae, producing a cordlike thickening which ulcerates.

Dramamine™ dimenhydrinate.*

drip *n* → intravenous.

drop attacks periodic falling because of sudden loss of postural control of the lower limbs, without vertigo or loss of consciousness. Usually followed by sudden return of normal muscle tone. → vertebrobasilar insufficiency.

droperidol (drō-pėr'-i-dol) *n* neuroleptic agent. Can be used as pre-operative medication. Induces a state of mental detachment without loss of consciousness or effect upon respiratory system. (Inapsine.)

dropsy *n* → edema—**dropsical** *adj*.

dry eye syndrome → Sjögren's syndrome.

Dubowitz score (dū'-bō-wits) assesses gestational age.

Duchenne muscular dystrophy (dū-shen') x-linked recessive disorder affecting only boys. Usually begins to show between 3 and 5 years, with progressive muscle weakness and loss of locomotor skills. Death usually occurs during the teens or early twenties from respiratory or cardiac failure.

Ducrey's bacillus (dū-krāz') *Haemophilus* * *ducreyi*.

duct *n* a tube or duct for carrying away secretions from a gland.

ductless glands endocrine* glands.

ductus arteriosus (duk'-tus ȧr-tēr-ē-ō'-sus) blood vessel connecting left pulmonary artery to the aorta, to bypass the lungs in the fetal circulation. At birth the duct closes, but if it remains open, it is called *persistent ductus arteriosus,* a congenital heart defect.

Duke's test the skin is pricked and blood continuously removed with absorbent paper until it ceases to flow; normal bleeding time is 3–5 min.

Dulcolax™ bisacodyl.*

"dumping syndrome" symptoms which sometimes follow partial gastrectomy: epigastric fullness and feeling of faintness and sweating after meals.

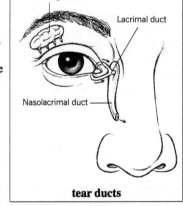

Lacrimal gland

Lacrimal duct

Nasolacrimal duct

tear ducts

duodenal ulcer ulcer* in the duodenal lining, caused by action of acid and pepsin. Pain occurs several hours after meals, but is relieved by food. The ulcer can bleed, leading to occult blood in stools, or it can perforate, constituting an abdominal emergency. Severe scarring following chronic ulceration may produce pyloric stenosis. Cimetidine* is drug of choice for uncomplicated duodenal ulcers.

duodenitis (dū-ō-den-ī'-tis) *n* inflammation of the duodenum.

duodenojejunal (dū-ō-dēn-ō-je-joo′-nàl) *adj* pertaining to duodenum and jejunum.

duodenopancreatectomy (dū-ō-dē′-nō-pan-krē-a-tek′-to-mē) *n* surgical excision of the duodenum and part of the pancreas, carried out in cases of cancer arising in the region of the head of the pancreas.

duodenoscope (dū-ō-dē′-nō-skōp) *n* a side-viewing flexible fiberoptic endoscope*—**duodenoscopic** *adj*, **duodenoscopy** *n*.

duodenostomy (dū-ō-dē-nos′-to-mē) *n* surgically made fistula between the duodenum and another cavity, e.g., cholecystoduodenostomy, a fistula between gallbladder and duodenum made to relieve jaundice in inoperable cancer of the head of the pancreas.

duodenum (dū-ō-dē′-num, dū-od′-e-num) *n* fixed, curved, first portion of the small intestine, connecting the stomach* above to the jejunum* below (→ Figure 18)—**duodenal** *adj*.

Dupuytren's contracture (dū′-pwi-trens) painless, chronic flexion of the digits of the hand, esp. the third and fourth, towards the palm. Etiology is uncertain but some cases are associated with hepatic cirrhosis.

Durabolin™ nandrolone* phenylpropionate.

dura mater (dū′-rà-mà′-ter) outer fibrous membrane of the meninges which surround the brain and spinal cord.

Duvoid™ bethanechol.*

dwarf *n* person of stunted growth. May be due to growth hormone deficiency. Also occurs in untreated congenital hypothyroidism (cretinism*) and juvenile hypothyroidism, achondroplasia and other conditions—**dwarfism** *n*.

Dyazide™ triamterene* and hydrochlorothiazide.*

dyflos (DFP) (dī′-flōs) *n* fluorine derivative with action similar to that of eserine and neostigmine.* Used mostly as 0.1% solution in oil for glaucoma, when a very long action is required. An organophosphorous compound, it is an insecticide in agriculture, with powerful and irreversible anticholinesterase action; potentially dangerous to man. (Floropryl.)

Dymelor™ acetohexamide.*

dynamometer (dī-nà-mom′-e-tèr) *n* apparatus to test strength of grip.

Dynapen™ cloxacillin.*

Dyrenium™ triamterine.*

dysarthria (dis-àrth′-rē-à) *n* neuromuscular disorder affecting the actual formation and articulation of words, and therefore the listener's understanding of such speech to varying degrees. Linguistic ability remains unimpaired. Generally, such speech is slow and monotonous with indistinct consonants and long intervals between words—**dysarthric** *adj*.

dyscalculia (dis-kal-kū'-lē-à) *n* impairment of ability to use numbers.

dyschezia (dis-kē'-zhà) *n* difficult or painful defecation.

dyschondroplasia (dis-kon-drō-plāz'-ē-à) *n* disorder of bone growth resulting in normal trunk, short arms and legs.

dyscoria (dis-kōr'-ē-à) *n* abnormality of the pupil of the eye.

dyscrasia (dis-krā'-zhà) *n* any abnormal condition of the body, esp. of blood.

dysentery (dis'-en-tèr-ē) *n* inflammation of the bowel with evacuation of blood and mucus, accompanied by tenesmus and colic. *amoebic dysentery* is caused by the protozoon *Entamoeba histolytica* → amoebiasis. *bacillary dysentery* is caused by *Shigella shigae, S. Flexneri* or *S. sonnei*. Disease results from poor sanitation; the housefly carries infection from feces to food—**dysenteric** *adj.*

dysesthesia (dis-es-thēz'-ē-à) *n* impairment of touch sensation.

dysfunction (dis-fungk'-shun) *n* abnormal functioning of any organ or part.

dysfunctional uterine bleeding any unusual uterine bleeding without organic uterine cause.

dysgammaglobulinemia (dis-gam'-mà-glob'-ū-lin-ē'-mē-à) *n* (*syn* antibody deficiency syndrome) disturbance of gammaglobulin production. Can be transient, congenital or acquired. Transient form occurs in neonates as mother-donated IgG level falls, leading to hypogammaglobulinemia with repeated respiratory infections. Injections of gammaglobulin are given until normal blood levels occur. Congenital agammaglobulinemia is a sex-linked recessive genetic variety and the commonest type of total deficiency, with abnormal lymph nodes and spleen. Males are solely affected, females being carriers of the abnormal gene. Disease usually presents in second or third year as severe, recurrent bacterial infections with high fever. Acquired agammaglobulinemia occurs at any age and in either sex. Cause unknown. Secondary agammaglobulinemia may occur in lymphoma, leukemia and myeloma, esp. after chemotherapy or radiation. Also found in bullous skin disorders such as pemphigus and eczema, and after burns, due to excessive loss of protein in exuded fluid.

dysgenesis (dis-jen'-e-sis) *n* malformation during embryonic development—**dysgenetic** *adj.*

dysgerminoma (dis-jèr-min-ō'-mà) *n* tumor of the ovary of low-grade malignancy. Not hormone secreting, as it develops from cells which date back to the undifferentiated state of gonadal development, i.e., before the cells have either male or female attributes.

dyshidrosis (dis-hīd-rō'-sis) *n* vesicular skin eruption, formerly thought to be caused by blockage of sweat ducts at their orifice; histologically an eczematous process.

dyskaryosis (dis-kār-ē-ōs'-is) *n* first stage of abnormality in a cervical smear. Follow-up tests may revert to normal, but some may become positive and demand biopsy.

dyskinesia (dis-kin-ēz'-ē-à) *n* impairment of voluntary movement. *tardive dyskinesia* uncontrollable movements often of the face and mouth which are a side-effect of antipsychotic medication—**dyskinetic** *adj*.

dyslalia (dis-lā'-lē-à) *n* difficulty in talking due to defect of speech organs. Immature articulation—**dyslalic** *adj*.

dyslexia (dis-leks'-ē-à) *n* condition affecting ability to read, write and spell in persons not lacking intelligence for such abilities. Can be acquired by brain injury or by early sensory/neural disorders which prevent consistency of sensory input at the "ab initio" stage of learning—**dyslexic** *adj*.

dysmelia (dis-mēl'-ē-à) *n* limb deficiency.

dysmenorrhea (dis-men-ōr-ē'-à) *n* painful menstruation. *spasmodic dysmenorrhea* during first day of a period, often within an hour or two of the start of bleeding; with spasms of acute colicky pain in lower abdomen, and sometimes in the back and inner part of the thighs. Spasms may be sharp enough to cause fainting and vomiting. *congestive dysmenorrhea* dull aching pain in lower abdomen beginning several days in advance of period, with increasing heaviness, perhaps constipation, nausea and lack of appetite. There may also be breast tenderness, headache and backache. Fluid retention at this time leads to typical edema and weight gain, ameliorated by diuretics.

dysmorphogenic (dis-mōr-fō-jen'-ik) *adj* now preferred to teratogenic when applied to drugs taken during pregnancy. → teratogen.

dysopia (dis-ō'-pē-à) *n* painful or defective vision.

dysorexia (dis-ōr-eks'-ē-à) *n* abnormal or unnatural appetite.

dyspareunia (dis-pār-ū'-nē-à) *n* painful or difficult coitus, experienced by the woman.

dyspepsia (dis-pep'-sē-à) *n* indigestion—**dyspeptic** *adj*.

dysphagia (dis-fā'-jà) *n* difficulty in swallowing—**dysphagic** *adj*.

dysphasia (dis-fā'-zhà) *n* disorder in which mental processes of language formulation and understanding are affected but not the physical production of speech. *expressive dysphasia* disturbance of the memory of motor speech pattern, resulting in difficulty in communicating thoughts even though comprehension is intact. Such speech is characterized by hesitancy, slowness and lack of grammar. Articulation and pronunciation are sometimes poor, thus may lead to an associated dysarthria.*

dysplasia (dis-plā'-zhà) *n* formation of abnormal tissue—**dysplastic** *adj*.

dyspnea (disp'-nē-à) *n* difficulty in, or labored, breathing; can be mainly of an inspiratory or expiratory nature—**dyspneic** *adj*.

dyspraxia (dis-prak'-sē-à) *n* lack of voluntary control over muscles, esp. the orofacial ones—**dyspraxic** *adj*.

dysrhythmia (dis-rith'-mē-à) *n* disordered rhythm, usually of heart, e.g., atrial fibrillation*—**dysrhythmic** *adj*.

dystaxia (dis-taks'-ē-à) *n* difficulty in controlling voluntary movements—**dystaxic** *adj*.

dystocia (dis-tōs'-ē-à) *n* difficult or slow labor.

dystrophy (dis'-tro-fē) *n* defective nutrition of an organ or tissue, usually muscle; applied to several unrelated conditions. → muscular dystrophy, Duchenne muscular dystrophy.

dysuria (dis-ūr'-ē-à) *n* painful micturition*—**dysuric** *adj*.

E

eardrum *n* → Figure 13.

Eaton agent (ē′-ton) *Mycoplasma* pneumoniae.*

Eaton-Lambert syndrome condition resembling myasthenia* gravis and due to IgG activity (→ immunoglobulins); often associated with presence of cancer.

EBV *abbr* Epstein* Barr virus.

Ebola (ē-bōl′-a) *n* a viral* hemorrhagic fever, usually transmitted by ticks.

ecbolic (ek-bol′-ik) *adj* describes any agent which stimulates contraction of the gravid uterus and hastens expulsion of its contents.

ECC *abbr* external cardiac compressions.

ecchondroma (ek-kon-drō′-mà) *n* benign tumor composed of cartilage that protrudes from the surface of the bone in which it arises—**ecchondromata** *pl.*

ecchymosis (ek-i-mō′-sis) *n* an extravasation of blood under the skin. → bruise—**ecchymoses** *pl.*

eccrine (ek′-rin) *adj* of ordinary, watery sweat; as compared to that of apocrine* glands, which contains substances produced within cells.

ECG *abbr* electrocardiogram,* → electrocardiograph. Also electrocorticography.*

Echinococcus (ek-īn′-ō-kok′-us) *n* genus of tapeworms; adults infect a primary host, e.g., a dog. In man (secondary host) encysted larvae cause "hydatid* disease."

echocardiography (ek-ō-kàr-dē-og′-raf-ē) *n* use of ultrasound as a diagnostic tool for studying structure and motion of the heart.

echoencephalography (ek-ō-en-sef-àl-og′-raf-ē) *n* passage of ultrasound waves across the head. Can detect abscess, blood clot, injury or tumor within brain.

echolalia (ek-ō-lā′-lē-à) *n* repetition, almost automatically, of words or phrases heard. Occurs most commonly in schizophrenia and dementia; sometimes in toxic delirious states. A characteristic of all infants' speech—**echolalic** *adj.*

echophony (ek′-ō-fō′-nē) *n* echo of a vocal sound heard during auscultation of the chest.

echopraxia (ek-ō-praks′-ē-à) *n* involuntary mimicking of another's movements.

echoviruses (ek'-ō-vī'-rus-es) *npl* "Enteric Cytopathic Human Orphan": group of viruses originally found in stools of diseaseless children. Echoviruses have caused meningitis and mild respiratory infection in children. At least 30 types identified.

eclampsia (e-klamp'-sē-à) *n* 1 severe manifestation of toxemia of pregnancy, associated with fits and coma. 2 a sudden convulsive attack—**eclamptic** *adj*.

ecmnesia (ek-nē'-zhà) *n* impaired memory for recent events with normal memory of remote ones. Common in old age and in early cerebral deterioration.

ecraseur (ā-krā-zūr') *n* instrument with a wire loop that can be tightened round the pedicle of a new growth to sever it.

ECT *abbr* → electroconvulsive therapy.

ecthyma (ek-thī'-mà) *n* crusted eruption of impetigo* contagiosa on the legs, producing necrosis of the skin, which heals with scarring. Similar condition occurs in syphilis.

ectoderm (ek'-tō-dèrm) *n* external primitive germ layer of the embryo. From it develop skin structures, nervous system, organs of special sense, pineal gland and part of the pituitary and adrenal glands—**ectodermal** *adj*.

ectodermosis (ek-tō-dèrm-ō'-sis) *n* disease of any organ or tissue derived from the ectoderm.

ectogenesis (ek-tō-jen'-e-sis) *n* growth of the embryo outside the uterus (in* vitro fertilization).

ectoparasite (ek-tō-pār'-a-sīt) *n* parasite that lives on exterior surface of its host—**ectoparasitic** *adj*.

ectopia (ek-tō'-pē-à) *n* malposition of an organ or structure, usually congenital. *ectopia vesicae* abnormally placed urinary bladder which protrudes through or opens on to the abdominal wall—**ectopic** *adj*.

ectopic beat (ek-top'-ik) → extrasystole.

ectopic pregnancy (ek-top'-ik) (*syn* tubal pregnancy) extrauterine gestation, the fallopian tube being most common site. At about the 6th week the tube ruptures, constituting a "surgical emergency."

ectozoa (ek-tō-zō'-à) *n* external parasites.

ectrodactyly (ek-trō-dak'-til-ē) *n* congenital absence of one or more fingers or toes or parts of them.

ectropion (ek-trō'-pē-on) *n* an eversion or turnover outward, esp. of the lower eyelid or of the pupil margin—*ectropion uveae*.

eczema (ek'-ze-mà) *n* skin reaction begining with erythema, then vesicles appear. These rupture, forming crusts or leaving pits which ooze serum—the exudative or weeping stage. In healing, the area becomes scaly. Some authorities limit the word "eczema" to the cases with internal (endogenous) causes while those caused by external (exogenous) contact factors are called dermatitis or eczematous dermatitis. → dermatitis—**eczematous** *adj*.

Edecrin™ ethacrinic* acid.

edema (e-dē'-mà) *n* abnormal infiltration of tissues with fluid. Many causes; may arise in the blood, or disease of cardiopulmonary system, urinary system or liver. → anasarca, angioneurotic edema, ascites—**edematous** *adj*.

edentulous (ē-dent'-ū-lus) *adj* without natural teeth.

edrophonium test (ed-rō-fō'-nē-um) in patients with myasthenia* gravis, a small intramuscular dose of edrophonium chloride immediately relieves symptoms, albeit temporarily, while quinine sulfate increases muscular weakness.

EDTA *abbr* ethylenediaminetetraacetic acid, a chelating agent, the calcium and sodium salts of which have been used to remove harmful metal ions from the body, e.g., lead, excess calcium and radioactive heavy metals. The stable chelate compounds are excreted in urine.

Edward syndrome an autosomal trisomy* associated with mental subnormality; cells have 47 chromosomes. Sometimes called trisomy E.

EEG *abbr* electroencephalogram,* → electroencephalograph.

EENT *abbr* eye, ear, nose and throat.

EFAs *abbr* → essential fatty acids.

effector *n* motor or secretory nerve ending in a muscle, gland or organ.

efferent (ef'-fėr-ent) *adj* carrying, conveying, conducting away from a center. → afferent *opp*.

effort syndrome form of anxiety neurosis, manifesting in a variety of cardiac symptoms, including precordial pain, for which no pathological explanation can be discovered.

effusion *n* extravasation of fluid into body tissues or cavities.

ejaculation (ē-jak-ū-lā'-shun) *n* sudden emission of semen from the erect penis at the moment of male orgasm.

ejaculatory duct → Figure 16.

EKG *abbr* electrocardiogram.*

Elavil™ amitriptyline.*

electrocardiogram (ECG, EKG) (ē-lek-trō-kàr'-dē-ō-gram) *n* recording of electrical activity of the heart on a moving paper strip, made by an electrocardiograph.*

electrocardiograph (ē-lek-tro-kàr'-dē-ō-graf) *n* instrument that records electrical activity of the heart from electrodes on limbs and chest—**electrocardiographic** *adj*, **electrocardiography** *n*.

electrocoagulation (ē-lek-trō-kō-ag-ū-lā'-shun) *n* technique of surgical diathermy.* Coagulation, esp. of bleeding points, by means of electrodes.

electrocochleography (ECoG) (ē-lek-trō-kō-klē-og'-raf-ē) *n* direct recording of the action potential generated following stimulation of cochlear nerve.

electroconvulsive therapy (ECT) (ē-lek-trō-kon-vul'-siv) a treatment still employed in depression, using an apparatus that delivers a definite voltage for a precise fraction of a second to electrodes placed on the head, producing a convulsion. *modified ECT* convulsive effects attenuated with an intravenous anesthetic and a muscle relaxant, thus reducing risk of unpleasant sequelae. ECT is currently invariably modified. *unilateral ECT* avoids the sequela of amnesia for recent events through application of ECT to right hemisphere only.

electrocorticography (ē-lek-trō-kor-ti-kog'-raf-ē) *n* direct recording from the cerebral cortex during operation—**electrocorticographic** *adj*, **electrocorticogram** *n*, **electrocorticograph** *n*.

electrodesiccation (ē-lek-trō-des-i-kā'-shun) *n* a technique of surgical diathermy,* with drying and subsequent removal of tissue, e.g., papillomata.

electrodiagnosis (ē-lek'-trō-dī-ag-nō'-sis) *n* use of graphic recording of electrical irritability of tissues in diagnosis—**electrodiagnostic** *adj*.

electroencephalogram (EEG) (ē-lek'-trō-en-sef'-al-ō-gram) *n* recording of electrical activity of the brain on a moving paper strip, made by electroencephalograph.*

electroencephalograph (ē-lek'-trō-en-sef'-al-ō-graf) *n* instrument by which electrical impulses derived from the brain are amplified and recorded on paper—**electroencephalographic** *adj*.

electrolysis (ē-lek-trol'-is-is) *n* **1** chemical decomposition by electricity. **2** term for destruction of individual hairs (epilation), eradication of moles, spider nevi, etc., using electricity.

electrolyte (ē-lek'-trō-līt) *n* liquid or solution of a substance which is capable of conducting electricity because it dissociates into ions. In medical usage refers to the ion itself, for example sodium, chloride and potassium ions in serum. Various diseases can cause serum electrolyte imbalance; deficiencies can be remedied orally or by intravenous drip; excesses can be removed by dialysis or by resins, taken by mouth or given by enema—**electrolytic** *adj*.

electromyography (ē-lek-trō-mī-og'-raf-ē) *n* use of an instrument which records electric currents generated in active muscle—**electromyographical** *adj*, **electromyogram** *n*, **electromyograph** *n*.

electro–oculography (ē-lek-trō–ok-ū-log'-raf-ē) *n* use of an instrument which records eye position and movement, and potential difference between front and back of the eyeball using electrodes placed on skin near socket. Can be used as an electrodiagnostic test—**electro-oculographical** *adj*, **electro-oculogram** *n*, **electro-oculograph** *n*.

electroretinogram (ERG) (ē-lek-trō-ret′-in-ō-gram) *n* graphic record of electrical currents generated in active retina.

electrosection *n* technique of surgical diathermy for cutting skin or parting soft tissues.

electroshock therapy electroconvulsive* therapy.

elephantiasis (el-ef-an-tī′-a-sis) *n* swelling of a limb, usually a leg, as result of lymphatic obstruction (lymphedema), followed by thickening of skin (pachydermia) and subcutaneous tissues. A complication of filariasis in tropical countries, or may be a result of syphilis or recurring streptococcal infection (elephantiasis nostras).

elimination *n* passage of waste from the body, usually reserved for urine and feces—**eliminate** *vt*.

ELISA *abbr* → enzyme-linked immunosorbent assay.

elixir *n* sweetened, aromatic solution of a drug, often containing an appreciable amount of alcohol. Elixirs differ from syrups in containing very little sugar and in requiring dilution before use.

elliptocytosis (ē-lip-tō-sī-tō′-sis) *n* anemia in which red blood cells are oval.

emasculation (ē-mas-kū-lā′-shun) *n* castration.*

embolectomy (em-bol-ek′-to-mē) *n* surgical removal of an embolus.* Usually a fine balloon catheter is used to extract the embolus.

embolism (em′-bol-izm) *n* condition with obstruction of a blood vessel by the impaction of a solid body (e.g., thrombi, fat globules, tumor cells) or an air bubble. → therapeutic embolization—**embolic** *adj*.

embologenic (em-bol-ō-jen′-ik) *adj* capable of producing an embolus.*

embolus (em′-bol-us) *n* solid body or air bubble transported in the circulation. → embolism—**emboli** *pl*.

embrocation (em-brō-kā′-shun) *n* liquid which is applied topically by rubbing.

embryo (em′-brē-ō) *n* the developing ovum during early months of gestation—**embryonic** *adj*.

embryology (em-brē-ol′-o-jē) *n* study of the development of an organism from fertilization to extrauterine life—**embryological** *adj*.

embryoma (em-brē-ōm′-à) *n* teratoma.*

embryopathy (em-brē-op′-à-thē) *n* disease or abnormality in the embryo. Includes "rubella* syndrome"—**embryopathic** *adj*.

embryotomy (em-brē-ot′-o-mē) *n* mutilation of the fetus to facilitate removal from womb, when natural birth is impossible.

emesis (em′-is-is) *n* vomiting.

emetic (ē-met′-ik) *n* any agent used to produce vomiting.

emetine (em′-i-tēn) *n* principal alkaloid of ipecacuanha.* Used in amoebic dysentery, often in association with other amoebicides.

emmetropia (em-met-rō′-pē-à) *n* normal or perfect vision—**emmetropic** *adj*.

emollient (ē-mol′-ē-ent) *adj, n* agent which softens and soothes skin or mucous membrane.

emphysema (em-fis-ēm′-à) *n* gaseous distension of the tissues. → crepitation, pulmonary, surgical emphysema—**emphysematous** *adj*.

empyema (em-pī-ēm′-à) *n* collection of pus in a cavity, hollow organ or space.

EMT *abbr* emergency medical technician.

emulsion *n* uniform suspension of fat or oil particles in an aqueous continuous phase (*O/W emulsion*) or aqueous droplets in an oily continuous phase (*W/O emulsion*).

enamel *n* hard, acellular external covering of the crown of a tooth.

encephalitis (en-sef-àl-ī′-tis) *n* inflammation of the brain.

encephalocele (en-sef-al′-ō-sēl) *n* protrusion of brain substance through the skull. Often associated with hydrocephalus when the protrusion occurs at a suture line.

encephalography (en-sef-àl-og′-ra-fē) *n* technique to examine the brain, to produce a printed or visible record of the investigation. → echoencephalography, electroencephalography, pneumoencephalography—**encephalogram** *n*.

encephaloma (en-sef-àl-ō′-mà) *n* tumor of the brain—**encephalomata** *pl*.

encephalomalacia (en-sef-àl-ō-mà-lā′-shà) *n* softening of the brain.

encephalomyelitis (en-sef-à-lō-mī-el-ī′-tis) *n* inflammation of brain and spinal cord.

encephalomyelopathy *n* disease affecting both brain and spinal cord—**encephalomyelopathic** *adj*.

encephalon (en-sef′-à-lon) *n* the brain.

encephalopathy (en-sef-à-lop′-à-thē) *n* any disease of the brain—**encephalo**pathic *adj*.

enchondroma (en-kon-drō′-mà) *n* a cartilaginous tumor—**enchondromata** *pl*.

encopresis (en-kō-prē′-sis) *n* involuntary passage of feces; usually reserved for fecal incontinence associated with mental illness—**encopretic** *adj, n*.

endarterectomy (end-àr-tèr-ek′-to-mē) *n* surgical removal of an atheromatous core from an artery, sometimes called disobliteration or "rebore." Carbon dioxide gas can be used to separate the occlusive core.

endarteritis (end-àr-tèr-īt′-is) *n* inflammation of the intima or inner lining coat of an artery. *endarteritis obliterans* intimal connective tissue fills the lumen.

endaural (end-ōr'-ål) *adj* pertaining to inner portion of the external auditory canal.

endemic (en-dem'-ik) *adj* recurring in an area. → epidemic.

endemiology (en-dē-mē-ol'-o-jē) *n* study of endemic diseases.

Endep™ amitriptyline.

endocardial mapping (en-dō-kår'-dē-al) recording of electrical potentials from various sites on the endocardium to determine origin of cardiac arrhythmia.

endocardial resection surgical removal of that part of the endocardium causing cardiac arrhythmia.

endocarditis (en-dō-kår-dī'-tis) *n* inflammation of the inner lining of the heart (endocardium*) due to infection by microorganisms (bacteria, fungi or *Rickettsia*), or to rheumatic fever. There may be temporary or permanent damage to the heart valves.

endocardium (en-dō-kår'-dē-um) *n* lining membrane of the heart, which covers the valves.

endocervical (en-dō-sėr'-vi-kål) *adj* pertaining to the inside of the cervix uteri.

endocervicitis (en-dō-sėr-vi-sī'-tis) *n* inflammation of the mucous membrane lining the cervix uteri.

endocrine (en'-dō-krin) *adj* secreting internally → exocrine

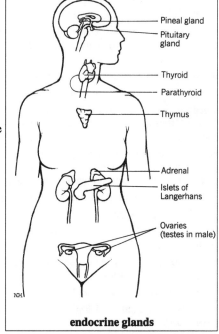

endocrine glands

opp. **endocrine glands** the ductless glands of the body; those which make an internal secretion or hormone which passes into the blood stream and influences general metabolic processes: e.g., the pineal, pituitary, thyroid, parathyroids, adrenals, ovaries, testes and pancreas—**endocrinal** *adj*.

endocrinology (en'-dō-krin-ol'-o-jē) *n* study of the ductless glands and their internal secretions.

endocrinopathy (en-dō-krin-op'-a-thē) *n* abnormality of one or more of the endocrine glands or their secretions.

endoderm (en'-dō-dėrm) *n* inner layer of cells which form during early development of the embryo—**endodermal** *adj*.

endogenous (en-do'-jen-us) *adj* originating within the organism. → ectogenous, exogenous *opp*.

endolymph (en'-dō-limf) *n* fluid contained in the membranous labyrinth of the internal ear.

endolymphatic shunt (en-dō-limf-at'-ik) drainage of excess endolymph* from vestibular labyrinth to the subarachnoid space, where it flows to join cerebrospinal fluid. Performed for Meniere's disease.

endolysin (en-dō-lī'-sin) *n* intracellular, leukocytic substance which destroys engulfed bacteria.

endometrioma (en-dō-mēt-rē-ō'-mȧ) *n* a tumor of misplaced endometrium. → chocolate cyst—**endometriomata** *pl*.

endometriosis (en-dō-mēt-rē-ō'-sis) *n* presence of endometrium in abnormal sites. → chocolate cyst.

endometritis (en-dō-mēt-rī'-tis) *n* inflammation of the endometrium.*

endometrium (en-dō-mēt'-rē-um) *n* lining mucosa of the uterus—**endometrial** *adj*.

endomyocardium (en-dō-mī-ō-kȧr'-dē-um) *n* relating to endocardium and myocardium—**endomyocardial** *adj*.

endoneurium (en-dō-nū'-rē-um) *n* delicate, inner connective tissue surrounding nerve fibers.

endoparasite (en-dō-pȧr'-ȧ-sīt) *n* any parasite living within its host—**endoparasitic** *adj*.

endophlebitis (en-dō-flē-bī'-tis) *n* inflammation of internal lining of vein. Can occur after prolonged intravenous infusion.

endophthalmitis (en-dof'-thal-mī'-tis) *n* internal infection of the eye, usually bacterial.

endorphins (en-dōr'-fins) *npl* group of neuropeptides elaborated by the pituitary gland; involved in both central and peripheral nervous functions and possess analgesic effect. They originate from a multifunctional prohormone that is the common precursor of adrenocorticotropic hormone and melanocyte-stimulating hormones. → encephalins.

endoscope (en'-dō-skōp) *n* instrument for visualization of body cavities or organs. May be of the tubular metal sort, or of the fiberoptic variety, smaller and more flexible. Permits examination, photography and biopsy of cavities or organs of a relaxed conscious person—**endoscopic** *adj*, **endoscopy** *n*.

endoscopic retrograde cholangiopancreatography (ERCP) (kōl-an'-jē-ō-pan'-krē-a-tog'-ra-fē) introduction of opaque medium into pancreatic and bile ducts via catheter from an endoscope located in the duodenum.

endospore (en'-dō-spōr) *n* bacterial spore, purely vegetative in function, so that metabolism is minimal and resistance to environmental conditions, esp. high temperature, desiccation and antibacterial drugs, is high. The only pathogenic spore-forming genera with pathogenic species are Bacillus and Clostridium.

endothelioid (en-dō-thē'-lē-oyd) *adj* resembling endothelium.*

endothelioma (en-dō-thē-lē-ō'-mà) *n* malignant tumor derived from endothelial cells.

endothelium (en-dō-thē'-lē-um) *n* lining membrane of serous cavities, heart, blood and lymph vessels—**endothelial** *adj*.

endotoxin (en-dō-tok'-sin) *n* a toxic product of bacteria released only in disintegration of the bacterial cell. → exotoxin *opp*—**endotoxic** *adj*.

endotracheal (en-dō-trāk'-ē-ál) *adj* within the trachea. *endotracheal anesthesia* administration of an anesthetic through a special tube passed into the trachea.

Enduron™ preparation of methyclothiazide.* → chlorothiazide.

Enduronyl™ preparation of methyclothiazide* and deserpidine.*

enema (en'-em-à) *n* introduction of a liquid into the bowel via the rectum, to be returned or retained. Evacuant* enemas are usually prepared commercially as disposable units; chemicals attract water into the bowel, promoting cleansing and peristatic contractions. Retained enemas are usually drugs, most common being cortisone. → barium enema—**enemas, enemata** *pl*.

enflurane (en'-flūr-ān) *n* halogenated ether, a volatilie liquid anesthetic agent. (Ethrane.)

enkephalins (en-kef'-à-lins) *n* two pentapeptides which are neuroleptic and relieve pain: *methionine-encephalin* and *isoleucine-encephalin*. Have been isolated in brain, gastrointestinal tract and pituitary gland. → endorphins.

enophthalmos (en-of-thal'-mus) *n* abnormal retraction of an eyeball within its orbit.

enostosis (en-os-tō'-sis) *n* bony growth within medullary canal of a bone.

ensiform (en'-si-fŏrm) *adj* sword shaped; xiphoid.

ENT *abbr* ear, nose and throat.

Entamoeba (ent-à-mē'-ba) *n* genus of protozoon parasites, three species infesting man: *E. coli* nonpathogenic, infesting intestinal tract; *E. gingivalis* nonpathogenic, infesting mouth; *E. hystolytica* pathogenic, causing amoebic* dysentery.

enteral (en'-tèr-ál) *adj* within the gastrointestinal tract. *enteral diets* those taken by mouth or through a nasogastric* tube; low residue enteral diets can be whole protein/polymeric, or amino acid/peptide. *enteral feeding* includes introduction of nutrients into gastrointestinal tract by modes other than eating. → gastrostomy, nasogastric.

enteric (en-tėr'-ik) *adj* pertaining to the small intestine. *enteric fever* includes typhoid* and paratyphoid* fever.

enteritis (en-tėr-ī'-tis) *n* inflammation of the intestines. The term "regional enteritis" currently preferred for Crohn's* disease.

enteroanastomosis (en'-tėr-ō-an-as-to-mō'-sis) *n* intestinal anastomosis.*

Enterobacter (en'-tėr-ō-bak'-tėr) *n* genus of aerobic, nonspore-bearing, Gram-negative bacilli of the family Enterobacteriaceae. Includes two species: *E. aerogenes* and *E. cloacae.*

enterobiasis (en'-tėr-ō-bī'-à-sis) *n* (*syn* oxyuriasis) infestation with *Enterobius* vermicularis (pinworm), causing irritation in the anal area. Female worm migrates to the anus to lay eggs, which may then cling to bedding, clothing, etc. Eggs reach the intestines after being inhaled or brought to the mouth by the hands (fecal-oral route). A single dose of mebendazole usually eliminates the parasite, though reinfestation is likely without thorough hygienic measures.

Enterobius vermicularis (pinworm) (en'-tėr-ō'-bī-us vėr-mik'-ū-lār'-is) nematode which infests large intestine.

enterocele (en'-tėr-ō-sēl) *n* prolapse* of intestine. Can be into upper third of vagina.

enteroclysis (en-tėr-ō-klī'-sis) *n* (*syn* proctoclysis) introduction of fluid into the rectum.

Enterococcus (en-tėr-ō-kok'-us) *n* Gram-positive coccus; occurs in short chains and is relatively resistant to heat. Enterococci belong to Lancefield's group D, and occur as commensals in human and warm-blooded animal intestines, and sometimes as pathogens in infections of urinary tract, ear, wounds and, more rarely, in endocarditis.

enterocolitis (en-tėr-ō-kō-lī'-tis) *n* inflammation of small intestine and colon. → necrotizing enterocolitis.

enterokinase (en-tėr-ō-kī'-nāz) *n* (*syn* enteropeptidase) an enzyme in intestinal juice. Proteolytic enzyme of pancreatic juice which converts inactive trypsinogen into active trypsin.

enterolith (en'-tėr-ō-lith) *n* an intestinal concretion.

enterolithiasis (en'-tėr-ō-lith-ī'-à-sis) *n* presence of intestinal concretions.

enteron (en'-tėr-on) *n* the gut.

enteropeptidase (en'-tėr-ō-pep'-ti-dāz) *n* → enterokinase.

enterostomy (en-tẻr-os'-to-mē) *n* surgically established fistula between small intestine and some other surface. → gastroenterostomy, ileostomy, jejunostomy—**enterostomal** *adj*.

enterotomy (en-tẻr-ot'-o-mē) *n* incision into the small intestine.

enterotoxin (en-tẻr-ō-toks'-in) *n* toxin which affects the gastrointestinal tract, causing vomiting, diarrhea and abdominal pain.

enteroviruses (en'-tẻr-ō-vī'-rus-es) *npl* viruses which enter via the alimentary tract; comprising poliomyelitis virus, coxsackie viruses and echo viruses, which tend to invade central nervous system.

enterozoa (en-tẻr-ō-zō'-ȧ) *npl* any animal parasites infesting the intestines—**enterozoon** *sing*.

entropion (en-trō'-pē-on) *n* inversion of an eyelid so that the lashes are in contact with the globe of the eye.

enucleation (ē-nū-klē-ā'-shun) *n* removal of an organ or tumor in its entirety, as of an eyeball from its socket.

enuresis (ē-nū-rē'-sis) *n* incontinence of urine, esp. bed-wetting. *nocturnal enuresis* bed wetting during sleep.

enzyme (en'-zīm) *n* soluble protein produced by living cells which acts as a catalyst,* usually with specific biochemical activity. *enzyme tests* since abnormal levels of particular enzymes can indicate specific underlying disease, tests for various enzymes can be a diagnostic tool—**enzymatic** *adj*.

enzyme-linked immunosorbent assay (ELISA) test for presence of certain antibodies or antigens using an indicator antibody that has been "tagged" with an enzyme, whose activity can be measured.

enzymology (en'-zīm-ol'-o-jē) *n* science dealing with structure and function of enzymes*—**enzymological** *adj*.

eosin (ē'-ō-sin) *n* red staining agent used in histology and laboratory diagnostic procedures.

eosinophil (ē-ō-sin'-ō-fil) *n* **1** cells having an affinity for eosin. **2** type of polymorphonuclear leukocyte containing eosin-staining granules—**eosinophilic** *adj*.

eosinophilia (ē-ō-sin-ō-fil'-ē-ȧ) *n* increased eosinophils in blood.

ependymoma (ep-end-im-ō'-mȧ) *n* neoplasm arising in the lining of cerebral ventricles or central canal of spinal cord. Occurs in all age groups.

ephedrine (ef-ed'-rin) *n* drug widely used in asthma and bronchial spasm for relaxant action on bronchioles; raises blood pressure by peripheral vasoconstriction. Useful in hay fever.

ephelides (e-fe'-līds) *npl* freckles, an increase in pigment granules with a normal number of pigment cells. → lentigo—**ephelis** *sing*.

epicanthus (ep-i-kan'-thus) *n* congenital occurrence of a fold of skin obscuring inner canthus of the eye—**epicanthal** *adj*.

epicardium (ep-i-kår'-dē-um) *n* visceral layer of the pericardium—**epicardial** *adj*.

epicondylitis (ep-i-kon'-di-lī'tis) *n* elbow inflammation caused by repetitive, forceful motions; also called "tennis elbow."

epicritic (ep-i-krit'-ik) *adj* describes cutaneous nerve fibers sensitive to fine variations of touch or temperature. → protopathic *opp*.

epidemic *n* simultaneously affecting many people in an area. → endemic.

epidemiology (ep-i-dēm-ē-ol'-o-jē) *n* study of the distribution of disease— **epidemiological** *adj*.

epidermis (ep-i-dėr'-mis) *n* external nonvascular layer of the skin (→ Figure 12); the cuticle—**epidermal** *adj*.

Epidermophyton (ep-i-dėr-mōf'-i-ton) *n* genus of fungi which affects skin and nails.

epidermophytosis (ep-i-dėr-mō-fī-tō'-sis) *n* infection with fungi of the genus *Epidermophyton*.

epididymectomy (ep-id-id-i-mek'-to-mē) *n* surgical removal of the epididymis.*

epididymis (ep-id-id'-i-mis) *n* small oblong body attached to posterior surface of the testes (→ Figure 16). Consists of the tubules which convey spermatozoa from testes to the vas deferens.

epididymitis (ep-id-id-i-mī'-tis) *n* inflammation of the epididymis.*

epididymoorchitis (ep-id-id-i-mō-ōr-kī'-tis) *n* inflammation of the epididymis* and testis.*

epidural (ep-i-dū'-rål) *adj* upon or external to the dura. *epidural block* single injection or intermittent injection through a catheter of local anesthetic for maternal analgesia during delivery or for surgical operations. *epidural space* region through which spinal nerves leave the spinal cord. Can be approached at any level of the spine, but administration of anesthetic is commonly done at the lumbar level or through the sacral cornua for caudal epidural block.

epigastrium (ep-i-gas'-trē-um) *n* abdominal region laying directly over the stomach—**epigastric** *adj*.

epiglottis (ep-i-glot'-tis) *n* thin leaf-shaped flap of cartilage behind the tongue which, in swallowing, covers the opening leading into the larynx. → Figure 6.

epiglottitis (ep-i-glot-ī'-tis) *n* inflammation of the epiglottis.*

epilation (ep-i-lā'-shun) *n* extraction or destruction of hair roots, e.g., by coagulation necrosis, electrolysis or forceps. → depilation—**epilate** *vi*.

epilatory (ep-il'-å-tōr-ē) *adj, n* agent which produces epilation.*

epilepsy (ep'-il-ep-sē) *n* correctly called the epilepsies, group of conditions resulting from disordered electrical activity of brain. Seizure is caused by an abnormal electrical discharge that disturbs cerebration and usually results in loss of consciousness. *major epilepsy* (*syn* grand mal), loss of consciousness with generalized convulsions. When patient does not regain consciousness between attacks the term status* epilepticus is used. *flicker epilepsy* one or more convulsions occurring as result of exposure to flickering light, particularly liable to occur with multicolored light. *focal epilepsy* (*syn* Jacksonian epilepsy) motor seizure begins in one part of body, can spread to other muscle groups, resembling clonic stage of major epilepsy. Fits can be sensory, i.e., abnormal *feeling* in one part that spreads to other parts. In *psychomotor epilepsy, temporal lobe epilepsy* "psychic" warning of seizure consists of feelings of unreality, deja vu; auditory, visual, gustatory or olfactory hallucinations. Jerking not as severe as in major epilepsy. *minor epilepsy* (*syn* petit mal) characterized by transitory interruption of consciousness without convulsions. Characteristic spike and wave pattern on EEG. Any seizure not conforming to this definition is not petit mal; the term is widely misused. All except petit mal can be symptomatic or idiopathic, but focal and temporal lobe epilepsy carry a higher incidence of symptomatic causes. Petit mal is always idiopathic. → akinetic.

epileptic (ep-il-ep'-tik) **1** *adj* pertaining to epilepsy. **2** *n* person with epilepsy. *epileptic aura* premonitory subjective phenomena (tingling in the hand or visual or auditory sensations) which precede an attack of major epilepsy. → aura. *epileptic cry* croak or shout heard from the epileptic person falling unconscious.

epileptiform (ep-il-ep'-ti-fōrm) *adj* resembling epilepsy.

epileptogenic (ep-il-ep'-tō-jen'-ik) *adj* capable of causing epilepsy.

epiloia (ep-il-oy'-ȧ) *n* → tuberous sclerosis.

epimenorrhea (ep-i-men-or-rē'-ȧ) *n* reduction of length of the menstrual cycle.

epinephrine (ep-in-ef'-rin) *n* hormone produced by the adrenal medulla in mammals; can be prepared synthetically. Solutions may darken in color and lose activity if stored for long periods. Applied locally in epistaxis; given by subcutaneous injection, invaluable in relieving serum sickness, asthmatic attacks, urticaria and other allergic states. Added to local anesthetic solutions to reduce diffusion and so prolong anesthetic effect. Also used in circulatory collapse, but only in dilute solution (1 to 100,000) by slow intravenous infusion. (*syn* adrenaline.)

epiphora (ē-pif'-ōr-ȧ) *n* pathological overflow of tears.

epiphysis (ē-pif'-i-sis) *n* the end of a growing bone. Separated from shaft by a plate of cartilage (epiphyseal plate) which ossifies when growth ceases— **epiphyses** *pl*, **epiphyseal** *adj*.

epiphysitis (e-pif-is-īt'-is) *n* inflammation of an epiphysis.*

epiploon (ep-i-plō′-on) *n* the greater omentum*—**epiploic** *adj*.

episclera (ep-i-sklér′-á) *n* loose connective tissue between the sclera and conjunctiva—**episcleral** *adj*.

episcleritis (ep-i-sklér-ī′-tis) *n* inflammation of the episclera.*

episiorrhaphy (ep-ēs-ē-ōr′-a-fē) *n* surgical repair of a lacerated perineum.

episiotomy (ep-ēs-ē-ot′-om-ē) *n* perineal incision made during childbirth, when vaginal orifice does not stretch sufficiently.

epispadias (ep-i-spā′-dē-ás) *n* congenital opening of urethra on the anterior (upper side) of the penis, often associated with ectopia* vesicae. → hypospadias.

epispastic (ep-i-spas′-tik) *n* a blistering agent.

epistaxis (ep-is-taks′-is) *n* bleeding from the nose—**epistaxes** *pl*.

epithelialization (ep-i-thēl′-ē-ál-īz-ā′-shun) *n* growth of epithelium over a raw area; final stage of healing.

epithelioma (ep-i-thēl′-ē-ō′-má) *n* malignant growth arising from squamous or transitional epithelium, usually the skin, esophagus or external genital organs.

epithelium (ep-i-thēl′-ē-um) *n* surface layer of cells covering cutaneous, mucous and serous surfaces. Classified according to arrangement and shape of the cells it contains—**epithelial** *adj*.

Epsom salts (ep′-som) → magnesium sulfate.

Epstein Barr virus (EBV) (ep′-stīn bar′) causative agent of infectious* mononucleosis. A versatile herpes virus which infects many people throughout the world; does not always produce symptoms. Cancer researchers have discovered EBV genome in malignant cells of Burkitt's lymphoma and nasopharyngeal carcinoma.

Epstein's pearls small white patches on the palate of the newborn.

epulis (e-pū′-lis) *n* tumor growing on or from the gums.

Equanil™ meprobamate.*

Erb's palsy (erbz) paralysis* involving shoulder and arm muscles from a lesion of the fifth and sixth cervical nerve roots. Arm hangs loosely at the side with forearm pronated ("waiter's tip position"). Most commonly a birth injury.

erectile (ē-rek′-tīl) *adj* upright; capable of being elevated; *erectile tissue* highly vascular tissue, which, under stimulus, becomes rigid and erect from hyperemia.

erector *n* muscle which achieves erection of a part. *erector spinae* → Figure 5.

erepsin (ē-rep′-sin) *n* a proteolytic enzyme in succus entericus (intestinal fluid).

ERG *abbr* → electroretinogram.

Ergomar™ ergotamine.*

ergometry (er-gom'-e-trē) *n* measurement of work done by muscles—**ergometric** *adj*.

ergonovine (ėr-gō-nō'-vēn) *n* main alkaloid of ergot.* Widely used in obstetrics to reduce hemorrhage and improve contraction of the uterus. (Ergotrate.)

ergosterol (ėr-gos'-tėr-ol) *n* provitamin present in subcutaneous fat of man and animals. On irradiation, converted into vitamin D_2, which has antirachitic properties.

ergot (ėr'-got) *n* a fungus found on rye. Widely used as ergonovine* for postpartum hemorrhage.

ergotamine (ėr-got'-à-mēn) *n* alkaloid of ergot* used in treatment of migraine. Early ergotamine treatment of an attack is more effective, esp. when combined with antiemetics. (Ergomar.)

ergotism (ėr'-got-izm) *n* poisoning by ergot,* which may cause gangrene, particularly of fingers and toes.

Ergotrate™ ergonovine.*

erosion *n* a wearing away or a kind of ulceration. *cervical erosion* destruction of tissue of the external layer of the cervix.

eructation (ē-ruk-tā'-shun) *n* → belching.

eruption *n* process by which a tooth emerges through the alveolar bone and gingiva.

erysipelas (e-ri-sip'-e-las) *n* acute, specific infectious disease, with a spreading, streptococcal inflammation of skin and subcutaneous tissues, accompanied by fever and constitutional disturbances.

erysipeloid (e-ri-sip'-é-loyd) *n* skin condition resembling erysipelas.* Occurs in butchers, persons who handle fish, or cooks. Infecting organism is the *Erysipelothrix* of swine erysipelas.

erythema (e-ri-thē'-mà) *n* reddening of the skin. *erythema induratum* Bazin's* disease. *erythema multiforme* form of toxic or allergic skin eruption which breaks out suddenly and lasts for days; lesions are violet-pink papules or plaques and suggest urticarial weals. Severe form called Stevens-Johnson syndrome. *erythema nodosum* eruption of painful red nodules on front of the legs. Occurs in young women, generally accompanied by rheumatoid pains. It may be a symptom of many diseases including tuberculosis, acute rheumatism, gonococcal septicemia, etc. *erythema pernio* → chilblain—**erythematous** *adj*.

erythrasma (e-rith-raz'-ma) *n* mild skin infection caused by *Corynebacterium minutissimum;* with patchy scaling in moist skin folds.

erythremia (er-ith-rē'-mē-à) *n* → polycythemia.

erythroblast (e-rith'-rō-blast) *n* a nucleated red blood cell found in red bone marrow, from which erythrocytes* are derived—**erythroblastic** *adj*.

erythroblastosis fetalis (e-rith′-rō-blast-ōs′-is) → hemolytic disease of the newborn. Immunization of women at risk, using immunoglobulin containing a high titer of anti-D, prevents the condition.

Erythrocin™ erythromycin.*

erythrocyanosis frigida (e-rith′-rō-sī-an-ōs′-is) *n* vasospastic disease with hypertrophy of arteriolar muscular coat—**erythrocyanotic** *adj*.

erythrocytes (e-rith′-rō-sītz) *npl* normal nonnucleated red cells of circulating blood; the red blood corpuscles. *erythrocyte sedimentation rate (ESR)* citrated blood is placed in a narrow tube; red cells fall, leaving a column of clear supernatant serum, which is measured at the end of an hour and reported in millimeters. Tissue destruction and inflammatory conditions cause an increase in ESR—**erythrocytic** *adj*.

erythrocythemia (e-rith′-rō-sī-thē′-mē-à) *n* overproduction of red cells. May be: (a) physiological response to a low atmospheric oxygen tension (high altitudes), or to need for greater oxygenation of tissues (congenital heart disease), in which case it is referred to as erythrocytosis; or (b) an idiopathic condition, polycythemia* vera—**erythrocythemic** *adj*.

erythrocytopenia (e-rith′-rō-sī-tō-pēn′-ē-à) *n* deficiency in number of red blood cells—**erythrocytopenic** *adj*.

erythrocytosis (e-rith′-rō-sī-tōs′-is) *n* → erythrocythemia.

erythroderma (e-rith′-rō-dėr-mà) *n* excessive redness of the skin.

erythrogenic (e-rith′-rō-jen′-ik) *adj* 1 producing or causing a rash. 2 producing red blood cells.

erythromycin (e-rith′-rō-mī′-sin) *n* orally active antibiotic, similar to penicillin* in range of action. Best reserved for use against organisms resistant to other antibiotics. Risk of jaundice, particularly with erythromycin estolate. (Erythrocin, Ilosone.)

erythropenia (e-rith′-rō-pē′-nē-à) *n* reduction in number of red blood cells; usually, but not necessarily, occurs in anemia.

erythropoiesis (e-rith′-rō-poy-ē′-sis) *n* production of red blood cells. → hemopoiesis.

erythropoietin (e-rith′-rō-poy′-e-tin) *n* hormone secreted by certain cells in the kidney in response to lowered oxygen content in blood. Acts on bone marrow, stimulating erythropoiesis.*

erythrosine (e-rith′-rō-sēn) *n* red dye used in dental disclosing tablets.

Esbach's albuminometer (es′-baks al-bū′-min-om′-me-tėr) graduated glass tube in which albumin in urine is precipitated by addition of Esbach's reagent (picric acid) and the result read after 24 h.

eschar (es'-kàr) *n* a slough, as results from a burn, application of caustics, diathermy etc.

escharotic (es-kàr-ot'-ik) *adj* describes any agent capable of producing a slough.

Escherichia (esh-ėr-ēk'-ē-à) *n* genus of bacteria. Motile, Gram-negative rods widely distributed in nature, esp. in intestinal tract of vertebrates. Some strains are pathogenic to man, causing enteritis, peritonitis, pyelitis, cystitis and wound infections. The type species is *E. coli*.

Esidrix™ hydrochlorothiazide.*

esophageal (ē-sof-a-jē'-al) *adj* pertaining to the esophagus.* *esophageal ulcer* ulceration of the esophagus due to gastroesophageal reflux caused by hiatus hernia.* *esophageal varices* varicosity of veins in the lower esophagus due to portal hypertension, often extending below the cardia into the stomach. In bleeding, they may cause a massive hematemesis, although it is uncommon. Patients may present with iron deficiency anemia or melena.

esophagectasis (ē-sof-a-jek'-ta-sis) *n* a dilated esophagus.*

esophagectomy (ē-sof-a-jek'-to-mē) *n* excision of most of the esophagus.*

esophagitis (ē-sof-a-gī'-tis) *n* inflammation of the esophagus.*

esophagoscope (ē-sof'-a-gō-skōp) *n* endoscope* for passage into the esophagus*—**esophagoscopy** *n*, **esophagoscopic** *adj*.

esophagostomy (ē-sof-a-gos'-to-mē) *n* surgically established fistula between esophagus and the skin in the root of the neck. Used temporarily for feeding after excision of the pharynx for malignant disease.

esophagotomy (ē-sof-a-got'-o-mē) *n* incision into the esophagus.

esophagus (ē-sof'-a-gus) *n* the musculomembranous canal. 23 cm in length, extending from pharynx* to the stomach* (→ Figure 18)—**esophageal** *adj*.

ESR *abbr* erythrocyte* sedimentation rate.

ESRD *abbr* end stage renal disease. → renal.

essence *n* solution of a volatile oil in rectified spirit.

essential fatty acids (EFAs) arachidonic, tinoleic and linolenic acids. Polyunsaturated acids which cannot be synthesized in the body. With diverse functions, most important being that as precursors of prostaglandins, they play a large role in fat metabolism and transfer, and are thought to prevent and break up cholesterol deposits on arterial walls. Present in natural vegetable oils and fish oils. Research suggests that deficiency contributes to premenstrual syndrome.

Estinyl™ ethinylestradiol.*

estradiol (es-trà-dī'-ol) *n* synthetic estrogen. Given in amenorrhea kraurosis, menopause and other conditions of estrogen deficiency, orally and by injection.

estriol (es'-trē-ol) *n* estrogen metabolite present in urine of pregnant women. Fetus and placenta are concerned in its production. Estriol excretion is an indicator of fetal well being.

estrogen (es'-trō-jen) *n* generic for ovarian hormones. Three "classical" ones: estriol, estrone, and estradiol. Urinary excretion of these substances increases throughout normal pregnancy—**estrogenic** *adj.*

estrone (es'-trōn) *n* an ovarian hormone.

Estrovis™ quinestrol.*

ethacrynic acid (eth-à-krin'-ik) loop diuretic with a wider range of effectiveness than thiazide group of saluretics. (Edecrin.) → diuretics.

ethambutol (eth-am'-bū-tol) *n* synthetic antituberculosis drug which can be taken by mouth. Highly effective when used with isoniazid.* (Myambutol.)

ethinylestradiol (eth'-in-il-es-trà-dī'-ol) *n* powerful, orally effective estrogen, usually well tolerated. (Estinyl.)

ethionamide (eth-ī-on'-à-mīd) *n* synthetic antitubercular compound. Hepatotoxicity guarded against by twice weekly SGOT tests. Like isoniazid,* ethionamide can be neurotoxic; may produce gastrointestinal side-effects. (Trecator.)

ethmoid (eth'-moyd) *n* a spongy bone forming lateral walls of the nose and upper portion of the bony nasal septum. → Figure 14.

ethmoidectomy (eth-moyd-ek'-to-mē) *n* surgical removal of part of the ethmoid bone, usually that forming the lateral nasal walls.

ethopropazine (eth-ō-prō'-pà-zēn) *n* antispasmodic used chiefly in rigidity of parkinsonism. May have more side-effects than other drugs. (Parsidol.)

ethosuximide (eth-ō-suks'-i-mīd) *n* anti-convulsant useful in minor epilepsy. (Zarontin.)

ethotoin (eth-ō-tō'-in) *n* antiepileptic drug useful in major, focal and psychomotor epilepsy. (Peganone.)

Ethrane™ enflurane.*

ethyl chloride (eth'-il) volatile general anesthetic for short operations, and a local anesthetic by reason of intense cold produced when applied to the skin; useful in sprains.

ethylestrenol (eth-il-es'-tren-ol) *n* an anabolic steroid; useful for treating severe weight loss, debility and osteoporosis.

ethylnorepinephrine (eth'-il-nōr-e-pin-ef'-rin) *n* bronchodilator useful for asthma. (Bronkephrine.)

ethynodiol diacetate (eth'-i-nō-dī'-ol dī-as'-e-tāt) controls uterine bleeding.

etiology (ē-tē-ol'-o-jē) *n* science dealing with the causation of disease— **etiological** *adj.*

etretinate (e-tre'-tin-āt) *n* vitamin A derivative used in severe psoriasis and some other serious skin disorders. Many adverse effects including fetal damage.

eucalyptus oil (ū-kȧ-lip'-tus) has mild antiseptic properties and sometimes used in nasal drops for catarrh.

euflavine (ū-flā'-vēn) *n* → acriflavine.

eugenics (ū-jen'-iks) *n* study of agencies and measures aimed at improving hereditary qualities of human generations—**eugenic** *adj*.

Eulexin™ flutamide.*

eunuch (ū'-nuk) *n* human male from whom the testes have been removed; a castrated male.

eupepsia (ū-pep'-sē-ȧ) *n* normal digestion.

Eurax™ crotamiton.*

eustachian tube (ūs-tāsh'-ē-ȧn) (*syn* pharyngotympanic tube) a canal, partly bony, partly cartilaginous, measuring 40–50 mm in length, connecting the pharynx with the tympanic cavity (→ Figure 13). Allows air to pass into middle ear, so that air pressure is kept even on both sides of the eardrum. *eustachian catheter* instrument for insufflating blocked eustachian tube.

euthanasia (ū-than-ā'-zhȧ) *n* **1** a good, inferring a painless, death. **2** frequently interpreted as the painless killing of a person suffering from incurable disease.

euthyroid state (ū-thī'-royd) denoting normal thyroid function.

eutocia (ū-tō'-shȧ) *n* natural and normal labor and childbirth without complications.

Eutonyl™ pargyline, a monoamine* oxidase inhibitor.

evacuant (ē-vak'-ū-ant) *n* agent which causes an evacuation; particularly of the bowel. → enema.

evacuator (ē-vak'-ū-ā-tor) *n* instrument for procuring evacuation, e.g., removal from the bladder of a stone, crushed by a lithotrite.

evaporating lotion one which, applied as a compress, absorbs heat in evaporating and so cools the skin.

eversion (ē-vėr'-zhun) *n* a turning outwards as of the upper eyelid to expose the conjunctival sac.

evisceration (ē-vis-ėr-ā'-shun) *n* removal of internal organs.

evulsion (ē-vul'-shun) *n* forcible tearing away of a structure.

Ewing's tumor (ū'-ingz) (*syn* reticulocytoma sarcoma) involving marrow of a long bone in a young person. May be difficult to distinguish from secondary bone deposit of malignant neuroblastoma.

exanthema (ex-an-thēm′-má) *n* a skin eruption—**exanthemata** *pl*, **exanthematous** *adj*.

excision *n* removal of a part by cutting—**excise** *vt*.

excoriation (eks-kōr-ē-ā′-shun) *n* → abrasion.

excrescence (eks-kres′-ens) *n* abnormal protuberance or growth of tissues.

excreta (eks-krē′-tá) *n* waste matter normally discharged from the body, particularly urine and feces.

excretion (eks-krē′-shun) *n* the elimination of waste material from the body, and also the matter so discharged—**excretory** *adj*, **excrete** *vt*.

exenteration (eks-en-tér-ā′-shun) *n* removal of the viscera from its containing cavity, e.g., the eye from its socket, the pelvic organs from the pelvis.

exfoliative cytology (eks-fō′-lē-à-tiv sī-tol′-o-jē) → cytology.

exfoliation (eks-fō-lē-a′-shun) *n* scaling off of tissues in layers—**exfoliative** *adj*.

Exna™ benzthiazide.*

exocrine (eks′-ō-krin) *adj* describes glands from which secretion passes via a duct; secreting externally. → endocrine *opp*—**exocrinal** *adj*.

exogenous (eks-o′-jen-us) *adj* of external origin. → endogenous *opp*.

exomphalos (eks-om′-fál-us) *n* condition present at birth and due to failure of the gut to return to the abdominal cavity during fetal development; intestines protrude through a gap in the abdominal wall, still enclosed in peritoneum.

exophthalmos (eks-of-thal′-mus) *n* protrusion of the eyeball—**exophthalmic** *adj*.

exostosis (eks-os-tō′-sis) *n* overgrowth of bone tissue forming a benign tumor.

exotoxin (eks′-ō-toks′-in) *n* any toxic product secreted by live bacteria. → endotoxin *opp*—**exotoxic** *adj*.

expected date of confinement (EDC) usually dated from first day of the last normal menstrual period, even though for the next 14 days there is really no pregnancy.

expectorant (eks-pek′-tōr-ant) *n* drug which promotes or increases expectoration.*

expectoration (eks-pek′-tōr-ā′-shun) *n* **1** elimination of secretion from the respiratory tract by coughing. **2** sputum*—**expectorate** *vt*.

expiration *n* act of breathing out air from the lungs—**expiratory** *adj*, **expire** *vt*, *vi*.

expression *n* **1** expulsion by force as of the placenta from the uterus; milk from the breast, etc. **2** facial disclosure of feelings, mood, etc.

expressive motor aphasia type of aphasia* in which patient is aware of what is said and wishes to reply, but is unable to assemble the symbols of language (speech) in any coherent order, thus giving impression of noncomprehension.

exsanguination (eks-sang-gwin-ā′-shun) *n* process of rendering bloodless— **exsanguinate** *vt*.

extension *n* **1** traction upon a fractured or dislocated limb. **2** straightening of a flexed limb or part.

extensor (eks-ten′-sor) *n* muscle which on contraction extends or straightens a part. → Figures 4, 5; flexor *opp*.

external cephalic version (ECV) → version.

external respiration → respiration.

extirpation *n* complete removal or destruction of a part.

extra-anatomic bypass (EAB) a prosthetic vascular graft is threaded subcutaneously to carry a limb-preserving blood supply from an efficient proximal part of an artery to a distal one, thus bypassing inefficient part of the artery.

extra-articular (eks′-trȧ-ȧr-tik′-ū-lȧr) *adj* outside a joint.

extracapsular (eks′-trȧ-kap′-sū-lȧr) *adj* outside a capsule. → intracapsular *opp*.

extracardiac (eks′-trȧ-kar′-dē-ak) *adj* outside the heart.

extracellular (eks′-trȧ-sel′-ū-lar) *adj* outside the cell membrane. → intracellular *opp*.

extracorporeal (eks-trȧ-kōr-pōr′-ē-ȧl) *adj* outside the body. *extracorporeal circulation* blood is directed through a machine ("heart-lung" or "artificial kidney") and returned to the general circulation.

extracorpuscular (eks-trȧ-kōr-pus′-kū-lȧr) *adj* outside corpuscles.

extraction *n* removal of a tooth. *extraction of lens* surgical removal of the lens. *extracapsular extraction* capsule is ruptured prior to delivery of the lens and preserved in part. *intracapsular extraction* the lens is removed within its capsule.

extradural (eks-trȧ-dū′-rȧl) *adj* external to the dura mater.

extragenital (eks-trȧ-jen′-i-tȧl) *adj* on areas of the body apart from genital organs. *extragenital chancre* primary ulcer of syphilis when it occurs on the finger, lip, breast, etc.

extrahepatic (eks-trȧ-hep-at′-ik) *adj* outside the liver.

extramural (eks′-trȧ-mūr′-al) *adj* outside the wall of a vessel or organ.

extraperitoneal (eks′-trȧ-per′-it-on-ē′-al) *adj* outside the peritoneum.

extrapleural (eks-trȧ-plū′-rȧl) *adj* outside the pleura, i.e., between the parietal pleura and the chest wall. → plombage.

extrapyramidal side-effects (eks'-trȧ-pir-am'-id-al) unwanted effects from drugs which interfere with function of the extrapyramidal* tracts.

extrapyramidal tracts those comprised of motor neurons from the brain to the spinal cord except for the fibers in the pyramidal* tracts. They are functional rather than anatomical units; control and coordinate postural, static mechanisms which cause contractions of muscle groups in sequence or simultaneously; maintain equilibrium and muscle tone, the neuromuscular "background."

extrarenal (eks-trȧ-rē'-nȧl) *n* outside the kidney.

extrasystole (eks-trȧ-sis'-to-lē) *n* premature beats (ectopic beats) in the pulse rhythm: the cardiac impulse is initiated in some focus apart from the sinoatrial node.

extrathoracic (eks-trȧ-thōr-as'-ik) *adj* outside the thoracic cavity.

extrauterine (eks-trȧ-ū'-tėr-in) *n* outside the uterus. *extrauterine pregnancy* → ectopic pregnancy.

extravasation (eks-trȧv-a-sā'-shun) *n* escape of fluid from its normal enclosure into surrounding tissues.

extravenous (eks-trȧ-vē'-nus) *adj* outside a vein.

extrinsic *adj* developing or having its origin from without; not internal. *extrinsic factor* now known to be vitamin B_{12}, absorbed in the presence of the intrinsic* factor secreted by the stomach.

extroversion (eks'-trō-vėr-shun) *n* turning inside out. *extroversion of the bladder* ectopia* vesicae.*

exudate (eks'-ū-dāt) *n* the product of exudation.*

exudation (eks-ū-dā'-shun) *n* the oozing out of fluid through capillary walls, or of sweat through pores of the skin—**exudate** *n,* **exude** *vt, vi.*

eyeteeth *npl* the canine teeth* in the upper jaw.

F

facet *n* a small, smooth, flat surface of a bone or a calculus. *facet syndrome* dislocation of some of the gliding joints between vertebrae causing pain and muscle spasm.

facial *adj* pertaining to the face. *facial nerve* seventh pair of the 12 pairs of cranial nerves which arise directly from the brain. *facial paralysis* paralysis of muscles supplied by the facial nerve.

facies (fā′-shēz) *n* appearance of the face, as in congenital syphilis with saddle nose, prominent brow and chin. *adenoid facies* open-mouthed, vacant expression due to deafness from enlarged adenoids. *facies hippocratica* drawn, pale, pinched appearance indicative of approaching death. *Parkinson facies* masklike appearance; saliva may trickle from corners of the mouth.

factor P one component of the complement system.

facultative (fak′-ul-tā-tiv) *adj* conditional; having the power of living under different conditions.

failure to thrive blanket term replacing marasmus.* Afflicted children do not progress because of malnutrition or difficulty in absorbing basic nutritional requirements.

falciform (fal′-si-fōrm) *adj* sickle-shaped.

fallopian tubes (fal-lō′-pē-ān) (*syn* oviducts, uterine tubes) two tubes opening out of the upper part of the uterus. Each measures 10 cm and the distal end is fimbriated (→ Fig. 17) and lies near the ovary. They convey ova into the uterus.

Fallot's tetralogy (fal-lōz′ tet-rol′-o-jē) congenital heart defect comprising interventricular septal defect, pulmonary stenosis, right ventricular hypertrophy and malposition of the aorta.

falx (falks) *n* sickle-shaped structure. *falx cerebri* that portion of the dura mater separating the two cerebral hemispheres.

Fanconi syndrome (fan-kōn′-ē) an inherited or acquired dysfunction of the proximal kidney tubules. Large amounts of amino acids, glucose and phosphates are excreted in urine, yet blood levels of these substances are normal. Symptoms may include thirst, polyuria, bone abnormalities and muscular weakness. → aminoaciduria, cystinosis.

farinaceous (far-i-nā′-shus) *adj* pertaining to cereal substances, i.e., made of flour or grain. Starchy.

farmer's lung form of alveolitis due to allergy to certain spores (e.g., *Micropolyspora faeni*) that occur in dust of moldy hay or other moldy vegetable produce. Recognized as an industrial disease.

far-sightedness *n* hyperopia.*

FAS *abbr* fetal* alcohol syndrome.

fascia (fashē'-à) *n* connective tissue sheath consisting of fibrous tissue and fat which unites the skin to the underlying tissues. Also surrounds and separates many of the muscles, and, in some cases, holds them together—**fascial** *adj*.

fasciculation (fas-ik-ū-lā'-shun) *n* visible flickering of muscle; can occur in the upper and lower eyelids.

fasciculus (fas-ik'-ū-lus) *n* a little bundle, as of muscle or nerve—**fascicular** *adj*, **fasciculi** *pl*.

fasciotomy (fash-ē-ot'-o-mē) *n* incision of a fascia.

fastigium (fas-tij'-ē-um) *n* highest point of a fever; period of full development of a disease.

fat *n* **1** an ester of glycerol with fatty acids which may be of animal or vegetable origin, and may be either solid or liquid. Vitamins A, D, E and K are fat-soluble. **2** adipose tissue, which acts as a reserve supply of energy and smooths out body contours—**fatty** *adj*.

fatty degeneration degeneration* of tissues that results in appearance of fatty droplets in cytoplasm; found esp. in disease of liver, kidney and heart.

fauces (faw'-sēz) *n* opening from the mouth into the pharynx, bounded above by the soft palate, below by the tongue. Pillars of the fauces anterior and posterior lie laterally and enclose the tonsil—**faucial** *adj*.

favism (fā'-vizm) *n* deficiency of enzyme G6PD (glucose-6-phosphate dehydrogenase), causing severe hemolytic anemia after eating fava beans.

favus (fā'-vus) *n* ringworm caused by *Trichophyton schoenleini*. Yellow cup-shaped crusts (scutula) develop, esp. on the scalp.

FDA *abbr* Food and Drug Administration.

febrile (fēb'-rīl) *adj* feverish; accompanied by fever.

fecalith (fē'-kà-lith) *n* concretion formed in the bowel from fecal matter; can cause obstruction and/or inflammation.

feces (fē'-sēz) *n* waste matter excreted from the bowel, consisting mainly of indigestible cellulose, unabsorbed food, intestinal secretions, water and bacteria—**fecal** *adj*.

fecundation (fe-kund-ā'-shun) *n* impregnation; fertilization.

fecundity (fe-kund'-it-ē) *n* the power of reproduction; fertility.

feed-back treatment physiological activities such as excessive muscle tension and raised blood pressure are measured graphically so that patients can observe, and learn to relax muscles and lower blood pressure.

Fehling's solution (fā′-lingz) alkaline copper solution used for detection and estimation of amount of sugars.

Feldene™ piroxicam.*

Felty syndrome (fel′-tē) enlargment of the liver, spleen and lymph nodes as a complication of rheumatoid* arthritis.

femoral artery (fem′-ōr-ȧl) → Figure 9.

femoral vein → Figure 10.

femoropopliteal (fem′-ėr-ō-pop-li-tē′-ȧl) *adj* usually, referring to the femoral and popliteal vessels.

femur (fē′-mur) *n* the thigh bone (→ Figures 2, 3); the longest and strongest bone in the body—**femora** *pl,* **femoral** *adj.*

fenestra (fen-es′-trȧ) *n* a windowlike opening. *fenestra ovalis* oval opening between the middle and internal ear. Below it lies the *fenestra rotunda* a round opening.

fenestration (fen-es-trā′-shun) *n* **1** surgical creation of an opening (of fenestra) in the inner ear for relief of deafness in otosclerosis. **2** (*syn* festination) type of walking seen in such nervous diseases as paralysis agitans: patient trots in bursts, getting faster and faster, stops and then starts off again.

fenfluramine (fen-flo͞or′-a-mēn) appetite suppressant; does not possess central stimulant effects of amphetamines. (Pondimin.)

fentanyl (fen′-tan-il) *n* morphinelike short-acting narcotic analgesic but of considerably higher potency. Can be used in conjunction with other drugs to promote anesthesia in children and the aged. (Sublimaze.)

fertilization *n* impregnation of an ovum by a spermatozoon.

festination (fes-tin-ā′-shun) *n* → fenestration.

fetal alcohol syndrome (FAS) stillbirth or fetal abnormality due to prenatal growth retardation caused by mother's consumption of alcohol during pregnancy.

fetal circulation circulation* of blood through the fetus, umbilical cord and placenta.

fetal monitor measures fetal heart rate either by external microphone or by application of an electrode to the fetal scalp, recording fetal ECG. Also measures maternal contractions.

fetishism (fet′-ish-izm) *n* condition in which a particular material object is regarded with irrational awe or a strong emotional attachment. Can have a psychosexual dimension in which such an object is repeatedly or exclusively used in achieving sexual excitement.

fetor (fē'-tor) *n* offensive odor, stench. *fetor oris* bad breath.

fetoscopy (fē-tos'-ko-pē) *n* direct visual examination of the fetus by using a suitable fiberglass endoscope.

fetus (fē'-tus) an unborn child. *fetus papyraceous* a dead fetus, one of a twin which has become flattened and mummified—**fetal** *adj*.

FEV *abbr* forced expiratory volume. → respiratory function tests.

fever *n* (*syn* pyrexia) elevation of body temperature above normal. Designates some infectious conditions, as paratyphoid fever, scarlet fever, typhoid fever, etc.

fibril (fī'-bril) *n* a component filament of a fiber; a small fiber.

fibrillation (fi-bril-lā'-shun) *n* uncoordinated quivering contraction of muscle; referring usually to atrial fibrillation in the myocardium wherein the atria beat very rapidly and are not synchronized with the ventricular beat. Result is a total irregularity of the pulse.

fibrin (fī'-brin) *n* matrix on which a blood clot forms; made of soluble fibrinogen* through catalytic (enzymatic) action of thrombin.* *fibrin foam* a white, dry, spongy material made from fibrinogen; used in conjunction with thrombin as a hemostatic in brain and lung surgery—**fibrinous** *adj*.

fibrinogen (fī-brin'-ō-jen) *n* soluble protein of the blood from which is produced the insoluble protein called fibrin,* essential to blood coagulation.

fibrinogenopenia (fī-brin'-ō-jen-ō-pē'-nē-à) *n* (*syn* fibrinopenia) lack of blood plasma fibrinogen.* Can be congenital or due to liver disease.

fibrinolysin (fī-brin-ō-lī'-sin) *n* blood-stream enzyme thought to dissolve fibrin* occurring after minor injuries. Has been administered intravenously in thrombosis.

fibrinolysis (fī-brin-ol'-is-is) *n* dissolution of fibrin* which can precede hemorrhage. There is normally a balance between blood coagulation and fibrinolysis in the body—**fibrinolytic** *adj*.

fibrinopenia (fī-brin-ō-pē-nē-à) *n* → fibrinogenopenia.

fibroadenoma (fī-brō-ad-en-ōm'-à) *n* benign tumor containing fibrous and glandular tissue.

fibroblast (fī'-brō-blast) *n* (*syn* fibrocyte) a cell which produces collagen, a major constituent of connective tissues—**fibroblastic** *adj*.

fibrocartilage (fī-brō-kàr'-ti-laj) *n* cartilage containing fibrous tissue—**fibrocartilaginous** *adj*.

fibrocaseous (fī-brō-kā'-sē-us) *adj* soft, cheesy mass infiltrated by fibrous tissue, formed by fibroblasts.

fibrochondritis (fī-brō-kon-drī'-tis) *n* inflammation of fibrocartilage.

fibrocyst (fī'-brō-sist) *n* a fibroma which has undergone cystic degeneration.

fibrocystic (fī-brō-sis'-tik) *adj* pertaining to a fibrocyst.* *fibrocystic disease of bone* cysts may be solitary or generalized. If generalized and accompanied by decalcification of bone, it is symptomatic of hyperparathyroidism. *fibrocystic disease of breast* breast feels lumpy due to presence of cysts, usually caused by hormone imbalance. *fibrocystic disease of pancreas* cystic* fibrosis.

fibrocyte (fī'-brō-sīt) *n* → fibroblast—**fibrocytic** *adj*.

fibroid (fī'-broyd) *n* fibromuscular benign tumor usually found in the uterus. An *interstitial uterine fibroid* is embedded in the wall of the uterus (intra-mural)—if extended to the outer surface it becomes a *subperitoneal fibroid* (subserous), if to the inner or endometrial surface, a *fibroid polypus*.

fibroma (fī-brō'-mà) *n* benign tumor composed of fibrous tissue—**fibromata** *pl*, **fibromatous** *adj*.

fibromuscular (fī-brō-mus'-kū-làr) *adj* pertaining to fibrous and muscle tissue.

fibromyoma (fī-brō-mī-ō'-ma) *n* benign tumor consisting of fibrous and muscle tissue—**fibromyomata** *pl*, **fibromyomatous** *adj*.

fibroplasia (fī-brō-plā'-zhà) *n* the production of fibrous tissue which is a normal part of healing. *retrolental fibroplasia* presence of fibrous tissue behind the lens, extending in an area from the ciliary body to the optic disk, causing blindness. Noticed shortly after birth, more commonly in premature babies who have had continuous oxygen therapy.

fibrosarcoma (fī-brō-sàr-kō'-mà) *n* a form of sarcoma; malignant tumor derived from fibroblastic cells—**fibrosarcomata** *pl*, **fibrosarcomatous** *adj*.

fibrosis (fī-brō'-sis) *n* formation of excessive fibrous tissues in a structure—**fibrotic** *adj*.

fibrositis (fī-brō-sī'-tis) *n* (*syn* muscular rheumatism) pain of uncertain origin which affects soft tissues of limbs and trunk; generally associated with muscular stiffness and local tender points—fibrositic nodules. Cause unknown; some disturbance in immunity may be a factor, as may be gout. Nonspecific factors include chill, postural trauma, muscular strain and psychological stress, esp. in tense, anxious people.

fibrovascular (fī-brō-vas'-kū-làr) *adj* pertaining to fibrous tissue which is well supplied with blood vessels.

fibula (fi'-bū-là) *n* one of the longest and thinnest bones of the body, situated on the outer side of the leg and articulating at the upper end with the lateral condyle of the tibia and at the lower end with the lateral surface of the talus (astragalus) and tibia (→ Figures 2, 3)—**fibular** *adj*.

Filaria (fi-lār'-ē-à) *n* genus of parasitic, threadlike worms, found mainly in the tropics and subtropics. Adults of *F. bancrofti* and *Brugia malayi* live in lymphatics, connective tissues or mesentery, where they may cause obstruction; embryos migrate to the blood stream. Completion of life cycle is dependent upon passage through a mosquito. → loiasis—**filarial** *adj.*

filariasis (fil-ar-ī'-á-sis) *n* infestation with *Filaria* → elephantiasis.

filaricide (fil-ār'-i-sīd) *n* agent which destroys *Filaria*.

filiform (fil'-i-form) *adj* threadlike. *filiform papillae* small projections ending in several minute processes; found on the tongue.

filix mas (fil'-iks mas) *n* male fern extract, used to expel taenia.*

filtrate *n* that part of a substance which passes through a filter.

filtration *n* process of straining through a filter under gravity, pressure or vacuum. Act of passing fluid through a porous medium. *filtration under pressure* occurs in the kidneys, due to the pressure of blood in the glomeruli.

filum (fī'-lum) *n* any filamentous or threadlike structure. *filum terminale* a strong, fine cord blending with the spinal cord above, and the periosteum of the sacral canal below.

fimbria (fim'-brē-á) *n* a fringe or frond; resembling the fronds of a fern; e.g., the fimbriae of the fallopian tubes (→ Figure 17)—**fimbriae** *pl,* **fimbrial, fimbriated** *adj.*

finger *n* a digit. *clubbed finger* swelling of terminal phalanx which occurs in many lung and heart diseases.

fissure *n* a split or cleft. *palpebral fissure* the opening between the eyelids. *anal fissure, anal ulcer* tear in wall of anal canal; often accompanied by pain and spasm, and bleeding at defecation. May be caused by hard or large stool; treated with stool softeners, but surgery required in non-self healing cases.

fistula (fis'-tū-lá) *n* an abnormal communication between two body surfaces or cavities, e.g., gastrocolic fistula between stomach and colon; colostomy, between the colon and the abdominal surface—**fistulae** *pl,* **fistular, fistulous** *adj.*

fixation *n* in optics, direct focusing of one or both eyes on an object so that image falls on the retinal disk.

flaccid (flas'-id) *adj* soft, flabby, not firm. *flaccid paralysis* results mainly from lower motor neuron lesions; with diminished or absent tendon reflexes—**flaccidity** *n.*

flagellum (fla-jel'-um) *n* a fine, hairlike appendage capable of lashing movement. Characteristic of spermatozoa, certain bacteria and protozoa—**flagella** *pl.*

Flagyl™ metronidazole.*

flail chest unstable thoracic cage due to fracture. → respiration.

flap *n* partially-removed tissue, retaining blood and nerve supply, used to repair defects in other parts of the body. Common in plastic surgery to treat burns and other injuries; skin flaps used to cover amputation stumps.

flat-foot *n* (*syn* pes planus) congenital or acquired deformity marked by depression of the longitudinal arches of the foot.

flat pelvis a pelvis in which the anteroposterior diameter of the brim is reduced.

flatulence (flat'-ū-lens) *n* gastric and intestinal distension with gas—**flatulent** *adj*.

flatus (flāt'-us) *n* gas in the stomach or intestines.

flavoxate (fla-voks'-āt) *n* oral urinary antiseptic useful for controlling urinary spasm. (Urispas.)

flecainide (flek'-ān-īd) *n* cardiac antiarrhythmic drug. (Tambocor.)

Flexeril™ cyclobenzaprine.*

flexibilitas cerea (fleks-i-bil'-i-tas sē'-rē-à) literally waxy flexibility. Condition of generallized hypertonia of muscles found in catatonic schizophrenia.* When fully developed, patient's limbs retain positions in which they are placed, remaining immobile for hours at a time. Occasionally occurs in hysteria as hysterical rigidity.

flexion (flek'-shun) *n* act of bending by which the shafts of long bones forming a joint are brought towards each other.

Flexner's bacillus (fleks'-nerz) *Shigella* *flexneri*.

flexor (fleks'-or) *n* muscle which on contraction flexes or bends a part. → Figures 4, 5; extensor *opp*.

flexure (fleks'-ūr) *n* a bend. *left colic (splenic) flexure* is situated at junction of the transverse and descending parts of the colon. It lies at a higher level than the *right colic* or *hepatic flexure* the bend between ascending and transverse colon, beneath the liver. *sigmoid flexure* S-shaped bend at lower end of the descending colon; continuous with the rectum below—**flexural** *adj*.

floaters *npl* floating bodies in the vitreous humor (of the eye), visible in field of view.

floating kidney abnormally mobile kidney. → nephropexy.

flocculation (flok-ūl-ā'-shun) *n* coalescence of colloidal particles in suspension, resulting in aggregation into larger discrete masses that are often visible to the naked eye as cloudiness. *flocculation test* serum is set up against various salts such as gold, thymol, cephalin or cholesterol; in presence of abnormal serum proteins results in cloudiness. Abnormal forms of albumin and globulin are produced by diseased liver cells.

flooding *n* popular term for excessive bleeding from the uterus.

floppy baby syndrome → amyotonia congenita.

flora (flōr'-à) *n* in medicine, the body's many normal indwelling microorganisms, mostly nonpathogenic, but which in particular circumstances can become pathogenic.

Florinef™ fludrocortisone.*

Floropryl™ dyflos.*

flu *n* influenza.*

fluctuation *n* a wavelike motion felt on digital examination of a fluid-containing tumor, e.g., abscess—**fluctuant** *adj*.

flucytosine (flū-sī'-tō-sēn) *n* antifungal agent effective against Candida and Cryptococcus. (Ancobon.)

Fludara™ fludarabine phosphate.*

fludarabine phosphate antileukemia drug; an antimetabolite, interferes with cell growth. (Fludara.)

fludrocortisone (floo-drō-kōr'-ti-sōn) *n* sodium-retaining tablets. Useful in some cases of Addison's disease. (Florinef.)

fluke *n* trematode worm of the order Digenea. The *European* or *sheep fluke (Fasciola hepatica)* usually ingested from watercress; causes fever, malaise, a large tender liver and eosinophilia. *Chinese fluke (Clonorchis sinensis)* usually ingested with raw fish; adult fluke lives in bile ducts and, while it may produce cholangitis, hepatitis and jaundice, it may be asymptomatic or be blamed for vague digestive symptoms. *lung fluke (Paragonimus)* usually ingested with raw crab, in China and Far East. Symptoms are those of chronic bronchitis, including blood in sputum.

fluocinolone (floo-ō-sin'-ō-lōn) *n* cortisone derivative for topical application. (Synalar.)

fluorescein (floor'-es-ēn) *n* red substance that forms a green fluorescent solution. Used as eye drops to detect corneal lesions, which stain green. Can be used in retinal angiography by injection into a vein, followed by viewing and photographing its passage through retinal blood vessels. *fluorescein string test* used to detect site of obscure upper gastrointestinal bleeding. Patient swallows a radioopaque knotted string; fluorescein is injected intravenously and after a few minutes the string is withdrawn. If staining has occurred the site of bleeding can be determined.

fluorescent treponemal antibody test (FTA) carried out for syphilis: virulent *Treponema pallidum* used as the antigen.

fluoride (floor'-īd) *n* ion sometimes present in drinking water. Can be incorporated into structure of bone, providing protection against dental caries, but in gross excess causes mottling of teeth. As a preventive measure added to water supply in a strength of 1 part fluoride in a million parts of water (fluoridation).

fluoroscopy (floor-os'-ko-pē) *n* X-ray examination of movement in the body, observed by means of fluorescent screen and TV system.

fluorouracil, 5-FU (floor-or'-à-sil) *n* antimetabolic cytotoxic agent. (Adrucil.)

Fluothane™ halothane.*

fluoxetine (floo-oks'-e-tēn) *n* popular antidepressant; not related to other drug groups, such as tricyclics, MAO inhibitors. (Prozac.)

fluphenazine (floo-fen'-à-zēn) *n* a phenothiazine* tranquilizer with anti-emetic properties. Can be given as a depot (slow-release) injection. A newer preparation is *fluphenazine deconoate* which is longer acting. (Permitil, Prolixin.)

flurazepam (floor-az'-e-pam) *n* drug chemically related to mitrazepam,* with basically similar properties. (Dalmane.)

flutamide (floot'-a-mīd) *n* drug that inhibits uptake of androgens; used in treatment of prostate cancer. (Eulexin.)

flux *n* any excessive flow of any body excretions.

folic acid (*syn* pteroylglutamic acid) a member of the vitamin* B complex that is abundant in green vegetables, yeast and liver. Absorbed from the small intestine; an essential factor for normal hemopoiesis and cell division generally. Used in treatment of megaloblastic anemias other than those due to vitamin B_{12} deficiency.

follicle (fol'-li-kl) *n* 1 a small secreting sac. 2 a simple tubular gland. *follicle stimulating hormone (FSH)* secreted by the anterior pituitary gland; trophic to the ovaries in the female, where it develops the ovum-containing (graafian) follicles; and to the testes in the male, where it is responsible for sperm production—**follicular** *adj*.

folliculitis (fol-li-kū-lī'-tis) *n* inflammation of follicles, such as the hair follicles. → alopecia.

folliculosis (fol-ik-ū-lō'-sis) *n* hypertrophy of follicles.

Folvite™ folic acid* and antianemia compounds especially for anemia in pregnancy.

fomentation (fō-men-tā'-shun) *n* a hot, wet application to produce hyperemia. When the skin is intact, strict cleanliness is observed (medical fomentation); when the skin is broken, aseptic technique is used (surgical fomentation).

fomite (fō'-mīt) *n* any article which has been in contact with infection and is capable of transmitting same.

fontanel (fon-tà-nel') *n* a membranous space between the cranial bones. The diamond-shaped anterior fontanel (bregma) is at junction of the frontal and two parietal bones. Usually closes in second year of life. The triangular posterior fontanel (lambda) is at junction of the occipital and two parietal bones; closes within a few weeks of birth.

food poisoning vomiting, with or without diarrhea, resulting from eating food contaminated with chemical poison, preformed bacterial toxin or live bacteria, or poisonous natural vegetation, e.g., berries, toadstools (fungi).

foot *n* that portion of the lower limb below the ankle. *foot drop* inability to dorsi-flex foot, as in severe sciatica and nervous disease affecting lower lumbar regions of the cord. Can be a complication of being bedfast.

foramen (fōr-ā'-men) *n* a hole or opening. Generally with reference to bones. *foramen magnum* opening in the occipital bone through which spinal cord passes. *foramen ovale* a fetal cardiac interatrial communication which normally closes at birth—**foramina** *pl*.

forced expiratory volume → forced vital capacity.

forced gut lavage fluid introduced via nasogastric tube for continuous perfusion of the large bowel lining.

forced vital capacity (FVC), forced expiratory volume maximum gas volume that can be expelled from the lungs in a forced expiration.

forceps (fōr'-seps) *n* surgical instruments with two opposing blades which are used to grasp or compress tissues, swabs, needles and many other surgical appliances. Blades are controlled by direct pressure on them (tonglike), or by handles (scissorlike). *obstetrical forceps* forceps used to extract fetal head during delivery.

forebrain *n* → Figure 1.

forensic medicine (*syn* medical jurisprudence) also called "legal medicine"; application of medical knowledge to questions of law.

foreskin *n* the prepuce or skin covering the glans* penis.

formaldehyde (fōr-mal'-de-hīd) *n* powerful germicide. Formalin* is a 40% solution; used mainly for room disinfection and preservation of pathological specimens.

formication (fōr-mi-kā'-shun) *n* sensation as of ants running over the skin. Occurs in nerve lesions, particularly in the regenerative phase.

formulary (fōr'-mū-lā-rē) *n* a collection of formulas. The *National Formulary* is published by the U.S. Pharmacopeial Convention and contains standards for drugs enforced by the U.S. government.

fornix (fōr'-niks) *n* an arch; particularly referred to the vagina, i.e., the space between the vaginal wall and the cervix of the uterus—**fornices** *pl*.

foscarnet (fos'-kar-net) *n* chelating drug, esp. for calcium and magnesium; action interferes with viral replication. Used in treatment of herpes group of viruses. (Foscavir.)

Foscavir™ foscarnet.*

fossa (fos'-så) *n* a depression or furrow—**fossae** *pl*.

fourchette (foor'-shet) *n* membranous fold connecting the posterior ends of the labia minora.

fovea (fō'-vē-à) *n* a small depression or fossa; particularly the fovea centralis retinae, the site of most distinct vision.

fracture *n* breach in continuity of a bone as result of injury. *Bennett's* fracture, closed fracture* no communication with external air. *Colles' fracture* → Colles'. *comminuted fracture* bone is broken into more than two pieces. *complicated fracture* with injury to surrounding organs and structures. *compression fracture* usually of lumbar or dorsal region due to hyperflexion of spine; the anterior vertebral bodies are crushed together. *depressed fracture* the broken bone presses on an underlying structure, such as brain or lung. *impacted fracture* one

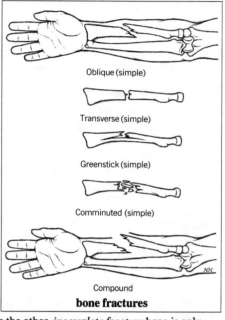

Oblique (simple)

Transverse (simple)

Greenstick (simple)

Comminuted (simple)

Compound

bone fractures

end of broken bone is driven into the other. *incomplete fracture* bone is only cracked or fissured—called "*green-stick fracture*" when it occurs in children. *open (compound) fracture* a wound permits communication of broken bone end with air. *pathological fracture* occurring in abnormal bone as result of force that would not break a normal bone. *spontaneous fracture* occurs without appreciable violence; may be synonymous with pathological fracture.

fragilitas (fra-jil'-i-tàs) *n* brittleness. *fragilitas ossium* congenital disease characterized by abnormal fragility of bone, multiple fractures and a china-blue coloring of the sclera.

frambesia (fram-bē'-zhē-à) *n* yaws.*

Freiberg's infarction (frī'-bergz) an aseptic necrosis of bone tissue; most commonly occurs in the head of the second metatarsal bone.

Frei test (frī) intradermal test using antigen from those infected with lymphogranuloma venereum and a control; positive skin reaction to the killed antigen confirms diagnosis.

French chalk talc.*

Frenkel's exercises (fren'-klz) special exercises for tabes* dorsalis to teach muscle and joint sense.

frenotomy (fren-ot'-o-mē) *n* surgical severance of a frenum, particularly for tongue-tie.

frenum (fren'-um) *n* a fold of membrane which checks or limits movement of an organ. *frenum linguae* from the undersurface of the tongue to the floor of the mouth.

friable (frī'-à-bl) *adj* easily crumbled; readily pulverized.

friction murmur heard through the stethoscope when two rough or dry surfaces rub together, as in pleurisy and pericarditis.

Friedlander's bacillus (frēd'-lan-dèrz) large Gram-negative rod bacterium occasionally found in the upper respiratory tract, in which it can cause inflammation.

Friedman's curve (frēd'-manz) graphic analysis of labor that correlates the length of labor with degree of cervical dilatation. Aids in evaluating normalcy of the progression of labor.

Friedreich's ataxia (frēd'-riks) progressive familial disease of childhood, with sclerosis of the sensory and motor columns in the spinal cord, and consequent muscular weakness and staggering (ataxia). Heart may also be affected.

frigidity *n* lack of normal sexual desire, esp. in relation to the female.

Frohlich's syndrome (fro'-liks) (*syn* adiposogenital dystrophy) uncommon syndrome resulting from anterior pituitary insufficiency secondary to hypothalamine neoplasm. Characterized by obesity, stunted growth, arrested sexual development and knock-knees.

frontal *adj* 1 pertaining to the front of a structure. 2 the forehead bone (→ Figure 14). *frontal sinus* a cavity at the inner aspect of each orbital ridge on the frontal bone (→ Figure 14).

frostbite *n* freezing of skin and superficial tissues resulting from exposure to extreme cold; lesion is similar to a burn and may become gangrenous. → trench foot.

frozen shoulder initial pain followed by stiffness, lasting several months. As pain subsides, exercises are intensified until full recovery. Cause unknown.

fructose (fruk'-tōs) *n* → evulose. *hereditary fructose intolerance* autosomal recessive defect causing inability to utilize fructose; the enzyme phosphofructoaldolase is absent. Symptoms are those of hypoglycemia, abstinence is sole remedy.

FSH *abbr* follicle* stimulating hormone.

FTA *abbr* fluorescent* treponemal antibody.

fulguration (ful-gūr-ā'-shun) *n* destruction of tissue by diathermy.

full-term *adj* mature—when pregnancy has lasted 40 weeks.

fulminant (ful'-min-ant) *adj* developing quickly and with an equally rapid termination.

Fulvicin™ griseofulvin.*

fumigation (fū-mi-gā'-shun) *n* disinfection by exposure to fumes of a vaporized disinfectant.

functional *adj* **1** in a general sense, pertaining to function. **2** of a disorder, of the function but not the structure of an organ. **3** as a psychiatric term, of neurotic origin, i.e., psychogenic, without primary organic disease.

fundoplication (fun-dō-plik-ā'-shun) *n* surgical folding of the gastric fundus to prevent reflux of gastric contents into the esophagus.

fundus (fun'-dus) *n* basal portion of a hollow structure; part which is distal to the opening. *fundus uteri* the top of the uterus between the openings to the fallopian tubes—**fundi** *pl,* **fundal** *adj.*

fungicide (fun'-ji-sīd) *n* agent lethal to fungi—**fungicidal** *adj.*

fungiform (fun'-ji-form) *adj* resembling a mushroom, like the fungiform papillae found chiefly in the dorsocentral area of the tongue.

fungistatic (fun-ji-stat'-ik) *adj* of an agent which inhibits growth of fungi.

Fungizone™ amphotericin B.

fungus *n* a low form of vegetable life including many microscopic organisms capable of producing superficial and systemic disease in man—**fungi** *pl,* **fungal** *adj.*

funiculitis (fū-nik-ū-lī'-tis) *n* inflammation of the spermatic cord.

funiculus (fū-nik'-ū-lus) *n* a cordlike structure.

funnel chest (*syn* pectus excavatum) congenital deformity in which breastbone is depressed towards the spine.

Furacin™ nitrofurazone.*

Furadantin™ nitrofurantoin.*

furazolidone (fūr-à-zol'-i-dōn) *n* used for nonspecific diarrheas, bacillary dysentery and bacterial food poisoning. (Furoxone.)

Furoxone™ furazolidone.*

furuncle (fur'-ung-kl) *n* → boil.

furunculosis (fur-un-kū-lō'-sis) *n* affliction due to boils.

furunculus orientalis (fur-un'-kū-lus ōr'-ē-ent-al'-is) oriental* sore.

fusiform (fū'-si-form) *adj* resembling a spindle.

FVC *abbr* forced* vital capacity. → respiratory function tests.

G

gait *n* manner or style of walking. *ataxic gait* incoordinate or abnormal gait. *cerebellar gait* reeling, staggering, lurching. *scissors gait* legs cross each other in progressing. *spastic gait* stiff, shuffling, the legs being held together. *tabetic gait* foot raised high then brought down suddenly, the whole foot striking the ground.

galactagogue (ga-lak′-ta-gog) *n* agent inducing or increasing the flow of milk.

galactocele (ga-lak′-tō-sēl) *n* a cyst containing milk, or fluid resembling milk.

galactorrhea (gal-ak-to-rē′-à) *n* excessive flow of milk. Usually reserved for abnormal or inappropriate secretion of milk.

galactose (ga-lak′-tōs) *n* monosaccharide found with glucose in lactose or milk sugar. *galactose test* after fasting, patient drinks 40 g of galactose dissolved in 500 ml of water. 5 hours later urine is collected; 2 g or more galactose indicates liver damage.

galactosemia (gal-ak-to-sēm′-ē-à) *n* excess of galactose in blood and other tissues. Normally lactase in small intestine converts lactose into glucose and galactose. In the liver another enzyme system converts galactose into glucose. Galactosemia is result of a congenital enzyme deficiency in this system (two types) and is one cause of mental subnormality—**galactosemic** *adj*.

gall *n* bile.*

gallbladder *n* pear-shaped bag on the undersurface of the liver (→ Figure 18); concentrates and stores bile.

gallipot (gal′-lē-pot) *n* small vessel for lotions.

gallstones *npl* concretions formed within the gallbladder or bile ducts; often multiple and faceted.

galvanocauterization (gal-van-ō-kaw′-tėr-ī-zā′-shun) *n* use of a wire heated by galvanic current to destroy tissue.

gamete (gam′-ēt) *n* a male or female reproductive cell. → ova, spermatazoon.

gammaencephalography (gam′-ma-en-sef-ål-og′-ra-fē) *n* use of small dose of isotope which concentrates in many cerebral tumors to detect presence and extent.

gammaglobulin (gam-mà-glo′-bū-lin) *n* group of plasma proteins (IgA, IgD, IgE, IgG and IgM) with antibody activity, referred to as immunoglobulins*; responsible for humeral aspects of immunity.

ganglion (gang'-lē-on) *n* **1** mass of nerve tissue forming a subsidiary nerve center which receives and sends out nerve fibers, e.g., ganglionic masses forming the sympathetic nervous system. **2** localized cystlike swelling near a tendon, sheath or joint. Contains a clear, transparent, gelatinous or colloid substance; sometimes occurs on back of the wrist due to strain, as excessive practice on the piano. **3** enlargement on the course of a nerve, as is found on receptor nerves at entry to spinal cord. *gasserian ganglion* deeply situated within the skull, on sensory root of fifth cranial nerve; involved in trigeminal neuralgia— **ganglia** *pl*, **ganglionic** *adj*.

ganglionectomy (gang-lē-on-ek'-to-mē) *n* surgical excision of a ganglion.

gangliosidosis (gang-lē-ō-sīd-ō'-sis) *n* → Tay-Sachs' disease.

gangrene (gang'-grēn) *n* death of body tissue, usually result of inadequate blood supply—often with consequent infection—but occasionally due to direct injury (traumatic gangrene) or primary infection. Deficient blood supply may result from pressure on blood vessels (e.g., tourniquets, tight bandages and swelling of a limb); from obstruction within healthy vessels (e.g., arterial embolism, frostbite with blocked capillaries); from spasm of vessel wall (e.g., ergot poisoning); or from thrombosis due to disease of the vessel wall (e.g., arteriosclerosis in arteries, phlebitis in veins). *dry gangrene* blood coagulates in affected tissues, which become shrunken and black. *gas gangrene* wound infection caused by anaerobic organisms of genus *Clostridium,* esp. *C. perfringens (welchii),* a soil microbe often harbored in intestines of man and animals. *moist gangrene* venous drainage is inadequate and tissues are swollen with fluid; associated with infection—**gangrenous** *adj*.

gangrenous stomatitis (gang'-gren-us stō-mà-tī'-tis) → cancrum oris.

Gantanol™ sulfamethoxazole.*

Ganser syndrome (gan'-sėr) (nonsense syndrome) hysterical condition in which approximate answers to questions are given which show that correct answers are known; e.g., a horse may be said to have six legs.

Gantrisin™ sulfisoxazole.*

Garamycin™ gentamicin.*

Gardenal™ phenobarbital.

gargoylism (gár'-goyl-izm) *n* (*syn* Hunter-Hurler syndrome) congenital disorder of mucopolysaccharide metabolism with recessive or sex-linked inheritance. The polysaccharides chondroitin sulfate "B" and hepan sulfate are excreted in urine. Characterized by skeletal abnormalities, coarse features, enlarged liver and spleen, mental subnormality. ACTH is useful.

gasserectomy (gas-sėr-ek'-to-mē) *n* surgical excision of the gasserian ganglion.*

gastralgia (gas-tral'-jà) *n* pain in the stomach.

gastrectomy (gas-trek'-to-mē) *n* removal of a part or all of the stomach. Often involves anastomosis, with loop of jejunum sutured to anterior of transverse colon. Total gastrectomy is carried out only for cancer of the stomach.

gastric (gas'-trik) *adj* pertaining to the stomach. *gastric crisis* → crisis. *gastric influenza* term used when gastrointestinal symptoms predominate. *gastric juice* acidic, and contains two proteolytic enzymes. *gastric suction* intermittent or continuous, to keep stomach empty after some abdominal operations. *gastric ulcer* ulcer in the gastric mucous membrane. Characteristically with pain shortly after eating, occasionally prompting inadequate nutrition and consequent weight loss. H_2 antagonists are drugs of choice. Can be complicated by hematemesis or perforation, constituting an abdominal emergency.

gastrin (gas'-trin) *n* hormone secreted by the gastric mucosa on entry of food, causing greater flow of gastric juice.

gastritis (gas-trī'-tis) *n* inflammation of the stomach, esp. the mucous membrane lining.

gastrocnemius (gas-trōk-nē'-mē-us) *n* large two-headed muscle of the calf (→ Figures 4, 5).

gastrocolic (gas-trō-kol'-ik) *adj* pertaining to stomach and colon.

gastroduodenal (gas-trō-dū-o-dēn'-ál) *adj* pertaining to stomach and duodenum.

gastroduodenostomy (gas-trō-dū-ō-dēn-os'-to-mē) *n* surgical anastomosis* between stomach and duodenum.

gastrodynia (gas-trō-dī'-nē-á) *n* pain in the stomach.

gastroenteritis (gas-trō-en-tér-ī'-tis) *n* inflammation of mucous membranes of the stomach and small intestine; although sometimes the result of dietetic error, cause is usually microbiological. Infant gastroenteritis is usually caused by viruses, esp. rotavirus, although enteropathic *Escherichia coli* is still a common cause. Infection spread via fecal-oral route, directly or indirectly.

gastroenterology (gas-trō-en-tér-ol'-o-jē) *n* study of the digestive tract, including liver, biliary tract and pancreas and their diseases—**gastroenterological** *adj*.

gastroenteropathy (gas-trō-en-tér-op'-a-thē) *n* disease of the stomach and intestine—**gastroenteropathic** *adj*.

gastroenteroscope (gas-trō-en'-tér-o-skōp) *n* endoscope* for visualization of stomach and intestine—**gastroenteroscopic** *adj*.

gastroenterostomy (gas-trō-en-tér-os'-to-mē) *n* surgical anastomosis* between the stomach and small intestine.

gastroesophageal (gas'-trō-ē-sof-á-jē'-ál) *adj* pertaining to the stomach and esophagus, as gastric reflux in heartburn.

gastroesophagostomy (gas'-trō-ē-sof-á-gos'-to-mē) *n* operation in which esophagus is joined to the stomach to bypass the natural juncture.

Gastrografin™ contrast medium composed of sodium and meglumine diatrizoate. Can be used early in patients with hematemesis. Its detergent and purgative effects are used in meconium ileus—given as an enema.

gastrointestinal (gas-trō-in-tes'-tin-ál) *adj* pertaining to stomach and intestine.

gastrojejunostomy (gas-trō-je-jūn-os'to-mē) *n* surgical anastomosis* between stomach and jejunum.

gastropathy (gas-trop'-a-thē) *n* any disease of the stomach.

gastropexy (gas'-trō-peks-ē) *n* surgical fixation of a displaced stomach.

gastrophrenic (gas-trō-fren'-ik) *adj* pertaining to the stomach and diaphragm.

gastroplasty (gas'-trō-plas-tē) *n* any plastic operation on the stomach, as for reconstruction of the cardiac orifice of the stomach, where fibrosis prevents replacement of the stomach below the diaphragm in cases of hiatus hernia.

gastroplication (gas-trō-plik-ā'-shun) *n* operation to cure dilated stomach by pleating the wall.

gastroptosis (gas-trop-tō'-sis) *n* downward displacement of the stomach.

gastropylorectomy (gas-trō-pī-lōr-ek'-to-mē) *n* excision of the pyloric end of the stomach.

gastroschisis (gas-trō-skiz'-is) *n* congenital incomplete closure of abdominal wall with consequent protrusion of the viscera uncovered by peritoneum.

gastroscope (gas'-trō-skōp) *n* → endoscope—**gastroscopic** *adj*, **gastroscopy** *n*.

gastrostomy (gas-tros'-to-mē) *n* surgically established fistula between the stomach and exterior abdominal wall; usually for artificial feeding.

gastrotomy (gas-trot'-o-mē) *n* incision into the stomach, as to remove a foreign body, to secure a bleeding blood vessel, or to approach the esophagus from below to pull down a tube through a constricting growth.

gastrula (gas'-trū-lá) *n* next stage after blastula in embryonic development.

Gaucher's disease (go'-shāz) rare familial disorder, mainly in Jewish children, characterized by a disordered lipoid metabolism (lipid reticulosis) and usually accompanied by very marked enlargement of the spleen. Diagnosis follows sternal marrow puncture and finding of typical Gaucher cells (distended with lipoid).

gavage feeding (ga-vazh') by custom refers to introducing fluid and nutrients into the stomach either by an esophageal tube passed orally or by a fine-bore nasogastric tube.

gemellus muscles (jem-el'-us) → Figure 5.

gene a specific unit, located at a specific place (locus) along a particular chromosome. Genes determine specific physical traits. Different forms of genes (alleles) may act as dominant, requiring only one (of the pair at every chromosomal locus) to express its encoded trait, or recessive, requiring the presence of two like alleles for expression. → heterozygous, homozygous.

generative (jen'-ėr-ȧ-tiv) *adj* pertaining to reproduction.

generic *adj* pertaining to a genus. *generic name* in reference to a drug, the distinctive, identifying name, not proprietary and not protected by a trademark.

genetic *adj* that which pertains to heredity. For example, of disorders arising from abnormalities of genetic material. → congenital.

genetic code information for all growth and function of an organism as determined by the precise ordering of nucleotide base pairs along strands of the DNA molecule.

genital *adj* pertaining to the organs of generation. *genital herpes* → herpes.

genitalia (jen-i-tā'-lē-ȧ) *n* external organs of generation.

genitourinary (jen-i-tō-ūr'-i-nār-ē) *adj* pertaining to the reproductive and urinary organs.

genome (jen'-ōm) *n* the basic set of chromosomes,* with the genes contained therein, equivalent to the sum total of gene types possessed by different organisms of a species.

genotype (jēn'-ō-tīp) *n* total genetic information encoded in chromosomes* of an individual (as opposed to the phenotype*). Also, the genetic constitution of an individual at a particular locus, namely the alleles* present at that locus.

gentamicin (jen-tȧ-mī'-sin) *n* antibiotic produced by *Micromonospora purpurea*. Antibacterial, esp. against *Pseudomonas* and staphylococci resistant to other antibiotics. Given intramuscularly and as eye and ear drops. Ototoxic and dangerous in renal failure. (Garamycin.)

gentian violet → crystal violet.

genu (jen'-ū) *n* the knee.

genu valgum (jen'-ū val'-gum) (knock-knee) abnormal incurving of legs, with a gap between the feet when the knees are in contact.

genu varum (jen'-ū vār'-um) (bowleg) abnormal outward curving of the legs resulting in separation of the knees.

Geopen™ carbenicillin.*

geophagia (jē-ō-fā'-jȧ) *n* the habit of eating clay or earth.

geriatrics (jer-ē-a'-triks) *n* branch of medical science dealing with old age and its diseases, and with the medical care and nursing required by "geriatric" patients—**geriatrician** *n*.

German measles → rubella.

gerontology (jer-on-tol′-o-jē) *n* scientific study of aging—**gerontological** *adj*.

gestation (jes-tā′-shun) *n* → pregnancy—**gestational** *adj*.

GFR *abbr* glomerular* filtration rate.

GH *abbr* growth hormone.

Ghon focus (gon) → primary complex.

giant cell arteritis → arteritis.

giardiasis (jē-ar-dī′-à-sis) *n* (*syn* lambliasis) infection with the flagellate *Giardia intestinalis*. Often symptomless, esp. in adults. Can cause diarrhea with steatorrhea. Treatment is quinacrine or metronidazole orally.

gigantism (jī-gan′-tizm) *n* an abnormal overgrowth, esp. in height. May be associated with anterior pituitary tumor if tumor develops before fusion of the epiphyses. Due to excess of growth hormone.

gingiva (jin′-ji-vȧ) *n* the gum; vascular tissue surrounding the necks of erupted teeth—**gingival** *adj*.

gingivectomy (jin-ji-vek′-to-mē) *n* excision of a portion of the gum, usually for pyorrhea.

gingivitis (jin-ji-vī′-tis) *n* inflammation of the gum or gingiva usually caused by irritation from dental plaque and calculus. Can occur with systemic use of some drugs, e.g., dilantin, and may be associated with pregnancy, due to hormone changes.

girdle *n* usually a bony structure of oval shape, as the shoulder and pelvic girdles.

gland *n* organ or structure capable of making an internal or external secretion. *lymphatic gland* (node) does not secrete, but is concerned with filtration of the lymph. → endocrine, exocrine—**glandular** *adj*.

glanders (glan′-dėrz) *n* contagious, febrile, ulcerative disease communicable from horses, mules and asses to man.

glandular fever → infectious mononucleosis.

glans (glanz) *n* the bulbous termination of the clitoris and penis. (→ Figure 16).

glaucoma (glaw-kō′-mȧ) *n* a condition in which intraocular pressure is raised. In the acute stage pain is severe; can result in blindness—**glaucomatous** *adj*.

glenohumeral (glē-nō-hū′-mėr-ȧl) *adj* pertaining to the glenoid cavity of scapula and the humerus.

glenoid (glē′-noyd) *n* a cavity on the scapula* into which the head of the humerus* fits to form the shoulder joint.

glia (glē′-à) *n* → neuroglia—**glial** *adj*.

glioblastoma multiforme (glē-o-blas-tō′-mȧ mul′-ti-form) a highly malignant brain tumor.

glioma (glē-ō'-mà) *n* a malignant growth which does not give rise to secondary deposits; arises from neuroglia. One form, occurring in the retina, is hereditary—**gliomata** *pl*.

gliomyoma (glē-ō-mī-ō'-mà) *n* tumor of nerve and muscle tissue—**gliomy-** omata *pl*.

glipizide (glip'-i-zīd) *n* orally active antidiabetic drug, a sulfonylurea. → tolbutamide. (Glucotrol.)

globin (glō'-bin) *n* protein which combines with hematin to form hemoglobin.

globulin (glob'-ū-lin) *n* the fraction of serum or plasma containing the immunoglobulins* A, D, E, G and M.

globulinuria (glob-ū-lin-ūr'-ē-à) *n* presence of globulin in urine.

globus hystericus (glōb'-us his-tėr'-i-kus) subjective feeling of a lump in the throat. Can also include difficulty in swallowing and is due to tension of muscles of deglutition. Occurs in hysteria, anxiety states and depression. Sometimes follows slight trauma to throat, e.g., scratch by foreign body.

globus pallidus (glōb'us pal'-i-dus) literally pale globe; situated deep within the cerebral hemispheres, lateral to the thalamus.

glomerular filtration rate (GFR) rate of filtration from blood in the glomerulus of renal capillaries to the fluid in Bowman's capsule. Usually 120 ml per min; a fine index of renal function.

glomerulitis (glom-ėr-ū-lī'-tis) *n* inflammation of the glomeruli, usually of the kidney. Use of electron microscopes and fluorescent staining of biopsy specimens has improved diagnosis and knowledge of the condition.

glomerulonephritis (glom-ėr-ū-lō-nef-rī'-tis) *n* term for several diseases having in common damage to the glomeruli of the renal cortex mediated through immune mechanisms. Proteinuria and microscopic hematuria are features but no bacteria appear in urine.

glomerulosclerosis (glom-ėr'-ū-lō-sklėr-ō'-sis) *n* fibrosis of the glomeruli of the kidney, usually the result of inflammation. *intercapillary glomerulosclerosis* common pathological finding in diabetics—**glomerulosclerotic** *adj*.

glomerulus (glom-ėr'-ū-lus) *n* coil of minute arterial capillaries held together by scanty connective tissue. It invaginates the entrance of the uriniferous tubules in the kidney cortex—**glomerular** *adj*, **glomeruli** *pl*.

glossa (glos'-sà) *n* the tongue—**glossal** *adj*.

glossectomy (glos-sek'-to-mē) *n* excision of the tongue.

glossitis (glos-ī'-tis) *n* inflammation of the tongue.

glossodynia (glos-ō-dī'-nē-à) *n* a painful tongue, but without visible change.

glossopharyngeal (glos-ō-fār-in-jē'-àl) *adj* pertaining to tongue and pharynx; of the ninth pair of the 12 pairs of cranial nerves arising directly from the brain.

glossoplegia (glos-ō-plē'-jȧ) *n* paralysis of the tongue.

glottis (glot'-tis) *n* that part of the larynx associated with voice production—**glottic** *adj*.

glucagon (gloo'-kȧ-gon) *n* hormone produced in alpha cells of pancreatic islets of Langerhans. Causes breakdown of glycogen into glucose, thus preventing blood sugar from falling too low during fasting. Can now be obtained commercially from the pancreas of animals. Given to accelerate breakdown of glycogen in the liver and raise blood sugar rapidly. As it is a polypeptide hormone, it must be given by injection.

glucocorticoid (gloo-kō-kōr'-ti-koyd) *n* any steroid hormone which promotes gluconeogenesis (i.e., formation of glucose and glycogen from protein) and which antagonizes action of insulin. Occurring naturally in the adrenal cortex as cortisone and hydrocortisone, and produced synthetically as, for example, prednisone and prednisolone.

glucogenesis (gloo-kō-jen'-e-sis) *n* production of glucose.

gluconeogenesis (gloo-kō-nē'-ō-jen'-e-sis) *n* (*syn* glyconeogenesis) formation of sugar from protein or fat when there is lack of available carbohydrate.

glucose (gloo'-kōs) *n* dextrose or grape sugar. A monosaccharide. The form in which carbohydrates are absorbed through the intestinal tract and circulated in blood. Stored as glycogen* in the liver. *glucose tolerance test* after a period of fasting, a measured quantity of glucose is taken orally; thereafter blood and urine samples are tested for glucose at intervals. Higher than normal levels are indicative of diabetes mellitus.

Glucotrol™ glipzide.*

glucuronic acid (gloo-kū-ron'-ik) an acid which acts on bilirubin* to form conjugate bilirubin.

glue ear accumulation of a gluelike substance in the middle ear which bulges the ear drum and impairs hearing.

glutaminase (gloo-tam'-in-ās) *n* an amino acid-degrading enzyme, being used in treatment of cancer.

gluteal (gloo'-tē-ȧl) *adj* pertaining to the buttocks.* → Figure 5.

gluten (gloo'-ten) *n* protein constituent of wheat flour insoluble in water but an essential component of the elastic "dough." It is not tolerated in celiac disease.*

gluten-induced enteropathy → celiac.

glutethimide (gloo-teth'-i-mīd) *n* hypnotic of medium action. Useful when an alternative to barbiturates is required. (Doriglute.)

gluteus muscles (gloo'-tē-us) → Figures 4,5.

glycine (glī'-sēn) *n* a nonessential amino* acid.

glycinuria (glī-sin-ūr'-ē-à) *n* excretion of glycine* in urine. Associated with mental subnormality.

glycogen (glī'-kō-jen) *n* main carbohydrate storage compound in animals; glucose molecules are linked in branched chains. *glycogen storage disease* metabolic, recessively inherited condition caused by various enzyme deficiencies—types 1–13 are now recognized. The liver becomes large and fatty due to excessive glycogen deposits. Hypoglycemia is a major problem. Body tends to metabolize fat rather than glucose, and ketosis and acidosis are prevalent.

glycogenase (glī-ko'-jen-āz) *n* enzyme necessary for conversion of glycogen into glucose.

glycogenesis (glī-kō-jen'-es-is) *n* glycogen formation from blood glucose.

glycogenolysis (glī-kō-jen-ol'-is-is) *n* breakdown of glycogen to glucose.

glycogenosis (glī-kō-jen-os'-is) *n* metabolic disorder leading to increased storage of glycogen.* Leads to glycogen myopathy.

glycolysis (glī-kol'-is-is) *n* hydrolysis of sugar in the body—**glycolytic** *adj.*

glyconeogenesis (glī-kō-nē-ō-jen'-es-is) → gluconeogenesis.*

glycopyrrolate (glī-kō-pī'-rol-āt) *n* synthetic, atropinelike drug; does not cause such extensive tachycardia as atropine.* (Robinul.)

glycosides (glī'-kō-sīdz) *npl* natural substances composed of a sugar with another compound. Nonsugar fragment is termed an "aglycone," and is sometimes of therapeutic value. Digoxin is a familiar example of a glycoside.

glycosuria (glī-kō-sū'-rē-à) *n* presence of large amounts of sugar in urine.

glycyrrhiza (glis-i-rī'-zà) *n* licorice root, demulcent, slightly laxative, expectorant and used as flavoring agent. Results in an increase in extracellular fluid, retention of sodium and increased excretion of potassium.

gnathalgia (nath-al'-jà) *n* pain in the jaw.

gnathoplasty (nath'-ō-plas-tē) *n* plastic surgery of the jaw.

goblet cells special secreting cells, shaped like a goblet, found in mucous membranes.

Goeckerman regime (gā'-kèr-man) a treatment for psoriasis: exposure to ultraviolet light alternating with application of a tar paste.

goiter (goy'-tèr) *n* an enlargement of the thyroid gland. In *simple goiter* patient does not show any signs of excessive thyroid activity. In *toxic goiter* enlarged gland secretes excess of thyroid hormone. Patient is nervous, loses weight and often has palpitations and exophthalmos. → colloid.

goitrogens (goy'-trō-jens) *npl* agents causing goiter. Some occur in plants, e.g., turnip, cabbage, brussels sprouts and peanuts.

golden eye ointment → mercuric oxide.

gold injection → aurothiomalate.

gonad (gō′-nad) *n* a male or female sex gland. → ovary, testis—**gonadal** *adj*.

gonadotropic (gō-nad-ō-trō′-pik) *adj* having an affinity for, or influence on, the gonads.

gonadotropin (gō-nad-ō-trō′-pin) *n* any gonad-stimulating hormone. → follicle stimulating hormone, human chorionic gonadotropin test, luteotropin.

gonioscopy (gō-nē-os′-ko-pē) *n* measuring angle of anterior chamber of eye with a gonioscope.

goniotomy (gō-nē-ot′-o-mē) *n* operation for glaucoma, incision through anterior chamber angle to the canal of Schlemm.

gonococcal complement fixation test (go-nō-kok′-al) specific serological test for diagnosis of gonorrhea.*

Gonococcus (gon-ō-kok′-us) *n* Gram-negative diplococcus (*Neisseria gonorrhea*), causative organism of gonorrhea. A strict parasite; occurs characteristically inside polymorphonuclear leukocytes in tissues—**gonococci** *pl*, **gonococcal** *adj*.

gonorrhea (gon-ōr-rē′-à) *n* sexually-transmitted disease in adults. In children infection is accidental, e.g., gonococcal ophthalmia of the newborn. Chief manifestations in males is purulent urethritis with dysuria, in females, urethritis, endocervicitis and salpingitis which may be symptomless. Incubation period is usually 2-5 days. *gonorrheal arthritis* a metastatic manifestation of gonorrhea. *gonorrheal ophthalmia* form of ophthalmia neonatorum—**gonorrheal** *adj*.

Goodpasture's syndrome association of hemorrhagic lung disorder with glomerulonephritis.

goserelin *n* analog of LHRH (luteinizing hormone releasing hormone); used in palliative treatment of prostate cancer. (Zoladex.)

gout *n* metabolic disorder in which sodium biurate is deposited in cartilages of joints, ears, and elsewhere. Big toe is classically involved, becoming acutely painful and swollen. Drugs which increase excretion of urates have largely controlled the disease.

graafian follicle (graf′-ē-àn) minute vesicles contained in the stroma of an ovary,* each holding a single ovum. When an ovum is extruded from a graafian follicle each month, the corpus luteum is formed under the influence of luteotropin from the anterior pituitary gland. If fertilization occurs, the corpus luteum persists for 12 weeks; if not, it only persists for 12–14 days.

gracilis muscle (gra-sil′-lis) → Figures 4, 5.

graft *n* tissue or organ transplanted to another part of the same animal (autograft), to another animal of the same species (homograft), or to another animal of a different species (heterograft).

gramicidin (gram-is'-i-din) *n* mixture of antibiotic substances obtained from tyrothricin.* Too toxic for systemic use, but valuable for topical application when local antibiotic therapy is required.

Gram's stain bacteriological stain for differentiation of microorganisms. Those retaining the blue dye are Gram-positive (+), those unaffected are Gram-negative (−).

grand mal (grahn' mahl) major epilepsy. → epilepsy.

granulation *n* outgrowth of new capillaries and connective tissue cells from the surface of an open wound. *granulation tissue* young, soft tissue so formed— **granulate** *vi*.

granulocyte (gran'-ū-lō-sīt) *n* a cell containing granules in its cytoplasm, as polymorphonuclear leukocytes, which have neutrophil, eosinophil or basophil granules.

granulocytopenia (gran'-ū-lō-sī-tō-pē'-nē-á) *n* decrease of granulocytes* (polymorphs) not sufficient to warrant the term agranulocytosis.*

granuloma (gran-ū-lō'-má) *n* tumor formed of granulation tissue. *granuloma* venereum lymphogranuloma* inguinale.

gravel *n* sandy deposit which,if present in bladder, may be passed with the urine.

Graves' disease (grāvz) → thyrotoxicosis.

gravid (gra'-vid) *adj* pregnant; carrying fertilized eggs or a fetus.

Gravindex test (grav'-in-deks) an immunological test for pregnancy.

Grawitz tumor (gra'-vits) → hypernephroma.

green monkey disease → Marburg disease.

Griffith's types (grif'-iths) antigenic subdivisions of Lancefield* group A streptococci by virtue of their characteristic M protein antigens.

grinder's asthma a popular name for silicosis* arising from inhalation of metallic dust.

grip *n* abdominal colic.

Grisactin™ griseofulvin.*

griseofulvin (gris-ē-ō-ful'-vin) *n* oral fungicide, useful in ringworm.* (Fulvicin, Grisactin.)

groin *n* junction of the thigh with the abdomen.

grommet *n* a ventilation tube inserted into the tympanic membrane. Frequently used in treatment of glue* ear. → myringotomy.

growth hormone (GH), growth hormone test (GHT) there is a reciprocal relationship between growth hormone (secreted by the pituitary* gland) and blood glucose. Blood is therefore estimated for GH during a standard 50 g oral glucose tolerance test. In acromegaly, not only is resting level of GH higher, but it does not show normal suppression with glucose.

guanethidine (gwan-eth'-i-dēn) *n* hypotensive, sympathetic blocking agent. Gives sustained reduction of intraocular pressure in glaucoma. Applied locally to block the sympathetic fibers to the eye in exophthalmos. (Ismelin.)

Guillain-Barré syndrome (gē-yan' bar-rā') (*syn* acute polyneuritis) polyneuritis accompanied by progressive muscular weakness.

guillotine (gil'-e-tēn) *n* surgical instrument for excision of the tonsils.

Guinea worm (gin'-ē) → *Dracunculus* * *medinensis*.

gullet *n* the esophagus.*

gumboil *n* lay term for an abscess of gum tissue and periosteum (dento-alveolar abscess); usually very painful.

gumma (gum'-mȧ) *n* localized area of vascular granulation tissue which develops in later stages (tertiary) of syphilis. Obstruction to blood supply results in necrosis, and gummata near a surface of the body tend to break down, forming chronic ulcers—**gummata** *pl*.

gut *n* the intestines, large and small. *gut decontamination* use of nonabsorbable antibiotics to suppress growth of microorganisms, to prevent endogenous infection in patients undergoing bowel surgery or those who are neutropenic or immunocompromised.

gynecography (gī-ne-cog'-rȧ-fē) *n* radiological visualization of internal female genitalia after pneumoperitoneum—**gynecographical** *adj*.

gynecoid (gī'-ne-koyd) *adj* resembling a woman. *gynecoid pelvis* normal-shaped female pelvis.

gynecology (gī-ne-kol'-o-jē) *n* science dealing with the diseases of the female reproductive system—**gynecological** *adj*, **gynecologist** *n*.

gynecomastia (gī-ne-kō-mas'-tē-ȧ) *n* enlargement of the male mammary gland.

gyrectomy (jī-rek'-to-mē) *n* surgical removal of a gyrus.*

gyrus (jī'-rus) *n* a convoluted portion of cerebral cortex.

H

habituation *n* means of acquiring or developing a pattern of behavior as a habit; often used in a negative sense. → drug dependence.

Haemophilus (hē-mof´-il-us) *n* genus of bacteria. Small Gram-negative rods with great variation in shape (pleomorphism). Strict parasites; accessory substances present in blood are usually necessary for growth. *H. aegyptius* causes a form of acute infectious conjunctivitis. *H. ducreyi* causes chancroid. *H. influenzae* (once mistakenly thought to cause flu) causes respiratory infections, influenza meningitis, conjunctivitis and septicemia. *H. pertussis* (now *Bordetella pertussis*) causes whooping cough.

hair *n* threadlike appendage present on all parts of human skin except palms, soles, lips, glans penis and that surrounding the terminal phalanges. The broken-off stump found at the periphery of spreading bald patches in alopecia areata is called an exclamation-mark hair. *hair bulb* → Figure 12. *hair follicle* sheath in which a hair grows. *hair root* → Figure 12. *hair shaft* → Figure 12.

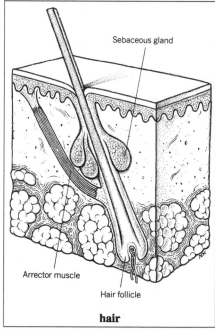

Sebaceous gland

Arrector muscle

Hair follicle

hair

Haldol™ haloperidol.*

halibut liver oil rich source of vitamins* A and D. Smaller dose required makes it more acceptable than cod liver oil.

halitosis (hal-i-tō´-sis) *n* foul-smelling breath.

hallucination (hal-lū-sin-ā′-shun) *n* a false perception occurring without any true sensory stimulus. Common symptom in severe psychoses including schizophrenia, paraphrenia and confusional states. Also common in delirium, during toxic states and following head injuries.

hallucinogen (hal-lū-sin′-ō-jen) *n* drug with ability to produce hallucinations,* as mescaline or LSD.

hallucinosis (hal-lū-sin-ō′-sis) *n* usually a subacute delirious state with auditory and visual hallucinations, but without mania or loss of mental faculty.

hallux (hal′-luks) *n* the great toe. *hallus valgus* → bunion. *hallux varus* displacement toward the other foot. *hallux rigidus* ankylosis of the metatarsophalangeal articulation caused by osteoarthritis.

haloperidol (hal-ō-pėr′-i-dol) *n* psychotropic agent used in treatment of schizophrenia and other psychotic disorders for its tranquilizing properties. Given orally or by injection. (Haldol.)

halothane (hal′-ō-thān) *n* clear colorless liquid used as an inhalation anesthetic. Non-explosive and nonflammable in all circumstances; odor is not unpleasant. (Fluothane.)

hammer toe permanent hyperextension of the first phalanx and flexion of second and third phalanges.

Hand-Schüller-Christian disease (hand shul′-ėr kris′-chan) rare condition usually manifesting in early childhood, with histiocytic granulomatous lesions affecting many tissues. Regarded as a form of histiocytosis X. Cause unknown and course relatively benign.

Hansen's bacillus → leprosy.

Hansen's disease synonym, often preferred, for leprosy.*

hantavirus (han′-tà-vī-rus) *n.* virus causing severe respiratory inflammation, sometimes fatal. Spread by contact with feces of certain field rodents, esp. of deer mice.

H₂ antagonist agent with selective action against H_2 histamine receptors and thereby decreases, for example, secretion of gastric juice.

haploid (hap′-loyd) *adj* refers to the chromosome complement of mature gametes (eggs and sperm) following meiosis (reduction division). This set represents the basic complement of 23 chromosomes in man. Its normal multiple is diploid, but abnormally three or more chromosome sets can be found (triploid, tetraploid).

harelip *n* congenital defect in the lip; a fissure extending from the margin of the lip to the nostril; may be single or double, and is often associated with cleft* palate.

Hartmann's solution (hàrt′-manz) electrolyte replacement solution. Contains sodium lactate and chloride, potassium chloride and calcium chloride.

Hartnup disease (hart'-nup) an inborn error of protein metabolism, associated with diffuse psychiatric symptoms or mild mental subnormality. It can be treated with nicotinamide and neomycin.

Hashimoto's disease (hash-ē-mō'-tōz) enlarged thyroid gland occurring in middle-aged females, and producing mild hypothyroidism. Result of sensitization of patient to her own thyroid protein, thyroglobulin.

haustration (haws-trā'-shun) *n* sacculation,* as of the colon—**haustrum** *sing*, **haustra** *pl*.

hay fever form of allergic rhinitis in which attacks of catarrh of the conjunctiva, nose and throat are precipitated by exposure to pollen.

Haygarth's nodes (hā'-gárths) swelling of joints sometimes seen in finger joints of patients suffering from arthritis.

HCG *abbr* human* chorionic gonadotropin.

healing *n* natural process of cure or repair of the tissues. *healing by first intention* when the edges of a clean wound are accurately held together, healing occurs with the minimum of scarring and deformity. *healing by second intention* when the edges of a wound are not held together, the gap is filled by granulation tissue before epithelium can grow over the wound—**heal** *vt, vi*.

health *n* World Health Organization definition, "Health is a state of complete physical, mental and social well-being and not merely the absence of disease or infirmity."

Health Maintenance Organization (HMO) a group medical practice that offers prepaid health care with an emphasis on complete care, including prevention.

heart *n* the hollow muscular organ which pumps blood round the body; situated

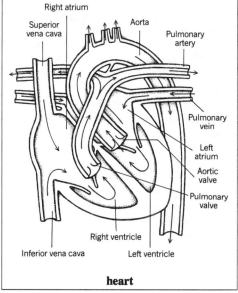

Right atrium
Superior vena cava
Aorta
Pulmonary artery
Pulmonary vein
Left atrium
Aortic valve
Pulmonary valve
Right ventricle
Inferior vena cava
Left ventricle

heart

behind the sternum, lying obliquely between the two lungs (→ Figure 6). *heart transplant* surgical transplantation of a heart from a suitable donor who has recently died. *heart block* partial or complete inhibition of conduction of electrical impulse from the atrium to the ventricle of the heart. Cause may be organic lesion or functional disturbance. In its mildest form, only detected electrocardiographically; in full manifestation, ventricles beat at their own slow intrinsic rate uninfluenced by the atria.

heartburn *n* → pyrosis.

heart-lung machine machine by means of which blood can be removed from a vein for oxygenation, after which it is returned to the vein.

heat exhaustion collapse, with or without loss of consciousness, suffered in conditions of heat and high humidity: largely resulting from loss of fluid and salt by sweating. If the surrounding air becomes saturated, heatstroke will ensue.

heatstroke *n* (*syn* sunstroke) final stage in heat exhaustion. When the body is unable to lose heat, hyperpyrexia occurs and death may ensue.

heavy chain diseases encompassing term for conditions in which certain immunoglobulins* are produced in abnormal forms. Can occur in association with several autoimmune diseases (as rheumatoid arthritis, SLE, myasthenia gravis) and tuberculosis. May enable serious bacterial infection.

hebephrenia (hē-be-frē′-nē-à) *n* common type of schizophrenia* characterized by general disintegration of the personality. Onset is sudden and usually occurs in the teenage years. Prognosis tends to be unfavorable—**hebephrenic** *adj*.

Heberden's disease (he′-bėr-denz) angina* pectoris. *Heberden's nodes* small osseous swellings at terminal phalangeal joints occurring in many types of arthritis.

Hegar's sign (hā′-gàrz) marked softening of the cervix in early pregnancy.

Heimlich maneuver (hīm′-lik) first-aid measure to dislodge a foreign body (e.g., food) obstructing the glottis, performed by holding the patient from behind and jerking the operator's clenched fists into the victim's epigastrium.

Heinz body (Hīnz) refractile, irregularly shaped body present in red blood cells in some hemoglobinopathies.

helix (hē′-liks) *n* outer edge of the external ear. → Figure 13. *double helix* double-stranded structure of the DNA molecule, consisting of two strands composed of alternating sugar-phosphate units, joined at intervals by four nitrogen bases: adenine, guanine, thymine and cytosine.

helminthagogue (hel-minth′-à-gog) *n* an anthelmintic.*

helminthiasis (hel-min-thī′-à-sis) *n* condition arising from infestation with worms.

helminthology (hel-min-thol′-o-jē) *n* study of parasitic worms.

hemagglutination tests for pregnancy are all based on the same principle and can be done rapidly. If urine from a pregnant woman contains certain antisera, it will prevent hemagglutination occurring between red cells pretreated with human chorionic gonadotropin, which confirms pregnancy.

hemangioma (hē-man-jē-ō'-mà) *n* malformation or proliferation of blood vessels which may occur in any part of the body—**hemangiomata** *pl*.

hemarthrosis (hē-mȧr-thrō'-sis) *n* presence of blood in a joint cavity—**hem**arthroses *pl*.

hematemesis (hē-mȧ-te-mē'-sis) *n* vomiting of blood, which may be bright red, if of recent origin, or of "coffee ground" appearance due to the action of gastric juice.

hematin (hē'-mȧ-tin) *n* an iron-containing constituent of hemoglobin. May crystallize in kidney tubules when there is excessive hemolysis.

hematinic (hē-mȧ-tin'-ik) *adj* any substance required for production of the red blood cell and its constituents.

hematite (hē'-mȧ-tīt) *n* (*syn* miner's lung) a form of silicosis* occurring in the hematite (iron ore) industry.

hematocolpos (hēm-ȧ-tō-kol'-pos) *n* retained blood in the vagina. → cryptomenorrhea.

hematocrit (hē-mȧt'-ō-krit) *n* proportion by volume of red blood cells (erythrocytes) in blood; part of complete blood* count. → Appendix.

hematogenous (hē-mȧ-toj'-en-us) *adj* **1** concerned with formation of blood. **2** carried by the blood stream.

hematology (hē-mȧ-tol'-o-je) *n* science dealing with formation, composition, functions and diseases of the blood—**hematological** *adj*.

hematoma (hē'-mȧ-tō'-mȧ) *n* a swelling filled with blood—**hematomata** *pl*.

hematometra (hē-mȧ-to-mē'-trȧ) *n* accumulation of blood (or menstrual fluid) in the uterus.

hematopoiesis (hē-mȧ-to-poy-ē'-sis) *n* → hemopoiesis.

hematoporphyrin test (hē-mȧ-tō-pōr'-fir-in) 1–3 h after injection, hematoporphyrin localizes in rapidly multiplying cells and fluoresces under ultraviolet light, facilitating detection of the extent of malignant or precancerous tissue.

hematosalpinx (hē-mȧ-tō-sal'-pinks) *n* (*syn* hemosalpinx) blood in the fallopian tube.

hematozoa (hē-mȧ-tō-zō'-ȧ) *n* parasites living in the blood—**hematozoon** *sing*.

hematuria (hē-mȧ-tū'-rē-ȧ) *n* blood in the urine; it may be from the kidneys, one or both ureters, the bladder or the urethra—**hematuric** *adj*.

hemeralopia (he-mȧr-ȧ-lō'-pē-ȧ) *n* defective vision in a bright light. Term has been incorrectly used for night* blindness.

hemianopia (hem-ē-à-nōp′-ē-à) *n* blindness in one half of the visual field of one or both eyes.

hemiatrophy (hem-ē-at′-rof-ē) *n* atrophy of one half or one side. *hemiatrophy facialis* a congenital condition or a manifestation of scleroderma* in which the structures on one side of the face are shrunken.

hemichorea (hem-ē-kōr-ē′-à) *n* choreiform movements limited to one side of the body. → chorea.

hemicolectomy (hem-ē-kō-lek′-to-mē) *n* removal of approximately half the colon.

hemicrania (hem-ē-krān′-ē-à) *n* unilateral headache, as in migraine.

hemidiaphoresis (hem-ē-dī-à-fōr-ē′-sis) *n* unilateral sweating of the body.

hemiglossectomy (hem-ē-glos-sek′-to-mē) *n* removal of approximately half the tongue.

hemiparesis (hem-ē-par-ē′-sis) *n* slight paralysis or weakness of one half of face or body.

hemiplegia (hem-ē-plē′-jà) *n* paralysis of one side of the body, usually resulting from cerebrovascular accident on the opposite side—**hemiplegic** *adj*.

hemispherectomy (hem-ē-sfèr-ek′-to-mē) *n* surgical removal of a cerebral hemisphere in the treatment of epilepsy. It may be either subtotal or total.

hemochromatosis (hē-mō-krō-mà-tō′-sis) *n* (*syn* bronzed diabetes) a congenital error in iron metabolism with increased iron deposition in tissues, resulting in brown pigmentation of the skin and cirrhosis of the liver—**hemochromatotic** *adj*.

hemoconcentration (hē-mō-kon-sen-trā′-shun) *n* relative increase of volume of red blood cells to volume of plasma, usually due to loss of the latter.

hemocytometer (hē-mō-sī-tom′-e-tèr) *n* instrument for measuring the number of blood corpuscles.

hemodialysis (hē-mō-dī-al′-i-sis) *n* removal of toxic solutes and excess fluid from the blood by dialysis*; performed through apparatus with a semipermeable membrane between the blood and a rinsing solution, called dialysate.* Necessary procedure in the end stage of renal failure (irreversible) or in acute renal failure (reversible).

hemodynamics (hē-mō-dī-nam′-iks) *npl* forces involved in circulating blood round the body.

hemofiltration (hē-mō-fil-trā′-shun) *n* mechanically similar to hemodialysis.* Cardiac output drives blood through a small, highly permeable filter, permitting separation of fluid and solutes. This hemofiltrate is measured, discarded, and replaced with an isotonic solution. When large amounts of hemofiltrate are removed, hemodialysis is unnecessary. Particularly useful for patients in acute renal failure, in congestive heart failure with diuretic-resistant overhydration and in hypernatremia resistant to drugs.

hemoglobin (hē'-mō-glō'-bin) *n* the respiratory pigment in the red blood corpuscles; composed of an iron-containing substance called "haem," combined with globin. Has the reversible property of combining with and releasing oxygen. At birth 45–90% of hemoglobin is of fetal type, which is replaced by adult hemoglobin by the end of the first year of life. → oxyhemoglobin.

hemoglobinemia (hē'-mō-glō-bin-ē'-mē-à) *n* unusually high hemoglobin level in the blood—**hemoglobinemic** *adj*.

hemoglobinometer (hē'-mō-glō-bin-om'-e-tėr) *n* instrument for estimating the percentage of hemoglobin in the blood.

hemoglobinopathy (hē'-mō-glō-bin-op'-ath-ē) *n* abnormality of the hemoglobin—**hemoglobinopathic** *adj*.

hemoglobinuria (hē'-mō-glō-bin-ū'-rē-à) *n* hemoglobin in the urine—**hemoglobinuric** *adj*.

hemolysin (hē-mō-lī'-sin) *n* an agent which causes disintegration of erythrocytes. → immunoglobulins.

hemolysis (hē-mol'-is-is) *n* disintegration of red blood cells, with liberation of contained hemoglobin—**hemolytic** *adj*.

hemolytic disease of the newborn (*syn* erythroblastosis fetalis) pathological condition in the newborn due to Rhesus incompatibility between infant's blood and that of the mother. Red blood cell destruction occurs with anemia, often jaundice and an excess of erythroblasts, or primitive red blood cells, in the circulating blood. Immunization of women at risk, using gammaglobulin containing a high titer of anti-D,* can prevent hemolytic disease of the newborn. Exchange transfusion of the infant may be essential.

hemolytic uremic syndrome (HUS) febrile illness resembling gastroenteritis and followed by intravascular hemolysis, which may also lead to hypertension and acute renal failure, manifested by oliguria. The longer this persists, the poorer the prognosis—which can be death or chronic renal failure. A third do not develop oliguria and make a good recovery. May be autoimmune in origin or an abnormal reaction to an uncommon virus.

hemopericardium (hē'-mō-pėr-i-kàr'-dē-um) *n* blood in the pericardial sac.

hemoperitoneum (hē'-mō-pėr-i-ton-ē'-um) *n* blood in the peritoneal cavity.

hemophilia (hē-mō-fil'-ē-a) *n* a group of conditions with congenital blood coagulation defects. In clinical practice the most commonly encountered defects are *hemophilia A*, factor VIII procoagulant deficiency and *hemophilia B* or Christmas disease factor IX procoagulant deficiency. Both are X-linked recessive disorders exclusively affecting males and resulting in abnormalities in the clotting mechanism only. Bleeding usually occurs into deep-lying structures, muscles and joints. → hemophilic arthropathy, von Willebrand's disease.

hemophilic arthropathy (hē-mō-fil'-ik árth-rop'-à-thē) the extent of joint damage, as staged from radiological findings: (a) synovial thickening, (b) epiphyseal overgrowth, (c) minor joint changes and cyst formation, (d) definite joint changes with loss of joint space, (e) end-stage joint destruction and secondary changes leading to deformity.

hemophthalmia (hē-mof-thal'-mē-à) *n* bleeding into the eyeball.

hemopneumothorax (hē-mō-nū-mō-thōr'-aks) *n* presence of blood and air in the pleural cavity.

hemopoiesis (hē-mō-poy-ē'-sis) *n* (*syn* hematopoiesis) the formation of blood. → erythropoiesis—**hemopoietic** *adj*.

hemoptysis (hē-mop'-tis-is) *n* coughing up of blood—**hemoptyses** *pl*.

hemorrhage (hem'-ōr-raj) *n, vi* escape of blood from a vessel; termed arterial, capillary, venous by site. *primary hemorrhage* that which occurs at time of injury or operation. *reactionary hemorrhage* that which occurs within 24 hours of injury or operation. *secondary hemorrhage* that which occurs within 7–10 days of injury or operation. *antepartum hemorrhage* → placental abruption. *intrapartum hemorrhage* that occurring during labor. *postpartum hemorrhage* excessive bleeding after delivery of child. In the US it must be at least 500 ml to qualify as hemorrhage. *secondary postpartum hemorrhage* excessive uterine bleeding more than 24 h after delivery—**hemorrhagic** *adj*.

hemorrhagic disease of the newborn characterized by gastrointestinal, pulmonary or intracranial hemorrhage occurring from the 2nd to the 5th day of life. Caused by a physiological variation in clotting power due to change in prothrombin content, which falls on 2nd day and returns to normal at end of first week, when colonization of gut with bacteria results in synthesis of vitamin K, thus permitting formation of prothrombin* by the liver. Responds to administration of vitamin K.

hemorrhagic fever → mosquito-transmitted hemorrhagic fevers, viral hemorrhagic fevers.

hemorrhoidal (hem-ōr-oyd'-al) *adj* 1 pertaining to hemorrhoids.* 2 applied to blood vessels and nerves in the anal region.

hemorrhoidectomy (hem-ōr-oyd-ek'-to-mē) *n* surgical removal of hemorrhoids.

hemorrhoids (hem'-ōr-oyds) *npl* (*syn* piles) varicosity of the veins around the anus. *external hemorrhoids* those outside anal sphincter, covered with skin. *internal hemorrhoids* those inside anal sphincter, covered with mucous membrane.

hemosalpinx (hē-mō-sal'-pinks) *n* → hematosalpinx.

hemosiderosis (hē-mō-sid-ėr-ōs'-is) *n* iron deposits in the tissues.

hemospermia (hē-mō-spėr'-mē-à) *n* discharge of bloodstained semen.

hemostasis (hē-mō-stā'-sis) *n* **1** arrest of bleeding. **2** stagnation of blood within its vessel—**hemostatic** *adj*.

hemothorax (hē-mō-thōr'-aks) *n* blood in the pleural cavity.

Henoch-Schonlein purpura (hen'-ok shān'-līn) a disorder mainly affecting children. Characterized by purpuric bleeding into the skin, particularly shins and buttocks, and from the wall of the gut, resulting in abdominal colic and melena; and bruising around joints. Recurrence is not uncommon.

hepar (hep'-ȧr) *n* the liver—**hepatic** *adj*.

heparin (hep'-ȧr-in) *n* an acid present in liver and lung tissue. Injected intravenously, inhibits coagulation of blood; widely used in treatment of thrombosis, often in association with orally active anticoagulants such as warfarin.*

heparinize (hep'-ȧ-rin-īz) *vt* to administer heparin therapeutically.

hepatectomy (hep-ȧ-tek'-to-mē) *n* excision of the liver, or more usually part of the liver.

hepatic (hep-at'-ik) *adj* pertaining to the liver. *hepatic coma* slow-developing coma associated with other signs of liver disease. Toxins, normally cleared from blood by a healthy liver, cause the condition. Term also refers to full syndrome of neuropsychiatric symptoms accompanying the disease, including diverse signs of impaired consciousness.

hepaticocholedochostomy (hep-at'-i-kō-kōl'-ē-dō-kos'-to-mē) *n* end-to-end union of the severed hepatic and common bile ducts.

hepaticoenteric (hep-at'-ik-ō-en-tėr'-ik) *adj* pertaining to the liver and intestine.

hepaticojejunostomy (hep-at'-i-kō-je-jūn-os'-to-mē) *n* anastomosis of the common hepatic duct to a loop of proximal jejunum.*

hepatitis (hep-ȧ-tī'-tis) *n* inflammation of the liver in response to toxins or infective agents. Usually accompanied by fever, gastrointestinal symptoms and itchy skin. *amoebic hepatitis* can occur as a complication of amoebic dysentery. *infective hepatitis* is caused by hepatitis-A virus spread by the fecal-oral route. Incubation period is 2–6 weeks, jaundice appearing after a brief influenzalike illness. *serum hepatitis* is caused by hepatitis-B virus and spread only by contact or inoculation with human blood and its products. Incubation period is 3–5 months; it is followed by three general patterns of clinical response: 30%–40% of adults develop clinically apparent hepatitis; the majority, 50%–60%, remain asymptomatic but show serological evidence of infection. But 5%–10% develop a chronic infection, the so-called chronic carrier state. Carrier populations are higher among drug addicts, male homosexuals and mentally subnormal patients in institutions. *viral hepatitis* includes infective and serum hepatitis, but other viruses including cytomegalovirus, Epstein-Barr virus, herpes simplex and rubella have also been implicated as causal agents. *hepatitis B immunoglobulin* a blood product for immunization against hepatitis B infection, recommended for at-risk populations.

hepatization (hep-à-tī-zā′-shun) *n* pathological changes in the tissues, which cause them to resemble liver. Occurs in the lungs in pneumonia.

hepatocirrhosis (hep-at′-ō-sèr-ō′-sis) *n* cirrhosis of the liver.

hepatolenticular degeneration → Wilson's disease.

hepatoma (hep-à-tō′-mà) *n* primary carcinoma of the liver—**hepatomata** *pl*.

hepatomegaly (hep-at′-ō-meg′-à-lē) *n* enlargement of the liver. It is palpable below the costal margin.

hepatosplenic (hep-at′-ō-splen′-ik) *adj* pertaining to the liver and spleen.

hepatosplenomegaly (hep-at′-ō-splen-ō-meg′-à-lē) *n* enlargement of liver and spleen, so that each is palpable below the costal margin.

hepatotoxic (hep-at′-ō-toks′-ik) *adj* having an injurious effect on liver cells—**hepatotoxicity** *n*.

Heptavax-B™ hepatitis* B immunoglobulin.

hereditary *adj* inherited, capable of being inherited.

hermaphrodite (hèr-maf′-rō-dīt) *n* individual possessing both ovarian and testicular tissue; approximate either to male or female type, but usually sterile from imperfect development of gonads.

hernia (hèr′-nē-à) *n* abnormal protrusion of an organ, or part of an organ, through an aperture in surrounding structures; commonly the protrusion of an abdominal organ through a gap in the abdominal wall. *diaphragmatic hernia* (*syn* hiatus hernia) protrusion through the diaphragm, most commonly involving the stomach at the esophageal opening. *femoral hernia* protrusion through the femoral canal, alongside the femoral blood vessels as they pass into the thigh. *inguinal hernia* protrusion through the inguinal canal in the male. *irreducible hernia* contents of the sac cannot be returned to the appropriate cavity without surgical intervention. *strangulated hernia* hernia in which blood supply to organ involved is impaired, usually due to constriction by surrounding structures. *umbilical hernia* (*syn* omphalocele) protrusion of a portion of intestine through the area of the umbilical scar.

hernioplasty (hèr′-nē-ō-plas′-tē) *n* operation for hernia in which an attempt is made to prevent recurrence by refashioning the structures to give greater strength—**hernioplastic** *adj*.

herniorrhaphy (hèr-nē-ōr′-raf-ē) *n* operation for hernia in which the weak area is reinforced by some of the patient's own tissues or by some other material.

herniotomy (hèr-nē-ot′-o-mē) *n* operation to cure hernia by the return of its contents to their normal position and removal of the hernial sac.

herpangina (hėr-pan-jī'-na) *n* minute vesicles and ulcers at the back of the palate. Short, febrile illness in children caused by coxsackievirus Group A.

herpes (hėr'-pēz) *n* vesicular eruption due to infection with herpes* simplex virus. *genital herpes* infection with the herpes* simplex virus (HSV) Type I or II; a sexually transmitted disease. In the female, ulcers and vesicles can occur on the cervix, vagina, vulva and labia. In the male, these occur on the glans, prepuce and penal shaft and less commonly on the scrotum. In both sexes lesions may be seen on the pharynx, thighs, buttocks and perianal regions. *herpes gestationis* a rare skin disease peculiar to pregnancy; clears in about 30 days after delivery. *herpes zoster* the virus attacks sensory nerves, with consequent severe pain, and appearance of vesicles along the distribution of involved nerves (usually unilateral).

herpes simplex virus (HSV) (hėr'-pēz sim'-pleks) consists of two biologically and immunologically distinct types designated Type I, which generally causes oral disease and lesions above the waist, and Type II, most commonly associated with genital disease and lesions below the waist. Recurrent episodes are common, as the virus remains latent in nerve ganglia after initial infection. → herpes.

herpetiform (hėr-pet'-i-form) *adj* resembling herpes.*

Herplex™ idoxuridine.*

Hess test (hes) a sphygmomanometer cuff is applied to the arm and inflated; petechial eruption in surrounding area after 5 min denotes weakness of capillary walls, characteristic of purpura.

heterologous (het-ėr-ol'-o-gus) *adj* of different origin; from a different species. → homologous *opp.*

heterophile (het'-ėr-ō-fil) *n* a product of one species which acts against that of another, for example, human antigen against sheep's red blood cells.

heteroplasty (het-ėr-ō-plas'-tē) *n* plastic operation using a graft from another individual—**heteroplastic** *adj.*

heterozygous (het-ėr-ō-zī'-gus) *adj* having different genes or alleles at the same locus on both chromosomes of a pair (one of maternal and the other of paternal origin). → homozygous *opp.*

hexachlorophene (heks-a-klōr'-ō-fēn) *n* antiseptic used in skin sterilization, and in some bactericidal soaps. Under suspicion as a possible cause of brain damage in babies. Any medicinal product containing hexachlorophene (irrespective of amount) must bear a warning on the container "not to be used for babies" or "not to be administered to a child under 2." (Phisohex.)

hexestrol (heks-es'-trol) *n* synthetic compound related to stilbestrol* and used for similar purposes.

hexose (heks'-ōs) *n* a class of simple sugars, monosaccharides containing six carbon atoms ($C_6H_{12}O_6$). Examples are glucose, mannose, galactose.

hiatus (hī-ā'-tus) *n* a space or opening. *hiatus hernia* → hernia—**hiatal** *adj*.

Hibiclens™ preparation of chlorhexidine* gluconate 4% in detergent base; esp. useful for preoperative baths.

hiccup (hi'-kup) *n* involuntary inspiratory spasm of the respiratory organs ending in a sudden closure of the glottis with production of characteristic sound.

hidrosis (hī-drō'-sis) *n* sweat secretion.

high density lipoprotein (HDL) a plasma protein relatively high in protein, low in cholestrol. It is involved in transporting cholesterol and other lipids from plasma to the tissues.

hilum (hī'-lum) *n* depression on the surface of an organ where vessels, ducts, etc., enter and leave. → adenitis—**hili** *pl*, **hilar** *adj*.

hindbrain (hīnd'-brān) *n* → Figure 1.

hip bone (innominate bone) formed by fusion of three separate bones—ilium, ischium and pubis. → Figures 2, 3.

Hirschsprung's disease (hirsh'-sproongz) congenital intestinal aganglionosis, leading to intractable constipation or even intestinal obstruction; with marked hypertrophy and dilation of the colon (megacolon) above the aganglionic segment. Commoner in boys and children with Down syndrome.

hirsute (hėr'-sūt) *adj* hairy or shaggy.

hirsuties, hirsutism (hėr'-sūt-ēz, hėr'-sūt-izm) *n* excessive growth of hair in sites in which body hair is normally found. → hypertrichosis.

hirudin (hi-roo'-din) *n* substance secreted by the medicinal leech,* which prevents clotting of blood by acting as an antithrombin.

hirudo (hi-roo'-dō) *n* → leech.

histamine (his'-tȧ-mēn) *n* a naturally occurring chemical substance in body tissues which, in small doses, has profound and diverse actions on muscle, blood capillaries, and gastric secretion. Sudden excessive release from the tissues, into the blood, is believed to be the cause of main symptoms and signs in anaphylaxis.* *histamine receptor cells* two types: H_1 in bronchial muscle, and H_2 in secreting cells in the stomach. *histamine test* designed to determine maximal gastric secretion of hydrochloric acid—**histaminic** *adj*.

histidinemia (his-ti-din-ē'-mē-ȧ) *n* genetically determined increase in histidine* in blood. Gives rise to speech defects without mental retardation.

histidine (his'-ti-dēn) *n* essential amino acid, widely distributed and present in hemoglobin; a precursor of histamine.*

histiocytes (his'-tē-ō-sīts) *npl* macrophages derived from reticuloendothelial cells; act as scavengers.

histiocytoma (his-tē-ō-sī-tō'-mȧ) *n* benign tumor of histiocytes.

histocompatibility antigens (his'-tō-kom-pat-i-bil'-i-tē) *n* antigens on nucleated cells which induce an allograft* response; important in organ transplantation. → major histocompatability complex (MHC).

histology (his-tol'-o-jē) *n* microscopic study of tissues—**histological** *adj*.

histolysis (his-tol'-is-is) *n* disintegration of organic tissue—**histolytic** *adj*.

histones (his'-tōns) *npl* special set of proteins closely associated with chromosomal DNA of higher organisms, which coils and supercoils around histone molecules.

histoplasmosis (his-tō-plaz-mō'-sis) *n* infection caused by inhaling spores of the fungus *Histoplasma capsulatum*. Primary lung lesion may go unnoticed or be accompanied by fever, malaise, cough and adenopathy. Progressive histoplasmosis can be fatal.

hives *npl* nettlerash; urticaria.*

hobnail liver firm nodular liver which may be found in cirrhosis.

Hodgkin's disease (hoj'-kinz) a malignant lymphoma* causing progressive enlargement of lymph nodes and involvement of reticuloendothelial tissues including bone marrow. Some cases show Pel-Ebstein* fever.

Hofmann reaction (hof'-man) chemical inactivation, without the activity of enzymes, of compounds which occur spontaneously in the blood.

holistic medicine (hōl-is'-tik) (wholistic) medical care which considers the patient as a whole, including physical, mental, emotional, social and economic needs.

Homans' sign (Hō'-manz) passive dorsiflexion of foot causes pain in calf muscles; indicative of incipient or established venous thrombosis of leg.

Homapin™ homatropine.*

homatropine (hōm-ȧ-trō'-pēn) *n* a mydriatic similar to atropine,* but with a more rapid and less prolonged effect. Often used as a 2% solution with a similar amount of cocaine,* which addition increases the mydriatic action and deadens pain. (Homapin.)

homeopathy (hō-mē-op'-ȧ-thē) *n* method of treating disease by prescribing minute doses of drugs which, in maximum dose, would produce symptoms of the disease. First adopted by Hahnemann—**homeopathic** *adj*.

homeostasis (hōm-ē-ō-stā'-sis) *n* physiological regulatory process whereby functions such as blood pressure, body temperature and electrolytes are maintained within a narrow range of normal.

homocystinuria (hō-mō-sis-tin-ū'-rē-ȧ) *n* excretion of homocystine (a sulfur-containing amino acid, homologue of cystine) in urine. Caused by an inborn recessively-inherited metabolic error. Gives rise to slow development or mental retardation of varying degree; lens may dislocate, and there is overgrowth of long bones with thrombotic episodes, which are often fatal in childhood— **homocystinuric** *adj*.

homograft (hō'-mō-graft) *n* tissue or organ which is transplanted from one individual to another of the same species. → allograft.

homologous (hom-ol'-o-gus) *adj* corresponding in origin and structure. → heterologous *opp. homologous chromosomes* those that pair during reduction cell division (meiosis) whereby mature gametes are formed. Of the two homologues, one is derived from the father, the other from the mother.

homonymous (hom-on'-i-mus) *adj* consisting of corresponding halves.

homotransplant (hō-mō-tranz'-plant) *n* (*syn* allotransplant) tissues or organ transplanted from nonidentical members of the same species.

homozygous (hō-mō-zī'-gus) *adj* having identical genes or alleles in the same locus on both chromosomes of a pair (one of maternal and the other of paternal origin). → heterozygous *opp*.

Honvol (hon'-vol) *n* stilbestrol diphosphate, broken down by prostatic tissue to release stilbestrol in situ, thus reducing systemic side-effects.

hookworm *n* → Ancylostoma.

hordeolum (hōr-dē'-ō-lum) *n* → sty.

hormone (hōr'-mōn) *n* specific chemical substance secreted by an endocrine gland and conveyed in the blood to regulate functions of tissues and organs elsewhere in the body.

hormonotherapy (hōr-mōn-ō-thėr'-à-pē) *n* treatment by hormones.

Horner syndrome (hōr'-nėr) clinical picture following paralysis of cervical sympathetic nerves on one side. There is myosis, slight ptosis with enophthalmos, and anhidrosis.

hospice (hos'-pis) *n* **1** homelike facility that provides physical, emotional, spiritual and social care to the dying and their families. **2** a program that provides this care to the dying in their own homes.

host *n* organic structure upon which parasites or bacteria thrive. *intermediate host* one in which the parasite passes its larval or cystic stage.

hourglass contraction circular constriction in the middle of a hollow organ (usually the stomach or uterus), dividing it into two portions following scar formation.

housemaid's knee → bursitis.

HSV *abbr* herpes* simplex virus.

human chorionic gonadotropin (HCG) (kōr-ē-on'-ik gō-nad'-ō-trō'-pin) a hormone arising from the placenta. Used for cryptorchism, and sometimes for female infertility. Presence of HCG in urine is detectable in an early morning specimen of urine from the 6th week of pregnancy. Result can be given in 2 min and confirmed in 2 h. (Pregnyl.)

Humatin™ paromomycin.*

humerus (hū'-mér-us) *n* the bone of the upper arm, between the elbow and shoulder joint (→ Figures 2, 3)—**humeri** *pl,* **humeral** *adj.*

humor *n* any fluid of the body. → aqueous, vitreous.

humoral immunity → immunity.

Humulin™ preparation of human insulin, completely free from animal insulin and pancreatic impurities.

Hunter-Hurler syndrome → gargoylism.

Hunter syndrome one of the mucopolysaccharidoses,* designated Type II. A sex-linked recessive condition.

Hunterian chancre (hun-tér'-ē-an shang'-ker) the hard sore of primary syphilis.

Huntington's chorea (hunt'-ing-tunz kōr-ē'-à) genetically determined inherited disease with slow progressive degeneration of nerve cells of basal ganglia and cerebral cortex. Affects both sexes, and due to a dominant gene of large effect. Develops in middle age, or later, and is associated with progressive dementia. → chorea.

Hurler syndrome one of the mucopolysaccharidoses*; designated Type II. Inherited as an autosomal recessive trait.

Hutchinson's teeth (huch'-in-sunz) defect of the upper central incisors (second dentition), which is part of the facies of the congenital syphilitic person. The teeth are broader at the gum than at the cutting edge, with the latter showing an elliptical notch.

hyaline (hī'-à-lin) *adj* like glass; transparent. *hyaline degeneration* degeneration of connective tissue, esp. that of blood vessels, in which tissue takes on a homogenous or formless appearance. *hyaline membrane disease* → respiratory distress syndrome.

hyalitis (hī-àl-ī'-tis) *n* inflammation of the optical vitreous* humor or its enclosing membrane. When the condition is degenerative rather than inflammatory, there are small opacities in the vitreous humor, and it is termed *asteroid hyalitis.*

hyaloid (hī'-à-loyd) *adj* resembling hyaline* tissue. *hyaloid membrane* → membrane.

hyaluronidase (hī-al-ūr-on'-id-āz) *n* an enzyme obtained from testes which, when injected subcutaneously, promotes the absorption of fluid. Given with or immediately before a subcutaneous infusion; 1000 units will facilitate absorption of 500–1000 ml of fluid. (Wydase.)

hydatid cyst (hī'-dat-id) *n* cyst formed by larvae of a tapeworm, *Echinococcus,* which is found in dogs. The encysted stage normally occurs in sheep but can occur in man. Cysts are commonest in the liver and lungs; they grow slowly and only do damage by the space they occupy. If they leak, or become infected, urticaria and fever supervene and "daughter" cysts can result. Treatment is surgical removal. → Casoni test.

hydatidiform (hī-dat-id'-i-form) *adj* pertaining to or resembling a hydatid* cyst. *hydatidiform mole* condition in which chorionic villi of the placenta undergo cystic degeneration and the fetus is absorbed. The villi penetrate and destroy only the decidual layer of the uterus, but a hydatidiform mole may progress to become an invasive mole in which the villi penetrate the myometrium and can destroy the uterine wall and metastasize to the vagina or even the lungs and brain; these regress after evacuation of the mole. Invasive mole is benign but may convert to choriocarcinoma.

hydralazine (hī-dral'-á-zēn) *n* synthetic compound which lowers blood pressure, mainly by peripheral vasodilator action. Response to treatment may be slow and use of diuretics* may enhance action. (Apresoline.)

hydramnios (hī-dram'-nē-os) *n* excess of amniotic fluid.

hydrarthrosis (hī-drár-thrō'-sis) *n* collection of synovial fluid in a joint cavity. *intermittent hydrarthrosis* afflicts young women; probably due to allergy. Synovitis develops spontaneously, lasts a few days and disappears as mysteriously.

hydrate (hī'-drāt) *vt* combine with water—**hydration** *n*.

hydremia (hī-drē'-mē-á) *n* a relative excess of plasma volume compared with cell volume of the blood; normally present in late pregnancy—**hydremic** *adj*.

hydroa (hī-drō'-á) *n* → dermatitis herpetiformis. *hydroa aestivale* 1 a vesicular or bullous disease occurring in atopic* children. Affects exposed parts and probably results from photosensitivity. 2 sun-induced dermatitis in some forms of porphyria. *hydroa vacciniforme* severe form, in which scarring ensues.

hydrocele (hī'-drō-sēl) *n* a swelling due to accumulation of serous fluid in the tunica vaginalis of the testis or in spermatic cord.

hydrocephalus (hī-drō-sef'-á-lus) *n* (*syn* "water on the brain") an excess of cerebrospinal fluid inside the skull due to an obstruction to normal CSF circulation. *external hydrocephalus* excess of fluid is mainly in the subarachnoid space. *internal hydrocephalus* excess of fluid is mainly in ventricles of the brain. A Spitz*-Holter valve is used in drainage operations for this condition—**hydrocephalic** *adj*.

hydrochloric acid (hī-drō-klōr'-ik) secreted by the gastric oxyntic cells and present in gastric juice (0.2%). The strong acid is caustic, but a 10% dilution is used orally in treatment of achlorhydria.

hydrochlorothiazide (hī′-drō-klōr-ō-thī′-à-zīd) *n* a thiazide diuretic. (Esidrex, HydroDiuril.) → diuretics.

hydrocortisone (hī-drō-kōr′-ti-sōn) *n* → cortisol.

hydrocyanic acid (hī-drō-sī-an′-ik) (*syn* prussic acid) the dilute acid (2%) has a sedative action on the stomach, and has been given with bismuth carbonate and other antacids in treatment of vomiting. In large doses, both the solution and its vapor are poisonous, and death may occur very rapidly from respiratory paralysis. Prompt treatment with intravenous injections of sodium nitrite, sodium thiosulfate and ketocyanor may be life-saving.

Hydro Diuril™ hydrochlorothiazide.*

hydroflumethiazide (hī-drō-floō-me-thī′-à-zīd) *n* a thiazide diuretic. (Diucardin.)

hydrolysis (hī-drol′-is-is) *n* the splitting into more simple substances by addition of water—**hydrolytic** *adj*, **hydrolyze** *vt*.

hydrometer (hī-drom′-é-tér) *n* instrument for determining specific gravity of fluids—**hydrometry** *n*.

hydrometria (hī-drō-mēt′-rē-à) *n* a collection of watery fluid within the uterus.

Hydromox™ quinethazone.*

hydronephrosis (hī-drō-nef-rō′-sis) *n* distension of the kidney pelvis with urine, from obstructed outflow. If unrelieved, pressure eventually causes atrophy of kidney tissue. Surgical operations include nephroplasty and pyeloplasty.

hydropericarditis (hī-drō-pér-ē-kár-dī′-tis) *n* pericarditis with effusion.

hydropericardium (hī-drō-pér-ē-kár′-dē-um) *n* fluid in the pericardial sac in the absence of inflammation. Can occur in heart and kidney failure.

hydroperitoneum (hī-drō-pér-it-on-ē′-um) *n* → ascites.

hydrophobia (hī-drō-fō′-bē-à) *n* → rabies.

hydrophylic (hī-drō-fil′-ik) *adj* having an affinity for water.

hydropneumopericardium (hī-drō-noō-mō-pér-i-kár′-dē-um) *n* presence of air and fluid in the membranous pericardial sac surrounding the heart; may accompany pericardiocentesis.*

hydropneumoperitoneum (hī-drō-noō′-mō-pér-i-ton-ē′-um) *n* presence of fluid and gas in the peritoneal cavity; may accompany paracentesis of that cavity, or perforation of the gut, or may be due to gas-forming microorganisms in the peritoneal fluid.

hydropneumothorax (hī-drō-noō-mō-thōr′-aks) *n* pneumothorax further complicated by effusion of fluid into pleural cavity.

hydrops (hī′-drops) *n* edema.* *hydrops fetalis* severe form of erythroblastosis fetalis*—**hydropic** *adj*.

hydrosalpinx (hī-drō-sal′-pinks) *n* distension of a fallopian tube with watery fluid.

hydrothorax (hī-drō-thōr′-aks) *n* presence of fluid in the pleural cavity.

hydroureter (hī-drō-ūr′-ė-tėr) *n* abnormal distension of the ureter with urine.

hydroxocobalamin (hī-droks′-ō-kō-bal′-à-min) *n* a longer-acting form of vitamin* B_{12}; given by injection. → cyanocobalamin.

hydroxybutyric dehydrogenase (hī-droks′-ē-bū-tėr′-ik dē-hī-droj′-en-āz) a serum enzyme: high concentrations are indicative of myocardial infarction.

hydroxychloroquine (hī-droks′-ē-klōr′-ō-kwin) *n* an antimalarial. → chloroquine. (Paquenil.)

hydroxyl (hī-droks′-il) *n* a monovalent ion (OH), consisting of a hydrogen atom linked to an oxygen atom.

hydroxyprogesterone caproate (hī-droks′-ē-prō-jest′-ėr-ōn kap′-rō-āt) given intramuscularly for recurrent and threatened abortion. (Delalutin.)

5-hydroxytryptamine (5-HT) (fīv-hī-droks′-i-trip′-ta-mēn) *n* → serotonin.

hydroxyurea (hī-droks′-i-ū-rē′-à) *n* simple compound given orally. Mode of action uncertain, may be of value in patients with chronic myeloid leukemia who no longer show a response to busulphan.*

hydroxyzine (hī-droks′-i-zēn) *n* antihistamine which is also a sedative; useful in treating nausea and vomiting. (Atarax, Vistaril.)

hygiene (hī′-jēn) *n* science dealing with maintenance of health—**hygienic** *adj*.

hygroma (hī-grō′-mà) *n* a cystic swelling containing watery fluid, usually situated in the neck and present at birth, sometimes interfering with birth—**hygromata** *pl*, **hygromatous** *adj*.

hygroscopic (hī-grō-skop′-ik) *adj* readily absorbing water, e.g., glycerine.

Hygroton™ chlorthalidone.*

hymen (hī′-men) *n* a membranous perforated structure stretching across the vaginal entrance. *imperforate hymen* congenital condition leading to hematocolpos. → cryptomenorrhea.

hymenectomy (hī-men-ek′-to-mē) *n* surgical excision of the hymen.

hymenotomy (hī-men-ot′-o-mē) *n* surgical incision of the hymen.

hyoid (hī′-oyd) *n* U-shaped bone at the root of the tongue → (Figure 6).

hyoscine (hī′-ō-sēn) *n* scopolamine.*

hyoscyamus (hī-ō-sī′-à-mus) *n* henbane leaves and flowers. Resembles belladonna in its properties. Sometimes given with potassium citrate for urinary tract spasm.

hyperacidity (hī-pėr-as-id′-it-ē) *n* excessive acidity. → hyperchlorhydria.

hyperaldosteronism (hī-pėr-al-dos'-tėr-ōn-izm) *n* production of excessive aldosterone. *primary hyperaldosteronism* Conn* syndrome. *secondary hyperaldosteronism* the adrenal responds to an increased stimulus of extra-adrenal origin.

hyperalgesia (hī-pėr-al-jē'-zhȧ) *n* excessive sensibility to pain—**hyperalgesic** *adj*.

hyperalimentation (hī-pėr-al-i-men-tā'-shun) *n* total parenteral* nutrition.

hyperbaric oxygen treatment carried out by inserting patient into a sealed cylinder, into which O_2 under pressure is introduced. Used for patients with carbon monoxide poisoning and gas gangrene.

hyperbilirubinemia (hī-pėr-bi'-lē-roo-bin-ēm'-ē-ȧ) *n* excessive bilirubin in blood. When it rises above $1-1.5$ mg per 100 ml, visible jaundice* occurs. Present in physiological jaundice of the newborn. → phototherapy—**hyperbilirubinemic** *adj*.

hypercalcemia (hī-pėr-kal-sē'-mē-ȧ) *n* excessive calcium in blood, usually arising from bone resorption as occurs in hyperparathyroidism, metastatic tumors of bone. Paget's disease and osteoporosis. Results in anorexia, abdominal pain, muscle pain and weakness. Accompanied by hypercalciuria and can lead to nephrolithiasis—**hypercalcemic** *adj*.

hypercalciuria (hī-pėr-kal-sē-ūr'-ē-ȧ) *n* greatly increased excretion of calcium in urine. Occurs in diseases which cause bone resorption. *idiopathic hypercalciuria* term used when there is no known metabolic cause. Hypercalciuria is of importance in the pathogenesis of nephrolithiasis—**hypercalciuric** *adj*.

hypercapnia (hī-pėr-kap'-nē-ȧ) *n* (*syn* hypercarbia) raised CO_2 tension* in arterial blood—**hypercapnic** *adj*.

hypercatabolism (hī-pėr-kat-ab'-ol-izm) *n* abnormal, excessive breakdown of complex substances into simpler ones within the body. Can occur in fevers and in acute renal failure—**hypercatabolic** *adj*.

hyperchloremia (hī-pėr-klōr-ēm'-ē-ȧ) *n* excessive chloride in blood. One form of acidosis*—**hyperchloremic** *adj*.

hyperchlorhydria (hī-pėr-klōr-hī'-drē-ȧ) *n* excessive hydrochloric acid in gastric juice—**hyperchlorhydric** *adj*.

hypercholesterolemia (hī'-pėr-kol-es'tėr-ol-ēm'-ē-ȧ) *n* excessive cholesterol in blood. Predisposes to atheroma and gallstones. Also found in myxedema—**hypercholesterolemic** *adj*.

hyperchromic (hī-pėr-krō'-mik) *adj* excessively colored or pigmented. Excessive hemoglobin in a red blood cell.

hyperemesis (hī-pėr-em'-es-is) *n* excessive vomiting. *hyperemesis gravidarum* a complication of pregnancy which may become serious.

hyperemia (hī-pėr-ēm'-ē-à) *n* excess of blood in an area. *active hyperemia* caused by increased flow of blood to a part, *passive hyperemia* by restricted flow of blood from a part—**hyperemic** *adj*.

hyperesthesia (hī-pėr-es-thē'-zhà) *n* excessive sensitivity of a part—**hyperesthetic** *adj*.

hyperextension (hī-pėr-eks-ten'-shun) *n* overextension.

hyperflexion (hī-pėr-flek'-shun) *n* excessive flexion.

hyperglycemia (hī-pėr-glī-sē'-mē-à) *n* excessive glucose in blood, usually indicative of diabetes mellitus. Discovery of isolated high blood glucose readings in an otherwise symptomless diabetic is of little value, but during illness raised blood glucose readings may signal need for higher insulin dosage—**hyperglycemic** *adj*.

hyperglycinemia (hī-pėr-glī-sin-ēm'-ē-à) *n* excess glycine in serum. Can cause acidosis and mental retardation—**hyperglycinemic** *adj*.

hyperhidrosis (hī-pėr-hī-drō'-sis) *n* excessive sweating—**hyperhidrotic** *adj*.

hyperinsulinism (hī-pėr-in'-sul-in-izm) *n* intermittent or continuous loss of consciousness, with or without convulsions, (a) due to excessive insulin from the pancreatic islets lowering blood sugar, (b) due to administration of excessive insulin.

hyperinvolution (hī'-pėr-in-vol-ū'-shun) *n* reduction to below normal size, as of the uterus after parturition.

hyperkalemia (hī-pėr-kal-ēm'-ē-à) *n* excessive potassium in blood, as occurs in renal failure; early signs are nausea, diarrhea and muscular weakness—**hyperkalemic** *adj*.

hyperkeratosis (hī-pėr-ker-à-tō'-sis) *n* hypertrophy of the horny layer of the skin—**hyperkeratotic** *adj*.

hyperkinesis (hī-pėr-kin-ē'-sis) *n* excessive movement—**hyperkinetic** *adj*.

hyperkinetic syndrome (hī-pėr-kin-et'-ik) first described as a syndrome in 1962; usually appears between the ages of 2 and 4 years. Child is slow to develop intellectually and displays a marked degree of distractability and a tireless unrelenting perambulation of the environment, together with aggressiveness (esp. towards siblings) even if unprovoked. Parents complain of cold unaffectionate character and destructive behavior.

hyperlipidemia (hī-pėr-lī-pi-dē'-mē-à) *n* excessive total fat in the blood—**hyperlipidemic** *adj*.

hyperlipoproteinemia (hī-pėr-lī'-pō-prō-tin-ēm'-ē-à) *n* hyperlipidemia* due to familially occurring lipid metabolism disorders; five types (I–V) are recognized.

hypermagnesemia (hī-pėr-mag-ne-sē'-mē-à) *n* excessive magnesium in blood, found in kidney failure and people who take excessive magnesium-containing antacids—**hypermagnesemic** *adj.*

hypermetabolism (hī-pėr-met-ab'-ol-izm) *n* production of excessive body heat. Characteristic of thyrotoxicosis—**hypermetabolic** *adj.*

hypermotility (hī-pėr-mō-til'-i-tē) *n* increased movement, as of peristalsis.

hypernatremia (hī-pėr-na-trē'-mē-à) *n* excessive sodium in blood, caused by excessive loss of water and electrolytes owing to polyuria, diarrhea, excessive sweating or inadequate fluid intake—**hypernatremic** *adj.*

hypernephroma (hī-pėr-nef-rō'-mà) *n* (*syn* Grawitz tumor) malignant neoplasm of the kidney whose structure resembles that of adrenocortical tissue— **hypernephromata** *pl,* **hypernephromatous** *adj.*

hyperonychia (hī-pėr-on-ik'-ē-à) *n* excessive growth of the nails.

hyperopia (hī-pėr-ōp'-ē-à) *n* longsightedness caused by faulty accommodation of the eye, with result that light rays are focused beyond, instead of on, the retina—**hyperopic** *adj.*

hyperosmolarity (hī-pėr-oz-mō-lãr'-it-ē) *n* (*syn* hypertonicity) condition of higher density of solution in one liquid with respect to another with which it is in contact through a semipermeable membrane, so that water passes from the lesser to the higher density solution. In medicine, the comparison is usually made with normal plasma.

hyperostosis (hī-pėr-os-tō'-sis) *n* exostosis.*

hyperoxaluria (hī-pėr-oks-al-ūr'-ē-à) *n* excessive calcium oxalate in urine— **hyperoxaluric** *adj.*

hyperparathyroidism (hī-pėr-pār-à-thī'-royd-izm) *n* overaction of the parathyroid* glands, with increase in serum calcium levels; may result in osteitis fibrosa cystica with decalcification and spontaneous fracture of bones. → hypercalcemia, hypercalciuria.

hyperperistalsis (hī-pėr-per-i-stal'-sis) *n* excessive peristalsis—**hyper-** peristaltic *adj.*

hyperphenylalaninemia (hī-pėr-fen-il-al'-à-nēn-ēm'-ē-à) *n* excess of phenylalanine in blood which results in phenylketonuria.*

hyperphagia (hī-pėr-fā'-jà) *n* overeating. → obesity.

hyperphosphatemia (hī-pėr-fos'-fà-tē'-mē-à) *n* excessive phosphates in blood—**hyperphosphatemic** *adj.*

hyperpiesis (hī-pėr-pī-ē'-sis) *n* hypertension.*

hyperpituitarism (hī-pėr-pi-too'-it-ar-izm) *n* overactivity of the anterior lobe of the pituitary,* producing gigantism or acromegaly.*

hyperplasia (hī-pėr-plā'-zhȧ) *n* excessive formation of cells—**hyperplastic** *adj*.

hyperpnea (hī-pėrp-nē'-ȧ) *n* rapid, deep breathing; panting; gasping—**hyperpneic** *adj*.

hyperpyrexia (hī-pėr-pī-reks'-ē-ȧ) *n* body temperature above 40–41° C (105° F). *malignant hyperpyrexia* inherited condition which presents during general anesthesia, with progressive rise in body temperature at a rate of 6° C per hour—**hyperpyrexial** *adj*.

hypersplenism (hī-pėr-splen'-izm) *n* describes depression of erythrocyte, granulocyte and platelet counts by enlarged spleen in presence of active bone marrow.

Hyperstat™ diazoxide.*

hypertelorism (hī-pėr-tel'-or-izm) *n* genetically determined cranial anomaly (low forehead and pronounced vertex) associated with mental subnormality.

hypertension (hī-pėr-ten'-shun) *n* abnormally high tension, by custom, abnormally high blood pressure involving systolic and/or diastolic levels. There is no universal agreement on upper limits of normal, esp. in increasing age. Many cardiologists consider a resting systolic pressure of 160 mmHg, and/or a resting diastolic pressure of 100 mmHg, to be pathological. Cause may be renal, endocrine, mechanical or toxic (as in toxemia of pregnancy) but often it remains unknown (essential hypertension). → portal* hypertension, pulmonary* hypertension—**hypertensive** *adj*.

hyperthermia (hī-pėr-thėr'-mē-ȧ) *n* very high body temperature. *whole body* hyperthermia is sometimes used in conjunction with chemotherapy for cancer—**hyperthermic** *adj*.

hyperthyroidism (hī-pėr-thī'-royd-izm) *n* thyrotoxicosis.*

hypertonia (hī-pėr-tō'-nē-ȧ) *n* increased tone in a muscular structure—**hypertonic** *adj*.

hypertonic (hī-pėr-ton'-ik) *adj* 1 pertaining to hypertonia. 2 pertaining to saline. *hypertonic saline* has a greater osmotic pressure than normal physiological (body) fluid. → hyperosmolarity—**hypertonicity** *n*.

hypertoxic (hī-pėr-toks'-ik) *adj* very poisonous.

hypertrichosis (hī-pėr-trik-ōs'-is) *n* excessive hairiness in sites not usually bearing prominent hair, e.g., the forehead.

hypertrophy (hī-pėr'-tro-fē) *n* increase in the size of tissues or structures, independent of natural growth. May be congenital, compensatory, complementary or functional. → stenosis—**hypertrophic** *adj*.

hyperuricemia (hī'-pėr-ūr-i-sē'-mē-ȧ) *n* excessive uric acid in blood, characteristic of gout. Occurs in untreated reticulosis, but is increased by radiotherapy, cytotoxins and corticosteroids. → Lesch-Nyhan disease—**hyperuricemic** *adj*.

hyperventilation (hī'-pėr-ven-til-ā'-shun) *n* increased breathing; may be active, as in salicylate poisoning or head injury, or passive, as when imposed as part of a technique of general anesthesia in intensive care.

hypervitaminosis (hī'-pėr-vī-tȧ-min-ōs'-is) *n* any condition arising from an excess of vitamins, esp. vitamin A and D.

hypervolemia (hī'-per-vol-ēm'-ē-ȧ) *n* increase in the volume of circulating blood.

hyphema (hī-fē'-mȧ) *n* blood in the anterior chamber of the eye.

hypnotic (hip-not'-ik) *adj* **1** pertaining to hypnotism. *n* **2** a drug which produces a sleep resembling natural sleep.

hypocalcemia (hī'-pō-kal-sēm'-ē-ȧ) *n* decreased calcium in the blood—**hypocalcemic** *adj*.

hypocapnia (hī-pō-kap'-nē-ȧ) *n* reduced CO_2 tension* in arterial blood; can be produced by hyperventilation—**hypocapnial** *adj*.

hypochloremia (hī-pō-klōr-ēm'-ē-ȧ) *n* reduced chlorides in circulating blood. A form of alkalosis*—**hypochloremic** *adj*.

hypochlorhydria (hī-pō-klōr-hī'-drē-ȧ) *n* decreased hydrochloric acid in gastric juice—**hypochlorhydric** *adj*.

hypochondria (hī-pō-kon'-drē-ȧ) *n* excessive anxiety about one's health. Common in depressive and anxiety states—**hypochondriac** *n, adj*, **hypochondriacal** *adj*, **hypochondriasis** *n*.

hypochondrium (hī-pō-kon'-drē-um) *n* the upper lateral region (left and right) of the abdomen, below the lower ribs—**hypochondriac** *adj*.

hypochromic (hī-pō-krō'-mik) *adj* deficient in coloring or pigmentation. Of a red blood cell, having decreased hemoglobin.

hypodermic (hī-po-dėr'-mik) *adj* below the skin; subcutaneous.

hypoesthesia (hī-pō-es-thē'-zhȧ) *n* diminished sensitivity of a part—**hypoesthetic** *adj*.

hypofibrinogenemia (hī-pō-fī-brin'-ō-jen-ēm'-ē-ȧ) *n* → acute defibrination syndrome—**hypofibrinogenemic** *adj*.

hypofunction (hī-pō-fung'-shun) *n* diminished performance.

hypogammaglobulinemia (hī-pō-gam-mȧ-glob'-ū-lin-ēm'-ē-ȧ) *n* decreased gammaglobulin in blood, occurring either congenitally or, more commonly, as a sporadic disease in adults. Lessens resistance to infection. → dysgammaglobulinemia—**hypogammaglobulinemic** *adj*.

hypogastrium (hī-pō-gas'-trē-um) *n* that area of the anterior abdomen which lies immediately below the umbilical region; flanked on either side by the iliac fossae—**hypogastric** *adj*.

hypoglossal (hī-pō-glos'-ál) *adj* under the tongue. *hypoglossal nerve* the 12th pair of the 12 pairs of cranial nerves which arise directly from the brain.

hypoglycemia (hī-pō-glī-sē'-mē-à) *n* decreased blood glucose, attended by anxiety, excitement, perspiration, delirium or coma. Hypoglycemia occurs most commonly in diabetes* mellitus, due either to insulin overdosage or inadequate intake of carbohydrate—**hypoglycemic** *adj*.

hypokalemia (hī-pō-kal-ēm'-ē-à) *n* abnormally low potassium level in blood. → potassium deficiency—**hypokalemic** *adj*.

hypomagnesemia (hī-pō-mag-nē-sēm'-ē-à) *n* decreased magnesium in blood—**hypomagnesemic** *adj*.

hypomania (hī-pō-mā'-nē-à) *n* a less intense form of mania, with mild elevation of mood, restlessness, distractability, increased energy and pressure of speech. The flight of ideas and grandiose delusions of frank mania* are usually absent—**hypomanic** *adj*.

hypometabolism (hī-pō-met-ab'-ol-izm) *n* decreased production of body heat. Characteristic of myxedema.*

hypomotility (hī-po-mō-til'-it-ē) *n* decreased movement, as of the stomach or intestines.

hyponatremia (hī-pō-nà-trē'-mē-à) *n* decreased sodium in blood—**hyponat-remic** *adj*.

hypo-osmolarity (hī-pō–oz-mo-lār'-it-ē) *n* (*syn* hypotonicity) condition of lower density of solution in one liquid with respect to another with which it is in contact through a semipermeable membrane, so that water passes from the lesser to the higher density solution. In medicine, the comparison is usually made with normal plasma.

hypoparathyroidism (hī-pō-pār-à-thī'-royd-izm) *n* underaction of the parathyroid* glands, with decrease in serum calcium levels, producing tetany.*

hypopharynx (hī-pō-fār'-inks) *n* that portion of the pharynx* lying below and behind the larynx, correctly called the laryngopharynx.

hypophoria (hī-pō-fōr'-ē-à) *n* state in which the visual axis in one eye is lower than the other.

hypophosphatemia (hī-pō-fos-fà-tēm'-ē-à) *n* decreased phosphates in blood—**hypophosphatemic** *adj*.

hypophysectomy (hī-pof-i-sek'-to-mē) *n* surgical removal of the pituitary gland.

hypophysis cerebri (hī-pof'-is-is sėr'-e-brē) *n* → pituitary gland—**hypophyseal** *adj*.

hypopiesis (hī-pō-pī-ē'-sis) *n* hypotension.*

hypopituitarism (hī'-pō-pit-ū'-it-ar-izm) *n* pituitary* gland insufficiency, esp. of the anterior lobe. Absence of gonadotropins leads to failure of ovulation, uterine atrophy and amenorrhea in women and loss of libido, pubic and axillary hair in both sexes. Lack of growth hormone in children results in short stature. Lack of corticotropin (ACTH) and thyrotropin (TSH) may result in lack of energy, pallor, fine dry skin, cold intolerance and sometimes hypoglycemia. Usually due to tumor of or involving pituitary gland or hypothalamus but sometimes cause is unknown. Occasionally due to postpartum infarction of the pituitary gland.

hypoplasia (hī-pō-plā'-zhà) *n* defective development of any tissue—**hypoplastic** *adj*.

hypoproteinemia (hī'-pō-prō-tin-ēm'-ē-à) *n* deficient protein in blood plasma, from dietary deficiency or excessive excretion (albuminuria*)—**hypoproteinemic** *adj*.

hypoprothrombinemia (hī-pō-prō-throm'-bin-ēm'-ē-à) *n* deficiency of prothrombin in blood, which retards clotting ability—**hypoprothrombinemic** *adj*.

hypopyon (hī-pō'-pē-on) *n* a collection of pus in the anterior chamber of the eye.

hyposmia (hī-poz'-mē-à) *n* decrease in the normal sensitivity to smell. Has been observed in patients following laryngectomy.

hypospadias (hī-pō-spā'-dē-ás) *n* congenital malformation of the male urethra. Subdivided into two types: (a) penile, the terminal urethral orifice opens at any point along the posterior shaft of the penis, (b) perineal, the orifice opens on the perineum and may give rise to problems of sexual differentiation—**epispadias** *opp*.

hypostasis (hī-pō-stā'-sis) *n* 1 a sediment. 2 congestion of blood in a part due to impaired circulation—**hypostatic** *adj*.

hypotension (hī-pō-ten'-shun) *n* low blood pressure (systolic below 110 mmHg, diastolic below 70 mmHg); may be primary, secondary (e.g., caused by bleeding, shock, Addison's disease) or postural. Can be produced by administration of drugs, to reduce bleeding in surgery—**hypotensive** *adj*.

hypothalamus (hī-pō-thal'-à-mus) *n* literally, below the thalamus. Forms ventral part of the diencephalon above the midbrain (→ Figure 1). It is the highest center of the autonomic nervous system and contains centers controlling various physiological functions such as emotion, hunger, thirst and circadian rhythms. Also has important endocrine function, producing hormones that act on the anterior pituitary and regulate the release of its hormones. Also produces oxytocin* and vasopressin,* which are released by the posterior pituitary.

hypothenar eminence (hī-poth'-en-ár) eminence on the ulnar side of the palm below the little finger.

hypothermia (hī-pō-thėr'-mē-á) *n* below normal body temperature, ascertained by a low-reading thermometer. Occurs particularly in the very young and in old people. An artificially induced hypothermia (30° C or 86° F) can be used in treatment of head injuries and in cardiac surgery. It reduces the oxygen consumption of tissues and thereby allows greater and more prolonged interference with normal blood circulation. *hypothermia of the newborn* failure of the newborn to adjust to external cold; may be associated with infection. *local hypothermia* has been tried in treatment of peptic ulcer.

hypothyroidism (hī-pō-thī'-royd-izm) *n* defines those clinical conditions that result from suboptimal circulating levels of one or both thyroid hormones; currently classified as: (a) overt, which if present at birth produces cretinism (later onset is myxedema*), (b) mild, (c) preclinical, (d) autoimmune thyroid disease (Hashimoto's* disease).

hypotonic (hī-pō-ton'-ik) *adj* 1 → hypo-osmolarity. 2 lacking in tone, tension, strength—**hypotonia, hypotonicity** *n*.

hypoventilation (hī-pō-ven-til-ā'-shun) *n* diminished breathing or underventilation.

hypovitaminemia (hī-pō-vī'-tá-min-ē'-mē-á) *n* deficiency of vitamins* in blood—**hypovitaminemic** *adj*.

hypovitaminosis (hī-pō-vī'-tá-min-ōs'-is) *n* any condition due to lack of vitamins.*

hypovolemia (hī-pō-vol-ēm'-ē-á) *n* → oligemia—**hypovolemic** *adj*.

hypoxemia (hī-poks-ēm'-ē-á) *n* diminished amount of oxygen in arterial blood, shown by decreased arterial oxygen tension* and reduced saturation—**hypoxemic** *adj*.

hypoxia (hī-poks'-ē-á) *n* diminished amount of oxygen in tissues. *anemic* hypoxia resulting from deficiency of hemoglobin. *histotoxic hypoxia* deficient function of cells in utilizing O_2, e.g., in cyanide poisoning. *hypoxic hypoxia* interference with pulmonary oxygenation. *stagnant hypoxia* a reduction in blood flow, as seen in the finger nails in surgical shock or in cold weather—**hypoxic** *adj*.

hysterectomy (his-tėr-ek'-to-mē) *n* surgical removal of the uterus. *abdominal* hysterectomy effected via lower abdominal incision. *subtotal hysterectomy* removal of the uterine body, leaving the cervix in the vaginal vault. Rarely performed because of risk of carcinoma developing in the cervical stump. *total* *hysterectomy* complete removal of the uterine body and cervix. *vaginal hysterectomy* carried out through the vagina. *Wertheim's hysterectomy* total removal of the uterus, adjacent lymphatic vessels and glands, with a cuff of the vagina.

hysteria (his-tėr'-ē-à) *n* a neurosis usually arising from mental conflict and repression, and characterized by production of diverse physical symptoms, e.g., tics, paralysis, anesthesia, etc. The disorder is characterized by dissociation*—**hysterical** *adj*.

hysterography (his-tėr-og'-rā-fē) *n* x-ray examination of the uterus— **hysterograph** *n*, **hysterogram** *n*, **hysterographical** *adj*.

hysterosalpingectomy (his'-tėr-ō-sal-pin-jek'-to-mē) *n* excision of the uterus and usually both fallopian tubes.

hysterosalpingography (his'-tėr-ō-sal-ping-og'-raf-ē) *n* → uterosalpingography.

hysterosalpingostomy (his'-tėr-ō-sal-ping-gos'-to-mē) *n* anastomosis* between a fallopian tube and the uterus.

hysterotomy (his-tėr-ot'-o-mē) *n* incision of the uterus to remove a pregnancy. The word is usually reserved for a method of abortion.*

hysterotrachelorraphy (his-tėr-ō-trāk-el-ōr'-à-fē) *n* repair of a lacerated cervix* uteri.

Hytakerol™ dihydrotachysterol.*

HZV *abbr* herpes zoster virus.

I

iatrogenic (ī-at-rō-jen'-ik) *adj* of a secondary condition arising from treatment of a primary condition..

ibuprofen (ī-bū-prō'-fen) *n* nonnarcotic analgesic. Can be irritant to gastrointestinal tract. (Motrin.)

ichthammol (ik'-tham-mol) *n* thick black liquid derived from destructive distillation of shale. Used as a mild antiseptic ointment for skin disorders and as a solution in glycerin to reduce inflammation. (Ichthyol.)

Ichthyol™ ichthammol.*

ichthyoses (ik-thē-ōs'-ēz) *npl* group of congenital conditions with dry, scaly skin. Fish skin. Xeroderma.* *ichthyosis hystrix* form of congenital nevus with patches of warty excrescences.

ICSH *abbr* interstitial*-cell stimulating hormone.

icterus (ik'-tėr-us) *n* → jaundice. *icterus gravis* acute diffuse necrosis of the liver. *icterus gravis neonatorum* a clinical form of hemolytic* disease of the newborn. *icterus neonatorum* excess of normal, or physiological, jaundice occurring in the first week of life as a result of excessive destruction of hemoglobin. → phototherapy. *icterus index* measurement of concentration of bilirubin in plasma. Used in diagnosis of jaundice.

ICU *abbr* intensive* care unit.

Idamycin™ idarubicin.*

idarubicin (ī-dȧ-roo'-bi-sin) *n* antineoplastic drug, related to daunorubicin,* that inhibits nucleic acid synthesis. (Idamycin.)

IDDM *abbr* insulin dependent diabetes mellitus.

ideomotor (id-ē-ō-mō'-tor) *n* mental energy, in the form of ideas, producing automatic movement of muscles, e.g., mental agitation producing agitated movement of limbs.

idiopathic (id-ē-ō-path'-ik) *adj* of a condition of unknown or spontaneous origin, e.g., some forms of epilepsy. *idiopathic respiratory distress syndrome* → respiratory.

idioventricular (id-ē-ō-ven-trik'-ū-lȧr) *adj* pertaining to cardiac ventricles* and not affecting the atria.

idoxuridine (ī-doks-ūr′-i-dēn) *n* 5-iodo-2-deoxyuridine; antiviral agent for corneal herpetic ulcers. Interferes with synthesis of DNA in herpes simplex virus and prevents it from multiplying. (Herplex.)

Ig *abbr* → immunoglobulins.

IgE one class of immunoglobulin* which binds to the surface of mast cells and basophils, involved in hay fever, asthma and anaphylaxis.

ileal bladder (il′-ē-al) → ileo-ureterostomy.

ileal conduit (il′-ē-al) → ileo-ureterostomy.

ileitis (il-ē-ī′-tis) *n* inflammation of the ileum.*

ileocecal (il-ē-ō-sē′-kål) *adj* pertaining to the ileum and the cecum.

ileocolic (il-ē-ō-kol′-ik) *adj* pertaining to the ileum and the colon.

ileocolitis (il-ē-ō-kō-lī′-tis) *n* inflammation of the ileum and the colon.

ileocolostomy (il-ē-ō-kol-os′-to-mē) *n* surgically made fistula between ileum and colon, usually the transverse colon. Most often used to bypass an obstruction or inflammation in the cecum or ascending colon.

ileocystoplasty (il-ē-ō-sis′-tō-plas-tē) *n* operation to increase size of urinary bladder—**ileocystoplastic** *adj*.

ileoproctostomy (il-ē-ō-prok-tos′-to-mē) *n* an anastomosis between ileum and rectum; used when disease extends to the sigmoid colon.

ileorectal (il-ē-ō-rek′-tål) *adj* pertaining to the ileum and the rectum.

ileosigmoidostomy (il-ē-ō-sig-moyd-os′-to-mē) *n* an anastomosis between ileum and sigmoid colon; used where most of the colon must be removed.

ileostomy (il-ē-os′-to-mē) *n* surgically made fistula between the ileum and the anterior abdominal wall; usually a permanent form of artificial anus when all of the large bowel has to be removed, e.g., in severe ulcerative colitis. *ileostomy bags* rubber or plastic bags used to collect liquid discharge from an ileostomy.

ileoureterostomy (il-ē-o-ū′-rē-tėr-os′-to-mē) *n* (*syn* ureteroileostomy) transplantation of lower ends of the ureters from the bladder to an isolated loop of small bowel (ileal bladder) which, in turn, is made to open on the abdominal wall (ileal conduit).

ileum (il′-ē-um) *n* lower three-fifths of the small intestine, lying between the jejunum* and the cecum*—**ileal** *adj*.

ileus (il′-ē-us) *n* intestinal obstruction. Usually restricted to paralytic as opposed to mechanical obstruction and characterized by abdominal distension, vomiting and the absence of pain. → meconium.

iliac artery (il′-ē-ak) → Figure 9.

iliococcygeal (il-ē-ō-kok-sij′-ē-ål) *adj* pertaining to the ilium and coccyx.

iliofemoral (il-ē-ō-fem′-or-ål) *adj* pertaining to the ilium and the femur.

iliopectineal (il-ē-ō-pek-tin'-ē-ǎl) *adj* pertaining to the ilium and the pubis.

iliopsoas (il-ē-ō-sō'-as) *n* consist of the ilium and the loin muscles.

iliotibial tract muscle (il-ē-ō-tib'-ē-ǎl) → Figure 5.

ilium (il'-ē-um) *n* upper part of the innominate (hip) bone; it is a separate bone in the fetus—**iliac** *adj*.

Ilosone™ erythromycin.*

Imferon™ iron dextran complex or parenteral iron therapy. Used as a total dose infusion for rapid response in marked iron deficiency anemia.

imipramine (im-ip'-ra-mēn) *n* tricyclic antidepressant with anticholinergic properties. Cardiotoxic in overdose. (Janimine, Tofranil.)

immersion foot → trench foot.

immune *adj* possessing capacity to resist infection. *immune body* immunoglobulin.*

immune reaction, response that which causes a body to reject a transplanted organ, to respond to bacterial disease, and to act against malignant cells; cell mediated immunity.*

immunity *n* intrinsic or acquired state of resistance to an infectious agent. *active immunity* is acquired, naturally, during an infection or artificially by immunization.* *cell mediated immunity* T lymphocyte-dependent responses which cause graft rejection, immunity to some infectious agents and tumor rejection. *humoral immunity* from immunoglobulin produced by B-lymphocytes. Immunity can be innate (from inherited qualities), or acquired, actively or passively, naturally or artificially. *passive immunity* is acquired naturally when maternal antibody passes to the child via the placenta or in the milk, or artificially by administering sera containing antibodies from animals or human beings.

immunization *n* administration of antigens to induce immunity.*

immunocompromised patients (*syn* immunosuppressed patients) patients with defective immune responses, often produced by treatment with drugs or irradiation. Also occurs in some patients with cancer and other diseases affecting the lymphoid system. Patients are liable to develop infections with opportunistic organisms, such as *Candida, Pneumocystis carinii* and *Cryptococcus neoformans*.

immunodeficiency *n* state of having defective immune responses, leading to increased susceptibility to infectious diseases.

immunodeficiency diseases inherited or acquired disorders of the immune system.

immunogenesis (im-mū-nō-jen'-es-is) *n* process of production of immunity—**immunogenetic** *adj*.

immunogenicity (im-mū-nō-jen-is′-it′-ē) *n* ability to produce immunity.*

immunoglobulins (Igs) (im-mū-nō-glob′-ū-lins) *npl* (*syn* antibodies) high molecular weight proteins produced by B lymphocytes that can combine with antigens such as bacteria and produce immunity or interfere with membrane signals to produce autoimmune disease, e.g., thyrotoxicosis. Gross classifications are IgA, IgD, IgE, IgG and IgM, with numerous subtypes. The basic Y-shaped immunoglobulin molecule is capable of expression in several million subtle variants, with "tailored" specificity for a myriad of antigens.

immunology *n* study of the lymphocytes, inflammatory cells and associated cells and proteins that affect response to antigens—**immunological** *adj*.

immunopathology *n* study of tissue injury involving the immune system.

immunosuppression *n* treatment which reduces immunological responsiveness—**immunosuppressive** *adj*.

immunotherapy *n* any treatment used to produce immunity.

immunotransfusion *n* transfusion of blood from a donor previously rendered immune by repeated inoculations with a given agent from the recipient.

Imodium™ loperamide.*

impacted *adj* firmly wedged, abnormal immobility, as of feces in the rectum; fracture; a fetus in the pelvis; a tooth in its socket or a calculus in a duct. → fracture.

imperforate (im-pėr′-fōr-āt) *adj* lacking a normal opening. *imperforate anus* congenital absence of an opening into the rectum. *imperforate hymen* a fold of mucous membrane at the vaginal entrance which has no natural outlet for the menstrual fluid. → hematocolpos.

impetigo (im-pe-tī′-gō) *n* inflammatory, pustular skin disease usually caused by *Staphylococcus*, occasionally by *Streptococcus impetigo contagiosa*, a highly contagious form of impetigo, commonest on the face and scalp, characterized by vesicles which become pustules and then honey-colored crusts. → ecthyma—**impetiginous** *adj*.

impotence *n* inability to participate in sexual intercourse, by custom, referring to the male. Can be due to lack of erection or premature ejaculation.

impregnate *vt* fill; saturate; render pregnant.

Imuran™ azathioprine.*

Inapsine™ droperidol.*

inassimilable (in-as-sim′-il-à-bl) *adj* not capable of absorption.

incarcerated (in-kár′-sėr-āt-ed) *adj* of the abnormal imprisonment of a part, as in a hernia which is irreducible or a pregnant uterus held beneath the sacral promontory.

incised wound one which results from cutting with a sharp knife or scalpel; if uninfected it heals by first intention.

incision *n* result of cutting into body tissue, using a sharp instrument— **incisional** *adj*, **incise** *vt*.

incisors (in-sī'-sorz) *npl* the teeth first and second from the midline, four in each jaw used for cutting food.

inclusion bodies minute particles found in some cells of pathological and normal tissues.

incompatibility *n* usually refers to the bloods of donor and recipient in transfusion, when antigenic differences in red cells result in reactions such as hemolysis or agglutination. Also, as of two or more medicaments that counteract or attenuate the desired effects of each other.

incompetence *n* inadequacy to perform natural function, e.g., mitral incompetence—**incompetent** *adj*.

incontinence (in-kon'-tin-ens) *n* inability to control evacuation of urine or feces. *overflow incontinence* dribbling of urine from an overfull bladder. *stress incontinence* occurs when intra-abdominal pressure is raised, as in coughing, giggling and sneezing; usually some weakness of the urethral sphincter muscle coupled with anatomical stretching and displacement of the bladder neck.

incubation (in-kū-bā'-shun) *n* **1** period from entry of infection to appearance of the first symptom. **2** process of development, of an egg, of a bacterial culture. **3** process to which a baby in an incubator is exposed.

incubator (in'-kū-bā-tor) *n* **1** an enclosed cradle kept at appropriate temperatures in which premature or delicate babies can be reared. **2** a low-temperature oven in which bacteria are cultured.

incus (in'-kus) *n* central bone of the middle ear. → Figure 13.

indapamide (in-dap'-à-mīd) *n* antihypotensive diuretic. (Lozol.)

Inderal™ propranolol.*

indican (in'-di-kan) *n* potassium salt excreted in urine as a detoxification product of indoxyl. → indicanuria.

indicanuria (in-di-kan-ū'-rē-à) *n* excessive potassium salt (indican*) in urine. There are traces in normal urine; high levels are suggestive of intestinal obstruction. → indole.

indicator *n* a substance which, when added in small quantities, is used to make visible the completion of a chemical reaction or attainment of a certain pH.

Indocin™ indomethacin.*

indole (in'-dōl) *n* a product of decomposition of tryptophan* in the intestines; oxidized to indoxyl in the liver and excreted in urine as indican. → indican, indicanuria.

indolent *adj* applied to a sluggish ulcer, generally painless and slow to heal.

indomethacin (in-dō-meth'-ă-sin) *n* prostaglandin inhibitor with analgesic and anti-inflammatory properties. Useful in rheumatic disorders. Can be given orally but, to prevent nausea, capsules should be taken with a meal or a glass of milk. Also available as suppositories. (Indocid.)

induction *n* act of bringing on or causing to occur, as applied to anesthesia and labor.

induration (in-dur-ā'-shun) *n* hardening of tissue, as in hyperemia, infiltration by neoplasm, etc.—**indurated** *adj*.

industrial disease (*syn* occupational disease) disease contracted by reason of occupational exposure to an industrial agent known to be hazardous, e.g., dust, fumes, chemicals, irradiation, etc., the notification of, safety precautions against and compensation for which are controlled by law.

inertia *n* inactivity. *uterine inertia* lack of contraction of parturient uterus; may be primary due to constitutional weakness, secondary due to exhaustion from frequent and forcible contractions.

in extremis (in eks-trē'-mis) at the point of death.

infant *n* a baby less than 1 year old.

infantile paralysis → poliomyelitis.

infantilism (in-fant'-il-izm) *n* general retardation of development with persistence of childlike characteristics into adolescence and adult life.

infarct (in'-făr-kt) *n* area of tissue affected when the end artery supplying it is occluded, e.g., in kidney or heart. Common complication of subacute endocarditis.

infarction (in-fărk'-shun) *n* death of a section of tissue because blood supply has been cut off. → myocardial infarction.

infection *n* successful invasion, establishment and growth of microorganisms in tissues of the host. May be of an acute or chronic nature. *autoinfection* infection resulting from commensals* becoming pathogenic, or when commensals or pathogens* are transferred from one part of the body to another, for example, by finger. *cross infection* occurs when pathogens are transferred from one person to another. *hospital-acquired (nosocomial) infection (HAI)* one which occurs in a patient who has been in hospital for at least 72 h and did not have signs and symptoms of such infection on admission: 10%–12% of hospital patients develop a hospital-acquired infection. Urinary tract infection is most common type. *opportunistic infection* serious infection by a microorganism with little or no normal pathogenic activity but which has been encouraged by compromised immune activity or by an imbalance in relative population, as through treatment for another disease or condition—**infectious** *adj*.

infectious disease disease caused by a specific, pathogenic organism and capable of being transmitted from one to another individual by direct or indirect contact.

infectious mononucleosis (mon'-ō-noo-klē-ōs'-is) (*syn* glandular fever) contagious self-limiting disease due to Epstein-Barr virus. Characterized by fever, sore throat, enlargement of superficial lymph nodes and appearance of atypical lymphocytes resembling monocytes. Specific antibodies to Epstein-Barr virus are present in blood as well as an abnormal antibody with "heterophile" activity directed against sheep's red blood cells—basis of the Paul*-Bunnell test, positive in infectious mononucleosis. One attack confers complete immunity. Usually virus particles are present in saliva, hence the synonym "kissing disease."

inferior *adj* lower; beneath.

infertility *n* lack of ability to reproduce. Psychological and physical causes can play a part.

infibulation (in-fib'-ū-lā'-shun) *n* → circumcision.

infiltration *n* penetration of surrounding tissues, the oozing or leaking of fluid into tissues. *infiltration anesthesia* analgesia produced by infiltrating tissues with a local anesthetic.

inflammation *n* reaction of living tissues to injury, infection, or irritation; characterized by pain, swelling, redness and heat. Degree of redness can be measured by a tintometer—**inflammatory** *adj*.

influenza (in-floo-en'-zà) *n* acute viral infection of the nasopharynx and respiratory tract which occurs in epidemic or pandemic form—**influenzal** *adj*.

infraspinatus muscle (in-fra spin-à'-tus) → Figure 5.

infundibulum (in-fun-dib'-ū-lum) *n* any funnel-shaped passage. *infundibulum with fimbriae* → Figure 17—**infundibula** *pl*, **infundibular** *adj*.

infusion *n* **1** fluid flowing by gravity into the body. **2** aqueous solution containing the active principle of a drug, made by pouring boiling water on the crude drug. **3** amniotic* fluid infusion.

ingrowing toenail spreading of the nail into the lateral tissue, causing inflammation.

inguinal (ing'-gwin-àl) *adj* of the groin. *inguinal canal* tubular opening through lower part of the anterior abdominal wall, parallel to and a little above the inguinal (Poupart's) ligament; measures 38 mm. In the male it contains spermatic cord; in the female, the uterine round ligaments. *inguinal hernia* → hernia.

INH *abbr* isoniazid.*

injected *adj* congested, with full vessels.

injection *n* 1 act of introducing a fluid (under pressure) into the tissues, a vessel, cavity or hollow organ. (Air can be injected into a cavity. → pneumothorax.) 2 the substance injected.

injector *n* device in which a high flow of fluid (gas or liquid) flows through a jet and sucks other fluid in fixed proportions from a side limb.

innervation (in-nėr-vā′-shun) *n* the nerve supply to a part.

innocent *adj* benign; not malignant.

innominate (in-nom′-in-āt) *adj* unnamed. → hip bone.

inoculation (in-ok-ū-lā′-shun) *n* 1 injection of substances, esp. vaccine, into the body. 2 introduction of microorganisms into culture medium for propagation.

inorganic *adj* neither animal nor vegetable in origin.

inositol nicotinate (in-os′-i-tol nik′-ō-tin-āt) vasodilator used in peripheral vascular disease.

inotropic (ī-nō-trō′-pik) *adj* affecting the force of muscle contraction, applied particularly to cardiac muscle. An inotrope is a drug which increases contractile force of the heart.

insemination (in-sem-in-ā′-shun) *n* introduction of semen into the vagina, normally by sexual intercourse. *artificial insemination* instrumental injection of semen into the vagina.

insensible *adj* without sensation or consciousness. Too small or gradual to be perceived, as insensible perspiration.

insertion *n* 1 act of setting or placing in. 2 the attachment of a muscle to the bone it moves.

in situ (in si′-tū) in the correct position, undisturbed. Also describes a cancer which has not invaded adjoining tissue.

insomnia (in-som′-nē-à) *n* sleeplessness.

inspiration *n* drawing of air into the lungs; inhalation—**inspiratory** *adj*, **inspire** *vt*.

inspissated (in′-spis-āt-ed) *adj* thickened, as by evaporation or withdrawal of water, applied to sputum and culture media used in the laboratory.

instep *n* arch of the foot on the dorsal surface.

instillation *n* insertion of drops into a cavity, e.g., conjunctival sac, external auditory meatus.

insufflation (in-su-flā′-shun) *n* blowing air along a tube (eustachian, fallopian) to establish patency; blowing powder into a body cavity.

insulin (in′-sul-in) *n* a pancreatic hormone, made in the islet cells of Langerhans, secreted into blood and having a profound influence on carbohydrate metabolism by stimulating transport of glucose into cells. Prepared commercially in several forms and strengths which vary in speed, length and potency of action and which are used in treatment of diabetes mellitus. *insulin dependent diabetes mellitus (IDDM)* → diabetes. *insulin pump* a 250 g, 20 mm-thick apparatus made of titanium, powered by a fluid freon, inserted usually into the abdomen; delivers insulin as needed. Refilled every 4–8 weeks via self-sealing valve under the skin. *insulin test* for determining the completeness or otherwise of surgical vagotomy. When the vagus nerve is intact, hypoglycemia, in response to an intravenous injection of insulin, produces secretion of acid from the stomach. Complete vagotomy abolishes this response.

insulinoma (in-sul-in-ō′-mȧ) *n* adenoma of the islets of Langerhans.

Intal™ cromolyn sodium.

integument (in-teg′-ū-ment) *n* a covering, esp. the skin.

intensive care unit (ICU) hospital unit in which highly specialized monitoring, resuscitation and therapeutic techniques are used.

intention tremor → tremor.

interarticular (in-tėr-ȧr-tik′-ū-lȧr) *adj* between joints.

interatrial (in-tėr-ā′-trē-ȧl) *adj* between the two atria of the heart.

intercellular (in-tėr-sel′-ū-lȧr) *adj* between cells.

intercostal (in-tėr-kos′-tal) *adj* between the ribs.

intercourse *n* **1** human communication. **2** coitus.*

intercurrent *adj* describes a second disease arising during the course of another disease.

interferon (in-tėr-fēr′-on) *n* any of a group of cytokines,* secreted by several lymphocytes and connective-tissue cells. Effective against some viruses; virus triggers cellular production of interferon, which interacts with surrounding cells and renders them resistant to virus attack. Interferon has caused regression of tumor in some cases of multiple myelomatosis.

interleukins (in-tėr-loo′-kinz) *npl* class of cytokines,* secreted principally by various lymphocytes, that mobilize immune response to antigenic challenge; they cause fever, inflammation and growth of T cell, B cell and mast cell populations.

interlobar (in-tėr-lō′-bȧr) *adj* between the lobes, e.g., interlobar pleurisy.

interlobular (in-tėr-lob′-ū-lȧr) *adj* between the lobules.

intermenstrual (in-tėr-mens′-trū-ȧl) *adj* between menstrual periods.

intermittent *adj* occurring at intervals. *intermittent claudication* → claudication. *intermittent peritoneal dialysis* → dialysis. *intermittent positive pressure* → positive pressure ventilation.

internal *adj* inside. *internal ear* that part of the ear which comprises the vestibule, semicircular canals and the cochlea. *internal respiration* → respiration.

internal secretions those produced by the ductless or endocrine glands and passed directly into the blood stream; hormones. *internal version* → version.

interosseous (in-tėr-os′-sē-us) *adj* between bones.

interphalangeal (in-tėr-fȧl-an′-jē-ȧl) *adj* between the phalanges.*

interposition operation surgical replacement of part or all of the chain of ossicles.

interserosal (in-tėr-sėr-ōs′-ȧl) *adj* between serous membrane, as in the pleural, peritoneal and pericardial cavities.

intersexuality *n* possession of both male and female characteristics. → Turner syndrome, Klinefelter syndrome.

interspinous (in-tėr-spīn′-us) *adj* between spinous processes, esp. those of the vertebrae.

intertrigo (in-tėr-trī′-gō) *n* superficial inflammation occurring in moist skin folds—**intertrigenous** *adj*.

intertrochanteric (in-tėr-trō-kan-tėr′-ik) *adj* between trochanters, usually referring to those on the proximal femur.

interventricular (in-tėr-ven-trik′-ū-lȧr) *adj* between ventricles, as those of the brain or heart.

intervertebral (in-tėr-vėr′-te-brȧl) *adj* between the vertebrae, as disks and foramina. → nucleus, prolapse.

intestine *n* a part of the alimentary canal extending from the stomach to the anus (→ Figure 18). Comprises the small intestine (gut) and the large intestine (bowel)—**intestinal** *adj*.

intima (in′-tim-ȧ) *n* internal coat of a blood vessel—**intimal** *adj*.

intra-abdominal (in-trȧ-ab-dom′-in-ȧl) *adj* inside the abdomen.

intra-amniotic (in-trȧ–am-nē-ot′-ik) *adj* within, or into the amniotic fluid.

intra-arterial (in-trȧ–ȧr-tēr′-ē-ȧl) *adj* within an artery.

intra-articular (in-trȧ–ȧr-tik′-ū-lȧr) *adj* within a joint.

intrabronchial (in-trȧ-brong′-kē-ȧl) *adj* within a bronchus.

intracanalicular (in-trȧ-kan-al-ik′-ū-lȧr) *adj* within a canaliculus.

intracapillary (in-trȧ-kap′-il-ār-ē) *adj* within a capillary.

intracapsular (in-trȧ-kap′-sū-lar) *adj* within a capsule, e.g., that of the lens or a joint. → extracapsular *opp*.

intracardiac (in-trȧ-kȧr′-dē-ak) *adj* within the heart.

intracaval (in-trȧ-kā′-vȧl) *adj* within the vena cava, by custom, referring to the inferior one.

intracellular (in-trȧ-sel′-ū-lȧr) *adj* within cells. → extracellular *opp*.

intracerebral (in-trȧ-sėr-ē′-brȧl) *adj* within the cerebrum.

intracorpuscular (in-trȧ-kōr-pus′-kū-lȧr) *adj* within a corpuscle.

intracranial (in-trȧ-krā′-nē-ȧl) *adj* within the skull.

intracranial pressure (ICP) maintained at a normal level by brain tissue; intracellular and extracellular fluid, cerebrospinal* fluid and blood.

intracutaneous (in-trȧ-kū-tā′-nē-us) *adj* within the skin tissues.

intradermal (in-trȧ-dėr′-mȧl) *adj* within the skin.

intradural (in-trȧ-dū′-rȧl *adj* inside the dura mater.

intragastric (in-trȧ-gas′-trik) *adj* within the stomach.

intragluteal (in-trȧ-glū′-te-ȧl) *adj* within the gluteal muscle comprising the buttock.

intrahepatic (in-trȧ-hep-at′-ik) *adj* within the liver.

Intralipid ™ emulsion of soybean oil suitable for intravenous drip infusion. Half a liter of 20% solution contains 1000 kcal. Antibiotics or other drugs must not be added to the infusion.

intralobular (in-trȧ-lob′-ū-lȧr) *adj* within the lobule, as the vein draining a hepatic lobule.

intraluminal (in-trȧ-lū′-min-ȧl) *adj* within the hollow of a tubelike structure.

intralymphatic (in-trȧ-lim-fat′-ik) *adj* within a lymphatic gland or vessel.

intramedullary (in-trȧ-med′-ū-lā-rē) *adj* within the bone marrow.

intramural (in-trȧ-mūr′-ȧl) *adj* within the layers of the wall of a hollow tube or organ.

intramuscular (in-trȧ-mus′-kū-lȧr) *adj* within a muscle.

intranasal (in-trȧ-nā′-zȧl) *adj* within the nasal cavity.

intranatal (in-trȧ-nā′-tȧl) *adj* → intrapartum.

intraocular (in-trȧ-ok′-ū-lȧr) *adj* within the globe of the eye.

intraoral (in-trȧ-ōr′-ȧl) *adj* within the mouth, as an intraoral appliance.

intraorbital (in-trȧ-ōr′-bit-ȧl) *adj* within the orbit.

intraosseous (in-trȧ-os′-ē-us) *adj* inside a bone.

intrapartum (in-trȧ-pȧr′-tum) *adj* (*syn* intranatal) at the time of birth; during labor, as asphyxia, hemorrhage or infection.

intraperitoneal (in-trȧ-pėr-it-on-ē′-ȧl) *adj* within the peritoneal cavity.

intrapharyngeal (in-trȧ-fȧr-in-jē′-ȧl) *adj* within the pharynx.

intraplacental (in-trȧ-plȧ-sen′-tȧl) *adj* within the placenta.

intrapleural (in-trȧ-ploo′-rȧl) *adj* within the pleural cavity.

intrapulmonary (in-trȧ-pul′-mon-ār-ē) *adj* within the lungs, as intrapulmonary pressure.

intraretinal (in-trȧ-ret′-in-ȧl) *adj* within the retina.

intraserosal (in-trȧ-sér-ōs'-ȧl) *adj* within a serous membrane.

intraspinal (in-trȧ-spī'-nȧl) *adj* within the spinal canal.

intrasplenic (in-trȧ-splen'-ik) *adj* within the spleen.

intrasynovial (in-trȧ-sin-ō'-vē-ȧl) *adj* within a synovial membrane or cavity.

intrathecal (in-trȧ-thē'-kȧl) *adj* within the meninges; into the subarachnoid space.

intrathoracic (in-trȧ-thōr-as'-ik) *adj* within the cavity of the thorax.

intratracheal (in-trȧ-trā'-kē-ȧl) *adj* within the trachea.

intratumor (in-trȧ-tū'-mor) *adj* within a tumor.

intrauterine (in-trȧ-ū'-tėr-in) *adj* within the uterus. *intrauterine contraceptive* device (*IUD*) device implanted in the cavity of the uterus to prevent conception. Over 60 different forms known by the International Planned Parenthood Federation. *intrauterine growth retardation* (*IUGR*) associated with a poor delivery of maternal blood to the placental bed, diminished placental exchange or a poor fetal transfer from the placental area. Serial ultrasonography is beneficial in high-risk mothers.

intravaginal (in-trȧ-vag'-in-ȧl) *adj* within the vagina.

intravascular (in-trȧ-vas'-kū-lȧr) *adj* within the blood vessels.

intravenous (in-trȧ-vē'-nus) *adj* within or into a vein. *intravenous infusion* commonly referred to as a "drip," the closed administration of fluids from a containing vessel into a vein for hydration, correcting electrolytic imbalance or introducing nutrients, *intravenous injection* introduction of drugs, including anesthetics, into a vein; not a continuous procedure.

intraventricular (in-trȧ-ven-trik'-ū-lȧr) *adj* within a ventricle, esp. a cerebral ventricle.

intrinsic (in-trin'-sik) *adj* inherent or inside; from within, real; natural. *intrinsic factor* a protein released by gastric glands, essential for satisfactory absorption of the extrinsic factor, vitamin B_{12}.

introitus (in-trō'-it-us) *n* any opening in the body; an entrance to a cavity, particularly, the vagina.

intubation (in-tū-bā'-shun) *n* insertion of a tube into a hollow organ. Tracheal intubation is used during anesthesia to maintain an airway and to permit suction of the respiratory tract. *duodenal intubation* a double tube is passed as far as the pyloric antrum under fluoroscopy. The inner tube is then passed along to the duodenojejunal flexure. Barium sulfate suspension can then be passed to outline the small bowel.

intussusception (in-tus-sus-sep'-shun) *n* condition in which one part of the bowel telescopes into another, causing severe colic and intestinal obstruction. Occurs most commonly in infants around the time of weaning.

intussusceptum (in-tus-sus-sep'-tum) *n* invaginated portion of an intussusception.

intussuscipiens (in-tus-sus-sip'-ē-ens) *n* receiving portion of an intussusception.

inunction (in-ungk'-shun) *n* rubbing an oily or fatty substance into the skin.

invagination (in-vaj-in-ā'-shun) *n* act or condition of being ensheathed; a pushing inward, forming a pouch—**invaginate** *vt., vi.*

Inversine™ mecamylamine.*

inversion *n* turning inside out, as inversion of the uterus. → procidentia.

invertase (in'-vėr-tāz) *n* (*syn* β- fructofuranosidase) a sugar-splitting enzyme in intestinal juice.

in vitro (in vē'-trō) in glass, as in a test tube. *in vitro fertilization* (*IVF*) human ova are fertilized in test tubes in laboratories specializing in the technique.

in vivo (in vē'-vō) in living tissue.

involucrum (in-vol-ū'-krum) *n* a sheath of new bone, which forms around necrosed bone, in such conditions as osteomyelitis. → cloaca.

involuntary *adj* independent of the will, as muscle of the thoracic and abdominal organs.

involution *n* **1** normal shrinkage of an organ after fulfilling its functional role, e.g., uterus after labor. **2** in psychiatry, the period of decline after middle life. → subinvolution—**involutional** *adj.*

iodine (ī'-ō-dīn) *n* powerful antiseptic used as a tincture for skin preparation and emergency treatment of small wounds. Solution must be fresh, as it can become contaminated with *Pseudomonas aeruginosa*. Orally it is antithyroid, i.e., decreases release of hormones from the thyroid gland. *povidone iodine* → povidone.

iodism (ī'-ō-dizm) *n* poisoning by iodine* or iodides*; symptoms are those of a common cold and the appearance of a rash.

iodized oil (ī'-ō-dīzed) poppy-seed oil containing 40% of organically combined iodine. Should be colorless or pale yellow; darker solutions have decomposed. Used as contrast agent in X-ray examination of bronchial tract, sinuses and other cavities.

iodoform (ī-ō'-dō-form) *n* antiseptic iodine compound of yellow color and characteristic odor. Now used chiefly as BIPP.*

iodopsin (ī-ō-dop'-sin) *n* protein substance which, within vitamin A, is a constituent of visual purple present in the rods of the retina.

iodoquinol (ī-ō'-dō-kwin-ol) *n* used chiefly in amoebic dysentery in association with emetine.* (Diquinol.)

Ionamin™ phentermine.*

iontophoresis (ī-on-tō-fōr-ēs'-is) *n* (*syn* iontherapy) treatment whereby ions of various soluble salts (e.g., zinc, chlorine, iodine, histamine) are introduced into tissues by means of a constant electrical current; a form of electro-osmosis.

iopanoic acid (ī-ō-pan-ō'-ik) complex iodine derivative of butyric acid, used as contrast agent in cholecystography. Side reactions are few. (Telepaque.)

ipecac (ip'-i-kak) *n* dried root of the ipecacuanha plant from Brazil and other South American countries. Principal alkaloid is emetine.* Has expectorant properties and is widely used in acute bronchitis and relief of dry cough. A safe emetic in larger doses.

IPPB *abbr* intermittent positive pressure breathing. → positive pressure ventilation.

ipsilateral (ip-si-lat'-ėr-àl) *adj* on the same side.

iridectomy (ir-id-ek'-to-mē) *n* excision of a part of the iris, thus forming an artificial pupil.

iridencleisis (ir-id-en-klī'-sis) *n* an older type of filtering operation. Scleral incision made at angle of anterior chamber; meridian cut in iris; either one or both pillars are left in scleral wound to contract as scar tissue. Decreases intraocular tension in glaucoma.*

iridocele (ir-id'-ō-sēl) *n* (*syn* iridoptosis) protrusion of part of the iris through a corneal wound (prolapsed iris).

iridocyclitis (ir-id-ō-sī-klī'-tis) *n* inflammation of the iris* and ciliary* body.

iridodialysis (ir-id-ō-dī-al'-is-is) *n* a separation of the iris from its ciliary attachment.

iridoplegia (ir-id-ō-plē'-jà) *n* paralysis of the iris.

iridoptosis (ir-id-op-tō'-sis) *n* → iridocele.

iridotomy (ir-id-ot'-o-mē) *n* an incision into the iris.

iris (ī'-ris) *n* circular colored membrane forming the anterior one-sixth of the middle coat of the eyeball (→ Figure 15). Perforated in the center by an opening, the pupil. Contraction of its muscle fibers regulates the amount of light entering the eyes. *iris bombe* bulging forward of the iris due to pressure of the aqueous* humor behind, when posterior synechiae are present around the pupil.

iritis (ī-rī'-tis) *n* inflammation of the iris.

iron gluconate (gloo'-kon-āt) an organic salt of iron, less irritant and better tolerated than ferrous sulfate.

irreducible *adj* unable to be brought to desired condition. *irreducible hernia* → hernia.

irritable *adj* capable of being excited to activity; responding easily to stimuli. *irritable bowel syndrome, spastic colon* unusual motility of both small and large bowel which produces discomfort and intermittent pain; no organic cause can be found—**irritability** *n*.

ischemia (is-kē'-mē-à) *n* deficient blood supply to any part of the body. → angina, Volkmann—**ischemic** *adj*.

ischemic heart disease (is-kē'-mik) deficient blood supply to cardiac muscle causes central chest pain of varying intensity which may radiate to arms and jaw. Lumen of the blood vessels is usually narrowed by atheromatous plaques. If treatment with vasodilator drugs is unsuccessful, bypass surgery may be considered. → angina pectoris, myocardial infarction.

ischiorectal (is-kē-ō-rek'-tál) *adj* pertaining to the ischium and the rectum, as an ischiorectal abscess which occurs between these two structures.

ischium (is'-kē-um) *n* lower part of the innominate bone of the pelvis; the bone on which the body rests when sitting—**ischial** *adj*.

islets of Langerhans (lāng'-ėr-hanz) collections of special cells scattered throughout the pancreas. They secrete insulin, which is absorbed directly into the blood stream.

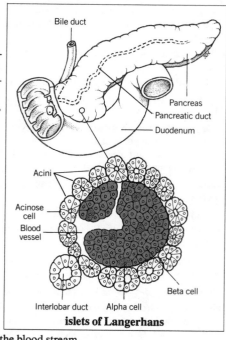

islets of Langerhans

Ismelin™ guanethidine.

isocarboxazid (ī-sō-kár-boks'-à-zid) *n* antidepressant. (Marplan.)

isoetharine (ī-sō-eth'-à-rēn) *n* smooth-muscle relaxant used as a bronchodilator. (Bronkosol.)

isoimmunization (ī-sō-im-mū-nī-zā'-shun) *n* development of anti-Rh agglutins in blood of an Rh-negative person who has been given an Rh-positive transfusion or who is carrying an Rh-positive fetus.

isoleucine (ī-sō-lū'-sēn) *n* one of the essential amino acids.

isoniazid (ī-sō-nī'-ȧ-zid) *n* derivative of isonicotinic acid; has a specific action against the tubercle bacillus and is widely employed in treatment of tuberculosis. Combined treatment with other tuberculostatic drugs, such as streptomycin* and PAS,* is not only more effective than any drug alone, but risk of bacterial resistance is also reduced. Can be neurotoxic, and some preparations include pyridoxine* to counteract this tendency. (Laniazid, Nydrazid.)

isopropamide (ī-sō-prōp'-ȧ-mīd) *n* drug which prevents spasm in digestive tract and helps to reduce acid secretion in the stomach. (Darbid.)

isoproterenol (ī-sō-prō-tēr'-en-ol) *n* epinephrine derivative that acts on beta-adrenergic receptors to relax bronchial smooth muscle; also acts as a cardiac stimulant. (Isuprel.)

isotonic (ī-sō-ton'-ik) *adj* equal tension; applied to any solution which has the same osmotic pressure as blood. *isotonic saline* (*syn* normal saline, physiological saline), 0.9% solution of salt in water.

isotopes (ī'-sō-tōps) *npl* two or more forms of the same element having identical chemical properties and the same atomic number but different mass numbers. Those isotopes with radioactive properties are used in medicine for research, diagnosis and treatment of disease.

isoxuprine (is-oks'-ū-prēn) *n* peripheral vasodilator and spasmolytic. Acts on myometrium, preventing contractions; thus useful in premature labor. (Vasodilan.)

isthmus (is'-thmus) *n* narrowed part of an organ or tissue such as that connecting the two lobes of the thyroid gland. *isthmus of the uterine tube* → Figure 17.

Isuprel™ isoproterenol.*

IUD *abbr* intrauterine* (contraceptive) device.

IV *abbr* intravenous.*

IVC *abbr* inferior vena cava.*

IVF *abbr* in* vitro fertilization.

IVP *abbr* intravenous pyelography. → urography.

IV push quick injection of medication intravenously.

J

Jacksonian epilepsy (jak-sōn'-ē-an) → epilepsy.

Jacquemier's sign (zhak'-mē-āz) blueness of the vaginal mucosa seen in early pregnancy.

Jakob-Creutzfeldt disease (jā'-kob–krutz'-feld) a recognized form of presenile dementia.*

Janimine™ imipramine.*

jaundice (jawn'-dis) *n* (*syn* icterus) condition characterized by raised bilirubin level in blood (hyperbilirubinemia). *latent jaundice* minor degrees are only detectable chemically; *overt* or *clinical jaundice* major degrees are visible in yellow skin, sclerae and mucosae. Jaundice may be due to (a) obstruction anywhere in the biliary tract (*obstructive jaundice*), (b) excessive hemolysis of red blood cells (*hemolytic jaundice*), (c) toxic or infective damage of liver cells (*hepatocellular jaundice*), (d) bile stasis (*cholestatic jaundice*). *acholuric jaundice* (*syn* spherocytosis*) jaundice without bile in the urine. *infective jaundice* most commonly due to a virus; infective hepatitis.* *leptospiral jaundice* → Weil's disease. *malignant jaundice* acute diffuse necrosis of the liver. *jaundice of the newborn* icterus* gravis neonatorum.

jawbone *n* either the maxilla (upper jaw) or mandible (lower jaw).

jejunostomy (je-joon-os'-to-mē) *n* surgically made fistula between the jejunum and the anterior abdominal wall; used temporarily for feeding in cases where passage of food through the stomach is impossible or undesirable.

jejunum (je-joo'-num) *n* that part of the small intestine between the duodenum* and the ileum*; about 2.44 m in length—**jejunal** *adj*.

joint *n* the articulation of two or more bones (arthrosis). Three main classes: (a) fibrous (synarthrosis), e.g., the sutures of the skull, (b) cartilaginous (*syn* chondrosis), e.g., between the manubrium and the body of the sternum, and (c) synovial, e.g., elbow or hip. → Charcot's joint.

jugular (jug'-ū-lar) *adj* pertaining to the throat. *jugular veins* two veins passing down either side of the neck (→ Figure 10).

junket *n* milk predigested by addition of rennet; curds and whey.

K

Kahn test serological test for diagnosis of syphilis.* Patient's serum reacts with a heterologous antigen prepared from mammalian tissue; flocculation occurs if syphilitic antibodies are present.

kala-azar (kȧ-lȧ–az′-ȧr) *n* generalized form of leishmaniasis* occurring in the tropics; with anemia, fever, splenomegaly and wasting. Caused by the parasite *Leishmania donovani* and spread by sandflies.

kanamycin (kan-ȧ-mī′-sin) *n* streptomycinlike antibiotic with basically similar actions and neurotoxic properties. (Kantrex.)

Kanner's syndrome (kan′-ėrz) autism.*

Kantrex™ kanamycin.*

kaolin (kā′-ō-lin) *n* natural aluminum silicate. When given orally absorbs toxic substances, hence useful in diarrhea, colitis and food poisoning. Also used as a dusting powder; when mixed with glycerin,* boric* acid, etc., used as a poultice.

Kaopectate™ antidiarrheal compound containing kaolin and pectin.

Kaposi's disease (kȧ-pō′-sēz) → xeroderma.

Kaposi's sarcoma (kȧ-pō′-sēz sȧr-kō′-mȧ) malignant, multifocal neoplasm of reticuloendothelial cells. First appears as brown or purple patches on the feet and spreads on the skin, metastasizing on the lymph nodes and viscera. Currently of interest because it can complicate acquired* immune deficiency syndrome.

Kaposi's varicelliform eruption occurs in eczematous children. Generalized bullous eczema; formerly fatal.

karyotype (kȧr′-ē-ō-tīp) *n* creation of an orderly array of chromosomes, usually derived from the study of cultured cells. Usually done for diagnostic purposes on abnormal persons, or persons prone to produce chromosomally abnormal children, or for prenatal detection of fetal abnormality in women at risk of producing chromosomally abnormal fetuses, for example, because of advancing age.

Kawasaki syndrome mucocutaneous* lymph node syndrome.

Kay Ciel™ potassium chloride.*

Keflex™ cephalexin* monohydrate.

Kegel exercises (ke'-gel) exercises for strengthening the female pelvic floor muscles.

Kell factor blood group factor found in about 10% of Caucasians; inherited according to Mendelian laws of inheritance. Anti-Kell antibodies can cross the placenta.

Kelly-Paterson syndrome → Plummer-Vinson syndrome.

keloid (kē'-loyd) *n* an overgrowth of scar tissue, which may produce a contraction deformity. Keloid scarring occurs in some heavily pigmented people; tends to get progressively worse.

Kemadrin™ procyclidine.*

Kenalog™ triamcinolone.*

keratectomy (kėr-à-tek'-to-mē) *n* surgical excision of a portion of the cornea.

keratin (kėr'-à-tin) *n* protein found in all horny tissue. Once used to coat pills given for intestinal effect, since keratin can withstand gastric juice.

keratinization (kėr'-àt-in-īz-ā'-shun) *n* conversion into horny tissue. Occurs as a pathological process in vitamin A deficiency.

keratitic precipitates (KP) (kėr-à-ti'-tik) large cells adherent to the posterior surface of the cornea*; present in inflammation of iris, ciliary body and choroid.

keratitis (kėr-à-tī'-tis) *n* inflammation of the cornea.*

keratoconjunctivitis (kėr'-à-tō-kon-jungk'-tiv-ī'-tis) *n* inflammation of cornea and conjunctiva. *epidemic keratoconjunctivitis* due to an adenovirus. Present as an acute follicular conjunctivitis with pre-auricular and submaxillary adenitis. *keratoconjunctivitis sicca* → Sjogren syndrome.

keratoconus (kėr-à-tō-kō'-nus) *n* a conelike protrusion of the cornea, usually due to a noninflammatory thinning.

keratoiritis (kėr'-à-tō-ī-rī'-tis) *n* inflammation of the cornea and iris.

keratolytic (kėr'-à-tō-li'-tik) *adj* having the property of breaking down keratinized epidermis.

keratoma (kėr-à-tō'-mà) *n* callosity*—**keratomata** *pl.*

keratomalacia (kėr'-à-tō-mal-ā'-sē-à) *n* softening of the cornea; ulceration may occur; frequently caused by lack of vitamin A.

keratome (kėr'-à-tōm) *n* a special knife with a trowel-like blade for incising the cornea.

keratopathy (kėr-à-top'-à-thē) *n* any disease of the cornea—**keratopathic** *adj.*

keratophakia (kėr'-à-tō-fāk'-ē-à) *n* surgical introduction of a biological "lens" into the cornea to correct hypermetropia.

keratoplasty (kėr-à-tō-plas'-tē) *n* → corneal graft—**keratoplastic** *adj.*

keratosis (kėr-à-tō'-sis) *n* thickening of the horny layer of the skin. Also referred to as hyperkeratosis. Has appearance of warty excrescences. *keratosis palmaris et plantaris* (*syn* tylosis) congenital thickening of horny layer of the palms and soles.

kerion (kē'-rē-on) *n* boggy suppurative mass of the scalp associated with ringworm.*

kernicterus (kėr-nik'-tėr-us) *n* bile staining of the basal ganglia in the brain that may result in mental deficiency; occurs in icterus* gravis neonatorum.

Kernig's sign (ker'-nigs) inability to straighten the leg at the knee joint when thigh is flexed at right angles to the trunk. Occurs in meningitis.

Ketalar™ ketamine.*

ketamine (ket'-à-mēn) *n* intravenous or intramuscular analgesic-anesthetic agent. Initial dose determined by patient's weight. Does not have muscular relaxation properties and is therefore unsuitable for intra-abdominal procedures. May cause hallucinations; postoperative absence of disturbance is important. (Ketalar.)

ketoacidosis (kē-tō-as-id-ōs'-is) *n* acidosis due to accumulation of ketones, intermediary products in the metabolism of fat—**ketoacidotic** *adj*.

ketoconazole (kē-tō-kon'-à-zōl) *n* antifungal agent. (Nizoral.)

ketogenic diet (kē-tō-jen'-ik) a high fat content producing ketosis (acidosis).

ketonemia (kē-tō-nē'-mē-à) *n* ketone bodies in blood—**ketonemic** *adj*.

ketones (kē'-tōns) *npl* organic compounds (e.g., ketosteroids) containing the carbonyl group, $C = 0$, bound to two other carbon atoms. *ketone bodies* (*syn* acetone bodies) term which includes acetone, acetoacetic acid and β-hydroxybutyric acid. → diabetes mellitus.

ketonuria (kē-tō-nū'-rē-à) *n* ketone bodies in urine—**ketonuric** *adj*.

ketoprofen (kē-tō-prō'-fen) *n* analgesic anti-inflammatory drug useful in arthritic and rheumatoid conditions. (Orudis.)

ketosis (kē-tō'-sis) *n* clinical picture arises from accumulation in blood stream of ketone bodies, β-hydroxybutyric acid, acetoacetic acid and acetone. Syndrome includes drowsiness, headache and deep respiration—**ketotic** *adj*.

ketosteroids (kē-tō-stėr'-oyds) *npl* steroid hormones which contain a carbonyl group, formed by addition of an oxygen molecule to the basic ring structure. The 17-ketosteroids (which have this oxygen at carbon-17) are excreted in normal urine and are present in excess in overactivity of the adrenal glands and the gonads.

kidney *n* gland situated one on either side of the vertebral column in the upper posterior abdominal cavity (→ Figures 19, 20). Main function is secretion of urine,* which flows into the ureters.* It secretes renin* and renal* erythropoietic factor. *horseshoe kidney* anatomical variation in which the inner lower border of each kidney is joined to give a horseshoe shape. Usually symptomless and only rarely interferes with drainage of urine into ureters. *kidney failure* → renal failure. *kidney machine* → dialyzer. *kidney transplant* surgical transplantation of a kidney from a previously tested suitable live donor or one who has recently died. Kidneys may also be transplanted from the renal bed to other sites in the same individual in cases of ureteric disease or trauma. *kidney function tests* various tests are available for measuring renal function. All require careful collection of urine specimens. Those in common use are para-aminohippuric acid clearance test for measuring renal blood flow; creatinine clearance test for measuring glomerular filtration rate; ammonium chloride test for measuring tubular ability to excrete hydrogen ions; urinary concentration and dilution tests for measuring tubular function.

Kimmelstiel-Wilson syndrome (kim'-el-stēl–wil'-son) intercapillary glomerulosclerosis* develops in diabetics who have hypertension, albuminuria and edema.

kinase (kī'-nāz) *n* enzyme activator which converts a zymogen to its active form; enzymes which catalyze the transfer of a high-energy group of a donor, usually adenosine triphosphate, to some acceptor, usually named after the acceptor (e.g., fructokinase).

kineplastic surgery (kin-ē-plas'-tik) operative measures whereby certain muscle groups are isolated and utilized to work certain modified prostheses.

kinesthesis (kin-es-thē'-sis) *n* muscle sense; perception of movement— **kinesthetic** *adj*.

kinetic (kin-et'-ik) *adj* pertaining to or producing motion.

Klebcil™ kanamycin.*

Klebsiella (kleb-sē-el'-à) *n* genus of bacteria. *K. pneumoniae* causes a rare form of severe pneumonia resulting in tissue necrosis and abscess formation.

Klebs-Loeffler bacillus (klebs–lef'-lér) *Corynebacterium* diphtheriae.

Klinefelter syndrome (klīn'-fel-tér) chromosomal abnormality affecting boys, usually with 47 chromosomes including XXY sex chromosomes. Puberty is frequently delayed, with small firm testes, often with gynecomastia. Associated with sterility, which may be the only symptom.

Klumpke's paralysis (kloomp'-kēz) paralysis and atrophy of muscles of forearm and hand, with sensory and pupillary disturbances due to injury to lower roots of brachial plexus and cervical sympathetic nerves. Clawhand results.

knee *n* hinge joint formed by the lower end of the femur and the head of the tibia. *kneecap* the patella.* *knee jerk* reflex contraction of the relaxed quadriceps muscle elicited by a tap on the patellar tendon; usually performed with the lower femur supported behind, knee bent and the leg limp. Persistent variation from normal usually signifies organic nervous disorder.

knuckles *npl* the dorsal aspect of any of the joints between the phalanges and the metacarpal bones, or between the phalanges.

Koch's bacillus (kōks) *Mycobacterium* tuberculosis.*

Koch-Weeks bacillus (kōk—wēks) *Haemophilus* aegyptius.*

Köhler's disease (ka'-lerz) osteochondritis* of the navicular bone. Confined to children of 3–5 years.

koilonychia (koyl-ō-nik'-ē-à) *n* spoon-shaped nails, characteristic of iron deficiency anemia.

Konakion™ phytonadione.*

Koplik's spots (kop'-liks) small white spots inside the mouth, during first few days of the invasion (prodromal) stage of measles.*

Korsakoff psychosis, syndrome (kōr'-sà-kof) alcoholic dementia; polyneuritic psychosis. A condition which follows delirium and toxic states. Often due to alcoholism. Mind is clear and alert, but patient is disoriented for time and place; memory is grossly impaired, esp. for recent events. Patient often confabulates to fill gaps in memory; afflicts more men than women in the 45–55 age group.

Krabbe disease (krab) genetically determined degenerative disease of the central nervous system associated with mental subnormality.

kraurosis vulvae (kraw-rō'-sis vul'-vē) degenerative condition of the vaginal introitus associated with postmenopausal lack of estrogen.

Kreb's cycle (krebs) citric acid cycle. Series of reactions in which a two-carbon substance is oxidized to form carbon dioxide and water, the end product of metabolism of carbohydrates, fats and proteins, producing energy as an end result.

Krukenberg tumor (Kruk'-en-berg) secondary malignant tumor of the ovary; primary growth is usually in the stomach.

kuru (koo'-roo) *n* slow virus disease of central nervous system. Probably transmitted by cannibalism. Rare and declining in incidence. Occurred exclusively among New Guinea highlanders.

kwashiorkor (kwash-ē-ōr'-kor) *n* nutritional disorder of infants and young children when diet is persistently deficient in essential protein; commonest where maize is the staple diet. Characteristic features are anemia, wasting, dependent edema and a fatty liver. Untreated, progresses to death.

Kwell™ lindane.*

KY jelly™ mucilaginous lubricating jelly.

kymograph (kī'-mō-graf) *n* apparatus for recording movements, e.g., of muscles, columns of blood. Used in physiological experiments—**kymographic** *adj*.

kypholordosis (kī-fō-lor-dō'-sis) *n* coexistence of kyphosis* and lordosis.*

kyphoscoliosis (kī-fō-skō-lē-ō'-sis) *n* coexistence of kyphosis* and scoliosis.*

kyphosis (kī-fō'-sis) *n* as in Pott's* disease, an excessive backward curvature of the dorsal spine—**kyphotic** *adj*.

L

labetalol (la-bet′-à-lol) *n* combined alpha-beta-blocking drug given by i.v. infusion in control of acute severe hypertension.* Also given orally in hypertension. (Normodyne, Trandate.)

labia (lā′-bē-à) *npl* lips. *labia majora* two large liplike folds extending from the mons veneris to encircle the vagina *labia minora* two smaller folds lying within the labia majora—**labium** *sing*, **labial** *adj*.

lability (la-bil′-it-ē) *n* instability. *emotional lability* rapid change in mood. Occurs esp. in mental disorders of old age—**labile** *adj*.

labioglossolaryngeal (lā′-bē-ō-glos′-ō-lar-in′-jē-àl) *adj* relating to the lips, tongue and larynx. *labioglossolaryngeal paralysis* nervous disease characterized by progressive paralysis of the lips, tongue and larynx.

labioglossopharyngeal (lā′-bē-ō-glos′-ō-far-in-jē-àl) *adj* relating to the lips, tongue and pharynx.

labor *n* (*syn* parturition) act of giving birth. First stage lasts from onset until full dilation of the cervical os; second stage lasts until baby is delivered; third stage until placenta is expelled.

labyrinth (lab′-i-rinth) *n* tortuous cavities of the internal ear. *bony labyrinth* that part directly hollowed out of the temporal bone. *membranous labyrinth* membrane that loosely lines the bony labyrinth—**labyrinthine** *adj*.

labyrinthectomy (lab-i-rin-thek′-to-mē) *n* surgical removal of part or all of membranous labyrinth of the internal ear. Sometimes carried out for Menière's disease.

labyrinthitis (lab-i-rin-thī′-tis) *n* inflammation of the internal ear.

lacerated wound one in which tissues are torn, usually by a blunt instrument or pressure; likely to become infected and to heal by second intention. → healing.

lacrimal, lachrymal, lacrymal (lak′-ri-mal) *adj* pertaining to tears. *lacrimal bone* a tiny bone at inner side of the orbital cavity. *lacrimal duct* connects lacrimal gland to upper conjunctival sac. *lacrimal gland* situated above the upper, outer canthus of the eye. → dacryocyst.

lacrimation (lak-ri-mā′-shun) *n* an outflow of tears; weeping.

lacrimonasal (lak-ri-mō-nā′-zàl) *adj* pertaining to the lacrimal and nasal bones and ducts.

lactagogue (lak′-tà-gog) *n* any substance given to stimulate lactation.

lactalbumin (lak-tal-bū'-min) *n* more easily digested of the two milk proteins. → caseinogen.

lactase (lak'-tāz) *n* (*syn* β-galactosidase) saccharolytic enzyme of intestinal juice; splits lactose* into glucose* (dextrose) and galactose.* *lactase deficiency* clinical syndrome of milk sugar intolerance. In severe congenital intolerance, infant may pass a liter or more of fluid stool per day. Temporary intolerance can follow neonatal alimentary tract obstructions, but rarely gives long-term problems. In non-Caucasian races a degree of intolerance develops at weaning.

lactate dehydrogenase (LDH) (dē-hī-dro'-jen-āz) (*syn* lactic dehydrogenase) an enzyme, of which there are five versions (isozymes), that catalyzes interconversion of lactate and pyruvate. LDH-1 is the one found in the heart; its blood level rises rapidly when heart tissues die, e.g., after a myocardial infarction. After heart transplant, rejection is imminent when LDH-1 activity is greater than that of its isozyme LDH-2 during the first four postoperative weeks. After 6 months this diagnostic indicator disappears. *lactate dehydrogenase test* when tissue of high metabolic activity dies the ensuing tissue necrosis is quickly reflected by an increase of the serum enzyme lactate dehydrogenase.

lactation (lak-tā'-shun) *n* **1** secretion of milk. **2** period during which child is nourished from the breast.

lacteals (lak'-tē-àls) *npl* the commencing lymphatic ducts in the intestinal villi; they absorb split fats and convey them to the receptaculum chyli.

lactic acid acid that causes souring of milk. Obtained by fermentation of lactose*; used as a vaginal douche, 1%. Sometimes added to milk to produce fine curds for treatment of gastroenteritis in infants.

lactiferous (lak-tif'-èr-us) *adj* conveying or secreting milk.

lactifuge (lak'-ti-fūj) *n* any agent which suppresses milk secretion.

Lactobacillus (lak'-tō-bà-sil'-us) *n* genus of bacteria. A large Gram-positive rod active in fermenting carbohydrates, producing acid. No members are pathogenic.

lactoflavin (lak'-tō-flā-vin) *n* riboflavin.*

lactogenic (lak-tō-jen'-ik) *adj* stimulating milk production.

lactose (lak'-tōs) *n* milk sugar, a disaccharide of glucose* and galactose.* Less soluble and less sweet than ordinary sugar. Used in infant feeding to increase carbohydrate content of diluted cow's milk. In some infants the gut is intolerant to lactose. → lactase.

lactosuria (lak-tō-sū'-rē-á) *n* lactose in urine—**lactosuric** *adj*.

lactulose (lak'-tū-lōs) *n* a sugar which is not metabolized, so that it reaches the colon unchanged. Sugar-splitting bacteria then act on it, promoting a softer stool. (Cephulac, Chronulac.)

lacuna (là-kū'-nà) *n* space between cells; usually used in description of bone—**lacunae** *pl*, **lacunar** *adj*.

lambliasis (lam-blī'-à-sis) *n* → giardiasis.

lamella (là-mel'-à) *n* **1** thin platelike scale or partition. **2** a gelatin-coated disk containing a drug; inserted under the eyelid—**lamellae** *pl*, **lamellar** *adj*.

lamina (lam'-in-à) *n* thin plate or layer, usually of bone—**laminae** *pl*.

laminectomy (lam-in-ek'-to-mē) *n* removal of vertebral laminae—to expose spinal cord nerve roots and meninges. Most often performed in lumbar region, for removal of degenerated intervertebral disk.

Lancefield's groups (lans'-fēlds) subdivision of the genus *Streptococcus* on the basis of antigenic structure. Members of each group have a characteristic capsular polysaccharide. Most dangerous to man belong to Group A.

Landry's paralysis (lan'-drēz) acute ascending condition accompanied by fever; may terminate in respiratory stasis and death. → paralysis.

Laniazid™ isoniazid.*

lanolin (lan'-ō-lin) *n* (*syn* adeps lanae hydrosus) wool fat containing 30% water. *Anhydrous lanolin* is that fat obtained from sheep's wool. Used in ointment bases, as such bases can form water-in-oil emulsions with aqueous constituents, and are readily absorbed by the skin. Contact sensitivity to lanolin products may occur.

Lanoxin™ digoxin.*

lanugo (lan-ū'-gō) *n* soft, downy hair sometimes present on newborn infants, esp. when premature. Usually replaced before birth by vellus hair.

laparoscopy (lap-àr-os'-ko-pē) *n* (*syn* peritoneoscopy) endoscopic examination of pelvic organs via transperitoneal route. A laparoscope is introduced through the abdominal wall after induction of a pneumoperitoneum.* For biopsy, aspiration of cysts and division of adhesions. Tubal ligation for sterilization and even ventrosuspension can be performed via the laparoscope—**laparoscopic** *adj*.

laparotomy (lap-àr-ot'-o-mē) *n* incision of the abdominal wall. Usually reserved for exploratory operation.

Larodopa™ levodopa.*

larvicide (làr'-vi-sīd) *n* any agent which destroys larvae—**larvicidal** *adj*.

laryngeal (lar-in-jē'-àl) *adj* pertaining to the larynx.

laryngectomy (lar-in-jek'-to-mē) *n* surgical removal of the larynx.

laryngismus stridulus (lar-in-jis'-mus strī'-dū-lus) momentary sudden attack of laryngeal spasm with a crowing sound on inspiration. Occurs in inflammation of the larynx, in connection with rickets, and as an independent disease.

laryngitis (lar-in-jī'-tis) *n* inflammation of the larynx.

laryngofissure (lar-ing'-gō-fish'-ūr) *n* operation of opening the larynx in midline.

laryngology (lar-ing-gol'-o-jē) *n* study of diseases affecting the larynx.

laryngoparalysis (lar-ing'-gō-par-al'-is-is) *n* paralysis of the larynx.

laryngopharyngectomy (lar-ing'-gō-far-in-jek'-to-mē) *n* excision of the larynx and lower part of pharynx.

laryngopharynx (lar-ing-gō-far'-ingks) *n* lower portion of the pharynx— **laryngopharyngeal** *adj*.

laryngoscope (lar-ing'-gō-skōp) *n* instrument for exposure and visualization of larynx, for diagnostic or therapeutic purposes or during the procedure of tracheal intubation—**larnygoscopy** *n*, **laryngoscopic** *adj*.

laryngospasm (lar-ing'-gō-spazm) *n* convulsive involuntary muscular contraction of the larynx, usually accompanied by spasmodic closure of the glottis.

laryngostenosis (lar-ing'-gō-sten-ōs'-is) *n* narrowing of the glottic aperture.

laryngotomy (lar-ing-got'-o-mē) *n* operation of opening the larynx.

laryngotracheal (lar-ing'-gō-trāk'-ē-ál) *adj* pertaining to the larynx* and trachea.*

laryngotracheitis (lar-ing'-gō-trāk-ē-ī'-tis) *n* inflammation of the larynx* and trachea.*

laryngotracheobronchitis (lar-ing'-gō-trāk'-ē-ō-brong-kī'-tis) *n* inflammation of the larynx,* trachea* and bronchi.*

laryngotracheoplasty (lar-ing'-gō-trāk'-ē-ō-plas'-tē) *n* operation to widen a stenosed airway—**laryngotracheoplastic** *adj*.

larynx (lar'-ingks) *n* the organ of voice, situated below and in front of the pharynx* and at the upper end of the trachea.* → Figure 6—**laryngeal** *adj*.

Lasen syndrome (las'-en) multiple joint dislocations.

Lassa fever (las'-så) a viral* hemorrhagic fever. Incubation period is 3–16 days; early symptoms resemble typhoid* and septicemia.* By the sixth day ulcers develop in mouth and throat; fever is variable, sometimes very high. Fatality rate in some areas is as high as 67%. Infected people must be nursed in strict isolation.

Lassar's paste (las'-sårz) contains zinc oxide, starch and salicylic acid in soft paraffin. Used in eczema and similar conditions as an antiseptic protective.

lateral (lat'-ér-ál) *adj* at or belonging to the side; away from the median line.

latissimus dorsi (lat-is'-i-mus dōr'-sī) → Figures 4, 5.

laudanum (lawd'-a-num) *n* old name for tincture of opium.*

laughing gas → nitrous oxide.

lavage (låv-åzh') *n* irrigation of or washing out a body cavity.

laxatives *npl* (*syn* aperients) drugs that produce peristalsis and promote evacuation of the bowel, usually to relieve constipation. More powerful laxatives are known as purgatives, and drastic purgatives are termed cathartics. Laxatives are further classified, relating to constituents or to function, as saline, vegetable, synthetic, bulk-increasers (bulking), or lubricators (lubricants).

LDH *abbr* lactate* dehydrogenase.

L-dopa *abbr* levodopa.*

LE *abbr* lupus* erythematosus. *LE cells* characteristic cells found in patients with lupus* erythematosus.

lead *n* soft metal with toxic salts. *lead and opium* applied as a compress to relieve bruises, pain and swelling. *lead colic* → colic. *lead lotion* weak solution of lead subacetate used as a soothing astringent lotion for sprains and bruises. *lead poisoning* (*syn* plumbism) acute poisoning is unusual, but chronic poisoning due to absorption of small amounts over a period is less uncommon. Can occur in young children by sucking articles made of lead alloys, or painted with lead paint. Where the water supply is soft, lead poisoning may occur because drinking water picks up lead from water pipes. In spite of legislation and safety precautions, industrial poisoning is still the commonest cause. Anemia, loss of appetite, and the formation of a blue line round the gums are characteristic. Nervous symptoms, including convulsions* are seen in severe cases.

lecithins (les'-i-thinz) *npl* group of phosphoglycerides esterified with the alcohol group of choline.* Found in animal tissues, mainly in cell membranes. *lecithin-sphingomyelin ratio* test which assesses fetal lung maturity. Below 20 is indicative of higher risk of respiratory* distress syndrome. Cortisone can be given to stimulate maturity of fetal lungs and so reduce risk of respiratory distress syndrome.

lecithinase (les'-i-thin-āz) *n* (*syn* phospholipase D) enzyme which catalyzes decomposition of lecithin (phosphatidylcholine) and occurs in toxin of *Clostridium perfringens*.

leech *n Hirudo medicinalis* aquatic worm which can be applied to the human body to suck blood; saliva contains hirudin,* an anticoagulant.

Lee-white clotting time blood coagulation test, used to detect severe bleeding disorders.

Legionella pneumophila (le-jun-el'-à nū-mof'-il-à) small Gram-negative non-acid-fast bacillus which causes legionnaire's* disease and Pontiac* fever.

legionnaires' disease severe and sometimes fatal disease caused by *Legionella* *pneumophilia*: with pneumonia, dry cough, myalgia and sometimes gastrointestinal symptoms. Can cause renal impairment and eventual cardiovascular collapse. → Pontiac fever.

Leishman-Donovan bodies (lēsh'-man–don'-o-van) rounded forms of the protozoa *Leishmania* found in endothelial cells and macrophages of patients suffering from leishmaniasis.*

Leishmania (lēsh-mā'-nē-à) *n* genus of flagellated protozoon. *L. donovani* responsible for disease of kala-azar* or leishmaniasis.*

leishmaniasis (lēsh-man-ī'-à-sis) *n* infestation by *Leishmania,* spread by sandflies. Generalized manifestation is kala-azar.* Cutaneous manifestation is such as oriental* sore.

lens *n* small biconvex crystalline body supported in the suspensory ligament immediately behind the iris of the eye (→ Figure 15). On account of its elasticity, the lens can alter in shape, enabling light rays to focus exactly on the retina.

lenticular (len-tik'-ū-làr) *adj* pertaining to or resembling a lens.*

lentigo (len-tī'-gō) *n* freckle with an increased number of pigment cells. → epiphelides—**lentigines** *pl.*

leontiasis (lē-on-tī'-à-sis) *n* enlargement of face and head giving a lionlike appearance; most often caused by fibrous dysplasia of bone.

leprology (lep-rol'-o-jē) *n* study of leprosy* and its treatment—**leprologist** *n.*

lepromata (le-prō'-mà-tà) *npl* the granulomatous cutaneous eruption of leprosy—**leproma** *sing,* **lepromatous** *adj.*

leprosy (lep'-ros-ē) *n* progressive and contagious disease, endemic in warmer climates and characterized by granulomatous formation in nerves or on skin. Caused by *Mycobacterium leprae* (Hansen's bacillus). BCG* vaccination conferred variable protection in different trials. Leprosy can be controlled but not cured by long-term treatment with sulfone drugs—**leprous** *adj.*

leptocytosis (lep-tō-sī-tō'-sis) *n* thin, flattened, circulating red blood cells (lepotocytes). Characteristic of thalassemia.* Also seen in jaundice, hepatic disease and sometimes after splenectomy.

leptomeningitis (lep-tō-men-in-jī'-tis) *n* inflammation of the covering membranes (arachnoid* and pia* mater) of brain or spinal cord.

Leptospira (lep-tō-spī'-rà) *n* genus of bacteria. Very thin, finely coiled bacteria which require dark ground microscopy for visualization. Common in water as saprophytes; pathogenic species are numerous in many animals and may infect man. *L. interrogans* serotype *icterohaemorrhagiae* causes Weil's* disease in man; *L. interrogans* serotype *canicola* "yellows" in dogs and pigs, transmissible to man. → leptospirosis.

leptospiral agglutination tests serological tests used in diagnosis of specific leptospiral infections, e.g., Weil's* disease.

leptospirosis (lep-tō-spī-rō'-sis) *n* infection of man by *Leptospira* from rats, dogs, pigs, foxes, mice, and possibly cats. With high fever, headache, conjunctival congestion, jaundice, severe muscular pains, and vomiting. As fever abates, in about a week, jaundice disappears. → Weil's disease.

Leptothrix (lep'-tō-thriks) *n* genus of bacteria. Gram-negative; found in water; nonpathogenic. Also used in medical bacteriology to describe filamentous bacteria resembling actinomycetes.*

Lesch-Nyhan disease (lesk–nī'-han) X-linked recessive genetic disorder. Overproduction of uric acid, associated with brain damage resulting in cerebral palsy and mental retardation. Victims are compelled, by a self-destructive urge, to bite away the sides of mouth, lips and fingers.

lesion (lē'-zhun) *n* pathological change in a bodily tissue.

leucine (loo'-sēn) *n* an amino acid. Leucine-induced hypoglycemia is a genetic metabolic disorder due to sensitivity to leucine.

leukemia (loo-kē'-mē-à) *n* malignant proliferation of the leukopoietic tissues usually producing an abnormal increase in leukocytes in blood. Proliferation of immature cells is acute leukemia, which is either myeloblastic or lymphoblastic. *acute myeloblastic leukemia* rapidly fatal if not treated; requires intensive in-patient chemotherapy. Average duration of first remission is 14 months. *acute lymphoblastic leukemia* has more favorable outlook and many children can expect to be cured after a 2-year course of treatment. Proliferation of mature cells is chronic leukemia, which is either myelocytic (granulocytic) or lymphocytic. *chronic myelocytic leukemia* may run a static course over several years but eventually acute phase supervenes (blast crisis). *chronic lymphocytic leukemia* occurs mainly in the elderly. Little active treatment is necessary and patients may live comfortably for many years—**leukemic** *adj.*

Leukeran™ chlorambucil.*

leukocidin (loo-kō-sī'-din) *n* bacterial exotoxin* which selectively destroys white blood cells.

leukocytes (loo'-kō-sīts) *npl* the white corpuscles of the blood, some of which are granular and some nongranular. In blood stream they are colorless, nucleated masses, and some are motile and phagocytic. → basophil, eosinophil, lymphocyte, mononuclear, polymorphonuclear—**leukocytic** *adj.*

leukocytolysis (loo-kō-sī-tol'-is-is) *n* destruction and disintegration of white blood cells—**leukocytolytic** *adj.*

leukocytosis (loo-kō-sī-tō'-sis) *n* increased number of leukocytes* in blood. Often a response to infection—**leukocytotic** *adj.*

leukoderma (loo-kō-dėr'-mà) *n* defective skin pigmentation, esp. when it occurs in patches or bands.

leukoma (loo-kō'-mà) *n* white opaque spot on the cornea—**leukomata** *pl,* **leukomatous** *adj.*

leukonychia (loo-kō-nik'-ē-à) *n* white spots on the nails.

leukopenia (loo-kō-pē'-nē-à) *n* decreased number of white blood cells in blood—**leukopenic** *adj*.

leukoplakia (loo-kō-plā'-kē-à) *n* white, thickened patch occurring on mucous membranes. Occurs on lips, inside mouth or on genitalia. Sometimes denotes precancerous change. Sometimes due to syphilis. → kraurosis vulvae.

leukopoiesis (loo-kō-poy-ēs'-is) *n* the formation of white blood cells—**leukopoietic** *adj*.

leukorrhoea (loo-kō-rē'-à) *n* sticky, whitish vaginal discharge—**leukorrhoeal** *adj*.

levallorphan (lev-al'-ōr-fan) *n* narcotic antagonist. (Lorfan.)

levator (lev-ā'-tor) **1** *adj* muscle which acts by raising a part. *levator ani* muscle which helps form the pelvic floor. *levator scapulae* → Figure 5. **2** *n* an instrument for lifting a depressed part.

levodopa (L-dopa) (le-vō-do'-pà) *n* synthetic anti-Parkinson drug. Treats inadequate dopamine* (a transmitter substance) in the basal ganglia. In these ganglia levodopa is converted into dopamine and replenishes stores. Unlike dopamine, levodopa can cross the blood-brain barrier. (Larodopa.) → carbidopa.

Levo-Dromoran™ levorphanol.*

levonorgestrel (le-vō-nōr-jes'-trel) *n* hormone widely used in oral contraceptives. In implant form, under the skin of forearm, effect lasts for 5 years. (Norplant.)

Levophed™ norepinephrine.*

levorphanol (le-vōr'-fan-ol) *n* synthetic substitute for morphine.* Less hypnotic than morphine but more extended action. Almost as effective by mouth as by injection. (Levo Dromoran.)

Levoprome™ methotrimeprazine.*

levothyroxine (le-vō-thī-roks'-ēn) *n* synthetic thyroxine, main hormone secreted by thyroid gland. Used for thyroxine replacement therapy.

levulose (lev'-ū-lōs) *n* fructose or fruit sugar, a monosaccharide found in many sweet fruits; the sugar in honey and, combined with glucose, major constituent of cane sugar. Sweeter and more easily digested than ordinary sugar; useful for diabetics. *levulose test* for hepatic function. A measured amount of levulose does not normally increase the level of blood sugar, except in hepatic damage.

LH *abbr* luteinizing hormone.

libido (li-bē'-dō) *n* though of fuller scope in psychoanalytic theory, loosely used in medicine to mean the sexual urge.

Librium™ chlordiazepoxide.*

lice *npl* → pediculus.

lichen (lī'-ken) *n* aggregations of papular skin lesions. *lichen nitidus* characterized by minute, shiny, flat-topped, pink papules of pinhead size. *lichen planus* eruption of unknown cause showing purple, angulated, shiny, flat-topped papules. *lichen scrofulosorum* a form of tuberculide. *lichen simplex* → neurodermatitis. *lichen spinulosus* disease of children characterized by very small spines protruding from follicular openings of the skin and resulting from vitamin A deficiency. *lichen urticatus* papular urticaria*—**lichenoid** *adj*.

lichenification (lī-ken'-i-fi-kā'-shun) *n* thickening of the skin, usually secondary to scratching. Skin markings become more prominent and the area affected appears to be composed of small, shiny rhomboids. → neurodermatitis.

licorice (lik'-ōr-ish) *n* → glycyrrhiza.

lidocaine (lī'-dō-kān) *n* local anesthetic with more powerful and prolonged action than procaine. Strength of solution varies from 0.5% for infiltration anesthesia to 2% for nerve block. Adrenalin* is usually added to delay absorption. Also effective for surface anesthesia as ointment (2%) and for urethral anesthesia as a 2% gel.(Xylocaine.)

lien (lī'-en) *n* the spleen.*

lienculus (lī-en'-kū-lus) *n* a small accessory spleen.

lienitis (lī-en-ī'-tis) *n* inflammation of the spleen.*

lienorenal (lī-en-ō-rē'-nál) *adj* pertaining to spleen* and kidney.* In *lienorenal* shunt, the splenic vein is anastomosed to the left renal vein to relieve portal hypertension.

ligament (lig'-à-ment) *n* strong band of fibrous tissue serving to bind bones or other parts together, or to support an organ. *ligament of ovary* → Figure 17—**ligamentous** *adj*.

ligate (lī'-gāt) *vt* to tie off blood vessels, etc., at operation—**ligation** *n*.

ligature (līg'-à-chūr) *n* material used for tying vessels or sewing tissues. Silk, horsehair, catgut, kangaroo tendon, silver wire, nylon, linen and fascia can be used.

lightening *n* commonly, relief of pressure on the diaphragm by the abdominal viscera, when presenting part of the fetus descends into the pelvis in the last 3 weeks of a primigravida's* pregnancy.

lightning pains symptomatic of tabes dorsalis. Occur as paroxysms of swift-cutting (lightning) stabs in lower limbs.

limbic system those parts of the brain concerned with controlling autonomic function and emotions.

lime water solution of calcium hydroxide (about 10–15%). Used in skin lotions, and with an equal volume of linseed or olive oil as a soothing application.

liminal (lim'-in-ål) *adj* of a stimulus, of the lowest intensity which can be perceived by the human senses. → subliminal.

Lincocin™ lincomycin.*

lincomycin (lin-kō-mī'-sin) *n* antibiotic for serious infections caused by Gram-positive pathogens; can induce severe colitis as a side-effect. (Lincocin.)

linctus (link'-tus) *n* sweet, syrupy liquid; should be slowly sipped.

lindane (lin'-dān) *n* used as shampoo for treatment of head lice. Less irritant than benzyl* benzoate for scabies; requires only one application. (Kwell.)

linea (lin'-ē-å) *n* a line. *linea alba* white line visible after removal of skin in the center of the abdomen, stretching from the ensiform cartilage to the pubis, its position on the surface being indicated by a slight depression. *linea nigra* pigmented line from umbilicus to pubis which appears in pregnancy. *lineae albicantes* white lines which appear on the abdomen after reduction of tension as after childbirth, tapping of the abdomen, etc.

lingua (ling'-gwå) *n* the tongue—**lingual** *adj*.

liniment *n* liquid to be applied to skin by gentle friction.

linolenic acid (lin-ō-lē'-nik) an unsaturated, essential fatty acid found in vegetable fats.

Lioresal™ baclofen.*

liothyronine (lī-ō-thī'-rō-nēn) *n* a secretion of thyroid gland, also known as triiodothyronine. Together with thyroxine* stimulates metabolism in body tissues. (Cytomel.)

lipase (lī'-pāz) *n* any fat-splitting enzyme. *pancreatic lipase* steapsin.*

lipid (lī'-pid) *n* any water-insoluble fat or fatlike substance extractable by nonpolar solvents such as alcohol. Lipids serve as a source of fuel and are an important constituent of cell membranes.

lipoid (lī'-poyd) *adj, n* substance resembling fats or oil. Serum lipoids are raised in thyroid deficiency.

lipoidosis (lī-poyd-ō'-sis) *n* disease due to disorder of fat metabolism—**lipoidoses** *pl*.

lipolysis (lī-pol'-is-is) *n* chemical breakdown of fat by lipolytic enzymes—**lipolytic** *adj*.

lipoma (lī-pō'-må) *n* benign tumor containing fatty tissue—**lipomata** *pl*, **lipomatous** *adj*.

lipoprotein (lī-pō-prō'-tēn) *n* lipid-protein compounds circulating in blood. Low-density lipoprotein (LDL) contains larger amounts of cholesterol than high* density lipoprotein (HDL), and higher levels (of LDL relative to HDL) are associated with cardiovascular disease.

lipotropic substances (lī-pō-trō′-pik) factors which cause removal of fat from the liver by transmethylation.

lipuria (lī-pū′-rē-à) *n* (*syn* adiposuria) fat in the urine—**lipuric** *adj*.

liquor *n* a solution. *liquor amnii* fluid surrounding the fetus. *liquor epispasticus* a blistering fluid. *liquor folliculi* fluid surrounding a developing ovum in a graafian follicle. *liquor sanguinis* fluid part of blood (plasma*).

Lithane™ lithium* carbonate.

lithiasis (li-thī′-à-sis) *n* any condition in which there are calculi.

lithium carbonate used in manic depressive illness. Possible side-effects include diarrhea, vomiting, drowsiness, ataxia, coarse tremor. Contraindicated in cardiac or renal disease. Regular blood serum levels of lithium are necessary and thyroid function should be assessed before and at regular intervals during treatment. (Lithane.)

litholapaxy (lith-ol-à-paks′-ē) *n* (*syn* lithopaxy) crushing a stone within the urinary bladder and removing the fragments by irrigation.

lithopedion (lith-ō-pē′-dē-on) *n* a dead fetus retained in the uterus, e.g., one of a pair of twins which dies and becomes mummified and sometimes impregnated with lime salts.

lithotomy (li-thot′-o-mē) *n* surgical incision of the bladder for removal of calculi.

lithotriptor (lith-ō-trip′-tor) *n* machine which sends sonic shock waves through renal calculi causing them to crumble and leave the body naturally in the urine.

lithotrite (lith′-ō-trīt) *n* instrument for crushing a stone in the urinary bladder.

lithuresis (lith-ūr-ēs′-is) *n* voiding of gravel* in the urine.

litmus (lit′-mus) *n* vegetable pigment used as an indicator of acidity (red) or alkalinity (blue). Often stored as paper strips impregnated with blue or red litmus; blue litmus paper turns red when in contact with an acid; red litmus paper turns blue when in contact with an alkali.

Little's disease diplegia* of spastic type causing "scissor leg" deformity. A congenital disease, with cerebral atrophy or agenesis.

liver *n* largest organ in the body, varying in weight but one-thirtieth of body weight (relatively much larger in the fetus). Situated in the right upper section of the abdominal cavity (→ Figure 18). Secretes bile,* forms and stores glycogen* and plays an important part in metabolism of proteins and fats. *liver transplant* surgical transplantation of a liver from a suitable donor who has recently died.

livid *adj* showing blue discoloration due to bruising, congestion or insufficient oxygenation.

lobe *n* rounded section of an organ, separated from neighboring sections by a fissure or septum, etc. → Figure 13—**lobar** *adj*.

lobectomy (lō-bek'-to-mē) *n* removal of a lobe, e.g., of the lung for lung abscess or localized bronchiectasis.

lobule (lōb'-ūl) *n* small lobe or subdivision of a lobe—**lobular, lobulated** *adj*.

lochia (lō'-kē-à) *n* vaginal discharge which occurs during the puerperium.* At first pure blood, later becomes paler, diminishes in quantity and finally ceases—**lochial** *adj*.

lockjaw *n* → tetanus.

locomotor (lō-kō-mō'-tor) *adj* applied to any tissue or system used in human movement. Usually refers to nerves and muscles. Sometimes includes bones and joints. *locomotor ataxia* disordered gait and loss of sense of position in the lower limbs, which occurs in tabes* dorsalis. Tabes dorsalis is still sometimes called "locomotor ataxia."

loculated (lok'-ū-lā-ted) *adj* divided into numerous cavities.

loiasis (lō-ī'-a-sis) *n* special form of filariasis (caused by the worm *Filaria loa*) which occurs in West Africa. The vector, a large horsefly, *Chrysops,* bites in the daytime. Larvae take 3 years to develop and may live in a man for 17 years. Accompanied by itching and eosinophilia.*

Lomotil™ mixture of diphenoxylate* and atropine* sulfate. Useful for loose colostomy and postvagotomy diarrhea. Reduces motility of gut and allows time for absorption of water from feces. A single dose lessens desire to defecate after 1 h, and is effective for 6 hours.

lomulizer (lom'-ū-lī-zer) *n* device which disperses fine powder (contained in a tiny plastic cartridge) through a mouthpiece.

lomustine (lō-mus'-tēn) *n* an alkylating cytotoxic agent.

Loniten™ minoxidil.

loperamide (lō-pèr'-à-mīd) *n* antidiarrheal agent especially useful in acute cases. (lmodium.)

lopressor™ metoprolol.*

lorazepam (lōr-az'-ė-pam) *n* tranquilizer similar to diazepam.* (Ativan.)

lordoscoliosis (lōr'-dō-skō-lē-ōs'-is) *n* lordosis* complicated by presence of scoliosis.*

lordosis (lōr-dō'-sis) *n* exaggerated forward, convex curve of the lumbar spine—**lordotic** *adj*.

Lorfan™ levallorphan.*

Lou Gehrig's disease amyotrophic* lateral sclerosis.

low back pain commonest cause seems to be posteriolateral prolapse of an intervertebral disk, putting pressure on the dura and cauda equina and causing the localized pain of lumbago. Can progress to trap the spinal nerve root, causing the nerve distribution pain of sciatica.

low birthweight term for a weight of 2.5 kg or less at birth, whether or not gestation was below 37 weeks—"small for dates."

lower respiratory tract infection (LRTI) → pneumonia.

Lozol™ indapamide.*

LPN *abbr* licensed practical nurse.

lubb-dupp (lub-dup′) words descriptive of the heart sounds as appreciated in auscultation.

lubricants (loo′-brik-ants) *npl* drugs which are emollient in nature and facilitate easy and painless evacuation of feces. → laxatives.

Ludwig's angina (lood′-vigz an-jī′-nà) → cellulitis.

Lugol's solution (loo′-golz) aqueous solution of iodine* and potassium* iodide. Used in preoperative stabilization of thyrotoxic patients.

lumbago (lum-bā′-gō) *n* incapacitating pain low down in the back.

lumbar (lum′-bàr) *adj* pertaining to the loin. *lumbar nerve* → Figure 11. *lumbar puncture* (*LP*) withdrawal of cerebrospinal fluid through a hollow needle inserted into the subarachnoid space in the lumbar region. Fluid can be examined for its chemical, cellular and bacterial content; its pressure can be measured by attachment of a manometer. The procedure is hazardous if pressure is high, but pressure in an adult has a wide range—50–200 mm water, so a better guide is examination of the optic fundi for papilledema. *lumbar sympathectomy* surgical removal of the sympathetic chain in the lumbar region; used to improve blood supply to lower limbs by allowing blood vessels to dilate. *lumbar vertebrae* → Figure 3.

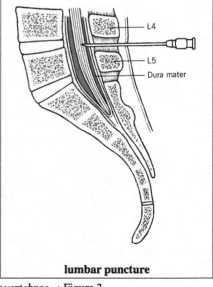

lumbar puncture

lumbocostal (lum-bō-kos′-tàl) *adj* pertaining to the loin and ribs.

lumbosacral (lum-bō-sā'-krål) *adj* pertaining to the loin or lumbar vertebrae and the sacrum.

Lumbricus (lum'-bri-kus) *n* genus of earthworms. → ascarides, ascariasis.

lumen (loo'-men) *n* space inside a tubular structure—**lumina** *pl*, **luminal** *adj*.

lumpectomy (lump-ek'-to-mē) *n* surgical excision of a tumor with removal of minimal surrounding tissue.

lungs *npl* the two main organs of respiration which occupy the greater part of the thoracic cavity; separated from each other by the heart and other contents of the mediastinum (→ Figures 6, 7). Together they weigh about 11.88 kg.

lunula (loon'-ū-lå) *n* semilunar pale area at the root of the nail.

lupus (loo'-pus) *n* several destructive skin conditions, with different causes. → collagen. *lupus erythematosus* (*LE*) an autoimmune process. Discoid variety is characterized by patulous follicles, adherent scales, telangiectasis and atrophy; commonest on nose, malar regions, scalp and fingers. The disseminated or systemic variety is characterized by large areas of erythema on the skin, pyrexia, toxemia, involvement of serous membranes (pleurisy, pericarditis) and renal damage. *lupus pernio* form of sarcoidosis. *lupus vulgaris* commonest variety of skin tuberculosis; ulceration occurs over cartilage (nose or ear) with necrosis and facial disfigurement.

luteotropin (loo'-tē-ō-trō'-pin) *n* secreted by the anterior pituitary gland; assists formation of the corpus luteum in the ovary. In males it acts on Leydig cells in the testis, which produce androgens.

luteum (loo'-tē-um) *n* yellow. *corpus luteum* yellow mass which forms in the ovary after rupture of a graafian follicle. Secretes progesterone* and persists and enlarges if pregnancy supervenes.

luxation (luks-ā'-shun) *n* partial dislocation.

lycopodium (lī-kō-pō'-dē-um) *n* a light, dry fungal spore; it is adsorbent and has been used for dusting the skin and excoriated surfaces. Once used as a coating for pills.

Lyme disease tick-borne spirochetal infection caused by *Borrelia burgdorferi;* with initial inflammation at bite followed in days or weeks by malaise, fatigue, fever and general flu-like symptoms. Neurologic, arthritic and cardiac symptoms can occur. Antibiotics are effective in treatment, but untreated disease may persist for weeks or months.

lymph (limf) *n* fluid contained in the lymphatic vessels. Transparent, colorless or slightly yellow. Unlike blood, lymph contains only one type of cell, the lymphocyte.* *lymph circulation* that of lymph collected from the tissue spaces; it then passes via capillaries, vessels, glands and ducts to be poured back into the blood stream. *lymph nodes* accumulations of lymphatic tissue at intervals along lymphatic vessels; mainly act as filters—**lymphatic** *adj*.

lymphadenectomy (lim-fad-en-ek'-to-mē) *n* excision of one or more lymph nodes.

lymphadenitis (lim-fad-en-ī'-tis) *n* inflammation of a lymph node.

lymphadenopathy (lim-fad-en-op'-à-thē) *n* any disease of the lymph nodes— **lymphadenopathic** *adj*.

lymphangiectasis (limf-an-jē-ek'-tà-sis) *n* dilation of the lymph vessels— **lymphangiectatic** *adj*.

lymphangiography (limf-an-jē-og'-raf-ē) *n* → lymphography.

lymphangioma (limf-an-jē-ōm'-à) *n* simple tumor of lymph vessels frequently associated with similar formations of blood vessels—**lymphangiomata** *pl*, **lymphangiomatous** *adj*.

lymphangioplasty (limf-an'-jē-ō-plas'-tē) *n* replacement of lymphatics by artificial channels (buried silk threads) to drain tissues. Relieves the "brawny arm" after radical mastectomy—**lymphangioplastic** *adj*.

lymphangitis (limf-an-jī'-tis) *n* inflammation of a lymph vessel.

lymphaticovenous (lim-fat-i-kō-vē'-nus) *adj* implies presence of both lymphatic vessels and veins to increase drainage from an area.

lymphedema (limf-e-dē'-mà) *n* excess of fluid in tissues from obstruction of lymph vessels. → elephantiasis, filariasis.

lymphoblast (lim'-fō-blast) *n* abnormal cell circulating in blood in acute lymphoblastic leukemia.* At one time thought to be a precursor of the lymphocyte.

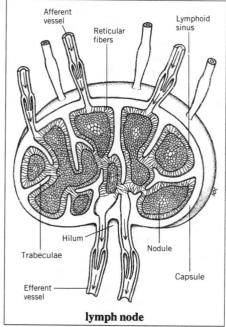

Afferent vessel

Reticular fibers

Lymphoid sinus

Hilum

Nodule

Trabeculae

Capsule

Efferent vessel

lymph node

lymphoblastoma (lim-fō-blast-ō'-mà) *n* malignant lymphoma in which single or multiple tumors arise from lymphoblasts* in lymph nodes. Sometimes associated with acute lymphatic leukemia.

lymphocyte (lim'-fō-sīt) *n* type of white blood cell. Lymphocytic stem cells undergo transformation to T lymphocytes (in the thymus) which can recognize the presence of antigens and attack them directly (→ T cells), and B lymphocytes which form antibodies and provide humoral immunity (→ B cells)—**lymphocytic** *adj*.

lymphocythemia (lim-fō-sī-thē'-mē-à) *n* excess of lymphocytes in blood.

lymphocytosis (lim-fō-sī-tō'-sis) *n* an increase in lymphocytes in the blood.

lymphoepithelioma (lim-fō-ep-i-thēl-ē-ōm'-à) *n* rapidly growing malignant pharyngeal tumor. May involve the tonsil. Often has metastases in cervical lymph nodes—**lymphoepitheliomata** *pl*.

lymphogranuloma venereum (lim-fō-gran-ū-lō'-mà ven-ėr'-ē-um) tropical venereal disease caused by a virus. Primary lesion on genitalia may be an ulcer or herpetiform eruption. Soon buboes appear in regional lymph nodes, forming a painful mass called poradenitis.* Further spread by lymphatics may cause severe periproctitis or rectal stricture in women. Patch skin test (lygranum) and a complement-fixation test of patient's serum are used in diagnosis.

lymphography (lim-fog'-ràf-ē) *n* X-ray examination of lymphatic system after it has been rendered radioopaque—**lymphographical** *adj*, **lymphogram** *n*, **lymphograph** *n*.

lymphoid (limf'-oyd) *adj* like or resembling lymph.*

lymphokines (limf'-ō-kīnz) *npl* chemical substances derived from stimulated T lymphocytes.

lymphoma (lim-fō'-mà) *n* benign tumor of lymphatic tissue. *malignant lymphoma* malignant tumors arising in lymph nodes—**lymphomata** *pl*, **lymphomatous** *adj*.

lymphorrhagia (lim-fōr-ā'-jà) *n* outpouring of lymph from a severed lymphatic vessel.

lymphosarcoma (lim-fō-sàr-kō'-mà) *n* malignant tumor arising from lymphatic tissue—**lymphosarcomata** *pl*, **lymphosarcomatous** *adj*.

lyophilization (lī'-ō-fil-īz-ā'-shun) *n* a method of preserving such biological substances as plasma, sera, bacteria and tissue.

lyophilized skin skin that has been subjected to lyophilization. Reconstituted and used for temporary skin replacement.

lypressin (lī-pres'-sin) *n* antidiuretic. → vasopressin. (Diapid.)

lysin (lī'-sin) *n* cell-dissolving substance in blood. → bacteriolysin, hemolysin.

lysine (lī'-sēn) *n* essential amino* acid, necessary for growth. Deficiency may cause nausea, dizziness and anemia. Destroyed by dry heating, as toasting bread.

lysis (lī'-sis) *n* **1** gradual return to normal, used esp. in relation to pyrexia. → crisis *opp*. **2** disintegration of the membrane of cells or bacteria.

lysozyme (lī'-sō-zīm) *n* basic enzyme which acts as an antibacterial agent and is present in various body fluids, such as tears and saliva.

lytic cocktail consists of promethazine* (Phenergan), meperidine* (Demerol) and chlorpromazine* (Thorazine) diluted in normal saline solution. Used during induction and maintenance of hypothermia. Abolishes shivering and convulsions.

M

Maalox™ aluminum hydroxide and magnesium hydroxide; an antacid.

maceration (mas-e-rā′-shun) *n* softening of the horny layer of the skin by moisture, e.g., in and below the toes (in tinea pedis), or in perianal area (in pruritus ani). Maceration reduces protective quality of the integument and so predisposes to penetration by bacteria or fungi.

Mackenrodt's ligaments (mak′-en-rod's) the transverse cervical or cardinal ligaments; the chief uterine supports.

macrisalb (mak′-ri-salb) *n* suspension of iodinated human albumin in the form of insoluble aggregates. After i.v. injection these aggregates are normally trapped by blood capillaries in lungs, thus can be detected by radioactivity. Low activity is an indication of reduced blood supply.

macrocephaly (mak-rō-sef′-å-lē) *n* excessive size of the head, not caused by hydrocephalus*—**macrocephalic** *adj*.

macrocheilia (mak-rō-kī′-lē-å) *n* excessive development of the lips.

macrocyte (mak′-rō-sīt) *n* a large red blood cell, found in association with a megaloblastic anemia, e.g., in pernicious anemia. *macrocytosis* an increased number of macrocytes—**macrocytic** *adj*.

macrodactyly (mak-rō-dak′-ti-lē) *n* excessive development of fingers or toes.

Macrodantin™ microfurantoin.*

Macrodex™ high molecular weight dextran* for plasma volume replacement in hypovolemic shock. Can be used as an anticoagulant when patients have to assume a particular position which increases the risk of deep vein thrombosis.

macroglossia (mak-rō-glos′-ē-å) *n* abnormally large tongue.

macromastia (mak-rō-mas′-tē-å) *n* abnormally large breast.

macrophages (mak′-rō-fāj-ez) *npl* mononuclear cells, which scavenge foreign bodies and cell debris. Part of the reticuloendothelial* system. → histiocytes.

macula (mak′-ū-lå) *n* a spot. *macula lutea* the yellow spot on the retina, area of clearest central vision—**macular** *adj*.

macule (mak′-ūl) *n* a nonpalpable localized area of change in skin color—**macular** *adj*.

maculopapular (mak-ū-lō-pap′-ū-lar) *adj* presence of macules and raised palpable spots (papules) on skin.

mafenide acetate (maf'-en-īd as'-e-tāt) *n* antiseptic dermatological cream used to treat burns.

magnesium carbonate powder widely used as an antacid in peptic ulcer and as a laxative.

magnesium hydroxide antacid and laxative; sometimes preferred to magnesium and other carbonates, as it does not liberate carbon dioxide in the stomach. Also used as an antidote in poisoning by mineral acids.

magnesium sulfate (*syn* Epsom salts) effective rapid-acting laxative, esp. when given in dilute solution on an empty stomach; used in 25% solution as a wet dressing for inflamed conditions of skin, and as a paste with glycerin for treatment of boils and carbuncles.

magnesium trisilicate (trī-sil'-i-kāt) tasteless white powder with mild but prolonged antacid action; used extensively in peptic ulcer, often combined with more rapidly acting antacids. Does not cause alkalosis, and large doses can be given without side-effects.

magnetic resonance imaging (MRI) (*syn* nuclear magnetic resonance, NMR) technique of imaging by computer using a strong magnetic field and radio frequency signals to examine thin slices through the body. Has advantage over computed* tomography that no X-rays are used, thus no biological harm.

major histocompatability complex (MHC) genetically determined molecules on the surface of all the body's nucleated cells (and platelets) which signify, to the immune system, the presence of "self" rather than "nonself." Leukocytes will attempt to destroy cells, such as bacteria, not bearing these "self" markers.

mal *n* disease. *mal de mer* seasickness. *grand mal* major epilepsy.* *petit mal* minor epilepsy.*

malabsorption (mal-ab-sorb'-shun) *n* poor or disordered absorption of nutrients from the digestive tract. *malabsorption syndrome* loss of weight and steatorrhea,* varying from mild to severe. Caused by: (a) lesions of small intestine, (b) lack of digestive enzymes or bile salts, (c) surgical operations.

malacia (mal-ā'-sē-à) *n* softening of a part. → keratomalacia, osteomalacia.

malaise (mal-āz') *n* feeling of illness and discomfort.

malalignment (mal-al-īn'-ment) *n* faulty alignment, as of teeth, or bones after a fracture.

malar (mā'-lår) *adj* relating to the cheek.

malaria (mà-lār'-ē-à) *n* tropical disease caused by one of the genus *Plasmodium* and carried by infected mosquitoes of the genus *Anopheles*. *P. falciparum* causes *malignant tertian malaria*. *P. vivax* causes *benign tertian malaria* and *P. malariae* causes *quartan malaria*. Signs and symptoms are caused by presence in the blood cells of the erythrocytic (E) stages of the parasite. In falciparum malaria *only* circulating blood-forms of the parasite exist. There is additional persistent infection in the liver (the extraerythrocytic or EE form) in vivax malaria, responsible for relapses. Clinical picture is one of recurring rigors, anemia, toxemia and splenomegaly—**malarial** *adj*.

malassimilation (mal-as-im-il-ā'-shun) *n* poor or disordered assimilation.

malignant *adj* virulent and dangerous; that which is likely to have a fatal termination. *malignant growth or tumor* → cancer, sarcoma; *malignant pustule* → anthrax—**malignancy** *n*.

malleolus (mal-lē'-o-lus) *n* part or process of a bone shaped like a hammer. *external malleolus* at the lower end of the fibula.* *internal malleolus* situated at the lower end of the tibia*—**malleoli** *pl*, **malleolar** *adj*.

malleus (mal'-ē-us) *n* hammer-shaped lateral bone of the middle ear (→ Figure 13).

malocclusion (mal-ok-klū'-shun) *n* failure of the upper and lower teeth to meet properly when the jaws are closed.

malposition *n* any abnormal position of a part.

malpresentation *n* any unusual presentation of the fetus in the pelvis.

Malta fever → brucellosis.

maltase (mawl'-tāz) *n* (*syn* α-glucosidase) a sugar-splitting (saccharolytic) enzyme, found esp. in intestinal juice.

maltose (mawl'-tōs) *n* malt sugar. A disaccharide produced by hydrolysis of starch by amylase during digestion. Used as a nutrient and sweetener.

malunion (mal-ūn'-yon) *n* union of a fracture in a bad position.

mamma (ma'-mà) *n* the breast—**mammae** *pl*, **mammary** *adj*.

mammaplasty (ma'-mà-plas-tē) *n* any plastic operation on the breast—**mammaplastic** *adj*.

mammilla (mam-il'-à) *n* **1** the nipple. **2** a small papilla—**mammillae** *pl*.

mammography (mam-og'-raf-ē) *n* radiographic demonstration of the breast by use of specially low-penetration (long wavelength) X-rays—**mammographic** *adj*.

mammotropic (mam-ō-trōp'-ik) *adj* having an effect upon the breast.

Mandelamine™ methenamine* mandelate.

mania *n* one phase of manic depressive psychoses in which prevailing mood is one of undue elation, with pronounced psychomotor overactivity and often pathological excitement. Flight of ideas and grandiose delusions are common—**maniac** *adj*.

manic depressive psychosis type of mental disorder which alternates between phases of excitement and phases of depression. Often between these phases are periods of complete normality.

manipulation *n* using the hands skillfully as in reducing a fracture or hernia, or changing the fetal position.

mannitol (man'-it-ol) *n* a natural sugar not metabolized in the body; acts as an osmotic diuretic. Esp. useful in some cases of drug overdose and in cerebral edema.

mannitol hexanitrate (man'-i-tol heks-à-nī'-trāt) long-acting vasodilator, used mainly for prophylactic treatment of angina pectoris. Prolonged administration may cause methemoglobinemia.

mannose (man'-ōs) *n* a fermentable monosaccharide.

manometer (man-om'-èt-ér) *n* instrument for measuring pressure exerted by liquids or gases.

Mantoux reaction (man'-too) intradermal injection of old tuberculin or PPD (purified protein derivative, a purified type of tuberculin) into the anterior aspect of forearm. Inspection after 48–72 h. If positive, there will be an area of induration and inflammation greater than 5 mm in diameter.

manubrium (ma-nū'-brē-um) *n* a handle-shaped structure; upper part of the breast bone or sternum.

MAOI *abbr* monoamine* oxidase inhibitor.

maple syrup urine disease genetic disorder of recessive familial type. Leucine,* isoleucine* and valine* are excreted in excess in urine giving the smell of maple syrup. Symptoms include spasticity, poor feeding and respiratory difficulties; severe damage to the CNS may occur. A diet low in the three amino acids may be effective if started sufficiently early, otherwise the disorder is rapidly fatal. Genetic counseling may be indicated. In the pregnant woman, investigation may reveal evidence of the disorder, and in such cases it may be wise to advise termination of pregnancy.

marasmus (mar-az'-mus) *n* wasting away of the body, esp. that of a baby, usually as a result of malnutrition. Currently preferred term is failure* to thrive—**marasmic** *adj*.

marble bones → osteopetrosis.

Marburg disease (mar'-berg) (*syn* green monkey disease) highly infectious viral disease characterized by sudden onset of fever, malaise, headache and myalgia. Between days 5 and 7 a rash appears. Treatment is symptomatic. Virus can persist in the body for 2–3 months after initial attack. Cross infection probably occurs by aerosol route. Incubation period believed to be 4–9 days and mortality rate in previous outbreaks has been around 30%.

Marcain™ bupivacaine.*

Marezine™ cyclizine.

Marfan's syndrome (mar'-fanz) hereditary genetic disorder of unknown cause: dislocation of the lens, congenital heart disease and arachnodactyly with hypotonic musculature and lax ligaments, occasionally excessive height and abnormalities of the iris.

Marion's disease hypertrophic stenosis of the internal urinary meatus at the neck of the bladder.

Marplan™ isocarboxozid.*

marrow *n* → bone marrow.

marsupialization (már-sū-pē-ál-īz-ā'-shun) *n* operation for cystic abdominal swellings that entails stitching the margins of an opening made into the cyst to the edges of the abdominal wound, thus forming a pouch.

mask of pregnancy → melasma.

massage *n* the soft tissues are kneaded, rubbed, stroked or tapped to improve circulation, metabolism and muscle tone, breaking down adhesions and generally relaxing the patient. *cardiac* *massage* done for cardiac arrest. With patient supine on a firm surface, lower portion of sternum is depressed 37–50 mm each second to massage the heart. → resuscitation.

mastalgia (mas-tal'-jà) *n* pain in the breast.

mastectomy (mas-tek'-to-mē) *n* surgical removal of the breast. → lumpectomy. *simple mastectomy* removal of the breast with the overlying skin. Combined with radiotherapy this operation is a treatment for carcinoma of the breast. *radical mastectomy* removal of the breast with the skin and underlying pectoral muscle together with all lymphatic tissue of the axilla: carried out for carcinoma when there has been spread to the glands.

mastication (mas-ti-kā'-shun) *n* act of chewing.

mastitis (mas-tī'-tis) *n* inflammation of the breast. *chronic mastitis* term formerly applied to nodular changes in the breast now usually called fibrocystic* disease.

mastoid (mas'-toyd) *adj* nipple-shaped. *mastoid air cells* extend in a backward and downward direction from the antrum. *mastoid antrum* air space within the mastoid process, lined by mucous membrane continuous with that of the tympanum and mastoid cells. *mastoid process* prominence of the mastoid portion of the temporal bone just behind the ear.

mastoidectomy (mas-toyd-ek'-to-mē) *n* drainage of the mastoid air cells and excision of diseased tissue. *cortical mastoidectomy* all the mastoid cells are removed, making one cavity which drains through an opening (aditus) into the middle ear. The external meatus and middle ear are untouched. *radical mastoidectomy* the mastoid antrum and middle ear are made into one continuous cavity for drainage of infection. Loss of hearing is inevitable.

mastoiditis (mas-toyd-ī'-tis) *n* inflammation of the mastoid air-cells.

mastoidotomy (mas-toyd-ot′-o-mē) *n* incision into the mastoid process of the temporal bone.

match test rough test of respiratory function: inability to blow out a lighted match held 10 cm from a fully open mouth confirms significant reduction in expiratory airflow.

materia medica (mat-ēr′-ē-à med′-i-kà) (*syn* pharmacology) science dealing with origin, action and dosage of drugs.

matrix (mā′-triks) *n* foundation substance in which tissue cells are embedded.

matter (gray and white) → Figure 1.

Matulane™ procarbazine.*

maxilla (maks-il′-à) *n* the jawbone; esp. the upper jaw—**maxillary** *adj*.

maxillofacial (maks-il-ō-fā′-shal) *adj* pertaining to the maxilla and face. A subdivision in plastic surgery.

Mazanor™ mazindol.*

mazindol (maz′-in-dol) *n* appetite depressant. (Mazanor, Sanorex.)

McBurney's point (mak-ber′-nēz) a point one-third of the way between the anterior superior iliac spine and the umbilicus, the site of maximum tenderness in cases of acute appendicitis.

measles *n* (*syn* morbilli) acute infectious disease caused by a virus. Characterized by fever, blotchy rash and catarrh of mucous membranes. Endemic and worldwide in distribution.

meatotomy (mē-a-tot′-o-mē) *n* surgery to the urinary meatus for meatal ulcer and stricture in men.

meatus (mē-ā′-tus) *n* an opening or channel—**meatal** *adj*.

mebendazole (me-ben′-da-zōl) *n* drug used to treat hookworm. (Vermox.)

mecamylamine (mek-am-il′-a-mēn) *n* orally effective ganglionic blocking agent used in treatment of hypertension. (Inversine.)

mechlorethamine (me-klōr-eth′-à-mēn) *n* cytotoxic agent. (Mustargen.)

Meckel's diverticulum (mek′-elz) a blind, pouchlike sac sometimes arising from the free border of the lower ileum. Occurs in 2% of population; usually symptomless. May cause gastrointestinal bleeding; may intussuscept or obstruct.

meclizine (mek′-li-zēn) *n* antihistamine.* (Sea Legs.)

meconium (me-kō′-nē-um) *n* bowel discharge of a newly born baby; a greenish-black, viscid substance. *meconium ileus* impaction of meconium in bowel, one presentation of cystic* fibrosis.

media 1 *n* middle coat of a vessel. 2 *npl* nutritive jellies used for culturing bacteria. → medium.

median *adj* the middle. *median line* imaginary line passing through the center of the body from a point between the eyes to between the closed feet. *median nerve* → Figure 11; *median vein* → Figure 10—**medial** *adj*.

mediastinum (mē-dē-as-tī'-num) *n* the space between the lungs—**mediastinal** *adj*.

mediastinoscopy (mē-dē-as'-tin-os'-ko-pē) *n* minor surgical procedure for visual inspection of the mediastinum. May be combined with biopsy of lymph nodes for histological examination.

medicine *n* **1** science or art of healing, esp. as distinguished from surgery* and obstetrics.* **2** a therapeutic substance—**medicinal** *adj*.

medicochirurgical (med-ik-ō-kī-rur'-ji-kàl) *adj* pertaining to both medicine and surgery.

mediolateral (mē-dē-ō-lat'-êr-àl) *adj* pertaining to the middle and one side.

Mediterranean anemia thalessemia.*

Mediterranean fever genetically inherited disease characterized by polyserositis.*

medium *n* substance used in bacteriology for the growth of organisms—**media** *pl*.

MEDLARS *abbr* Medical Literature Analysis and Retrieval System; computerized bibliography service of the U.S. Library of Medicine.

medrogestone (med-rō-jest'-ōn) *n* a female hormone, given orally or by injection. Shrinks diseased prostate gland.

Medrol™ methyl* prednisolone.

medroxyprogesterone (med-roks-ē-prō-jest'-er-ōn) *n* hormone product useful for threatened and recurrent abortion, functional uterine bleeding, secondary amenorrhea, endometrial carcinoma, endometriosis and short-term contraception.

medroxyprogesterone acetate long-acting (90 days) contraceptive given by injection. (Depo-Provera, Provera.)

medulla (me-dul'-là) *n* **1** marrow in the center of a long bone. **2** soft internal portion of glands, e.g., kidneys, adrenals, lymph nodes, etc. *medulla oblongata* upper part of spinal cord between the foramen magnum of the occipital bone and the pons cerebri (Figure 1)—**medullary** *adj*.

medullated (med'-ū-lā-ted) *adj* containing or surrounded by a medulla* or marrow, particularly referring to nerve fibers.

medulloblastoma (med-ū-lō-blas-tō'-mà) *n* malignant, rapidly growing tumor occurring in children; appears in the midline of the cerebellum.

mefenamic acid (mef-en-am'-ik) analgesic. Also has anti-inflammatory and antipyretic actions. As a prostaglandin inhibitor, effective in dysmenorrhea and menorrhagia in some women using intrauterine* contraceptive devices. (Ponstel.)

megacephalic (meg-à-sef-al′-ik) *adj* (*syn* macrocephalic, megalocephalic) large-headed.

megacolon (meg-à-kō′-lon) *n* dilatation and hypertrophy of the colon. *aganglionic megacolon* due to congenital absence of ganglionic cells in a distant segment of the large bowel, with loss of motor function resulting in hypertrophic dilatation of the normal proximal colon. *acquired megacolon* associated with chronic constipation in the presence of normal ganglion cell innervation; can accompany amoebic or ulcerative colitis.

megakaryocyte (meg-à-kār′-ē-ō-sīt) *n* large multinucleated cells of the marrow which produce blood platelets.

megaloblast (meg′-à-lō-blast) *n* large, nucleated, primitive red blood cell formed where there is a deficiency of vitamin B_{12} or folic acid—**megaloblastic** *adj*.

megalocephalic (meg-à-lō-sef-al′-ik) *adj* → megacephalic.

meibomian cyst (mī-bō′-mē-an) cyst* on the edge of the eyelid from retained secretion of the meibomian glands.

meibomian glands (mī-bō′-mē-an) sebaceous glands lying in grooves on the inner surface of the eyelids, their ducts opening on the free margins of the lids.

Meigs syndrome (mīgs) benign, solid ovarian tumor associated with ascites* and hydrothorax.*

meiosis (mī-ōs′-is) *n* process which, through two successive cell divisions, leads to formation of mature gametes—ova* and sperm.* Begins in the pairing of partner chromosomes, which then separate from each other at the meiotic divisions, so that the diploid* chromosome number (23 pairs in humans) is halved to 23 chromosomes, only one member of each original pair; this set constitutes the haploid complement. → mitosis, germ cells.

melancholia (mel-an-kō′-lē-à) *n* term reserved in psychiatry to mean severe forms of depression—**melancholic** *adj*.

melanin (mel′-an-in) *n* brownish-black pigment found in hair, skin and the choroid of the eye.

melanoma (mel-an-ō′-mà) *n* tumor arising from pigment-producing cells of the deeper layers in the skin, or of the eye—**melanomata** *pl*, **melanomatous** *adj*.

melanosarcoma (mel′-an-ō-sàr-kō′-mà) *n* form of malignant melanoma—**melanosarcomata** *pl*, **melanosarcomatous** *adj*.

melanosis (mel-an-ōs′-is) *n* dark pigmentation of surfaces, as in sunburn, Addison's disease—**melanotic** *adj*.

melanuria (mel-an-ūr′-ē-à) *n* melanin* in the urine—**melanuric** *adj*.

melasma (mel-az'-má) *n* blotchy brownish coloring over forehead and cheeks occurring during pregnancy, the "mask of pregnancy."

melatonin (mel-á-tōn'-in) *n* catecholamine hormone produced by the pineal gland; appears to inhibit numerous endocrine functions.

melena (mel'-e-ná, mel-ē'-ná) *n* black, tarry stools, evidence of gastrointestinal bleeding.

melitensis (mel-i-ten'-sis) *n* → brucellosis.

Mellaril™ thioridazine.*

melphalan (mel'-fa-lan) *n* alkylating cytotoxic agent of the nitrogen* mustard group. Effective orally for multiple myelomatosis; can be given intravenously, and in treatment of malignant melanoma is perfused via intra-arterial route. (Alkaran.)

membrane *n* thin lining or covering substance. *basement membrane* thin layer beneath the epithelium of mucous surfaces. *hyaloid membrane* transparent capsule surrounding the vitreous humor of the eye. *mucous membrane* contains glands which secrete mucus; lines cavities and passages that communicate with exterior of the body. *serous membrane* lubricating membrane lining the closed cavities, and reflected over their enclosed organs. *synovial membrane* membrane lining intra-articular parts of bones and ligaments; does not cover the articular surfaces. *tympanic membrane* the eardrum (→ Figure 13)—**membranous** *adj*.

menadiol (men-á-dī'-ol) *n* water-soluble analogue of vitamin* K; given orally or by injection in hypothrombinemia and neonatal hemorrhage. (Synkayvite.)

menarche (men-ar'-kē) *n* when the menstrual periods commence and other bodily changes occur.

Mendelson syndrome (men'-del-son) inhalation of regurgitated stomach contents, which can cause immediate death from anoxia, or may produce extensive lung damage or pulmonary edema with severe bronchospasm.

Meniere's disease (man'-ē-ārz') distention of membranous labyrinth of inner ear from excess fluid. Pressure causes failure of function of nerve of hearing and balance, with fluctuating deafness, tinnitus and repeated attacks of vertigo.

meninges (men-in'-jēz) *npl* surrounding membranes of the brain and spinal cord, three in number: (a) dura mater (outer), (b) arachnoid membrane (middle), (c) pia mater (inner)—**meninx** *sing*, **meningeal** *adj*.

meningioma (men-in-jē-ō'-má) *n* slowly growing fibrous tumor arising in the meninges—**meningiomata** *pl*, **meningiomatous** *adj*.

meningism (men'-in-jism) *n* (*syn* meningismus) condition presenting with signs and symptoms of meningitis (e.g., neck stiffness); meningitis does not develop.

meningitis (men-in-jī′-tis) *n* inflammation of the meninges. An epidemic form is known as cerebrospinal fever, the infecting organism is *Neisseria* meningitidis* (meningococcus). The term *meningococcal meningitis* is now preferred. → leptomeningitis, pachymeningitis—**meningitides** *pl*.

meningocele (men-ing′-gō-sēl) *n* protrusion of the meninges through a bony defect; forms a cyst filled with cerebrospinal fluid. → spina bifida.

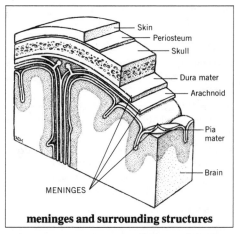

Skin
Periosteum
Skull
Dura mater
Arachnoid
Pia mater
Brain
MENINGES

meninges and surrounding structures

meningococcus (men-ing-go-kok′-us) *n Neisseria* meningitidis*—**meningococcal** *adj*.

meningoencephalitis (men-ing′-gō-en-sef-ȧ-lī′-tis) *n* inflammation of the brain and the meninges—**meningoencephalitic** *adj*.

meningomyelocele (men-ing′-gō-mī′-el-ō-sēl) *n* (*syn* myelomeningocele) protrusion of a portion of the spinal cord and its enclosing membranes through a bony defect in the spinal canal. Differs from a meningocele* in being covered with a thin, transparent membrane, which may be granular and moist.

meniscectomy (men-is-ek′-to-mē) *n* removal of a semilunar* cartilage of the knee joint, following injury and displacement. Medial cartilage is damaged most commonly.

meniscus (men-is′-kus) *n* **1** semilunar* cartilage, esp. in the knee joint. **2** the curved upper surface of a column of liquid—**menisci** *pl*.

menopause (men′-ō-pawz) *n* end of the period of possible sexual reproduction, as evidenced by cessation of menstrual periods, normally between ages of 45 and 50 years. Other bodily and mental changes may occur. *artificial menopause* an earlier menopause induced by radiotherapy or surgery—**menopausal** *adj*.

menorrhagia (men-ōr-ā′-jȧ) *n* excessive regular menstrual flow.

menorrhea (men-ōr-ē′-ȧ) *n* normal menstrual flow.

menotropins (men-ō-trō′-pins) *n* gonadotropin used to stimulate follicle growth and maturation for inducing ovulation in anovulatory women. (Pergonal.)

menses (men′-sēz) *npl* sanguineous fluid discharged from the uterus during menstruation; menstrual flow.

menstrual (men'-stroo-ǎl) *adj* relating to the menses.* *menstrual cycle* cyclical chain of events that eventuates a flow of blood (menstrual flow) for 4–5 days every 28 days. Cycle is governed by hormones from the anterior pituitary gland and ovaries.

menstruation (men-stroo-ā'-shun) *n* flow of blood from the uterus once a month in the female. Commences about the age of 13 years and ceases about 45 years.

menthol (men'-thol) *n* mild analgesic obtained from oil of peppermint. Used in liniments and ointments for rheumatism, and as an inhalation or drops for nasal catarrh.

mentoanterior (men-tō-an-tē'-rē-or) *adj* forward position of the fetal chin in the maternal pelvis in a face presentation.

mentoposterior (men-tō-post-ē'-rē-or) *adj* backward position of the fetal chin in the maternal pelvis in a face presentation.

meperidine (me-pėr'-i-dēn) *n* synthetic analgesic and spasmolytic. Widely used for pre-and post-operative and obstetrical anesthesia instead of morphine. May produce physical and/or psychological dependence. (Demerol.)

mepivacaine (me-piv'-ȧ-kān) *n* local anesthetic. More potent and less toxic than procaine. Used for nerve block.

meprobamate (mep-rō-bam'-āt) *n* mild tranquilizer which, by central nervous action, produces mental relaxation. (Equanil, Miltown.)

mercaptopurine (mer-kap'-tō-pū'-rēn) *n* used in treatment of acute leukemia in children. Prevents synthesis of nucleic acid. (Purinethol.)

mercurialism (mer-kūr'-ē-al-izm) *n* toxic effects on human body of mercury—the ancient cure for syphilis. May result from use of calomel-containing teething powders or calomel (as an abortifacient). Symptomatology includes stomatitis, loosening of teeth, gastroenteritis and skin eruptions.

mercurochrome (mer-kūr'-ō-krōm) *n* red dye containing mercury in combination. Has antiseptic properties.

mesarteritis (mes-ȧrt-ėr-ī'-tis) *n* inflammation of the middle coat of an artery.

mesencephalon (mes-en-sef'-ȧ-lon) *n* the midbrain.*

mesentery (mes'-en-ter-ē) *n* large slinglike fold of peritoneum passing between a portion of the intestine and the posterior abdominal wall—**mesenteric** *adj*.

mesoderm (mes'-ō-dėrm) *n* middle layer of cells which form during early development of the embryo. The other two layers are the ectoderm and the endoderm—**mesodermal** *adj*.

mesothelioma (mes-ō-thēl'-ē-ōm'-ȧ) *n* rapidly fatal tumor that spreads over the mesothelium of the pleura, pericardium or peritoneum. Of current interest because of its association with the absestos industry.

Mestinon™ pyridostigmine.*

metabolic (met-à-bol'-ik) *adj* pertaining to metabolism. *basal metabolic rate* (*BMR*) expression of basal metabolism in terms of kJ per sq m of body surface per hour.

metabolism (met-ab'-ol-izm) *n* continuous series of chemical changes by which life is maintained. Food and tissues are broken down (catabolism), new substances are created for growth and rebuilding (anabolism) and energy made available. → adenosine diphosphate, adenosine triphosphate. *basal metabolism* minimum energy expended in maintenance of respiration, circulation, peristalsis, muscle tonus, body temperature and other vegetative functions of the body—**metabolic** *adj*.

metabolite (met-ab'-ol-īt) *n* any product of or substance taking part in metabolism. *Essential metabolites* are those necessary for normal metabolism, e.g., vitamins.

metacarpophalangeal (met-à-kàr'-pō-fal-an'-jē-àl) *adj* pertaining to the metacarpus* and the phalanges.*

metacarpus (met-à-kar'-pus) *n* five bones which form that part of the hand between wrist and fingers (→ Figures 2, 3)—**metacarpal** *adj*.

Metamucil™ psyllium.*

metaproterenol (met-à-prō-ter'-en-ol) *n* bronchodilator for relief of bronchospasm. Derivative of epinephrine*; available as tablets or aerosol. (Alupent.)

metaraminol (met-àr-am'-in-ol) *n* vasopressor agent used in hypotensive shock. (Aramine.)

metastasis (met-as'-tas-is) *n* spread of tumor cells from one part of the body to another, usually by blood or lymph. A secondary growth—**metastases** *pl*, **metastatic** *adj*, **metastasize** *vi*.

metatarsalgia (met-à-tàr-sal'-jà) *n* pain under the metatarsal heads. *Morton's* metatarsalgia neuralgia caused by a neuroma on the digital nerve, most commonly that supplying the third toe cleft.

metatarsophalangeal (met-à-tàr'-sō-fal-an'-jē-àl) *adj* pertaining to the metatarsus and the phalanges.

metatarsus (met-à-tàr'-sus) *n* five bones of the foot between the ankle and the toes (→ Figure 2)—**metatarsal** *adj*.

metazoa (met-à-zō'-à) *npl* multicellular animal organisms with differentiation of cells to form tissues—**metazoal** *adj*.

meteorism (mē'-tē-ōr-izm) *n* → tympanites.

methacycline (meth-à-sī'-klin) *n* antibiotic particularly useful in exacerbations of chronic bronchitis.

methadone (meth'-à-dōn) *n* synthetic morphinelike analgesic, but with reduced sedative action. Given orally or by injection. Particularly valuable in visceral pain and useful in treatment of unproductive cough. May cause addiction if treatment is prolonged. Can be used in withdrawal programs for heroin addicts. (Dolophine.)

methandrostenolone (meth-an-drō-sten'-o-lōn) *n* anticatabolic agent, useful in muscle wasting occurring as a result of the body's attempt to restore nitrogen balance, as when protein nitrogen is lost in serum from a large wound or pressure sore, and in senile debility.

methantheline (meth-an'-thel-ēn) *n* anticholinergic* used in peptic ulcer and gastritis. (Banthine.)

methemalbumin (meth-ēm-al-bū'-min) *n* abnormal compound in blood from combination of haem with plasma albumen.

methemoglobin (meth-ēm'-ō-glō-bin) *n* form of hemoglobin consisting of globin combined with oxidized haem, containing ferric iron. This pigment is unable to transport oxygen. May be formed following administration of a variety of drugs, including sulfonamides.* May be present in blood as result of a congenital abnormality.

methemoglobinemia (meth-ēm'-ō-glō-bin-ēm'-ē-à) *n* methemoglobin in blood. If large quantities are present, individuals may show cyanosis, but otherwise no abnormality except, in severe cases, breathlessness on exertion, because methemoglobin cannot transport oxygen—**methemoglobinemic** *adj*.

methemoglobinuria (meth-ēm'-ō-glō-bin-ūr'-ē-à) *n* methemoglobin in urine—**methemoglobinuric** *adj*.

methenamine (meth-en'-a-mēn) *n* a urinary antiseptic. (Mandelamine.)

methicillin (meth-i-sil'-in) *n* semisynthetic penicillin given by injection; active against pencillin-resistant staphylococci. The emergence of resistant strains of staphylococci has led to preference for more potent derivatives, such as cloxacillin.* (Staphcillin.)

methionine (meth-ī'-on-ēn) *n* one of the essential sulfur-containing amino* acids. Occasionally used in hepatitis, paracetamol overdose and other conditions associated with liver damage.

methocarbamol (meth-ō-kàr'-bà-mol) *n* skeletal muscle relaxant useful in muscle injury. (Robaxin.)

methohexital sodium (meth-ō-heks'-i-tol) ultrashort-acting barbiturate given i.v. pre-operatively as induction agent for anesthesia. (Brevital.)

methotrexate (meth-ō-treks'-āt) *n* a folic acid antagonist, useful in treatment of acute lymphoblastic leukemia, some lymphomas and sometimes resistant psoriasis.

methotrimeprazine (meth-ō-trī-mep'-rȧ-zēn) *n* chlorpromazinelike drug with tranquilizing and analgesic properties useful in schizophrenia and terminal illness. (Levoprome.)

methoxamine (meth-oks'-ȧ-mēn) *n* pressor drug used to restore blood pressure during anesthesia; few cardiac or CNS side-effects. Given intravenously or intramuscularly. (Vasoxyl.)

methsuximide (meth-suks'-i-mīd) *n* anticonvulsant used for control of temporal lobe epilepsy and petit mal. (Celontin.)

methylated spirit (meth'-il-āt-ed) alcohol containing 5% of wood naphtha, to make it nonpotable.

methylcellulose (meth-il-sel'-ū-lōs) *n* compound which absorbs water and gives bulk to intestinal contents, thus encouraging peristalsis. (Cologel.)

methyldopa (meth-il-dō'-pȧ) *n* inhibitor of dopa decarboxylase. Hypotensive agent. Action increased with thiazide diuretics.* (Aldomet.)

methylene blue (meth'-il-ēn) antiseptic dye formerly used in urinary infections, often with hexamine.* Intramuscular injection of 2.5% solution has been used in renal function test.

methylphenidate (meth-il-fen'-i-dāt) *n* cerebral stimulant, chemically similar to amphetamine. Has a paradoxical calming effect on hyperkinetic children. (Ritalin.)

methylprednisolone (meth-il-pred-ni'-so-lōn) *n* steroid suitable for rheumatoid arthritis, inflammatory and allergic conditions. Sometimes injected locally for exophthalmos. (Medrol.)

methylsalicylate (meth-il-sal-is'-il-āt) *n* (oil of Wintergreen) used externally as a mild counterirritant and analgesic in rheumatic and similar conditions. Supplied as ointment or liniment.

methyltestosterone (meth-il-tes-tos'-tėr-ōn) *n* orally active form of testosterone.* Given as sublingual tablets.

methyprylon (meth-il-prī'-lon) *n* nonbarbiturate hypnosedative. (Noludar.)

methysergide (meth-i-sėr'-jīd) *n* drug of value in long-term prophylaxis of migraine. Can cause retroperitoneal fibrosis, requiring immediate withdrawal, esp. in patients with cardiovascular disease, hypertension, and liver or renal dysfunction. (Sansert.)

metoclopramide (me-tō-klō'-prȧ-mīd) *n* gastric sedative and antiemetic; given orally or by injection. Given in high doses to control vomiting due to cytotoxic drugs. Not so effective in vomiting of labyrinthine origin. (Reglan.)

metolazone (met-ol'-a-zōn) *n* diuretic. (Diulo, Zaroxolyn.)

Metopirone™ metyrapone.* *Metopirone test* a test of pituitary and adrenal function: urinary excretion of 17-hydroxycorticosteroids is estimated before and after oral administration of Metopirone. Disease of the pituitary or adrenal cortex produces abnormal result.

metoprolol (met-ō-prō'-lol) *n* beta-adrenergic blocking agent for treatment of hypertension. By reducing rate and force of cardiac contraction and decreasing rate of conduction of impulses through the conducting system, it reduces the response to stress and exercise. (Lopressor.)

metritis (me-trī'-tis) *n* inflammation of the uterus.

metronidazole (me-trō-nid'-a-zōl) *n* antimicrobial agent esp. useful for treating anaerobic bacterial pathogens. Given intravenously and orally. Also drug of choice for amoebiasis, trichomonas and Vincent's infection. (Flagyl.)

metropathia hemorrhagica (met-rō-path'-ē-à hem-ō-ra'-jik-à) irregular episodes of anovular uterine bleeding due to excessive and unopposed estrogens* in the blood stream. Usually associated with follicular cyst in the ovary.

metrorrhagia (met-rō-rā'-jà) *n* uterine bleeding between menstrual periods.

metyrapone (me-tir'-à-pōn) *n* drug with indirect diuretic action by inhibiting secretion of aldosterone in the adrenal cortex. Usually given in conjunction with spironolactone* or a thiazide* drug. (Metopirone.) → Metopirone test.

metyrosine (me-tir'-ō-sēn) *n* an inhibitor of catecholamine* synthesis. Used in preoperative control of pheochromocytoma. (Demser.)

mexiletine (meks-il'-e-tēn) *n* antiarrhythmic agent. Controls ventricular arrhythmia occurring after myocardial infarction and can be used as a prophylactic. (Mexitil.)

Mexitil™ mexiletine.*

Mezlin™ mezlocillin.*

mezlocillin (mez-lō-sil'-lin) *n* broad-spectrum antibiotic similar to ampicillin.* (Mezlin.)

MHC *abbr* major* histocompatability complex.

miconazole (mī-kon'-à-zōl) *n* antifungal agent used as a pessary and cream for treatment of vulvovaginal candidiasis. (Monistat Cream.)

microangiopathy (mī-krō-an-jē-op'-àth-ē) *n* thickening and reduplication of the basement membrane in blood vessels. Occurs in diabetes mellitus, collagen diseases, infections and cancer. Common manifestations are kidney failure and purpura.

microbe (mī'-krōb) *n* → microorganism—**microbial, microbic** *adj*.

microcephalic (mī-krō-sef-ál'-ik) *adj* pertaining to an abnormally small head.

microcirculation *n* arterioles, blood capillaries and venules involved in tissue respiration.

Micrococcus (mī-krō-kok'-us) *n* genus of bacteria. Gram-positive spherical bacteria occurring in irregular masses. They comprise saprophytes, parasites and pathogens.

microcyte (mī'-krō-sīt) *n* undersized red blood cell found esp. in iron deficiency anemia. *microcytosis* increased number of microcytes—**microcytic** *adj*.

microcytosis (mī-krō-sī-tō'-sis) *n* increased number of microcytes in circulating blood.

microfilaria (mī-krō-fil-ār'-ē-à) *n* genus of tiny worms which cause filariasis.*

micrognathia (mī-krō-nath'-ē-à) *n* small jaw, esp. the lower one.

micronor (mī'-krō-nōr) *n* a mini-pill or progestin-only oral contraceptive containing low dose of norethindrone.*

micronutrients *npl* trace* elements.

microorganism (mī-krō-ōr'-gan-izm) *n* (*syn* microbe) a microscopic cell. Often synonymous with bacterium but includes virus, protozoon, rickettsia, fungus, alga and lichen.

Microsporum (mī-krō-spōr'-um) *n* genus of fungi. Parasitic, living in keratin-containing tissues of man and animals. *M. audouini* commonest cause of scalp ringworm.*

microsurgery *n* use of binocular operating microscope during performance of operations—**microsurgical** *adj*.

microvilli (mī-krō-vil'-lī) *npl* microscopic hairlike projections from the free surface of cell membranes.

micturition (mik-tur-i'-shun) *n* (*syn* urination) act of passing urine.

Midamor™ amiloride.*

midbrain *n* → Figure 1.

Midol™ combination of aspirin and ephedrine, used for relief of symptoms of dysmenorrhea.

Midrin™ dichloralphenazone.*

MIE *abbr* meconium* ileus equivalent.

mifepristone (mi-fe-pris'-tōn) *n* progesterone blocking contraceptive, a "morning* after" pill. Some side-effects. (RU 486.)

migraine (mī'-grān) *n* recurrent localized headaches which are often associated with vomiting and visual and sensory disturbances (the aura); caused, it is thought, by intracranial vasoconstriction—**migrainous** *adj*.

Migralan™ preparation containing ergotamine,* cyclizine* and caffeine.* Useful in early treatment of migraine.

Milkulicz disease (mik'-ū-lich) chronic hypertrophic enlargement of the lacrimal and salivary glands. Now thought to be an autoimmune process.

miliaria (mil-i-ār'-ē-à) *n* prickly heat common in the tropics; affects waistline, cubital fossae and chest, with vesicular and erythematous eruption, caused by blocking of sweat ducts and their subsequent rupture, or their infection by fungi or bacteria.

miliary (mil'-i-ār-ē) *adj* resembling a millet seed. *miliary tuberculosis* → tuberculosis.

milium (mil'-i-um) *n* condition in which tiny, white, cystic excrescences appear on the face, esp. about the eyelids; associated with seborrhea.*

Milontin™ phensuximide.*

Miltown™ meprobamate.*

mineralocorticoid (min-ér-àl'-ō-kōr'-ti-koyd) *n* → aldosterone.

miner's lung → hematite.

Minims™ range of ophthalmic drugs presented in single-use eyedroppers.

Minipress™ prazosin.*

Minocin™ minocycline.*

minocycline (min-ō-sī'-klēn) *n* a tetracycline that is absorbed from the stomach in the presence of food and so can be taken at a time convenient to the patient; rarely it causes skin sensitivity to sunlight. (Minocin.)

minoxidil (min-oks'-i-dil) *n* used in severe hypertension resistant to other drugs.

Mintezol™ thiabendazole.*

miosis (myosis) (mī-ōs'-is) *n* excessive contraction of the pupil of the eye.

Miostat™ carbachol.*

miotic (myotic) (mī-ot'-ik) *adj* pertaining to or producing miosis.*

miscarriage *n* termination of pregnancy before fetus has reached viability.

mistura (mis-tū'-rà) *n* a fluid for oral administration in which there may be soluble or suspended insoluble substances. Should always be well shaken before use.

Mithracin™ plicamycin.*

mitochondrion (mī-tō-kon'-drē-on) *n* a highly specialized structure within cell cytoplasm; an important site of ATP synthesis.

mitomycin (mī-tō-mī'-sin) *n* cytotoxic antibiotic used in cancer of the breast and upper gastrointestinal tract. May cause lung damage and delayed bone marrow toxicity. (Mutamycin.)

mitosis (mī-tō'-sis) *n* the ordinary type of nuclear (cell) division, preceded by faithful replication of chromosomes. Through this process, daughter cells, derived from division of a mother cell, retain the diploid chromosome number, 46 in humans. → meiosis—**mitotic** *adj*.

mitral (mī'-tràl) *adj* miter-shaped, as the valve between left atrium and ventricle of the heart (bicuspid valve). *mitral incompetence* defect in closure of the mitral valve whereby blood tends to flow backwards into the left artium from the left ventricle. *mitral stenosis* narrowing of the mitral orifice, usually due to rheumatic fever. *mitral valvulotomy (valvotomy)* operation for splitting the cusps of a stenosed mitral valve.

mittelschmerz (mit'-el-shmerts) *n* abdominal pain midway between menstrual periods, at time of ovulation.

Moduretic™ mixture of amiloride* and hydrochlorothiazide.*

mold *n* multicellular fungus.

molding *n* compression of fetal head during its passage through the birth canal in labor.

mole *n* a pigmented area on the skin, usually brown. Some moles are flat, some are raised and occasionally have hairs growing from them. Malignant changes can occur in them.

mollities (mol'-it-ēz) *n* softness. *mollities ossium* osteomalacia.*

molluscum (mo-lus'-kum) *n* a soft tumor. *molluscum contagiosum* infectious condition, common in infants, caused by a virus. Tiny translucent papules with a central depression are formed. *molluscum fibrosum* superficial tumors of von* Recklinghausen's disease.

monarticular (mon-àr-tik'-ū-làr) *adj* relating to one joint.

Mönckeberg's sclerosis (menk'-ē-bergz) senile degenerative change resulting in calcification of the median muscular layer in arteries, esp. of the limbs; leads to intermittent claudication and, rarely, to gangrene, if atherosclerosis coexists.

mongolism (mong'-gol-izm) *n* → Down syndrome—**mongoloid** *adj*, **mongol** *n*.

Monilia (mon-il'-ē-à) *n* → Candida.

moniliasis (mon-il-ī'-à-sis) *n* → candidiasis.

Monistat Cream™ miconazole.*

monoamine oxidase (mon'-ō-à-mēn oks'-i-dāz) enzyme which inhibits breakdown of serotonin* and catecholamines* in the brain. *monoamine oxidase inhibitor (MAOI)* substance which, by inhibiting action of monoamine oxidase, increases level of serotonin and catecholamines in the brain; useful for relief of exogenous or reactive depression. Increases effects of many drugs, esp. alcohol and barbiturates, and requires caution in intake of tyramine-containing food and drugs (esp. overripe fruits, aged cheese, wines, reserpine, OTC decongestants, among others). (Eutonyl.)

monocular (mon-ok'-ū-làr) *adj* pertaining to one eye.

monocyte (mon'-ō-sīt) *n* a mononuclear* cell—**monocytic** *adj*.

mononuclear (mon-ō-noo'-klē-ar) *adj* with a single nucleus. Usually refers to a type of blood cell (monocyte), the largest of cells in normal blood, with a round, oval or indented nucleus.

mononucleosis (mon-ō-noo-klē-ō'-sis) *n* increase in number of circulating monocytes (mononuclear* cells) in blood. *infectious mononucleosis* → infectious.*

monoplegia (mon-ō-plē'-jà) *n* paralysis of only one limb—**monoplegic** *adj*.

monorchidism (mon-ōr'-kid-izm) *n* condition in which only one testis is descended, the other may be absent or undescended.

monosaccharide (mon-ō-sak'-à-rīd) *n* simple sugar carbohydrate with the general formula CH_2O. Examples are glucose,* fructose* and galactose.*

monosodium glutamate (mon-ō-sō'-dē-um glū'-tà-māt) chemical sometimes added to food as a flavor enhancer; can cause Chinese* restaurant syndrome.

monosomy (mon'-o-sō-mē) *n* state resulting from absence of a chromosome from the normal diploid* (paired) chromosome complement.

monovular (mon-ov'-ū-lar) *adj* → uniovular.

mons veneris (mons ven-ėr'-is) eminence formed by the pad of fat which lies over the pubic bone in the female.

Mooren's ulcer (moor'-enz) gutterlike excoriation of the peripheral cornea with a tendency to spread.

morbidity *n* state of being diseased—**morbid** *adj*.

morbilli (mōr-bil'-lī) *n* → measles.

morbilliform (mōr-bil'-i-fōrm) *adj* describes a rash resembling that of measles.*

moribund (mōr'-i-bund) *adj* in a dying state.

morning after pill series of pills begun 24–72 hours after sexual intercourse to prevent pregnancy. Contains high doses of estrogens, progesterone, or a combination of both. If pregnancy does occur, use of these pills may cause birth defects.

Moro reflex (mō'-rō) on being startled a baby throws arms outwards, then brings them together in an embracing movement.

morphine (mōr'-fēn) *n* active principle of opium* and a most valuable analgesic. Widely used in pain due to spasm, in hemorrhage and shock. May cause some respiratory depression, esp. in full doses.

morphea (mōr'-fē-à) *n* → scleroderma.

mortality *n* number or frequency of deaths. *mortality rate* the death rate; ratio of number of deaths to total population.

mortification *n* death of tissue. → gangrene.

Morton's metatarsalgia (mōr'-tonz met-å-tår-sal'-jē-å) → metatarsalgia.

mosquito-transmitted hemorrhagic fevers infections occur mainly in the tropics, with bleeding particularly into joints, muscles and skin. Chief diseases are dengue, Rift valley fever and yellow fever.

motile (mō'-til) *adj* capable of spontaneous movement—**motility** *n*.

motor *adj* pertaining to action. → neuron. *motor nerve* → Figure 1. *motor endplate* terminal of motor axon, in contact with striated muscle; release of acetylcholine at this synapse causes muscle contraction. *motor neuron disease* progressive degenerative disease of the motor part of the nervous system; occurs in middle age and results in increasing muscle weakness and wasting.

Motrin™ ibuprofen.*

mottling *n* discoloration of the skin.

mountain sickness symptoms of sickness, tachycardia and dyspnea caused by low oxygen content of rarefied air at high altitude.

mouth-to-mouth resuscitation → resuscitation.

MS *abbr* multiple sclerosis.

mucilage (mū'-si-laj) *n* solution of a gum in water—**mucilaginous** *adj*.

mucin (mū'-sin) *n* mixture of glycoproteins found in and secreted by many cells and glands—**mucinous** *adj*.

mucinase (mū'-sin-āz) *n* specific mucin-dissolving substance contained in some aerosols. Useful in cystic fibrosis.

mucinolysis (mū-sin-ol'-is-is) *n* dissolution of mucin*—**mucinolytic** *adj*.

mucocele (mū'-kō-sēl) *n* distension of a cavity with mucus.*

mucocutaneous (mū-kō-kū-tān'-ē-us) *adj* pertaining to mucous membrane* and skin. *mucocutaneous lymph node syndrome (MLNS)* disease affecting mainly babies and children, first noticed in Japan in the late 1960s. Characterized by fever, dry lips, red mouth and strawberrylike tongue. A rash in a glove-and-stocking distribution is followed by desquamation. There is cervical adenitis, polymorphonuclear leukocytosis and a raised ESR.

mucoid (mū'-koyd) *adj* resembling mucus.*

mucolytics (mū-kō-li'-tiks) *npl* drugs which reduce viscosity of secretion from the respiratory tract.

Mucomyst™ acetylcysteine.*

mucopolysaccharidoses (mū'-kō-pol-ē-sak'-å-rīd-ōs'-ez) *npl* group of inherited neurometabolic conditions in which genetically determined, specific enzyme defects lead to accumulation of abnormal amounts of mucopolysaccharides. → gargoylism, Hunter syndrome.

mucopurulent (mū-kō-pū'-ru-lent) *adj* containing mucus and pus.

mucopus (mū'-kō-pus) *n* mucus containing pus.

mucosa (mū-kō'-så) *n* a mucous membrane*—**mucosae** *pl*, **mucosal** *adj*.

mucositis (mū-kō-sī'-tis) *n* inflammation of a mucous membrane.*

mucous (mū'-kus) *adj* pertaining to or containing mucus.* *mucous colitis* also called mucomembranous colitis. Possibly a functional disorder, manifested by passage of mucus in the stool, obstinate constipation and occasional colic. *mucous polypus* a growth (adenoma) of mucous membrane which becomes pedunculated. *mucous membrane* → membrane.

mucoviscidosis (mū-kō-vis-i-dō'-sis) *n* cystic* fibrosis.

mucus (mū'-kus) *n* viscid fluid secreted by mucous glands—**mucous, mucoid** *adj*.

multigravida (mul-ti-grav'-id-å) *n* (*syn* multipara) woman who has had more than one pregnancy—**multigravidae** *pl*.

multilobular (mul-ti-lob'-ū-lar) *adj* possessing many lobes.

multilocular (mul-ti-lok'-ū-lar) *adj* possessing many small cysts, loculi or pockets.

multinuclear (mul-ti-noo'-klē-ar) *adj* possessing many nuclei—**multinucleate** *adj*.

multipara (mul-tip'-a-rå) *n* → multigravida—**multiparae** *pl*.

multiple sclerosis (MS) (*syn* disseminated sclerosis) variably progressive disease of the nervous system, most commonly first affecting young adults. Patchy, degenerative changes occur in nerve sheaths in the brain, spinal cord and optic nerves, followed by sclerosis.* Presenting symptoms can be diverse, ranging from diplopia to weakness or unsteadiness of a limb; disturbances of micturition are common.

mumps *n* (*syn* infectious parotitis) acute, specific inflammation of the parotid* glands, caused by a virus.

Munchausen syndrome (mun-chow'-zen) patients consistently produce false stories to obtain needless medical tests, operations and treatments. *Munchausen syndrome by proxy* mother produces false stories for her child.

mural *adj* pertaining to the wall of a cavity, organ or vessel.

murmur *n* (*syn* bruit) abnormal sound heard on auscultation of heart or great vessels. *presystolic murmur* characteristic of mitral stenosis in regular rhythm.

muscle *n* strong, contractile tissue that produces movement in the body (→ Figures 2, 3). *cardiac muscle* makes up the middle wall of the heart; it is involuntary, striated and innervated by autonomic nerves. *skeletal muscle* surrounds the skeleton; it is voluntary, striated and innervated by peripheral nerves of the central nervous system. *visceral* (*internal*) *muscle* nonstriated and involuntary, and innervated by autonomic nerves. *muscle relaxants* group of drugs widely used in surgery, in tetanus to prevent spasm, in mechanically aided respiration and in convulsive shock therapy for mental disorder. Two types: depolarizing and nondepolarizing; the latter are reversed by anticholinesterases, e.g., neostigmine.* Muscle relaxants paralyze all skeletal muscles, including those of breathing. They have no sedative action—**muscular** *adj*.

muscular dystrophies (dis'-trō-fēz) group of genetically transmitted diseases; all characterized by progressive atrophy of different groups of muscles, with loss of strength and increasing disability and deformity. Pseudohypertrophic or Duchenne type is the most severe. Presents in early childhood and runs a malignant course. → Duchenne muscular dystrophy.

muscular rheumatism → fibrositis.

musculature (mus'-kū-là-chur) *n* the muscular system, or any part of it.

musculocutaneous (mus-kū-lō-kū-tā'-nē-us) *adj* pertaining to muscle and skin.

musculoskeletal (mus-kū-lō-skél'-e-tàl) *adj* pertaining to the muscular and skeletal systems.

mustard *n* crushed seeds of the mustard plant which have been used orally as an emetic or externally as a counterirritant.

mustargen (mus'-tàr-jen) *n* a nitrogen* mustard, mechlorethamine.

mutagen (mū'-tà-jen) *n* agent which induces gene or chromosome mutation.

mutagenesis (mū-tà-jen'-es-is) *n* production of mutations—**mutagenic,** mutagenetic *adj*.

mutagenicity (mū-tà-jen-is'-it-ē) *n* capacity to produce gene mutations or chromosome aberrations.

Mutamycin™ mitomycin.*

mutant *n* a cell (or individual) that carries a genetic change or mutation.

mutation *n* an alteration in genes or chromosomes of a living cell giving rise to genetic change, thus altering character of the cell. The change is heritable. *induced mutation* gene mutation produced by known agents outside the cell that affect and may alter chromosome structure or number, as ionizing radiation and mutagenic chemicals, ultraviolet radiation, etc. *spontaneous mutation* genetic mutation taking place without apparent influence from outside the cell.

mute 1 *adj* unable to speak. 2 *n* a person who is unable to speak.

mutism (mū'-tizm) *n* (*syn* dumbness) inability or refusal to speak. May be due to congenital causes, the most common being deafness; may be result of physical disease, the most common being a stroke, and it can be a manifestation of mental disease.

myalgia (mī-al'-jà) *n* pain in the muscles. *epidemic myalgia* → Bornholm disease—**myalgic** *adj*.

Myambutol™ ethambutol.*

myasthenia (mī-as-thē'-nē-à) *n* muscular weakness. *myasthenia gravis* disorder characterized by marked fatiguability of voluntary muscles, esp. those of the eye. Caused by biochemical defect associated with abnormal behavior of acetylcholine* at neuromuscular junctions. There is considerable evidence for an autoimmune process—**myasthenic** *adj*.

myasthenic crisis sudden deterioration with weakness of respiratory muscles due to an increase in severity of myasthenia. Distinguished from cholinergic* crisis by giving edrophonium chloride 10 mg intravenously. Marked improvement confirms myasthenic crisis. → edrophonium test.

myatonia (mī-à-tō'-nē-à) *n* absence of muscle tone. *myatonia congenita* form of congenital muscular dystropy in infancy. Child is unable to support weight of head—**myatonic** *adj*.

mycelium (mī-sēl'-ē-um) *n* mass of branching filaments (hyphae) of molds or fungi—**mycelial** *adj*.

Mycobacterium (mī-kō-bak-tēr'-ē-um) *n* genus of rod-shaped acid-fast bacteria. *M. avium* → avian. *M. leprae* causes leprosy and *M. tuberculosis* causes tuberculosis.

mycology (mī-kol'-o-jē) *n* study of fungi—**mycological** *adj*, **mycologist** *n*.

Mycoplasma (mī-kō-plaz'-mà) *n* genus of microscopic organisms considered the smallest free-living organisms. Some are parasites, some are saprophytes and others are pathogens. *M. pneumoniae* causes primary atypical pneumonia, previously called viral pneumonia. *M. hominis* associated with inflammatory disease of the female upper genital tract and *Ureaplasma* with nongonococcal urethritis.

mycosis (mī-kō'-sis) *n* disease caused by any fungus. *mycosis fungoides* chronic and usually fatal lymphomatous disease, not fungal in origin; manifested by generalized pruritus, followed by skin eruptions of diverse character which become infiltrated and finally develop into granulomatous ulcerating tumors—**mycotic** *adj*.

Mycostatin™ nystatin.*

mycotoxins (mī-kō-toks'-ins) *npl* secondary metabolites of molds or microfungi. About 100 chemical substances have been identified as mycotoxins, many capable of causing cancer as well as other diseases—**mycotoxic** *adj*.

Mydriacyl™ tropicamide.*

mydriasis (mid-rī'-à-sis) *n* abnormal dilation of the pupil of the eye.

mydriatics (mid-rē-at'-iks) *npl* drugs which cause mydriasis.*

myelin (mī'-e-lin) *n* white, fatty substance constituting the medullary sheath of a nerve.

myelitis (mī-el-ī'-tis) *n* inflammation of the spinal cord.

myeloblasts (mī′-el-ō-blasts) *npl* the earliest identifiable cells which after several stages become granulocytic white blood cells—**myeloblastic** *adj*.

myelocele (mī′-el-ō-sēl) *n* an accompaniment to spina* bifida wherein development of the spinal cord itself has been arrested, and the central canal of the cord opens on the skin surface discharging cerebrospinal fluid.

myelocytes (mī′-el-ō-sīts) *npl* precursor cells of granulocytic white blood cells normally present only in bone marrow—**myelocytic** *adj*.

myelofibrosis (mī′-el-ō-fī-brō′-sis) *n* formation of fibrous tissue within the bone marrow cavity. Interferes with formation of blood cells.

myelogenous (mī-el-o′-jen-us) *adj* produced in or by bone marrow.

myelography (mī-el-og′-raf-ē) *n* radiographic examination of spinal canal by injection of contrast medium into the subarachnoid space—**myelographic** *adj*, **myelogram** *n*, **myelograph** *n*.

myeloid (mī′-el-oyd) *adj* pertaining to the granulocyte precursor cells in bone marrow.

myeloma (mī-el-ō′-må) *n* malignant condition arising from plasma cells, usually in bone marrow. *multiple myeloma* formation of a number of myelomata in bones—**myelomata** *pl*, **myelomatous** *adj*.

myelomatosis (mī′-el-ō-må-tō′-sis) *n* plasma cell neoplasia. Crowding of bone marrow by abnormal plasma cells, suppression of normal blood cells leading to anemia, thrombocytopenia and neutropenia. Consequent immunosuppression invites infection. May produce changes in serum globulins and Bence-Jones proteinuria.

myelomeningocele (mī-el-ō-men-in′-gō-sēl) *n* → meningomyelocele.

myelopathy (mī-el-op′-å-thē) *n* disease of the spinal cord. Can be a serious complication of cervical spondylosis—**myelopathic** *adj*.

Mylanta™ aluminum hydroxide and magnesium hydroxide suspension, an antacid.

Myleran™ busulfan.*

myocardial infarction (mī-ō-kår′-dē-ål in-fårk′-shun) death of a part of the myocardium* from deprivation of blood. The deprived tissue becomes necrotic and requires time for healing. Patient experiences a "heart attack" with sudden intense chest pain which may radiate to arms and jaws. Because of danger of ventricular fibrillation many patients are nursed in a coronary care or intensive care unit. → angina (pectoris), ischemic heart disease.

myocarditis (mī-ō-kår-dī′-tis) *n* inflammation of the myocardium.*

myocardium (mī-ō-kår′-dē-um) *n* middle layer of the heart wall. → muscle—**myocardial** *adj*.

myocele (mī′-ō-sēl) *n* protrusion of a muscle through its ruptured sheath.

myoclonus (mī-ō-klō'-nus) *n* clonic contractions of individual or groups of muscles.

Myochrysine™ aurothiomalate.*

myoelectric (mī-ō-ē-lek'-trik) *adj* pertaining to electrical properties of muscle.

myofibril (mī-ō-fī'-bril) *n* small fiber of muscular tissue.

myofibrosis (mī-ō-fī-brō'-sis) *n* excessive connective tissue in muscle. Leads to inadequate functioning of part—**myofibroses** *pl*.

myogenic (mī-ō-jen'-ik) *adj* originating in or starting from muscle.

myoglobin (mī'-ō-glō-bin) *n* a muscle protein resembling a single subunit of hemoglobin and thus of much lower molecular weight. Combines with oxygen released by erythrocytes, stores and transports it to muscle cell mitochondria where energy is generated for synthesis and heat production.

myoglobinuria (mī-ō-glō-bin-ūr'-ē-a) *n* excretion of myoglobin in urine, as in crush syndrome.

myohemoglobin *n* myoglobin.*

myokymia (mī-ō-kī'-mē-à) *n* muscle twitching. *facial myokymia* may result from long use of phenothiazine* drugs; has also been observed in patients with multiple sclerosis.

myoma (mī-ō'-mà) *n* tumor of muscle tissue—**myomata** *pl*, **myomatous** *adj*.

myomalacia (mī-ō-mal-ā'-shà) *n* softening of muscle, as occurs in the myocardium after infarction.

myomectomy (mī-ō-mek'-to-mē) *n* enucleation of uterine fibroid(s).*

myometrium (mī-ō-mē'-trē-um) *n* thick muscular wall of the uterus.

myoneural (mī-ō-noo'-ràl) *adj* pertaining to muscle and nerve.

myopathy (mī-op'-à-thē) *n* any disease of the muscles. → glycogenosis—**myopathic** *adj*.

myope (mī'-ōp) *n* a shortsighted person—**myopic** *adj*.

myopia (mī-ōp'-ē-à) *n* shortsightedness. Light rays come to a focus in front of, instead of on, the retina—**myopic** *adj*.

myoplasty (mī'-ō-plas-tē) *n* plastic surgery of muscles—**myoplastic** *adj*.

myosarcoma (mī-ō-sàr-kō'-mà) *n* malignant tumor derived from muscle—**myosarcomata** *pl*, **myosarcomatous** *adj*.

myosin (mī'-ō-sin) *n* a main protein of muscle; reacts with actin in the muscle cell to cause contraction.

myosis (mī-ōs'-is) *n* → miosis—**myotic** *adj*.

myositis (mī-ō-sī'-tis) *n* inflammation of a muscle. *myositis ossificans* deposition of active bone cells in muscle, resulting in hard swellings.

myotomy (mī-ot'-o-mē) *n* cutting or dissection of muscle tissue.

myotonia (mī-ō-tō′-nē-à) *n* an increase in muscle tone at rest. *myotonia congenita* genetically-determined form of congenital muscular weakness, usually presenting in infancy and due to degeneration of anterior horn cells in the spinal cord. Fibrillation of affected muscles is characteristic—**myotonic** *adj*.

myringa (mir-ing′-gà) *n* the eardrum or tympanic membrane.

myringitis (mir-in-jī′-tis) *n* inflammation of the eardrum* (tympanic membrane).

myringoplasty (mir-ing′-gō-plas′-tē) *n* operation to close a defect in the tympanic membrane. Grafts are frequently used—**myringoplastic** *adj*.

myringotome (mir-ing′-gō-tōm) *n* delicate instrument for incising the eardrum* (tympanic membrane).

myringotomy (mir-ing-got′-o-mē) *n* incision into the eardrum* (tympanic membrane). Performed for drainage of pus or fluid from the middle ear. Middle ear ventilation maintained by insertion of a grommet or Teflon tube.

Mysoline™ for primidone.*

Mysteclin F™ combination of tetracycline* and an antifungal powder.

myxedema (miks-e-dē′-mà) *n* clinical syndrome of hypothyroidism.* Patient becomes slow in movement and dull mentally, with bradycardia, low temperature, dry skin and swelling of limbs and face. Associated with low serum thyroxine and raised thyrotropin levels. *pretibial myxedema* violaceous indurated areas of skin, usually on foreleg, in some cases of thyrotoxicosis.* May be associated with exophthalmos and clubbing of fingers. *myxedema coma* impaired level of consciousness in severe myxedema. Mortality rate high from hypothermia, heart failure, cardiac arrhythmias or bronchopneumonia—**myxedematous** *adj*.

myxoma (miks-ō′-mà) *n* connective tissue tumor composed largely of mucoid material—**myxomata** *pl*, **myxomatous** *adj*.

myxosarcoma (miks-ō-sàr-kō′-mà) *n* malignant tumor of connective tissue with a soft, mucoid consistency—**myxosarcomata** *pl*, **myxosarcomatous** *adj*.

myxoviruses (miks-ò-vī′-rus-es) *npl* the influenza group of viruses.

N

nabothian follicles (nȧ-both′-ē-ȧn) cystic distension of chronically inflamed cervical glands of uterus, where the duct of the gland has become obliterated by a healing epithelial covering and normal mucus cannot escape.

Naegele's obliquity (na′-ge-lēz ob-lik′wit-ē) (*syn* asynclitism) tilting of fetal head to one side to decrease the transverse diameter presented to the pelvic brim.

nafcillin (naf-sil′-in) *n* penicillin used for treating infections caused by penicillinase-producing staphylococci. (Unipen.)

nalidixic acid (nal-i-diks′-ik) chemotherapeutic agent esp. useful for urinary infections. (NegGram.)

naloxone (nȧ-loks′-ōn) *n* narcotic antagonist; reverses all actions of narcotics and has no analgesic action itself. Lasts about half an hour. (Narcan.)

nandrolone phenylpropionate (nan′-dro-lōn fen′-il-prō′-pē-on-āt) agent with similar protein-forming and tissue building functions to testosterone but without masculinizing effects on women; used for patients who have extensive tissue damage from any cause, or wasting diseases. (Durabolin.)

nape *n* back of the neck; the nucha.

naphazoline (nȧf-az′-ō-lēn) *n* decongestive substance used in allergic nasal conditions, and in rhinitis; 1 in 2000 to 1 in 1000 solution as spray or drops.

Naprosyn™ naproxen.*

naproxen (nȧ-proks′-en) *n* relieves pain, reduces inflammation and eases joint stiffness without causing gastric bleeding. (Naprosyn.)

Narcan™ naloxone.*

narcoanalysis (nȧr-kō-an-al′-is-is) *n* analysis of mental content under light anesthesia, usually an intravenous barbiturate—**narcoanalytic** *adj*.

narcolepsy (nȧr′-kō-lep-sē) *n* an irresistible tendency to fall asleep. More usual to speak of the narcolepsies rather than of narcolepsy for sudden, repetitive attacks of sleep occurring in the daytime; arise in diverse clinical conditions—**narcoleptic** *adj*.

narcosis (når-kō'-sis) *n* unconsciousness produced by a drug. *carbon dioxide* narcosis full bounding pulse, muscular twitchings, mental confusion and eventual coma due to increased CO_2 in blood. *continuous narcosis* prolonged sleep induced by spaced administration of narcotics. Used occasionally in mental illness to cut short attacks of excitement or for severe emotional upset.

narcotic *n, adj* describes a drug which produces abnormally deep sleep. Strong analgesic narcotics, morphine and opiates, cause profound respiratory depression which is reversible by narcotic antagonists.*

Nardil™ phenelzine.*

nares (nar'-ēz) *npl* (*syn* choanae) the nostrils. *anterior nares* the pair of openings from exterior into the nasal cavities. *posterior nares* the pair of openings from the nasal cavities into the nasopharynx*—**naris** *sing*.

nasal *adj* pertaining to the nose.

nasogastric (nā-zō-gas'-trik) *adj* pertaining to nose and stomach, as passing a *nasogastric tube* via this route, usually for suction, lavage or feeding. → enteral.

nasojejunal (nā-zō-je-jū'-nål) *adj* pertaining to the nose and jejunum, usually referring to a tube passed via the nose into the jejunum. → gavage feeding.

nasolacrimal (nā-zō-lak'-ri-mål) *adj* pertaining to the nose and lacrimal apparatus.

nasopharyngitis (nā-zō-far-in-jī'-tis) *n* inflammation of the nasopharynx.*

nasopharyngoscope (nā-zō-far-ing'-gō-skōp) *n* endoscope for viewing nasal passages and postnasal space—**nasopharyngoscopic** *adj*.

nasopharynx (nā-zō-far'-inks) *n* portion of the pharynx above the soft palate—**nasopharyngeal** *adj*.

nasosinusitis (nā-zō-sī'-nus-ī'-tis) *n* inflammation of the nose and adjacent sinuses.

natamycin (nat-a-mī'-sin) *n* antifungal antibiotic, active against candidal infection. (Natacyn.)

Naturetin™ bendroflumethazide.*

naturopathy (nā-chūr-op'-ath-ē) *n* system of therapeutics based on natural foods grown without chemical fertilizers, and medicines which are prepared from herbs, spices and plants—**naturopathic** *adj*.

nausea *n* feeling of impending vomiting—**nauseate** *vt*.

Navane™ thiothixene.*

navel *n* → umbilicus.

navicular (na-vik'-ū-lår) *adj* shaped like a canoe.

Nebcin™ tobramycin.*

nebula (neb'-ū-lá) *n* a greyish corneal opacity.

NebuPent™ pentamidine.*

Necator (nē-kā'-tor) *n* genus of hookworms.*

necropsy (ne-krop'-sē) *n* the examination of a dead body.

necrosis (ne-krō'-sis) *n* localized death of tissue—**necrotic** *adj*.

necrotizing enterocolitis (NEC) condition occurring primarily in preterm or low birth-weight neonates. Parts of the gut wall become necrotic, leading to intestinal obstruction and peritonitis. Probably caused by a combination of ischemia and infection.

needling *n* → discission.

NegGram™ nalidixic acid.*

Negri bodies a diagnostic feature in rabies,* eosinophilic inclusions found in infected neurons.

Neisseria (nī-ser'-ē-á) *n* genus of bacteria. Gram-negative cocci, usually arranged in pairs, found as commensals of man and animals, as *N. catarrhalis*, or pathogens to man. *N. gonorrheae* causes gonorrhea and *N. meningitidis* causes meningitis.

Nelaton's line (nel'-a-tonz) imaginary line joining anterior superior iliac spine to the ischial tuberosity. The greater trochanter of the femur normally lies on or below this line.

Nelson syndrome associated with a pituitary tumor. Skin changes color, that is, white becomes black and black becomes white.

nematodes (nē'-má-tōdz) *npl* wormlike creatures that have two sexes and an intestinal canal. Some species are parasitic to man; can be divided into two groups: (a) those that mainly live in the intestine, e.g., hookworms, and whipworm (b) those that are mainly tissue parasites, e.g., guinea worms, filiarial worms.

Nembutal™ pentobarbital.*

neoarthrosis (nē-ō-ár-thrō'-sis) *n* abnormal articulation; a false joint, as at the site of a fracture.

neomycin (nē-ō-mī'-sin) *n* antibiotic frequently used with corticosteroids in treatment of inflamed and infected skin conditions. Sometimes given orally for intestinal infections. (Cortisporin.)

neonatal jaundice → icterus.

neonatal period first 28 days of life in a baby. *neonatal mortality* death rate of babies in first month of life. *neonatal herpes* comparatively rare disease acquired during vaginal delivery from a mother actively shedding herpes simplex virus; a devastating illness with a 75% mortality rate and a high incidence of severe neurological sequelae among survivors.

neonate (nē'-ō-nāt) *n* newborn baby up to 4 weeks old.

neonatology (nē-ō-nā-tol'-o-jē) *n* scientific study of the newborn.

neonatorum (nē-ō-nā-tōr'-um) *adj* pertaining to the newborn.

neoplasia (nē-ō-plā'-zē-à) *n* literally, the formation of new tissue. By custom, refers to the pathological process in tumor formation—**neoplastic** *adj*.

neoplasm (nē'-ō-plazm) *n* a new growth; a tumor which is either cancerous or noncancerous—**neoplastic** *adj*.

Neosporin™ ophthalmic drops containing polymyxin,* neomycin* and gramicidin.*

neostigmine (nē-ō-stig'-mēn) *n* synthetic compound used in myasthenia gravis; as a curarine antagonist; and in postoperative ileus and urinary retention. Given orally and by injection. Can cause excess bronchial secretion. (Prostigmin.)

Neo-Synephrine™ xylometazoline.*

nephralgia (nef-ral'-jà) *n* pain in the kidney. → Dietl's crisis.

nephrectomy (nef-rek'-to-mē) *n* surgical removal of a kidney.

nephritis (nef-rī'-tis) *n* term embracing a group of conditions with inflammation, focal or diffuse, of the kidneys. → glomerulonephritis, glomerulosclerosis, nephrotic syndrome, renal failure—**nephritic** *adj*.

nephroblastoma *n* → Wilms' tumor.

nephrocalcinosis (nef-rō-kal-sin-ō'-sis) *n* multiple areas of calcification within the kidney.

nephrocapsulectomy (nef-rō-kap-soo-lek'-to-mē) *n* surgical removal of the kidney capsule. Occasionally done for polycystic* renal disease.

nephrogenic (nef-rō-jen'-ik) *adj* arising in or produced by the kidney.

nephrography (nef-rog'-ra-fē) *n* technique of imaging renal shadow following injection of opaque medium, demonstrated in aortograph series—**nephrographical** *adj*, **nephrogram** *n*, **nephrograph** *n*.

nephrolithiasis (nef-rō-li-thī'-à-sis) *n* the presence of stones in the kidney.

nephrolithotomy (nef-rō-li-thot'-o-mē) *n* removal of a stone from the kidney by incision through the kidney substance.

nephrology (nef-rol'-o-jē) *n* special study of the kidneys and diseases which afflict them.

nephron (nef'-ron) *n* the basic unit of the kidney, comprising a glomerulus,* Bowman's capsule, proximal and distal convoluted tubules, with the loop of Henle connecting them; a straight collecting tubule follows via which urine is conveyed to the renal pelvis.

nephropathy (nef-rop'-à-thē) *n* kidney disease. May be of vasomotor origin, when it is often reversible—**nephropathic** *adj*.

nephropexy (nef'-rō-peks-ē) *n* surgical fixation of a floating* kidney.

nephroplasty (nef-rō-plas'-tē) *n* any plastic operation on the kidney, esp. for large aberrant renal vessels, which are dissected off the urinary tract and the kidney folded laterally upon itself. → hydronephrosis.

nephroptosis (nef-rop-tō'-sis) *n* downward displacement of the kidney; word sometimes used for a floating* kidney.

nephropyosis (nef-rō-pī-ōs'-is) *n* pus formation in the kidney.

nephrosclerosis (nef-rō-sklêr-ō'-sis) *n* renal insufficiency from hypertensive vascular disease, developing into a clinical picture identical with that of chronic nephritis. → renal failure—**nephrosclerotic** *adj*.

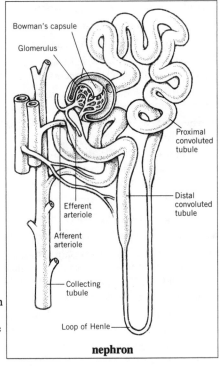

nephron

nephroscope (nef'-rō-skōp) *n* endoscope* for viewing kidney tissue. Can be designed to create a continuous flow of irrigating fluid and provide an exit for fluid and accompanying debris—**nephroscopic** *adj*.

nephrosis (nef-rō'-sis) *n* any degenerative, noninflammatory change in the kidney—**nephrotic** *adj*.

nephrostomy (nef-ros'-to-mē) *n* surgically established fistula from pelvis of the kidney to the body surface.

nephrotic syndrome (nef-rot'-ik) characterized by reduction in blood plasma albumen, albuminuria and edema, usually with hyperlipemia; minimal histological changes in the kidneys. May occur in other conditions, such as amyloid disease and glomerulosclerosis* complicating diabetes.

nephrotomogram (nef-rō-tō'-mō-gram) *n* a tomograph* of the kidney.

nephrotomy (nef-rot'-o-mē) *n* an incision into the kidney substance.

nephrotoxic (nef-rō-toks'-ik) *adj* of a substance which inhibits or prevents function of kidney cells, or causes their destruction—**nephrotoxin** *n*.

nephroureterectomy (nef-rō-ūr-ē'-tėr-ek'-to-mē) *n* removal of the kidney along with a part or all of the ureter.

nerve *n* an elongated bundle of fibers which serves for transmission of impulses between the periphery and the nerve centers. *afferent nerve* one conveying impul-

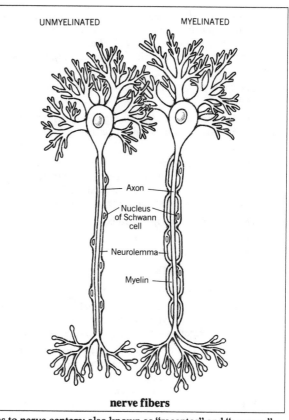

UNMYELINATED   MYELINATED

Axon

Nucleus of Schwann cell

Neurolemma

Myelin

nerve fibers

ses from the tissues to nerve centers; also known as "receptor" and "sensory" nerves. *efferent nerve* one which conveys impulses outwards from nerve centers; also known as "effector," "motor," "secretory," "trophic," "vasoconstrictor," "vasodilator," etc., according to function and location.

nervous *adj* **1** relating to nerves or nerve tissue. **2** referring to a state of restlessness or timidity. *nervous system* structures controlling the actions and functions of the body; comprises the brain and spinal cord and their nerves (central nervous system), and the ganglia and fibers forming the autonomic* system (→ Figure 11, peripheral, sympathetic).

nettle rash (*syn* hives) urticaria; weals of the skin.

network *n* a netlike structure of fibers, a reticulum.

neural (noo'-rȧl) *adj* pertaining to nerves. *neural canal* → vertebral canal. *neural tube* formed from fusion of the neural folds from which the brain and spinal cord arise. *neural tube defect* any of a group of congenital malformations involving the neural tube, including anencephaly,* hydrocephalous* and spina* bifida.

neuralgia (noo-ral'-jȧ) *n* pain along the distribution of a sensory nerve—**neuralgic** *adj*.

neurapraxia (noo-rȧ-praks'-ē-ȧ) *n* temporary loss of function in peripheral nerve fibers. Most commonly due to crushing or prolonged pressure. → axonotmesis.

neurasthenia (noo-ras-thē'-nē-ȧ) *n* a frequently misused term, the precise meaning of which is an uncommon nervous condition consisting of lassitude, inertia, fatigue and loss of initiative. Restless fidgeting, over-sensitivity, undue irritability and often an asthenic physique are also present—**neurasthenic** *adj*.

neurectomy (noo-rek'-to-mē) *n* excision of part of a nerve.

neurilemma (noo-ri-lem'-ȧ) *n* thin membranous outer covering of a nerve fiber surrounding the myelin sheath.

neuritis (noo-rī'-tis) *n* inflammation of a nerve—**neuritic** *adj*.

neuroblast (noo'-rō-blast) *n* a primitive nerve cell.

neuroblastoma (noo-rō-blas-tō'-mȧ) *n* malignant tumor arising in adrenal medulla from tissue of sympathetic origin. Most cases show a raised urinary catecholamine excretion—**neuroblastomata** *pl*, **neuroblastomatous** *adj*.

neurodermatitis (noo-rō-dėr-mȧ- tī'-tis) *n* (*syn* lichen simplex) leathery, thickened patches of skin secondary to pruritus and scratching. As skin thickens, irritation increases and continued scratching causes further thickening. Patches develop characteristically as a thickened sheet dissected into small, shiny, flat-topped papules. Common manifestation of atopic* dermatitis.

neurofibroma (noo-rō-fī-brō'-mȧ) *n* tumor arising from connective tissue of nerves—**neurofibromata** *pl*, **neurofibromatous** *adj*.

neurofibromatosis (noo-rō-fī-brō-mȧ-tō'-sis) *n* genetically determined condition with many fibromata. → Recklinghausen's disease.

neurogenic (noo-rō-jen'-ik) *adj* originating within or forming nervous tissue. *neurogenic bladder* interference with nerve control of the urinary bladder causing either retention of urine, which presents as incontinence, or continuous dribbling without retention. When necessary the bladder is emptied by exerting manual pressure on the anterior abdominal wall.

neuroglia (noo-rōg'-lē-ȧ) *n* (*syn* glia) supporting tissue of the brain and spinal cord—**neuroglial** *adj*.

neuroglycopenia (noo-rō-glī-kō- pē'-nē-à) *n* shortage of glucose in nerve cells, which is the immediate cause of brain dysfunction when it occurs in hypoglycemia—**neuroglycopenic** *adj*.

neuroleptics (noo-rō-lep'-tiks) *npl* drugs acting on the nervous system. Includes the major antipsychotic tranquilizers.

neurology (noo-rol'-o-jē) *n* **1** science and study of nerves—their structure, function and pathology. **2** branch of medicine dealing with diseases of the nervous system—**neurologist** *n*, **neurological** *adj*.

neuromuscular (noo-ro-mus'-kū-lar) *adj* pertaining to nerves and muscles.

neuron (noo'-ron) *n* basic structural unit of the nervous system, comprising fibers (dendrites) that convey impulses to the nerve cell; the nerve cell itself, and the fibers (axons) which convey impulses from the cell. → motor neuron disease. *lower motor neuron* cell is in the spinal cord and axon passes to skeletal muscle. *upper motor neuron* cell is in the cerebral cortex and axon passes down the spinal cord to arborize with a lower motor neuron—**neuronal, neural** *adj*.

neuropathic (noo-rō-path'ik) *adj* relating to disease of the nervous system—**neuropathy** *n*.

neuropathology (noo-rō-pa-thol'-o-jē) *n* branch of medicine dealing with diseases of the nervous system—**neuropathological** *adj*.

neuropeptides (noo-rō-pep'-tīds) *npl* chemical substances secreted continually in the brain, and associated with moods and states. They include the endorphins.*

neuropharmacology (noo-rō-fàr-mà- kol'-o-jē) *n* branch of pharmacology dealing with drugs that affect the nervous system—**neuropharmacological** *adj*.

neuroplasticity (noo-rō-plas-tis'-i-tē) *n* capacity of nerve cells to regenerate.

neuroplasty (noo'-rō-plas-tē) *n* surgical repair of nerves—**neuroplastic** *adj*.

neuropsychiatry (noo-rō-sī-kī'-à-trē) *n* combination of neurology and psychiatry. Specialty dealing with organic and functional disease—**neuropsychiatric** *adj*.

neurorrhaphy (noo-ror'-à-fē) *n* suturing the ends of a divided nerve.

neurosis (noo-rō'-sis) *n* (*syn* psychoneurosis) a functional (i.e., psychogenic*) disorder consisting of a symptom or symptoms caused, though usually unknown to the patient, by mental disorder. Four commonest are anxiety state, reactive depression, hysteria and obsessional neurosis. Distinguished from psychosis* in that neurosis arises as a result of stresses and anxieties in patient's environment. *institutional neurosis* apathy, withdrawal and nonparticipation occurring in long-stay patients as a result of the environment. May be indistinguishable from signs and symptoms for which patient was admitted to the institution—**neurotic** *adj*.

neurosurgery (noo-rō-sėr'-jėr-ē) *n* surgery of the nervous system—**neuro**-surgical *adj*.

neurosyphilis (noo-rō-sif'-il-is) *n* infection of brain or spinal cord, or both, by *Treponema pallidum*. The variety of clinical pictures produced is large, but two common syndromes encountered are tabes* dorsalis and general* paralysis of the insane (GPI). Basic pathology is disease of blood vessels, with later development of pathological changes in meninges and underlying nervous tissue. Very often symptoms of the disease do not arise until 20 years or more after primary infection. → Argyll Robertson pupil—**neurosyphilitic** *adj*.

neurotmesis (noo-rot-mē'-sis) *n* → axonotmesis.

neurotomy (noo-rot'-o-mē) *n* surgical cutting of a nerve.

neurotoxic (noo-rō-toks'-ik) *adj* poisonous or destructive to nervous tissue— **neurotoxin** *n*.

neurotropic (noo-rō-trō'-pik) *adj* with predilection for the nervous system. *Treponema pallidum* often produces neurosyphilitic complications. Neurotropic viruses (rabies, poliomyelitis, etc.) attack cells of the nervous system.

neutropenia (noo-trō-pē'-nē-à) *n* shortage of neutrophils, i.e., less than 500 circulating neutrophils per μl blood, but not sufficient to warrant the description agranulocytosis*—**neutropenic** *adj*.

neutrophil (noo'-trō-fil) *n* most common form of granulocyte in blood, in which the granules are neither strongly basophilic nor strongly eosinophilic.

nevoid amentia (nē'-voyd ā-men'-sha) → Sturge-Weber syndrome.

nevus (nē'-vus) *n* a mole; a circumscribed lesion of the skin arising from pigment-producing cells (melanoma) or due to developmental abnormality of blood vessels (angioma)—**nevi** *pl,* **nevoid** *adj*.

NGU *abbr* nongonococcal* urethritis.

niacin (nī'-à-sin) *n* → nicotinic acid.

niclosamide (ni-klō'-sà-mīd) *n* causes expulsion of adult tapeworm. Given in a single dose of 2 g. No starvation or purgation necessary. (Nicloside.)

Nicloside™ niclosamide.*

nicotinamide (ni-ko-tin'-à-mīd) *n* derivative of nicotinic* acid useful when vasodilator action of that drug is not desired, as in treatment of pellegra.

nicotinic acid (ni-kō-tin'-ik) (*syn* niacin) an essential food factor of the vitamin B complex. Vasodilator action is useful in chilblains, migraine, etc.

nictitation (nik-ti-tā'-shun) *n* rapid and involuntary blinking of the eyelids.

nidation (nī-dā'-shun) *n* implantation of the early embryo in the uterine mucosa.

nidus (nī'-dus) *n* the focus of an infection. A septic focus.

Niemann-Pick disease (nē'-man–pik) lipoid metabolic disturbance, chiefly in female Jewish infants. Now thought to be due to absence or inadequacy of enzyme sphingomyelinase; with enlargement of liver, spleen and lymph nodes with mental subnormality. Now classified as a lipid reticulosis.

night blindness (*syn* nyctalopia) sometimes occurs in vitamin A deficiency; a maladaptation of vision to darkness.

night cry a shrill noise, uttered during sleep. May be of significance in hip disease when pain occurs in the relaxed joint.

night sweat profuse sweating, usually during sleep; typical of tuberculosis.*

Nikolsky's sign (ni-kol'-skēz) slight pressure on the skin causes "slipping" of apparently normal epidermis, in the way that a rubber glove can be moved on a wet hand. Characteristic of pemphigus.*

Nipent™ pentostatin.*

nipple *n* conical eminence in the center of each breast, containing the outlets of the milk ducts.

nitrofurantoin (nī-trō-fūr'-an-tō-in) *n* urinary antiseptic, of value in Gram-positive and Gram-negative infections. Unrelated to sulfonamides or antibiotics. (Furadantin.)

nitrofurazone (nī-trō-fūr'-à-zōn) *n* antibacterial agent available as ointment and solution for topical application. (Furacin.)

nitrogen (nī'-trō-jen) *n* gaseous element; chief constituent of the atmosphere. Only dietary sources (fixed nitrogen) can be utilized. Nitrogen is present in all proteins and in many other substances synthesized by the body. *nitrogen balance* daily intake of nitrogen from proteins equal to daily excretion of nitrogen: a negative balance occurs when excretion of nitrogen exceeds daily intake. Nitrogen is excreted mainly as urea in the urine; ammonia, creatinine and uric acid account for a further small amount. Less than 10% total nitrogen excreted in feces. *nitrogen mustards* a group of cytotoxic drugs, derivatives of mustard gas—**nitrogenous** *adj*.

nitroglycerin (nī-tro-glis'-er-in) *n* vasodilator used chiefly in angina pectoris. Given mainly as tablets to be chewed, or dissolved under the tongue; or transdermally by application as a gel to the skin. (TransdermNitro.)

nitrous oxide (*syn* laughing gas) widely used inhalation gaseous anesthetic.

Nizoral™ ketoconazole.*

NMR *abbr* → magnetic resonance imaging.

nocardiosis (nō-kȧr-dē-ō'-sis) *n* infection by Gram-positive bacteria *Nocardia* asteroides, an actinomycete found in soil. With respiratory symptoms, fever, chills, weakness, weight loss. Disease may spread to brain, and is often fatal, esp. without antibiotic treatment.

nocturia (nok-tū'-rē-á) *n* passing urine at night.

node *n* a protuberance or swelling. A constriction. *atrioventricular node* the commencement of the bundle of His in the right atrium of the heart. *node of Ranvier* the construction in the neurilemma of a nerve fiber. *sinoatrial node* situated at the opening of the superior vena cava into the right atrium; the wave of contraction begins here, then spreads over the heart.

nodule (nod'-ūl) *n* a small node—**nodular** *adj.*

Noludar™ methyprylon.*

Nolvadex™ tamoxifen.*

non compos mentis (non kom'-pōs men'tis) of unsound mind.

nongonococcal urethritis (NGU) (non-gon-ō-kok'-ál ū-rē-thrī'-tis) (*syn* nonspecific urethritis—NSU) common sexually transmitted disease. About half of cases are caused by *Chlamydia;* other causatory organisms are *Ureaplasma* and *Mycoplasma genitalium.*

non-Hodgkin's lymphoma (non-hoj'-kinz) disease of lymphoid tissue, which can infiltrate into any organ or tissue. Cytotoxic drugs are effective but eventual prognosis is poor.

noninsulin dependent diabetes mellitus (NIDDM) → diabetes.

noninvasive *adj* describes any diagnostic or therapeutic technique that does not require penetration of skin or of any cavity or organ.

nonprotein nitrogen (NPN) nitrogen derived from all nitrogenous substances other than protein, i.e., urea, uric acid, creatinine, creatine and ammonia.

nonsense syndrome →Ganser syndrome.

nonspecific urethritis (NSU) nongonococcal* urethritis.

nonsteroidal anti-inflammatory drugs (NSAID) class of drugs useful in rheumatological diseases but which can produce gastric ulceration and bleeding from alimentary mucous membrane.

nonstress test (NST) test of fetal well-being performed by applying an external fetal monitor to a pregnant woman and recording fetal heart baseline and variability.

Noonan syndrome (noo'-nan) (*syn* Bonnevie-Ullrich syndrome) in either males or females, with eyes set apart (hypertelorism) and other ocular and facial abnormalities; short stature, sometimes with neck webbing (and other Turner*-like features). Commonest and most characteristic cardiac abnormality is congenital pulmonary stenosis.

Norcuron™ vecuronium.*

norepinephrine (nor-ep-in-ef'-rin) *n* endogenous norepinephrine is a neuro-humoral transmitter released from adrenergic nerve endings. Although small amounts are associated with epinephrine in the adrenal medulla, its role as a hormone is a secondary one. Has intense peripheral vasoconstrictor action; given by slow intravenous injection in shock and peripheral failure. (Levophed.)

norethindrone (nōr-eth'-in-drōn) *n* a progestogen; suppresses gonadotropin production by the pituitary; used in oral contraceptives.

Norflex™ orphenadrine.*

normoblast (nōr'-mō-blast) *n* a normal-sized nucleated red blood cell, the precursor of the erythrocyte—**normoblastic** *adj*.

normocyte (nōr'-mō-sīt) *n* red blood cell of normal size—**normocytic** *adj*.

Normodyne™ labetalol.*

normoglycemic (nōr-mō-glī-sē'-mik) *adj* having a normal amount of glucose in the blood—**normoglycemia** *n*.

normotension (nōr-mō-ten'-shun) *n* normal tension, by current custom, alluding to blood pressure—**normotensive** *adj*.

normothermia (nōr-mō-thėr'-mē-a) *n* normal body temperature, as opposed to hyperthermia* and hypothermia*—**normothermic** *adj*.

normotonic (nōr-mō-ton'-ik) *adj* normal strength, tension, tone; by current custom, referring to muscle tissue. Spasmolytic drugs induce normotonicity in muscle, and can be used before radiography—**normotonicity** *n*.

Norpace™ disopyramide.*

Norplant™ levonorgestrel.*

Norpramin™ desipramine.*

nortriptyline (nōr-trip'-til-in) *n* antidepressant similar to amitriptyline.* (Aventyl, Pamelor.)

Norvasc™ amlodipine* besylate.

Norwalk agent virus; leading cause of so-called "intestinal flu."

nose *n* → Figures 6, 14.

nosocomial (nō-sō-kō'-mē-ál) *adj* pertaining to a hospital. → infection.

nostrils *npl* the anterior openings in the nose; the anterior nares, choanae.

Novocain™ procaine.*

NSU *abbr* → nonspecific urethritis.

nucha (nū'-kà) *n* nape* of the neck—**nuchal** *adj*.

nuclear magnetic resonance (NMR) → magnetic resonance imaging.

nucleoproteins (nū'-klē-ō-prō'-tēns) *npl* proteins found esp. in nuclei of cells. They consist of a protein conjugated with nucleic acid and are broken down during digestion. Among the products are the purine and pyrimidine bases. End product of nucleoprotein metabolism is uric acid, excreted in urine.

nucleotoxic (nū-klē-ō-toks'ik) *adj* poisonous to cell nuclei. Term may be applied to chemicals and viruses—**nucleotoxin** *n*.

nucleus (nū'-klē-us) *n* **1** the inner part of a cell which contains the chromosomes. Genes, located on the chromosomes, control activity and function of the cell by specifying the nature of enzymes and structural proteins for that cell. **2** a circumscribed accumulation of nerve cells in the central nervous system associated with a particular function. *nucleus pulposus* soft core of an intervertebral disk, which can prolapse into the spinal cord and cause sciatica*—**nuclei** *pl*, **nuclear** *adj*.

nullipara (nul-ip'-a-rà) *n* a woman who has not borne a child—**nulliparous** *adj*, **nulliparity** *n*.

nummular (num'-ū-lar) *adj* coin-shaped; resembling rolls of coins, as the sputum in phthisis.

Nupercaine™ dibucaine.*

nutation (nū-tā'-shun) *n* nodding; applied to uncontrollable head shaking.

nutrient *n, adj* substance serving as or providing nourishment. *nutrient artery* one which enters a long bone. *nutrient foramen* hole in a long bone which admits the nutrient artery.

nutrition *n* sum total of processes by which a living organism receives and utilizes materials necessary for survival, growth and repair of worn-out tissues.

nux vomica (nuks vom'-ik-à) nut from which strychnine* is obtained. Occasionally used with other bitters as a gastric stimulant.

nyctalgia (nik-tal'-jà) *n* pain occurring during the night.

nyctalopia (nik-tà-lō'-pē-à) *n* night blindness.

nycturia (nik-tū'-rē-à) *n* incontinence of urine at night.

Nydrazid™ isoniazid.*

nymphae (nim'-fē) *npl* the labia* minora.

nystagmus (nis-tag'-mus) *n* involuntary and jerky repetitive movement of the eyeballs.

nystatin (nī-stat'-in) *n* antifungal antibiotic effective in treatment of candidiasis. Prevents intestinal fungal overgrowth during broad spectrum antibiotic treatment. (Mycostatin.)

O

OA *abbr* occipito-anterior.*

oat cell carcinoma malignant epithelial bronchogenic neoplasm which spreads along submucosal lymphatics. One-third of all long tumors are of this type. Prognosis is poor.

OB *abbr* obstetrics.

obesity *n* deposition of excessive fat around the body, particularly in subcutaneous tissue. Intake of food is in excess of body's energy requirements.

objective *adj* pertaining to things external to one's self. → subjective *opp. objective signs* those which an observer notes, as distinct from the symptoms of which patient complains.

obligate *adj* characterized by the ability to survive only in a particular set of environmental conditions, e.g., an obligate parasite cannot exist other than as a parasite.

oblique (ō-blēk′) *adj* of external and internal muscles. → Figures 4,5.

obstetrics (ob-stet′-riks) *n* science dealing with care of the pregnant woman during antenatal, parturient and puerperal stages; midwifery—**obstetrician** *n*.

obturator (ob′-tū-rā-tor) *n* that which closes an aperture. *obturator foramen* the opening in the innominate bone which is closed by muscles and fascia *obturator infernus* → Figure 5. *obturator nerve* → Figure 11.

occipital (ok-sip′-it-al) *adj* pertaining to the back of the head. *occipital bone* characterized by a large hole through which the spinal cord passes.

occipitoanterior (ok-sip′-it-ō-an-tē′-rē-or) *adj* describes fetal presentation with fetal occiput lying in the anterior half of maternal pelvis.

occipitofrontal (ok-sip′-it-ō-front′-ȧl) *adj* pertaining to the occiput* and forehead.

occipitoposterior (ok-sip′-it-ō-pos-tēr′-ē-or) *adj* describes fetal presentation with fetal occiput in posterior half of the maternal pelvis.

occiput (ok′-sip-ut) *n* posterior region of the skull.

occlusion (ok-kloo′-zhun) *n* the closure of an opening, esp. of ducts or blood vessels. In dentistry, the fit of the teeth as two jaws meet—**occlusal** *adj*.

occupational disease → industrial disease.

occupational therapy teaching/learning crafts to exercise particular sets of muscles as therapy and prevention of boredom; also includes assessment of and helping with patient activities of daily living (ADLs).

ocular (ok'-ū-lår) *adj* pertaining to the eye.

oculentum (ok-ū-len'-tum) *n* eye ointment—**oculenta** *pl.*

oculogenital (ok-ū-lō-jen'-it-ål) *adj* pertaining to the eye and genital region, as the virus TRIC,* found in male and female genital canals and in the conjunctival sacs of the newborn.

oculogyric (ok-ū-lō-jī'-rik) *adj* referring to movements of the eyeball.

oculomotor (ok-ū-lō-mō'-tor) *n* the third cranial nerve, which moves the eye and supplies the upper eye lid.

OD *abbr* oculus dexter, right eye.

odontalgia (ō-don-tal'-jå) *n* toothache.

odontic (ō-don'-tik) *adj* pertaining to teeth.

odontitis (ō-don-tī'-tis) *n* inflammation of the teeth.

odontoid (ō-don'-toyd) *adj* resembling a tooth.

odontolith (ō-don'-tō-lith) *n* tartar; the concretions which are deposited around teeth.

odontology (ō-don-tol'-o-jē) *n* dentistry.

odontoma (ō-don-tō'-må) *n* tumor developing from or containing tooth structures—**odontomatous** *adj.*

odontotherapy (ō-don-tō-thér'-å-pē) *n* treatment of diseases of the teeth.

Ogen™ piperazine.*

OL *abbr* oculus laevus, left eye.

olecranon process (ō-lek'-ra-non) large process at the upper end of the ulna; forms tip of the elbow when the arm is flexed. *olecranon bursitis* → bursitis.

oleum ricini (ō'-lē-um ri-sin'-ē) castor* oil.

olfactory (ōl-fak'-tō-rē) *adj* pertaining to sense of smell. *olfactory bulb* → Figure 14. *olfactory nerve* nerve supplying olfactory region of the nose; the first cranial nerve. *olfactory organ* the nose. → Figure 14—**olfaction** *n.*

oligohydramnios (ol-i-gō-hī-dram'-nē-os) *n* deficient amniotic fluid.

oligomenorrhea (ol-i-gō-men-ōr-rē'-å) *n* infrequent menstruation; normal cycle prolonged beyond 35 days.

oligophrenia (ol-i-gō-frē'-nē-å) *n* mental deficiency—**oligophrenic** *adj.*

oligospermia (ol-i-gō-spér'-mē-å) *n* reduction in number of spermatozoa in semen.

oliguria (ol-i-gūr'-ē-å) *n* deficient urine secretion—**oliguric** *adj.*

omentum (ō-men'-tum) *n* slinglike fold of peritoneum. *gastrosplenic omentum* connects stomach and spleen; functions are protection, repair and fat storage. *greater omentum* fold which hangs from the lower border of the stomach and covers the front of the intestines. *lesser omentum* a smaller fold, passing between the transverse fissure of the liver and the lesser curvature of the stomach—**omental** *adj*.

Omnipen™ ampicillin.*

omphalitis (om-fǎl-īt'-is) *n* inflammation of the umbilicus.*

omphalocele (om-fǎl'-ō-sēl) *n* → hernia.

Onchocerca (ong-kō-sėr'-kȧ) *n* genus of filarial worms.

onchocerciasis (ong-kō-sėr-kī'-ȧ-sis) *n* infestation with *Onchocerca*. Adult worms encapsulated in subcutaneous connective tissue. Can cause "river blindness" if larvae migrate to the eyes.

oncogenes (on'-kō-gēns) *n* mutated genes, which when activated, can direct cells into uncontrollable cancerous growth.

oncogenic (on-kō-jen'-ik) *adj* capable of tumor production.

oncology (on-kol'-o-jē) *n* scientific and medical study of neoplasms—**oncological** *adj*.

oncolysis (on-kol'-is-is) *n* destruction of a neoplasm. Sometimes used to describe reduction in size of tumor—**oncolytic** *adj*.

Oncovin™ vincristine.*

onychia (ō-nik'-ē-ȧ) *n* acute inflammation of the nail matrix; suppuration may spread beneath the nail, causing it to become detached and fall off.

onychocryptosis (on-ik-ō-krip-tō'-sis) *n* ingrowing of the nail.

onychogryposis (on-ik-ō-grī-pō'-sis) *n* a ridged, thickened deformity of the nails, common in the elderly.

onycholysis (on-ik-ol'-is-is) *n* loosening of toe or finger nail from nail bed—**onycholytic** *adj*.

onychomycosis (on-ik-ō-mī-kō'-sis) *n* fungal infection of the nails.

oocyte (ō'-e-sīt) *n* an immature ovum.

oogenesis (ō-e-jen'-e-sis) *n* production and formation of ova* in the ovary—**oogenetic** *adj*.

oophorectomy (ō-e-fōr-ek'-to-mē) *n* (*syn* ovariectomy, ovariotomy) excision of an ovary.*

oophoritis (ō'-e-fōr-ī'-tis) *n* (*syn* ovaritis) inflammation of an ovary.*

oophoron (ō-ef'-ōr-on) *n* an ovary.*

oophorosalpingectomy (ō'-e-fōr-ō-sal-ping-jek'-to-mē) *n* excision of an ovary and its associated fallopian tube.

oosperm (ō'-e-spėrm) *n* a fertilized ovum.

operating microscope illuminated binocular microscope enabling surgery on delicate tissues, as nerves and blood vessels. Some models incorporate a beam splitter and a second set of eyepieces to enable a second person to view the operation site.

ophthalmia (of-thal'-mē-à) *n* (*syn* ophthalmitis) inflammation of the eye. *ophthalmia neonatorum* purulent discharge from the eyes of a neonate; variety of causative organisms and viruses. Can become epidemic in nurseries. *sympathetic ophthalmia* iridocyclitis of one eye secondary to injury or disease of the other.

ophthalmic (of-thal'-mik) *adj* pertaining to the eye.

ophthalmitis (of-thal-mī'-tis) *n* → ophthalmia.

ophthalmology (of-thal-mol'-o-jē) *n* science that deals with structure, function and diseases of the eye—**ophthalmological** *adj*, **ophthalmologist** *n*.

ophthalmoplegia (of-thal-mō-plē'-jà) *n* paralysis of one or more muscles which move the eye—**ophthalmoplegic** *adj*.

ophthalmoscope (of-thal'-mo-skōp) *n* instrument fitted with a lens and illumination for examining interior of the eye—**ophthalmoscopic** *adj*.

ophthalmotonometer (of-thal'-mō-ton-om'-e-tėr) *n* instrument for determining intraocular pressure.

opioid (ō'-pē-oyd) *adj* like opium* or an opiate* in pharmacological action.

opisthotonos (op-is-tho-tō'-nus) *n* extreme extension of the body occurring in tetanic spasm—**opisthotonic** *adj*.

opium (ō'-pē-um) *n* dried juice of opium poppy capsules. Contains morphine,* codeine,* and other alkaloids. Valuable analgesic, but more constipating than morphine. Also used as tincture of opium and as paregoric (camphorated tincture of opium). Use is not permitted in the U.S.

opsonic index (op-son'-ik) figure obtained by experiment which indicates the ability of phagocytes to ingest foreign bodies such as bacteria.

opsonin (op-son'-in) *n* an antibody which unites with an antigen, usually part of intact cells, rendering cells more susceptible to phagocytosis.* → immunoglobulins—**opsonic** *adj*.

optic *adj* pertaining to sight. *optic chiasma* → chiasma. *optic disk* point at which optic nerve enters the eyeball. *optic nerve* → Figure 15.

optician (op-tish'-un) *n* one who prescribes glasses to correct refractive errors.

optometry (op-tom'-e-trē) *n* measurement of visual acuity.

orabase™ gel product which protects lesions on mucous membranes.

oral *adj* pertaining to the mouth—**orally** *adj*.

Orap™ pimozide.*

orbicular (ōr-bik′-ū-lår) *adj* resembling a globe; spherical or circular.

orbit *n* bony socket containing the eyeball and its append-ages—**orbital** *adj*.

orchidectomy (ōr-ki-dek′-to-mē) *n* excision of a testis.*

orchidopexy (ōr-kid-ō-peks′-ē) *n* operation to bring an unde-scended testis* into the scro-tum,* and fix it in this position.

orchis (ōr′-kis) *n* the testis.

orchitis (ōr-kī′-tis) *n* inflam-mation of a testis.

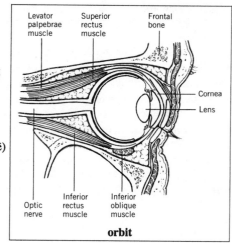

Levator palpebrae muscle — Superior rectus muscle — Frontal bone — Cornea — Lens — Optic nerve — Inferior rectus muscle — Inferior oblique muscle

orbit

orf (ōrf) *n* skin lesion caused by a virus normally affecting sheep.

organic *adj* pertaining to an organ. Associated with life, *organic brain syndrome* → dementia. *organic disease* one in which there is structural change.

organism *n* living cell or group of cells differentiated into functionally distinct parts which are interdependent.

orgasm (ōr′-gazm) *n* climax of sexual excitement.

oriental sore form of cutaneous leishmaniasis* producing papular, crusted, granulomatous eruptions of the skin. A disease of the tropics and subtropics.

orifice (ōr′-if-is) *n* a mouth or opening.

Orinase™ tolbutamide.*

ornithine (ōr′-ni-thēn) *n* amino acid, obtained from arginine* by splitting off urea.*

ornithosis (ōr-ni-thō′-sis) *n* human illness resulting from disease of birds. → Chlamydia.

orogenital (ōr-ō-jen′-i-tål) *adj* pertaining to the mouth and the external genital area.

oropharynx (ōr-ō-far′-inks) *n* that portion of the pharynx below the level of the soft palate and above the level of the hyoid bone.

oropharyngeal (ōr-ō-far-in-jē′-ål) *adj* pertaining to the mouth and pharynx.

orphenadrine (ōr-fen'-à-drēn) *n* anticholinergic agent used in Parkinson's disease. May reduce drug-induced parkinsonism caused by tranquilizers. (Norflex.)

OrthoDienestrol™ dienestrol.*

orthodontics (ōr-thō-don'-tiks) *n* branch of dentistry dealing with prevention and correction of irregularities of the teeth.

orthodox sleep lasts approximately one hour in each sleep* cycle; metabolic rate and therefore oxygen consumption is lowered.

Ortho-Novum™ oral contraceptive containing estrogen combined with progestogen.

orthopedics (ōr-thō-pēd'-iks) *n* branch of surgery dealing with all conditions affecting the locomotor system.

orthopnea (ōr-thop'-nē-à) *n* breathlessness necessitating an upright, sitting position for relief—**orthopneic** *adj*.

orthoptics (ōr-thop'-tiks) *n* study and treatment of muscle imbalances of eye (squint*).

orthosis (ōr-thō'-sis) *n* device which can be applied to or around the body in the care of physical impairment or disability. → prosthesis—**orthoses** *pl*, **orthotic** *adj*.

orthostatic (ōr-thō-stat'-ik) *adj* caused by the upright stance. *orthostatic albuminuria* occurs in some healthy subjects only in the upright position. When lying in bed urine is normal.

orthotics (ōr-tho'-tiks) *n* scientific study and manufacture of devices that can be applied to or around the body in the care of physical impairment or disability.

Ortolani's sign (ōr-to-la'-nēz) test performed shortly after birth to discern dislocation of the hip.

Orudis™ ketoprotein.*

os (os) *n* a mouth *external os* opening of the cervix into the vagina (→ Figure 17). *internal os* opening of the cervix into uterine cavity—**ora** *pl*.

oscillometry (os-il-om'-e-trē) *n* measurement of vibration, using a special apparatus (oscillometer). Measures the magnitude of the pulse wave more precisely than palpation.

Osler's nodes (os'-lerz) small painful areas in pulp of fingers or toes, or palms and soles, caused by emboli and occurring in subacute bacterial endocarditis.

osmosis (os-mō'-sis) *n* passage of pure solvent across a semipermeable membrane under the influence of osmotic* pressure.

osmotic pressure (os-mot'-ik) pressure with which solvent molecules are drawn across a semipermeable membrane separating two concentrations of solute (such as sodium chloride, sugars, urea) dissolved in the same solvent, when the membrane is impermeable to the solute but permeable to the solvent.

osseous (os'-ē-us) *adj* pertaining to or resembling bone.

ossicles (os'-ik-ls) *npl* small bones, particularly those contained in the middle ear: malleus, incus and stapes.

ossification (os-if-ik-ā'-shun) *n* conversion of cartilage, etc., into bone—**ossify** *vt, vi*.

osteitis (os-tē-ī'-tis) *n* inflammation of bone *osteitis deformans* → Paget's disease *osteitis fibrosa* cavities form in the interior of bone; cysts may be solitary or the disease may be generalized (which may result from excessive parathyroid secretion and absorption of calcium from bone).

osteoarthritis (os'-tē-ō-ȧr-thrī'-tis) *n* degenerative arthritis, may be primary, or may follow injury or disease involving articular surfaces of synovial joints. Articular cartilage becomes worn, osteophytes form at the periphery of joint surface and loose bodies may result. → arthropathy, spondylosis deformans—**osteoarthritic** *adj*.

osteoblast (os'-tē-ō-blast) *n* a bone-forming cell—**osteoblastic** *adj*.

osteochondritis (os-tē-ō-kon-drī'-tis) *n* originally an inflammation of bone cartilage. Usually applied to nonseptic conditions, esp. avascular necrosis involving joint surfaces, e.g., osteochondritis dissecans, in which a portion of joint surface may separate to form a loose body in the joint. → Scheuermann's disease. Köhler's disease.

osteochondroma (os-tē-ō-kon-drō'-mà) *n* benign bony and cartilaginous tumor.

osteoclasis (os-tē-ō-klā'-sis) *n* therapeutic fracture of a bone.

osteoclast (os'-tē-ō-klast) *n* bone destroyer, the cell which dissolves or removes unwanted bone.

osteoclastoma (os-tē-ō-klas-tō'-mà) *n* a tumor of the osteoclasts. May be benign, locally recurrent, or frankly malignant. Usual site is near the end of a long bone. → myeloma.

osteocyte (os'-tē-ō-sīt) *n* a bone cell.

osteodystrophy (os'-tē-ō-dis'-tro-fē) *n* faulty growth of bone.

osteogenic (os-tē-ō-jen'-ik) *adj* bone-producing *osteogenic sarcoma* malignant tumor originating in cells which normally produce bone.

Osteogenesis imperfecta (os-tē-ō-jen'-e-sis im-pėr-fek'-tà) hereditary disorder usually transmitted by an autosomal dominant gene. Disorder may be congenital or develop during childhood; congenital form is much more severe and may lead to early death, as affected child's bones are extremely fragile and may fracture after mildest trauma.

osteolytic (os-tē-ō-li′-tik) *adj* destructive of bone, e.g., osteolytic malignant deposits in bone.

osteoma (os-tē-ōm′-à) *n* benign tumor of bone which may arise in compact tissue (*ivory osteoma*) or in the cancellous tissue. May be single or multiple.

osteomalacia (os-tē-ō-mal-ā′-sē-à) *n* demineralization of mature skeleton, with softening and bone pain. Commonly caused by insufficient dietary intake of vitamin D or lack of sunshine, or both.

osteomyelitis (os-tē-ō-mī-el-ī′-tis) *n* inflammation commencing in the marrow of bone—**osteomyelitic** *adj*.

osteopathy (os-tē-op′-à-thē) *n* theory which attributes a wide range of disorders to mechanical derangements of skeletal system, which it is claimed can be rectified by suitable manipulations—**osteopathic** *adj*, **osteopath** *n*.

osteopetrosis (os-tē-ō-pet-rō′-sis) *n* (*syn* Albers-Schönberg disease, marble bones) congenital abnormality giving rise to very dense bones that fracture easily.

osteophony (os-tē-of′-ō-nē) *n* conduction of sound waves to the inner ear by bone.

osteophyte (os′-tē-ō-fīt) *n* a bony outgrowth or spur, usually at margins of joint surfaces, e.g., in osteoarthritis—**osteophytic** *adj*.

osteoplasty (os-tē-ō-plas′-tē) *n* reconstructive operation on bone—**osteoplastic** *adj*.

osteoporosis (os-tē-ō-por-ōs′-is) *n* loss of bone density caused by excessive absorption of calcium and phosphorus from bone, due to progressive loss of the protein matrix of bone which normally carries the calcium deposits—**osteoporotic** *adj*.

osteosarcoma (os-tē-ō-sàr-kō′-mà) *n* sarcomatous tumor growing from bone—**osteosarcomata** *pl*, **osteosarcomatous** *adj*.

osteosclerosis (os-tē-ō-sklér-ōs′-is) *n* increased density or hardness of bone—**osteosclerotic** *adj*.

osteotome (os′-tē-o-tōm) *n* instrument for cutting bone; similar to a chisel but bevelled on both sides of the cutting edge.

osteotomy (os-tē-ot′-o-mē) *n* division of bone followed by realignment of the ends to encourage union by healing.

ostium (os′-tē-um) *n* opening or mouth of any tubular passage—**ostia** *pl*, **ostial** *adj*.

OT *abbr* occupational* therapist.

otalgia (ō-tal′-jà) *n* earache.

OTC *abbr* over-the-counter, refers to medicines sold without a prescription.

otitis (ō-tī'-tis) *n* inflammation of the ear. *otitis externa* inflammation of skin of external auditory canal. *otitis media* inflammation of middle ear cavity. The effusion tends to be serous, mucoid or purulent. Nonpurulent effusions in children are often called glue* ear. → grommet.

otolaryngology (ot-ō-lar-ing-gol'-o-jē) *n* science dealing with structure, function and diseases of the ear and larynx, each of which can be a separate speciality. → otology, laryngology.

otoliths (ō'-tō-liths) *npl* tiny calcareous deposits within the membranous labyrinth of the internal ear.

otology (ō-tol'-o-jē) *n* science dealing with structure, function and diseases of the ear—**otologist** *n*.

otomycosis (ō-tō-mī-kō'-sis) *n* a fungal (*Aspergillus*, *Candida*) infection of the external auditory meatus—**otomycotic** *adj*.

otorhinolaryngology (ō-tō-rī-nō-lar-ing-gol'-o-jē) *n* science dealing with structure, function and diseases of the ear, nose and throat; each may be considered a specialty. → rhinology, laryngoly, otology.

otorrhea (ō-tō-rē'-à) *n* discharge from the external auditory meatus.

otosclerosis (ō-tō-sklér-ōs'-is) *n* new bone formation affecting primarily the footplate of the stapes* and a common cause of progressive deafness—**otosclerotic** *adj*.

otoscope (ō'-tō-skōp) *n* instrument used for examination of the ear.

ototoxic (ō-tō-toks'-ik) *adj* having a toxic action on the ear.

ova (ō'-và) *npl* female reproductive cells—**ovum** *sing*.

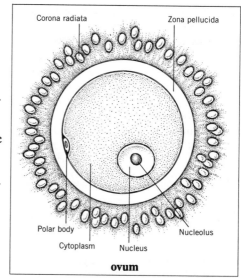

Corona radiata — Zona pellucida — Polar body — Cytoplasm — Nucleus — Nucleolus

ovum

ovarian (ō-vär'-ē-àn) *adj* pertaining to ovaries. *ovarian cyst* a tumor of the ovary, usually containing fluid—may be benign or malignant. Can reach large size and twist on its stalk creating an acute emergency surgical condition.

ovariectomy (ō-vär-ē-ek'-to-mē) *n* → oophorectomy.

ovariotomy (ō-vār-ē-ot′-o-mē) *n* literally, incision of an ovary, but usually applies to removal of an ovary (oophorectomy).

ovaritis (ō-var-ī′-tis) *n* → oophoritis.

ovary (ō′-var-ē) *n* one of two small oval bodies situated on either side of the uterus on the posterior surface of the broad ligament (→ Figure 17). Structures in which the ova* are developed. *cystic ovary* retention cysts in ovarian follicles. Cysts contain estrogen-rich fluid which causes menorrhagia—**ovarian** *adj*.

overbite *n* overriding of the upper front teeth over the lower teeth when jaw is closed.

oviduct (ō′-vi-dukt) *n* → fallopian tube.

Ovral™ oral contraceptive containing both estrogen and progestogen.

ovulation (ov′-ū-lā′-shun) *n* maturation and rupture of a graafian* follicle with discharge of an ovum.

oxacillin (oks-à-sil′-in) *n* an isoxazole penicillin active against penicillinase-producing strains of staphylococcus aureus. (Bactocill.)

oxaluria (oks-à-lū′-rē-à) *n* excretion of urine containing calcium oxalate crystals; associated often with dyspepsia.

oxazepam (oks-az′-e-pam) *n* mild tranquilizer; e.g., benzodiazepine.* (Serax.)

oxidase (oks′-i-dāz) *n* any enzyme which promotes oxidation.

oximeter (oks-im′-ė-tėr) *n* instrument attached to the ear to "sense" oxygen saturation of arterial blood. An accurate noninvasive technique.

oxprenolol (oks-pren′-o-lol) *n* beta-adrenergic blocking agent used in treatment of hypertension. (Trasicor.)

oxtriphylline (oks′-trif′-il-in) *n* resembles aminophylline* in general effects, but less erratic in action. Incidence of gastric irritation is much less, and response more reliable. (Choledyl.)

oxycodone (oks-i-kō′-dōn) *n* narcotic analgesic obtained from an opium alkaloid, can produce drug dependency. (Percodan.)

oxygenation (oks-i-jen-ā′-shun) *n* saturation of a substance (particularly blood) with oxygen. Arterial oxygen tension* indicates degree of oxygenation; reference range 90–100 mmHg (*c* 130 kPa)—**oxygenated** *adj*.

oxygenator (oks′-i-jen-ā-tor) *n* artificial "lung" as used in heart surgery.

oxyhemoglobin (oks-ē-hē′-mō-glō-bin) *n* oxygenated hemoglobin, unstable compound formed from hemoglobin on exposure to alveolar gas in the lungs.

oxymetazoline (oks-ē-met-az-ōl′-ēn) *n* nasal vasoconstrictor; gives quick relief but action is short-lived; danger of rebound congestion after repeated use.

oxymetholone (oks-ē-meth′-o-lōn) *n* an anabolic steroid. → anabolic compound. (Anadrol.)

oxyntic (oks-in′-tik) *adj* producing acid. *oxyntic cells* cells in gastric mucosa that produce hydrochloric acid.

oxyphenbutazone (oks-ē-fen-bū′-ta-zōn) *n* anti-inflammatory, analgesic, anti-arthritic drug. Because of toxicity, no longer used except as an eye ointment. (Tanderil.)

oxytetracycline (oks-ē-tet-ri-sī′-klin) *n* orally effective antibiotic with a wide range of activity. May be given by slow intravenous injection in severe infections. Prolonged use may cause candidal overgrowth in intestinal tract. (Terramycin.)

oxytocic (oks-ē-tō′-sik) *adj, n* hastening parturition; an agent promoting uterine contractions.

oxytocin (oks-ē-tō′-sin) *n* one of the posterior pituitary hormones. Contracts muscle in milk ducts and hence causes milk ejection. Preparations of pituitary extract (Syntocinon, Pitocin) can cause uterine contractions, and so are useful in postpartum hemorrhage. Given intramuscularly, subcutaneously, orally, nasally, or intravenously in titration method with a positive pressure peristaltic pump.

Oxyuris (oks-ē-ūr′-is) *n* genus of nematodes, commonly called threadworms.

ozena (ō-zē′-nȧ) *n* atrophic* rhinitis.

ozone (ō′-zōn) *n* allotropic form of oxygen. O_3. Has powerful oxidizing properties and is therefore antiseptic and disinfectant. Both irritating and toxic in the pulmonary system.

P

pacemaker *n* region of the heart which initiates atrial contraction and thus controls heart rate. The natural pacemaker is the sinoatrial node, at the opening of the superior vena cava into the right atrium; the wave of contraction begins here, then spreads over the heart. *artificial pacemaker* → cardiac.

pachyblepharon (pak-i-blef'-à-ron) *n* thick eyelids.

pachycephalia (pak-i-sef-àl'-ē-à) *n* a thick skull.

pachychilia (pak-i-kī'-lē-à) *n* thick lip(s).

pachydermia (pak-i-der'-mē-à) *n* thick skin. → elephantiasis.

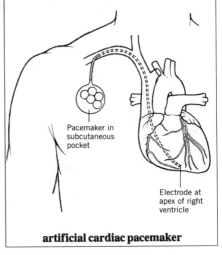

Pacemaker in subcutaneous pocket

Electrode at apex of right ventricle

artificial cardiac pacemaker

pachymeningitis (pak-i-men-in-jī'-tis) *n* inflammation of the dura mater (pachymeninx).

paclitaxel (pak-li-taks'-l) *n* unusual drug which disturbs microtubule formation in certain growing tumors, esp. during mitosis; used principally in treatment of ovarian cancer. Substance was originally obtained from Pacific yew tree, but has been synthesized. (Taxol.)

Paget-Schroetter syndrome (pa'-jet–shrō'-ter) axillary or subclavian vein thrombosis, often associated with effort in fit young persons.

Paget's disease (pa'-jets) **1** (*syn* osteitis deformans) excess of the enzyme alkaline phosphatase causes too rapid bone formation; consequently bone is thin. There is loss of stature, crippling deformity, enlarged head, collapse of vertebrae and neurological complications can result. Sufferers are particularly susceptible to sarcoma of bone. If auditory nerve is involved, there is impairment of hearing. Calcitonin* is drug of choice. **2** erosion of the nipple caused by invasion of the dermis by intraduct carcinoma of the breast.

palate (pal'-at) *n* roof of the mouth (→ Figure 14). *cleft palate* congenital failure of fusion between right and left palatal processes. Often associated with harelip.* *hard palate* front part of the roof of the mouth formed by the two palatal bones. *soft palate* situated at the posterior end of the palate and consisting of muscle covered by mucous membrane—**palatal, palatine** *adj*.

palatine (pal'-à-tīn) *adj* pertaining to the palate. *palatine arches* bilateral double pillars or archlike folds formed by the descent of the soft palate as it meets the pharynx.

palatoplegia (pal-à-tō-plē'-jà) *n* paralysis of the soft palate—**palatoplegic** *adj*.

palliative (pal'-ē-à-tiv) *adj, n* describes anything which serves to alleviate but cannot cure a disease—**palliation** *n*.

pallidectomy (pal-i-dek'-to-mē) *n* destruction of a predetermined section of globus pallidus. → chemopallidectomy, stereotactic surgery.

pallidotomy (pal-i-dot'-o-mē) *n* surgical severance of the fibers from the cerebral cortex to the corpus striatum.

palmar (pal'-mar) *adj* pertaining to the palm* of the hand. *palmar arches* → Figure 9.

palmaris longus (pal-mar'-is long'us) → Figure 4.

palpation (pal-pā'-shun) *n* the act of manual examination—**palpate** *vt*.

palpebra (pal-pē'-brà) *n* an eyelid—**palpebrae** *pl*, **palpebral** *adj*.

palpitation (pal-pi-tā'-shun) *n* rapid forceful beating of the heart of which the patient is conscious.

palsy (pal'-sē) *n* paralysis,* but retained only in compound forms—Bell's* palsy, cerebral* palsy and Erb's* palsy.

Pamelor™ nortriptyline.*

Panadol™ acetaminophen.*

panarthritis (pan-àrth-rī'-tis) *n* inflammation of all the structures of a joint.

pancarditis (pan-kàr-dī'-tis) *n* inflammation of all the structures of the heart.

pancreas (pan'-krē-as) *n* tongue-shaped glandular organ lying below and behind the stomach (→ Figure 18). Its head is encircled by the duodenum and its tail touches the spleen; about 18 cm long and weighs about 100 g. Secretes the hormone insulin,* and also pancreatic juice, which contains enzymes involved in digestion of fats and proteins in the small intestine.

pancreatectomy (pan-krē-à-tek'-to-mē) *n* excision of part or all of the pancreas.

pancreatic function test Levin's tubes are positioned in the stomach and second part of duodenum. Response of the pancreatic gland to various hormonal stimuli can be measured by analyzing the duodenal aspirate. → selenomethionine.

pancreatin (pan'-krē-à-tin) *n* mixture of enzymes obtained from the pancreas. Used in pancreatic diseases and deficiency. Standard and triple-strength products are available.

pancreatitis (pan-krē-à-tī'-tis) *n* inflammation of the pancreas.* Lipase level of blood and urine is used as an indicator of pancreatitis. → diastase.

pancreatotropic (pan-krē-à-tō-trō'-pik) *adj* having an affinity for or an influence on the pancreas. Some anterior pituitary hormones have a pancreatotropic action.

pancreozymin (pan-krē-ō-zī'-min) *n* hormone secreted by the duodenal mucosa; stimulates flow of pancreatic enzymes, esp. amylase.

pancuronium bromide (pan-kū-rō'-nē-um) nondepolarizing muscle relaxant. Produces neuromuscular block by competing with acetylcholine at the neuromuscular junction. Complete paralysis is induced but without alteration in consciousness. (Pavulon.)

pancytopenia (pan-sī-tō-pē'-nē-à) *n* describes peripheral blood picture when red cells, granular white cells and platelets are reduced as occurs in suppression of bone marrow function.

pandemic (pan-dem'-ik) *n* an infection spreading over a whole country or the world.

pannus (pan'-us) *n* corneal vascularization, often associated with conjunctival irritation.

panophthalmitis (pan-of-thal-mī'-tis) *n* inflammation of all tissues of the eyeball.

panosteitis (pan-os-tē-ī'-tis) *n* inflammation of all constituents of a bone— medulla, bony tissue and periosteum.

pantothenic acid (pan-tō-then'-ik) constituent of the vitamin B complex.

PAO *abbr* peak acid output. → pentagastrin test.

PaO2 *abbr* pulmonary arterial oxygen saturation and tension.

Pap test (Papanicolaou) a smear of epithelial cells taken from the cervix, stained and examined under microscope to detect early stages of cancer.

papaverine (pa-pà-vėr'-ēn) *n* a less important alkaloid of opium*; a relaxant in spasm, asthma and peripheral vascular disorders. (Pavabid.)

papilla (pa-pil'-là) *n* a minute nipple-shaped eminence. *renal papilla* → Figure 20—**papillae** *pl*, **papillary** *adj*.

papilledema (pap-il-e-dē'-mà) *n* (*syn* choked disk) edema of the optic disk; suggestive of increased intracranial pressure.

papillitis (pap-il-ī'-tis) *n* **1** inflammation of the optic disk. **2** inflammation of a papilla. Can arise in the kidney after excessive phenacetin* intake.

papilloma (pap-il-ō'-må) *n* simple tumor arising from a nonglandular epithelial surface—**papillomata** *pl,* **papillomatous** *adj.*

papillomatosis (pap-il-ō-må-tō'-sis) *n* growth of benign papillomata on skin or a mucous membrane. Removal by laser ensures fewer recurrences.

papule (pap'-ūl) *n (syn* pimple) small circumscribed elevation of the skin— **papular** *adj.*

papulopustular (pap'-ū-lō-pus'-tū-lår) *adj* pertaining to both papules* and pustules.*

paraaminobenzoic acid (par-å-å-mēn'-ō-benz-ō'-ik) filters ultraviolet rays from the sun; cream or lotion protects skin from sunburn.

paraaortic (par-å-ā-ōr'-tik) *adj* near the aorta.*

paracasein (par-å-kās'-ēn) *n →* casein.

paracentesis (par-å-sen-tē'-sis) *n →* aspiration—**paracenteses** *pl.*

Paradione™ paramethadione.*

paradoxical sleep *(syn* REM sleep) constitutes about a quarter of sleeping time. Characterized by rapid eye movements during which dreaming occurs.

paraesophageal (par-å-ē-sof-å-jē'-ål) *adj* near the esophagus.

paraganglioma (par-å-gang-glē-ō'-må) *n →* pheochromocytoma.

parainfluenza virus (par-å-in-flū-en'-zå) *n* causes acute upper respiratory infection. One of the myxoviruses.

paraldehyde (par-al'-de-hīd) *n* liquid with sedative properties similar to chloral.* Given orally, by intramuscular injection or rectally as a solution in olive oil. Now rarely used.

paralysis (par-al'-is-is) *n* complete or incomplete loss of nerve function to a part of the body. *paralysis agitans →* parkinsonism.

paralytic (par-å-lit'-ik) *adj* pertaining to paralysis. *paralytic ileus* paralysis of intestinal muscle, so that bowel content cannot pass onwards even though there is no mechanical obstruction. *→* aperistalsis.

paramedian (par-å-mēd'-ē-an) *adj* near the middle.

paramedic (par-å-med'-ik) *n* a non-physician trained to do rescue work or to be a physician's assistant.

paramenstruum (par-å-men'-strū-um) *n* the four days before the start of menstruation and the first four days of the period itself.

paramethadione (par-a-meth'-å-dī'-ōn) *n* anticonvulsant compound, useful in petit mal seizures. (Paradione.)

paramethasone (par-a-meth'-å-sōn) *n* a corticosteroid.

parametritis (par-å-mē-trī'-tis) *n →* cellulitis.

parametrium (par-à-mē'-trē-um) *n* connective tissues immediately surrounding the uterus—**parametrial** *adj*.

paranasal (par-à-nā'-zàl) *adj* near the nasal cavities, as the various sinuses.

paraneoplastic (par-à-nē-ō-plas'-tik) *adj* describes syndromes associated with malignancy but not caused by the primary growth or its metastases.

paranoia (par-à-noy'-à) *n* a mental disorder characterized by insidious onset of delusions of persecution—**paranoid** *adj*.

paraphimosis (par-à-fī-mō'-

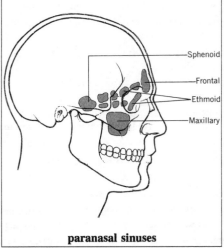

paranasal sinuses

sis) *n* retraction of the prepuce* behind the glans* penis so that the tight ring of skin interferes with blood flow in the glans.

paraphrenia (par-à-frē'-nē-à) *n* psychiatric illness in the elderly characterized by well-circumscribed delusions, usually of a persecutory nature—**paraphrenic** *adj*.

paraplegia (par-à-plē'-jà) *n* paralysis of lower limbs, usually including bladder and rectum—**paraplegic** *adj*.

pararectal (par-à-rek'-tàl) *adj* near the rectum.

parasite *n* an organism which obtains food or shelter from another organism, the "host"—**parasitic** *adj*.

parasitemia (par-à-sī-tēm'-ē-à) *n* parasites in the blood—**parasitemic** *adj*.

parasympathetic (par-à-sim-pà-thet'-ik) *adj* describes portion of autonomic nervous system derived from some of the cranial and sacral nerves belonging to the central nervous system.

parasympatholytic (par-à-sim-path'-ō-lit'-ik) *adj* capable of neutralizing the effect of parasympathetic stimulation, e.g., atropine* and scopolamine.*

parathormone (par-àth-ōr'-mōn) *n* → parathyroid glands.

parathyroid glands (par-à-thī'-royd) four small endocrine glands lying close to or embedded in posterior surface of the thyroid* gland. They secrete a hormone, parathormone, which mobilizes calcium from bone when blood levels are low.

parathyroidectomy (par-à-thī-royd-ek′-to-mē) *n* excision of one or more parathyroid* glands.

paratracheal (par-à-trā′-kē-àl) *adj* near the trachea.

paratyphoid fever (par-à-tī′-foyd) variety of enteric fever, less severe and prolonged than typhoid* fever. Caused by *Salmonella paratyphi A* and *B*, and more rarely *C*. → TAB.

paraurethral (par-à-ū-rē′-thràl) *adj* near the urethra.

paravaginal (par-à-vaj′-in-àl) *adj* near the vagina.

paravertebral (par-à-vėr′-te-bràl) *adj* near the spinal column. *paravertebral* block anesthesia is induced by infiltration of local anesthetic around spinal nerve roots as they emerge from the intervertebral foramina. *paravertebral injection* of local anesthetic into sympathetic chain, can be used as a test in ischemic limbs to see if sympathectomy will be of value.

paregoric (par-e-gōr′-ik) *n* camphorated tincture of opium used for diarrhea. Only treats symptoms, may mask signs of underlying disease.

parenchyma (par-eng-kī′-mà) *n* parts of an organ which, in contradistinction to its interstitial tissue, are concerned with its function—**parenchymal, parenchymatous** *adj*.

parenteral (par-en′-tėr-àl) *adj* not via the alimentary tract. *parenteral feeding* is necessary when it is impossible to provide adequate nutrition via the gastrointestinal tract. A sterile solution of nutrients is infused into a silicone catheter inserted into a large peripheral or, more usually, a large central vein (e.g., the vena cava). An infusion pump regulates the number of drops per minute.

paresis (pa-rē′-sis) *n* partial or slight paralysis; weakness of a limb—**paretic** *adj*.

paresthesia (par-es-thē′-zhà) *n* any abnormality of sensation.

pareunia (par-ūn′-ē-à) *n* coitus.*

parietal (par-ī′-et-àl) *adj* pertaining to a wall. *parietal bones* two bones which form sides and vault of the skull.

parkinsonism (pàr′-kin-son-izm) *n* syndrome of masklike expression, shuffling gait, tremor of the limbs and pill-rolling movements of the fingers. Can be drug-induced. Postencephalitic type may develop many years after illness, often in the 30–40 age group (sporadic type). Degenerative type of parkinsonism (paralysis agitans) develops during middle life. Arteriosclerotic type affects mainly the elderly; characterized by distinctive clinical pattern of tremor and rigidity. *Parkinson's disease,* which is a degenerative process associated with aging, is usually distinguished from parkinsonism, the causes of which are multiple and include such factors as injury, stroke, atherosclerosis, various toxic agents and the viral infection encephalitis lethargica.

Parlodel™ bromocriptine.*

Parnate™ tranylcypromine.*

paromomycin (par-ō-mō-mī'-sin) *n* an amebicide administered orally only. Useful for temporary or long-term suppression of bowel flora, treatment of various forms of acute enteritis. (Humatin.)

paronychia (par-o-nik'-ē-à) *n* (*syn* whitlow) inflammation around a fingernail; may be bacterial or fungal. Herpes simplex may also cause multiple vesicles over inflamed skin—*herpetic paronychia.*

parotidectomy (par-ot'-id-ek'-to-mē) *n* excision of a parotid* gland.

parotid gland (par-ot'-id) salivary gland, situated in front of and below the ear on either side.

parotitis (par-ō-tī'-tis) *n* inflammation of a parotid* gland. *infectious parotitis* mumps.* *septic parotitis* refers to ascending infection from the mouth via the parotid duct; parotid abscess may result.

parous (par'us) *adj* having borne a child or children.

paroxysm (par'-oks-izm) *n* sudden, temporary attack.

paroxysmal (par-oks-iz'-mál) *adj* coming on in attacks or paroxysms. *paroxysmal dyspnea* occurs mostly at night in patients with cardiac disease. *paroxysmal fibrillation* occurs in the atrium of the heart and is associated with a ventricular tachycardia and total irregularity of pulse rhythm. *paroxysmal tachycardia* may result from ectopic impulses arising in the atrium or in the ventricle itself.

Parrot's nodes (par'-rots) bossing of frontal bones in the congenital syphilitic. → pseudoparalysis.

Parsidol™ ethopropazine.*

parturient (pàr-tū'-rē-ent) *adj* pertaining to childbirth.

parturition (pàr-tū-ri'-shun) *n* → labor.

Pasteurella (pas-tūr-el'-a) *n* genus of bacteria. Short Gram-negative rods, staining more deeply at the poles (bipolar staining). Pathogenic in man and animals.

pasteurization (pas-tūr-ī-zā'-shun) *n* process whereby pathogenic organisms in fluid (esp. milk) are killed by heat. *flash method of pasteurization* (HT, ST—high temperature short time); fluid heated to 72° C, maintained at this temperature for 15 s, then rapidly cooled. *holder method of pasteurization* fluid heated to 63–65.5° C maintained at this temperature for 30 min, then rapidly cooled.

Patau's syndrome (pa-tōz') autosomal trisomy of chromosome 13. Closely associated with mental subnormality. There are accompanying physical defects.

patch test skin test for identifying reaction to allergens, which are incorporated in an adhesive patch applied to the skin. Allergy is apparent by redness and swelling.

patella (pa-tel'-à) *n* a triangular, sesamoid bone; the kneecap (→ Figure 2)—**patellae** *pl,* **patellar** *adj.*

patellectomy (pa-tel-ek'-to-mē) *n* excision of the patella.*

patent *adj* open; not closed or occluded. *patent ductus arteriosus* failure of ductus arteriosus to close soon after birth, so that the abnormal shunt between pulmonary artery and aorta is preserved. *patent interventricular septum* a congenital defect in dividing wall between right and left ventricle of the heart—**patency** *n.*

pathogen (path'-ō-jen) *n* a disease-producing agent, usually restricted to a living agent—**pathogenic** *adj,* **pathogenicity** *n.*

pathogenesis (path-ō-jen'-e-sis) *n* the origin and development of disease—**pathogenetic** *adj.*

pathogenicity (path-ō-jen-is'-i-tē) *n* capacity to produce disease.

pathognomonic (path-og-nō-mon'-ik) *adj* characteristic of or peculiar to a disease.

pathology (pa-thol'-o-jē) *n* science dealing with the cause and nature of disease—**pathological** *adj.*

pathophysiology (path-ō-fiz'-ē-ol'-o-jē) *n* science dealing with abnormal biological functioning of the human being—**pathophysiological** *adj.*

patulous (pat'-ū-lus) *adj* opened out; expanded.

Paul-Bunnell test (pawl-bun-el') serological test used in diagnosis of infectious mononucleosis. Antibodies in infected patients agglutinate sheep's erythrocytes.

Paul tube a flanged glass tube used to collect the contents after the bowel has been opened on the surface of the abdomen.

Pavabid™ papaverine.*

Pavulon™ pancuronium* bromide.

Pawlik's grip (paw'-liks) method of determining the engagement or otherwise of the fetal head in the maternal pelvic brim.

PBI *abbr* protein-bound iodine. Iodine combined with protein as part of thyroid hormone. Low, in thyroid deficiency.

PBZ™ tripelennamine.*

PDR *abbr* Physician's* Desk Reference.

peak-expiratory flow rate measured amount of air in a forced exhalation over one second.

peau d'orange (pō dōr-ongzh') appearance of skin over the breast in acute inflammation or in advanced carcinoma, when lymphedema causes the orifices of hair follicles to appear as dimples, resembling pits in the skin of an orange.

pectineus muscle (pek-tin-ē'-us) → Figure 4.

pectoral (pek'-tor-ȧl) *adj* pertaining to the breast.

pectus (pek'-tus) *n* the chest. *pectus carinatum* → pigeon chest. *pectus excavatum* → funnel chest.

pedal (pē'-dȧl) *adj* pertaining to the foot.

pediatrics (pē-dē-at'-riks) *n* branch of medicine dealing with children and their diseases—**pediatric** *adj*, **pediatrician** *n*.

pedicle (ped'-i-kl) *n* a stalk, e.g., the narrow part by which a tumor is attached to surrounding structures.

pediculosis (ped-ik-ū-lō'-sis) *n* infestation with lice (pediculi).

Pediculus (ped-ik'-ū-lus) *n* genus of parasitic insects (lice) important as vectors of disease (relapsing fever and typhus). *P. capitis* the head louse. *P. corporis* the body louse. *P.* (more correctly, *Phthirius*) *pubis* the pubic or crab louse.

peduncle (ped-ungk'-l) *n* a stalklike structure, often acting as a support—**peduncular, pedunculated** *adj*.

pegademase bovine enzyme used to replace lacking adenosine deaminase (ADA) in severe combined immunodeficiency (SCID). (Adagen.)

Peganone™ ethotoin.*

Pel-Ebstein fever (pel–eb'-stīn) regularly recurring bouts of pyrexia found in lymphadenoma (Hodgkin's disease).

Pelizaeus-Merzbacher disease (pel-ēz'-ē-us–merz'-bak-er) genetically determined degenerative disease associated with mental subnormality.

pellagra (pel-ā'-grȧ) *n* deficiency disease caused by lack of vitamin B complex and protein. Syndrome includes glossitis, dermatitis, peripheral neuritis and spinal cord changes (even producing ataxia), anemia and mental confusion.

pelvic floor a mainly muscular partition with the pelvic cavity above and perineum below. In the female, weakening of these muscles can contribute to urinary incontinence and uterine prolapse.

pelvic girdle the bony pelvis, comprising two innominate bones, the sacrum and coccyx.

pelvic inflammatory disease (PID) inflammatory process that results from other pelvic diseases; may result from gonorrhea, tuberculosis, or postpartal infection.

pelvic pain syndrome (PPS) pelvic pain which occurs in women but for which no pathological cause is evident, consequently, there is no effective treatment.

pelvimeter (pel-vim′-ėt-ėr) *n* instrument to measure the pelvic diameters for obstetric purposes—**pelvimetry** *n*.

pelvis (pel′-vis) *n* **1** a basin-shaped cavity, e.g., pelvis of the kidney (→ Figure 20). **2** large bony basin-shaped cavity formed by the innominate bones and sacrum, containing and protecting bladder, rectum and, in the female, the organs of generation. *contracted pelvis* one in which one or more diameters are smaller than normal; may result in difficulties in childbirth. *false pelvis* wide expanded part of the pelvis above the brim. *true pelvis* that part of the pelvis below the brim—**pelvic** *adj*.

pemphigoid (pem′-fi-goyd) *n* allied to pemphigus,* a bullous eruption in the latter half of life which is of autoimmune cause. Histological examination of the base of a blister differentiates it from pemphigus.

pemphigus (pem′-fig-us) *n* skin conditions with bullous (blister) eruptions, but more correctly used of a group of dangerous diseases called pemphigus vulgaris, pemphigus vegetans and pemphigus erythematosus. The latter two are rare. *pemphigus neonatorum* (a) a dangerous form of impetigo* occurring as an epidemic in the hospital nursery; (b) bullous eruption in congenital syphilis of the newborn. *pemphigus vulgaris* a bullous disease of middle-age and later, of autoimmune etiology. Edema of the skin results in blister formation in the epidermis, with resulting secondary infection and rupture, so that large raw areas develop. Bullae develop also on mucous membranes. Death is from malnutrition or intercurrent disease.

pendulous (pen′-dū-lus) *adj* hanging down. *pendulous abdomen* a relaxed condition of the anterior wall, allowing it to hang down over the pubis.

penetrating ulcer ulcer* which is locally invasive and may erode a blood vessel causing hematemesis or melena in gastric or duodenal ulcer respectively.

penicillamine (pen-is-il′-a-mēn) *n* a degradation product of penicillin* used in treatment of heavy metal intoxication, Wilson's* disease and lead poisoning; occasionally useful in rheumatoid arthritis when symptoms are not relieved by other drugs. (Cuprimine.)

penicillin (pen-i-sil′-in) *n* the first antibiotic, also known as "penicillin G" or "benzyl penicillin." Several variants, widely used by injection in many Gram-positive infections. High blood levels are obtained rapidly, and can be supplemented by injections of the slower acting procaine-penicillin or longer acting benethamine penicillin. Dose varies widely according to severity of infection, the largest being given in bacterial endocarditis (2,000,000 units). (Bicillin, Wycillin.)

penicillin V antibiotic of penicillin* family, also called phenethicillin. (Pen-Vee, V-Cillin.)

penicillinase (pen-is-il′-in-āz) *n* an enzyme which destroys penicillin.*

Penicillium (pen-i-sil'-ē-um) *n* a genus of molds. The hyphae bear spores characteristically arranged like a brush. A common contaminant of food. *P. chrysogenum* is now used for commercial production of the antibiotic. *P. notatum* is a species shown by Fleming (1928) to produce penicillin.

penis (pē'-nis) *n* male organ of copulation (→ Figure 16)—**penile** *adj.*

pentaerythritol tetranitrate (pen-ta-er-ith'-rit-ol tet-rá-nī'-trāt) coronary vasodilator. (Peritrate.)

pentagastrin (pen-tá-gas'-trin) *n* synthetic hormone which has largely replaced histamine as the stimulant of choice for evoking maximal acid secretion in gastric function tests. *pentagastrin test* when injected, pentagastrin causes parietal cells in the stomach to secrete acid to their utmost capacity, expressed as mEq H + in 1 h, for the peak 30 min after injection—PAO (peak acid output).

pentamidine (pen-tam'-i-dēn) *n* synthetic compound used in trypanosomiasis, kala-azar and leishmaniasis. (NebuPent.)

pentazocine (pen-taz'-ō-sēn) *n* used for relief of moderate pain. In the presence of bradycardia or hypertension pentazocine is better than morphine.* Can be given orally, intramuscularly, intravenously. (Talwin.)

Penthrane™ methoxyflurane.*

pentobarbital (pen-tō-bár'-bi-tol) *n* a short-acting barbiturate.* Often used for premedication in children. (Nembutal.)

pentose (pen'-tōs) *n* a class of monosaccharides.

pentostatin *n* antileukemia (esp. hairy cell type) drug; inhibits the enzyme adenosine deaminase (ADA). (Nipent.)

pentosuria (pen-tō-sū'-rē-á) *n* pentose* in the urine. Can be due to metabolic disorder—**pentosuric** *adj.*

Pentothal™ thiopental.*

Pen-Vee™ penicillin* V.

pepsin (pep'-sin) *n* proteolytic enzyme of the gastric juice which hydrolyzes proteins to polypeptides. It has an optimum pH of 15–20 and a specificity for peptide bonds involving the aromatic amino acids, although other bonds are split.

pepsinogen (pep-sin'-ō-jen) *n* a zymogen secreted mainly by the chief cells in the gastric mucosa and converted into pepsin by contact with hydrochloric acid (gastric acid) or pepsin itself.

peptic (pep'-tik) *adj* pertaining to pepsin or to digestion generally. *peptic ulcer* a nonmalignant ulcer* in those parts of the digestive tract which are exposed to gastric secretions; hence usually in the stomach or duodenum but sometimes in the lower esophagus or with Meckel's diverticulum.

peptides (pep'-tīdz) *npl* low molecular weight compounds which yield two or more amino acids on hydrolysis, e.g., dipeptides, tripeptides and polypeptides.

peptones (pep'-tōnz) *npl* substances produced when a proteolytic enzyme (e.g., pepsin) or an acid acts upon a native protein during the first stage of protein digestion.

peptonuria (pep-tōn-ūr'-ē-à) *n* peptones in the urine—**peptonuric** *adj*.

Percodan™ oxycodone* plus aspirin.

percussion *n* tapping to determine resonance or dullness of the area examined. Normally a finger of the left hand is laid on the skin and middle finger of the right hand (plexor) is used to strike the left finger.

percutaneous (pèr-kū-tā'-nē-us) *adj* through the skin. → cholangiography.

perforation (pèr-fōr-ā'-shun) *n* a hole in an intact sheet of tissue, as in perforation of the tympanic membrane, or the wall of the stomach or gut (perforating ulcer,* constituting a surgical emergency).

Pergonal™ menotropins.*

Periactin™ cyproheptadine.*

periadenitis (pèr-ē-ad-en-ī'-tis) *n* inflammation in soft tissues surrounding glands. Responsible for the "bull" neck in rubella.

perianal (pèr-ē-ā'-nàl) *adj* surrounding the anus.

periarterial (pèr-ē-àr-tēr'-ē-àl) *adj* surrounding an artery.

periarteritis (pèr-ē-àr-ter-ī'-tis) *n* inflammation of the outer sheath of an artery and the periarterial tissue. *periarteritis nodosa* → polyarteritis.

periarthritis (pèr-ē-àr-thrī'-tis) *n* inflammation of structures surrounding a joint. Sometimes applied to frozen* shoulder.

perarticular (pèr-ē-àr-tik'-ū-làr) *adj* surrounding a joint.

pericardectomy (pèr-ē-kàr-dek'-to-mē) *n* surgical removal of the pericardium,* thickened from chronic inflammation (pericarditis) and embarrassing the heart's action.

pericardiocentesis (pèr-ē-kàr'-dē-ō-sen-tē'-sis) *n* aspiration of the pericardial sac.

pericarditis (pèr-ē-kàr-dī'-tis) *n* inflammation of the outer, serous covering of the heart. It may or may not be accompanied by an effusion and formation of adhesions between the two layers. → Broadbent's sign, pericardectomy.

pericardium (pèr-ē-kàr'-dē-um) *n* double membranous sac which envelops the heart. Layer in contact with the heart is called "visceral"; that reflected from the sac is called "parietal." Between them is the pericardial cavity, which normally contains a small amount of serous fluid—**pericardial** *adj*.

perichondrium (pèr-ē-kon'-drē-um) *n* membranous covering of cartilage— **perichondrial** *adj*.

pericolic (pėr-ē-kōl'-ik) *adj* around the colon.

pericranium (pėr-ē-krā'-nē-um) *n* periosteal covering of the cranium— **pericranial** *adj*.

perifollicular (pėr-ē-fol-ik'-ū-lȧr) *adj* around a follicle.

perilymph (pėr'-ē-limf) *n* the fluid contained in the internal ear, between the bony and membranous labyrinth.

perimetrium (pėr'-ē-mē'-trē-um) *n* peritoneal covering of the uterus— **perimetrial** *adj*.

perinatal (pėr-ē-nā'-tȧl) *adj* the weeks before a birth, the birth and succeeding few weeks.

perinatology (pėr-ē-nā-tol'-o-jē) *n* medical specialty which includes events before, during and immediately after the birth of an infant.

perineometer (pėr-in-ē-om'-ė-tėr) *n* pressure gauge inserted into the vagina to register strength of contraction in the pelvic floor muscles.

perineorraphy (pėr-in-ē-ōr'-af-ē) *n* operation to repair a torn perineum.

perineotomy (pėr-in-ē-ot'-o-mē) *n* episiotomy.*

perinephric (pėr-ē-nef'-rik) *adj* surrounding the kidney.

perineum (pėr-in-ē'-um) *n* portion of the body at the outlet of the pelvis— **perineal** *adj*.

periodic breathing period of apnea in a newborn of 5–10 seconds followed by a period of hyperventilation at a rate of 50–60 breaths a minute, for a period of 10–15 seconds; overall respiratory rate remains between 30 and 40 breaths per minute.

periodontal disease (pėr-ē-ō-don'-tȧl) commonly an inflammatory disease of the periodontal tissues resulting in gradual loss of the supporting membrane and bone around the root of a tooth and a deepened gingival sulcus* or periodontal pocket. → pyorrhea.

perionychia (pėr-ē-ō-nik'-ē-ȧ) *n* red and painful swelling around nail fold. Common in hands that are much in water or have poor circulation. Due to infection from the fungus *Candida*. Secondary infection can occur.

perioral (pėr-ē-ōr'-ȧl) *adj* around the mouth. *perioral dermatitis* a red scaly or papular eruption around the mouth. Common in young adult females; thought due to use of corticosteroids* on the face.

periosteum (pėr-ē-os'-te-um) *n* membrane which covers a bone. In long bones only the shaft as far as the epiphysis is covered. Protective and essential for regeneration—**periosteal** *adj*.

periostitis (pėr-ē-os-tī'-tis) *n* inflammation of the periosteum.* *diffuse periostitis* that involving periosteum of long bones. *hemorrhagic periostitis* that accompanied by bleeding between periosteum and bone.

periostosis (pėr-ē-os-tō′-sis) *n* inflammatory hypertrophy of bone.

peripartum (pėr-ē-pàr′-tum) *n* at the time of delivery. A precise word for what is more commonly called perinatal.

peripheral (pėr-if′-ėr-àl) *adj* pertaining to the outer parts of an organ or of the body. *peripheral nervous system* those nerves which supply the musculoskeletal system and surrounding tissues, as opposed to the autonomic nervous* system. *peripheral neuropathy* sensory loss due to disease of one or more peripheral nerves; syndrome can progress to muscular weakness and wasting. Causes are legion, including trauma, infection, poisoning, overmedication. *peripheral resistance* force exerted by arteriolar walls, an important factor in control of normal blood pressure. *peripheral vascular disease (PVD)* any abnormal condition arising in blood vessels outside the heart, the main one being atherosclerosis,* which can lead to thrombosis and occlusion, resulting in gangrene. *peripheral vision* that surrounding the central field of vision.

periportal (pėr-ē-pōr′-tàl) *adj* surrounding the portal vein.

periproctitis (pėr-ē-prok-tī′-tis) *n* inflammation around rectum and anus.

perirenal (pėr-ē-rē′-nàl) *adj* around the kidney.

perisplenitis (pėr-ē-splen-ī′-tis) *n* inflammation of peritoneal coat of the spleen and of adjacent structures.

peristalsis (pėr-is-tal′-sis) *n* characteristic movement of the intestines by which the contents are moved along the lumen; consists of alternating contraction and relaxation waves—**peristaltic** *adj*.

peritomy (pėr-it′-o-mē) *n* excision of a portion of conjunctiva at the edge of the cornea to prevent vascularization of a corneal ulcer.

peritoneal dialysis (per-it-on-ē′-àl dī-al′-is-is) → dialysis.

peritoneoscopy (pėr-it-on-ē-os′-kop-ē) *n* → laparoscopy.

peritoneum (pėr-it-on-ē′-um) *n* the delicate serous membrane which lines abdominal and pelvic cavities and also covers the organs contained in them—**peritoneal** *adj*.

peritonitis (pėr-it-on-ī′-tis) *n* inflammation of the peritoneum, usually secondary to disease of one of the abdominal organs.

peritonsillar abscess (quinsy) (pėr-ē-ton′-sil-àr) acute inflammation of the tonsil and surrounding loose tissue, with abscess formation.

Peritrate™ pentaerythritol* tetranitrate.

periurethral (pėr-ē-ū-rē′-thràl) *adj* surrounding the urethra, as a periurethral abscess.

perivascular (pėr-ē-vas′-kū-làr) *adj* around a blood vessel.

perleche (pėr-lesh′) *n* lip licking. An intertrigo* at the angles of the mouth with maceration, fissuring, or crust formation. May result from use of poorly fitting dentures, bacterial infection, thrush infestation, vitamin deficiency, drooling or thumbsucking.

Permitil™ fluphenazine.*

pernicious anemia (per-nish'-us) → anemia.

perniosis (per-nē-ōs'-is) *n* chronic chilblains; smaller arteioles go into spasm readily from exposure to cold.

peromelia (pėr-ō-mē'-lē-à) *n* teratogenic malformation of a limb.

peroneal nerve (pėr-ō-nē'-àl) → Figure 11.

peroneus muscles (per-on-ē'-us) → Figures 4, 5.

peroral (per-ōr'-àl) *adj* through the mouth, as biopsy of the small bowel.

perphenazine (pėr-fen'-à-zēn) *n* tranquilizing and antiemetic agent. (Trilafon.)

Persantine™ dipyridamole.*

perseveration (pėr-sev'-ėr-ā'-shun) *n* constant repetition of a meaningless word or phrase.

perspiration *n* the excretion from sweat glands through skin pores. *insensible perspiration* (*syn* percutaneous water loss) that water which is lost by evaporation through the skin other than by sweating; greatly increased in inflammed skin. *sensible perspiration* visible drops of sweat on the skin.

Perthes disease (pėr'-tēz) (*syn* pseudocoxalgia) avascular degeneration of the upper femoral epiphysis; revascularization occurs, but residual deformity of the femoral head may subsequently lead to arthritic changes.

Pertofrane™ despiramine.*

pertussis (pėr-tus'-sis) *n* (*syn* whooping cough) infectious disease of children, with attacks of violent coughing ending in an inspiratory whoop. Organism responsible is *Bordetella* pertussis*. Prophylactic vaccination has reduced case incidence.

pes (pes) *n* a foot or footlike structure. *pes cavus* → claw-foot. *pes planus* → flatfoot.

pessary (pes'-sàr-ē) *n* **1** instrument inserted into the vagina to correct uterine displacements. A *ring* or *shelf pressary* is used to support a prolapse; a *hodge pessary* corrects a retroversion. **2** a medicated suppository used to treat vaginal infections, or as a contraceptive.

petechia (pe-tē'-kē-à) *n* a small, hemorrhagic spot—**petechiae** *pl*, **petechial** *adj*.

petit mal (pe'-tē mal) minor epilepsy. → epilepsy.

petrissage (pā-tri-sahzh') *n* kneading, as massage of a muscle or tendon.

petrous (pet'-rus) *adj* resembling stone.

Peyer's patches (pī′érz) flat patches of lymphatic tissue situated in the small intestine but mainly in the ileum; the seat of infection in typhoid fever; also known as "aggregated lymph nodules."

Peyronie's disease (pay-ron-ēz′) deformity and painful erection of penis due to fibrous tissue formation, cause unknown. Often associated with Dupuytren's* contracture.

pH *abbr* concentration of hydrogen ions expressed as a negative logarithm. A neutral solution has a pH 7.0; pH falls with increasing acidity and rises with increasing alkalinity.

phacoemulsification (fā′-kō-ē-muls-if-i-kā′-shun) *n* ultrasonic vibration to liquefy mature lens fibers.

phagocyte (fag′-ō-sīt) *n* cell capable of engulfing bacteria and other particulate material—**phagocytic** *adj*.

phagocytosis (fag-ō-sī-tō′-sis) *n* engulfment by phagocytes of bacteria or other particles.

phalanges (fàl-an′-jēz) *npl* the small bones of the fingers and toes (→ Figures 2, 3)—**phalanx** *sing*, **phalangeal** *adj*.

phallus (fal′-us) *n* the penis*—**phallic** *adj*.

phantom limb sensation that a limb is still attached to the body after it has been amputated. Pain may seem to come from the amputated limb.

phantom pregnancy → pseudocyesis.

pharmaceutical (fàr-mà-soo′-ti-kàl) *adj* relating to drugs.

pharmacokinetics (fàr-mà-kō-kin-et′-iks) *n* study of the way in which drugs are absorbed, distributed and excreted from the body.

pharmacology (fàr-mà-kol′-o-jē) *n* the science dealing with drugs—**pharmacological** *adj*.

pharyngeal pouch (far-in-jē′-al) pathological dilatation of lower part of the pharynx.

pharyngectomy (far-in-jek′-to-mē) *n* surgical removal of part of the pharynx.

pharyngismus (far-in-jis′-mus) *n* spasm of the pharynx.

pharyngitis (far-in-jī′-tis) *n* inflammation of the pharynx.*

pharyngolaryngectomy (far-ing′-gō-lar-in-jek′-to-mē) *n* surgical removal of the pharynx and larynx.

pharyngoplasty (far-ing′-gō-plas′-tē) *n* any plastic operation to the pharynx.

pharyngotomy (far-ing-got′-o-mē) *n* the operation of opening into the pharynx.

pharyngotympanic tube (far-ing′-gō-tim-pan′-ik) → eustachian tube.

pharynx (far′-ingks) *n* cavity at the back of the mouth (→ Figures 6, 14): cone shaped, ranges in length (average 75 mm), and lined with mucous membrane.

At lower end it opens into the esophagus.* The eustachian tubes pierce its lateral walls and the posterior nares pierce its anterior wall. The larynx lies immediately below it and in front of the esophagus—**pharyngeal** *adj.*

phenazopyridine (fen-àz'-ō-pī'-ri-dēn) *n* urinary tract sedative, esp. useful in cystitis. (Pyridium.)

phenelzine (fen'-el-zēn) *n* antidepressant, a monoamine oxide inhibitor. (Nardil.)

Phenergan™ promethazine.*

phenmetrazine (fen-met'-rà-zēn) *n* appetite depressant; danger of addiction and psychosis of a paranoid nature. (Preludin.)

phenobarbital (fēn-ō-bàrb'-it-ol) *n* long-acting barbiturate and anticonvulsant. Used as a general sedative, and in epilepsy. (Donnatal.)

phenol (fē'-nol) *n* (*syn* carbolic acid) the first disinfectant; paved the way to aseptic surgery. It has been replaced for most purposes by more active and less toxic compounds. Still used in calamine lotion for its local anesthetic effect in relieving itching.

phenolphthalein (fē-nol-thal'-ēn) *n* powerful nontoxic purgative, often given with liquid paraffin.

phenothiazines (fē-nō-thī'-à-zēnz) *npl* powerful tranquilizing drugs, represented by chlorpromazine.*

phenotype (fēn'-ō-tīp) *n* physical characteristics of an organism, based on the interplay between its genetic makeup (genotype) and environment.

phenoxybenzamine (fē-noks-ē-ben'-zà-mēn) *n* peripheral vasodilator used in Raynaud's disease, and in the symptomatic relief of benign prostatic hypertrophy. (Dibenzyline.)

phensuximide (fen-suks'-i-mīd) *n* anticonvulsant used in treating petit mal seizures. (Mitontin.)

phentermine (fen'-tėr-mēn) *n* an appetite suppressant. (Ionamin.)

phentolamine (fen-tol'-à-mēn) *n* adrenaline antagonist, used mainly by injection in diagnosis and surgery of pheochromocytoma, to control excessive variation of blood pressure. Occasionally used orally in vasospasm. (Regitine.)

phenylalanine (fen-l-al'-à-nēn) *n* an essential amino* acid. Inability to metabolize it causes phenylketonuria.*

phenylbutazone (fen-l-bū'-tà-zōn) *n* analgesic with powerful, prolonged action. Toxic effects are common; now used only in hospital for ankylosing spondylitis. (Azolid.)

phenylephrine (fen-l-ef'-rin) *n* vasoconstrictor and pressor drug similar to epinephrine,* but more stable. Given intramuscularly or subcutaneously. Used mainly as eyedrops (0.5–10%) and as nasal spray (0.25%).

phenylketonuria (PKU) (fen-l-kē-tō-nū'-rē-à) *n* metabolites of phenylalanine* (phenylketones among them) in urine. Occurs in hyperphenylalaninemia, owing to lack or inactivity of phenylalanine hydroxylase enzyme in the liver, which converts dietary phenylalanine into tyrosine.* Autosomal recessive disease, resulting in mental subnormality unless discovered by screening and treated from birth with appropriate diet—**phenylketonuric** *adj*.

phenytoin (fen-i-tō'-in) *n* anticonvulsant used in major epilepsy, sometimes with phenobarbital.* (Dilantin.)

pheochromocytoma (fē-ō-krō-mō-sī-tō'-mà) *n* (*syn* paraganglioma) tumor of the adrenal medulla, or of structurally similar tissues associated with the sympathetic chain. It secretes adrenaline and allied hormones; symptoms are due to excess of these substances. Etiology unknown. → Rogitine test.

phimosis (fī-mō'-sis) *n* tightness of the prepuce so that it cannot be retracted over the glans penis.

pHisoHex™ antiseptic and antibacterial skin cleansing agent combining a detergent, 3% hexachlorophene, lanolin, cholesterols and petrolatum in an emulsion with the same pH as skin.

phlebectomy (fle-bek'-to-mē) *n* excision of a vein. *multiple cosmetic phlebectomy (MCP)* removal of varicose veins through little stab incisions which heal without scarring.

phlebitis (fle-bī'-tis) *n* inflammation of a vein—**phlebitic** *adj*.

phlebography (fle-bog'-raf-ē) *n* → venography.

phlebolith (fleb'-ō-lith) *n* concretion which forms in a vein.

phlebothrombosis (fleb-ō-throm-bō'-sis) *n* thrombosis in a vein due to sluggish flow of blood rather than to inflammation in the vein wall, occurring chiefly in bedridden patients and affecting deep veins of lower limbs or pelvis. A loosely attached thrombus may break off and lodge in the lungs as an embolus.

phlebotomy (fle-bot'-o-mē) *n* → venesection.

phlegm (flem) *n* secretion of mucus expectorated from the bronchi.

phlyctenula (flik-ten'-ū-là) *n* a minute blister (vesicle) usually occurring on the conjunctiva or cornea—**phlyctenular** *adj*.

phobia (fō'-bē-à) *n* morbid fear—**phobic** *adj*.

phocomelia (fō-kō-mē'-lē-à) *n* teratogenic malformation. Arms and feet attached directly to trunk giving a seal-like appearance. An epidemic in the 1960s was caused by pregnant women taking the sedative drug thalidomide.

phonation (fō-nā'-shun) *n* the production of voice by vibration of the vocal cords.

phonocardiography (fō-nō-kȧr-dē-og′-raf-ē) *n* graphic recording of heart sounds and murmurs. Fetal heart rate and its relation to uterine contraction can be measured continuously—**phonocardiographic** *adj*, **phonocardiogram** *n*.

phosphaturia (fos-fȧ-tū′-rē-ȧ) *n* excess of phosphates in urine—**phosphaturic** *adj*.

phospholine iodide (fos′-fō-lēn ī′-ō-dīd) anticholinesterase drug, a powerful miotic.

phospholipase D (fos-fō-lī′-pāz dē) → lecithinase.

phosphorylation (fos′-for-il-ā′-shun) *n* metabolic process of introducing a phosphatic group into an organic molecule.

photalgia (fō-tal′-jȧ) *n* pain in the eyes from exposure to intense light.

photochemical (fō-tō-kem′-i-kȧl) *adj* chemically reactive in the presence of light.

photocoagulation (fō-tō-kō-ag′-ū-lā′-shun) *n* burning of tissues with a powerful, focused light source.

photoendoscope (fō-tō-en′-dō-skōp) *n* endoscope to which a camera is attached for making a permanent record—**photoendoscopic** *adj*, **photoendoscopy** *n*.

photophobia (fō-tō-fō′-bē-ȧ) *n* inability to expose the eyes to light—**photophobic** *adj*.

photosensitive (fō-tō-sens′-i-tiv) *adj* sensitive to light, as the pigments in the eye.

phototherapy (fō-tō-thėr′-ȧ-pē) *n* exposure to artificial blue light. In hyperbilirubinemia, it dehydrogenates bilirubin to biliverdin. Used for mild neonatal jaundice and to prevent jaundice in premature infants.

phren (fren) *n* the diaphragm—**phrenic** adj.

phrenicotomy (fren-i-kot′-o-mē) *n* division of phrenic nerve to paralyze one half of the diaphragm.

phrenoplegia (fren-ō-plē′-jē-ȧ) *n* paralysis of the diaphragm—**phrenoplegic** *adj*.

phthisis (thī′-sis) *n* an old term for pulmonary tuberculosis.*

physician (fi-zish′-un) *n* person licensed as a medical doctor.

Physician's Desk Reference (PDR) a yearly publication of current drugs, with descriptions and information on their usage.

physiological (fiz-ē-ō-loj′-i-kȧl) *adj* in accordance with natural processes of the body. Often used to describe a normal process or structure, to distinguish it from an abnormal or pathological feature. *physiological saline* → isotonic. *physiological solution* a fluid isotonic* with the body fluids and containing similar salts—**physiology** *n*.

physostigmine (fī-sō-stig′-mēn) *n* alkaloid used in glaucoma as drops (0.5–1%), and to reverse the action of atropine.* Occasionally used in paralytic ileus.

phytonadione (fī-tō-nȧ-dī′-ōn) *n* vitamin* K₁. Used mainly in overdose and hemorrhage following synthetic anticoagulants such as warfarin,* and in vitamin K deficiency in the newborn. (Aquamephyton, Konakion.)

pia, pia mater (pē′-ȧ mȧ′-tėr) innermost of the meninges; the vascular membrane which lies in close contact with the substance of the brain and spinal cord.

pica (pī′-kȧ) *n* desire for extraordinary articles of food, a feature of some pregnancies.

Pick's disease 1 syndrome of ascites, hepatic enlargement, edema and pleural effusion occurring in constrictive pericarditis. **2** type of cerebral atrophy which produces mental changes similar to presenile dementia.*

picornavirus (pī-kōr-nȧ-vī′-rus) *n* from pico (very small) and RNA (ribonucleic acid). Small RNA viruses. Group includes polio, coxsackie, echo and rhinoviruses. → virus.

PID *abbr* pelvic* inflammatory disease.

pigeon chest (*syn* pectus carinatum) a narrow chest, bulging anteriorly in the breastbone region.

piles *npl* → hemorrhoids.

pilocarpine (pī-lō-kȧr′-pēn) *n* alkaloid used in 0.5–1% solution as a miotic in glaucoma. Stimulates salivary glands and is occasionally used in high dose atropine* therapy. *pilocarpine iontophoresis* introduction of pilocarpine ions into tissues through the skin by means of electricity. Used as a test for cystic fibrosis.

pilomotor nerves (pī-lō-mō′-tor) tiny nerves attached to the hair follicle; innervation causes hair to stand upright and give the appearance of "goose flesh."

pilonidal (pī-lō-nī′-dȧl) *adj* hair-containing. *pilonidal sinus* sinus containing hairs usually found in hirsute people in the cleft between the buttocks; potential site of infection.

pilosebaceous (pī-lō-se-bā′-shus) *adj* pertaining to the hair follicle and sebaceous gland opening into it.

pilosis (pī-lō′-sis) *n* an abnormal growth of hair.

pimozide (pī′-mō-zīd) *n* long-acting neuroleptic and powerful antischizophrenic drug. Often considered a first-choice drug for apathetic patients. (Orap.)

pimple *n* → papule.

pineal body (pin'-ē-ȧl) small reddish-grey conical structure on the dorsal surface of the midbrain (→ Figure 1). Function is not fully understood, but some evidence is that it secretes melatonin,* which appears to inhibit secretion of the luteinizing hormone.

pinguecula (pin-gwek'-ū-lȧ) *n* a yellowish, slightly elevated thickening of the bulbar conjunctiva near the lid aperture. Associated with the aging eye.

pink disease → erythredema polyneuritis.

pinkeye *n* popular name for acute contagious conjunctivitis.*

pinna (pin'-ȧ) *n* that part of the ear which is external to the head; the auricle (→ Figure 13).

pinta (pin'tȧ) *n* color changes in patches of skin due to *Treponema pinta,* identical to those of syphilis* and yaws.*

pinworm *n* → enterobiasis.

piperacillin (pī-pėr-ȧ-sil'-in) *n* antibiotic with wide activity, low toxicity and high stability. Inactive orally. (Pipracil.)

piperazine citrate (pī-pėr'-a-zēn sī'-trāt) anthelmintic. Piperazine therapy can be followed by incidents of unsteadiness and falling—"worm wobble." (Ogen.)

Pipracil™ piperacillin.*

piriformis muscle (pir'-i-form-is) → Figure 5.

piroxicam (pir-oks'-i-kam) *n* nonsteroidal anti-inflammatory agent. (Feldene.)

Pitocin™ synthetic oxytocin.*

Pitressin (pi-tres'-in) *n* a synthetic preparation of vasopressin.*

pitting 1 *adj* making an indentation in edematous tissue. 2 *n* depressed scars left on the skin, esp. after smallpox.

pituitary gland (pi-tū'-it-ār'-ē) (*syn* hypophysis cerebri) a small oval endocrine gland lying in the pituitary fossa of the sphenoid bone (→ Figure 5). The anterior lobe secretes several hormones: growth hormone, corticotropin, thyrotropin, luteotropin, follicle stimulating hormone and prolactin. Controlled by the hypothalamus.* The overall function of pituitary hormones is to regulate growth and metabolism.

Pituitrin™ extract of the posterior pituitary.

pityriasis (pit-i-rī'-ȧ-sis) *n* scaly (branny) eruption of the skin. *pityriasis alba* a common eruption in children, characterized by scaly hypopigmented macules on cheeks and upper arms. *pityriasis capitis* dandruff. *pityriasis rosea* slightly scaly eruption of ovoid erythematous lesions, widespread over the trunk and proximal parts of the limbs, with mild itching. A self-limiting condition. *pityriasis rubra pilaris* a chronic skin disease characterized by tiny red papules of perifolicular distribution. *pityriasis versicolor,* also called "tinea versicolor," is a yeast infection which produces buff-colored patches on the chest.

Pityrosporum (pit-i-ros'-spōr-um) *n* genus of yeasts. *P. orbiculare (Malassezia furfur)* is associated with pityriasis versicolor.

PKU *abbr* phenylketonuria.*

placebo (plă-sē'-bō) *n* a harmless substance given as medicine. In experimental research, an inert substance identical in appearance with material being tested. Neither physician nor patient knows which is which.

placenta (plă-sen'-tă) *n* the afterbirth, a vascular structure developed about the third month of pregnancy and attached to the inner wall of the uterus. Through it the fetus is supplied with nourishment and oxygen, and is ridded of its waste products. In normal labor it is expelled within an hour of birth. When this does not occur it is termed a *retained placenta* and may be an *adherent placenta*. The placenta is usually attached to the upper segment of the uterus; should it lie in the lower uterine segment it is called a *placenta previa* and usually causes placental* abruption—**placental** *adj*.

placental abruption (plă-sent'-al ab-rup'-shun) (*syn* antepartum hemorrhage) premature separation of the placenta from the uterine wall, accompanied by severe abdominal pain, rigid abdomen, and hemorrhage.

placental insufficiency inadequacy of the placenta. Can occur due to maternal disease or postmaturity of fetus, giving rise to a "small for dates" baby.

placentography (plă-sen-tog'-raf-ē) *n* X-ray examination of the placenta after injection of opaque substance.

plague (plāg) *n* very contagious epidemic disease caused by *Yersinia pestis,* and spread by infected rats. Transfer of infection from rat to man is through fleas. Main clinical types are bubonic, septicemic or pneumonic.

plantar (plan'-tăr) *adj* pertaining to the sole of the foot. *plantar arch* union of the plantar and dorsalis pedis arteries in the sole of the foot. *plantar flexion* downward movement of the big toe.

plantaris muscle (plan-tar'-is) → Figure 5.

plaque (plak) *n* → dental plaque.

Plaquenil™ hydroxychloroquine.* → chloroquine.

plasma (plaz'-mă) *n* the fluid fraction of blood. *blood plasma* is used for infusion in cases of hemoconcentration of the patient's blood, as in severe burns. *dried plasma* is in the form of a yellow powder which must be "reconstituted" before use for infusion. Various plasma substitutes are available, e.g., Dextran, Plasmosan. *plasma cell* a normal cell with an eccentric nucleus produced in the bone marrow and reticuloendothelial system, and concerned with the production of antibodies; abnormally produced in myelomatosis.

plasmapheresis (plaz-mă-fĕr-ēs'-is) *n* taking blood from a donor, removing desired fractions, then returning the red cells. Used in treatment of some diseases which are caused by antibodies or immune complexes circulating in the patient's plasma. Removing the plasma and replacing it with human plasma protein fraction (PPF) or a plasma* substitute can improve the prognosis of the disease and prevent or delay onset of renal failure.

plasmin (plaz-min) *n* a fibrinolysin.*

plasminogen (plaz-min'-ō-jen) *n* precursor of plasmin.* Release of activators from damaged tissue promotes the conversion of plasminogen into plasmin.

Plasmodium (plaz-mō'-dē-um) *n* a genus of protozoa. Parasites in the blood of warm-blooded animals which complete their sexual cycle in blood-sucking arthropods. Four species cause malaria* in man—**plasmodial** *adj.*

plastic *adj* capable of taking a form or mold. *plastic surgery* transfer of healthy tissue to repair damaged area and to restore and create form.

platelet (plāt'-let) *n* → thrombocyte. *platelet stickiness test* the stickiness of platelets is increased in multiple sclerosis and rapidly growing tumors. May be consequent on degradation of neural tissue, as it is rich in phospholipid, fractions of which have been shown to be potent aggregators of platelets in a suspension.

platyhelminth (pla-tē-hel'-minth) *n* flat worm; fluke. → schistosomiasis.

platypelloid (pla-tē-pel'-oyd) *adj* having a broad pelvis.

platysma muscle (plat-iz'-mà) → Figure 4.

pleomorphism (plē-ō-mōr'-fizm) *n* denotes a wide range in shape and size of individuals in a bacterial population—**pleomorphic** *adj.*

plethysmograph (ple-thiz'-mō-graf) *n* instrument which accurately measures blood flow in a limb—**plethysmographic** *adj.*

pleura (ploo'-rà) *n* serous membrane covering the surface of the lung (visceral pleura), diaphragm, mediastinum and chest wall (parietal pleura)—**pleural** *adj.*

pleurisy, pleuritis (ploo'-ri-sē, ploo-rī'-tis) *n* inflammation of the pleura.* May be fibrinous (dry), associated with an effusion (wet), or complicated by empyema—**pleuritic** *adj.*

pleurodesis (ploo-rō-dē'-sis) *n* adherence of the visceral to the parietal pleura. Can be achieved therapeutically by using iodized talc.

pleurodynia (ploo-rō-dī'-nē-à) *n* intercostal myalgia or muscular rheumatism (fibrositis); a feature of Bornholm disease.

pleuropulmonary (ploo-rō-pul'-mon-ār-ē) *adj* pertaining to the pleura and lung.

plexus (pleks'-us) *n* a network of vessels or nerves (→ Figure 11).

plicamycin (plī-kà-mī'-sin) *n* antibiotic with cytotoxic activity; now used mainly in hypercalcemia associated with malignant disease. Given intravenously. (Mithracin.)

plication (plī-kā'-shun) *n* surgical procedure of making tucks or folds to decrease the size of an organ—**plica** *sing*, **plicae** *pl*, **plicate** *adj, vt*.

plombage (plom-bazh') *n* extrapleural compression of a tuberculous lung cavity.

plumbism (plum'-bizm) *n* → lead poisoning.

Plummer-Vinson syndrome (plum'-er-vin'-son) (*syn* Kelly-Paterson syndrome) combination of severe glossitis with dysphagia and nutritional iron deficiency anemia. Iron taken orally usually leads to complete recovery.

pluriglandular (ploo-ri-glan'-dū-lår) *adj* pertaining to several glands, as mucoviscidosis.

PMS *abbr* premenstrual* syndrome.

pneumaturia (nū-må-tū'-rē-å) *n* passage of flatus with urine; usually result of vesico-colic (bladder-bowel) fistula.

pneumococcus (nū-mō-kok'-us) *n Strept. pneumoniae,* a coccal bacterium arranged characteristically in pairs. A common cause of lobar pneumonia and other infections—**pneumococcal** *adj*.

pneumoconiosis (nū'-mō-kō-nē-ō'-sis) *n* (*syn* dust disease) fibrosis of the lung caused by long continued inhalation of dust in industrial occupations. Most important complication is occasional superinfection with tuberculosis. *rheumatoid pneumoconiosis* fibrosing alveolitis occurring in patients suffering from rheumatoid arthritis. → anthracosis, asbestosis, byssinosis, siderosis, silicosis—**pneumoconioses** *pl*.

Pneumocystis carinii (nū-mō-sis'-tis kar-ē'-nē-ī) a microorganism which causes pneumonia. Usual victims are infants, debilitated and immunosuppressed patients; mortality is high.

pneumocytes (nū'-mō-sīts) *npl* special cells which line the alveolar walls in the lungs. Type I are flat. Type II are cuboidal and secrete surfactant.

pneumoencephalography (nū'-mō-en-sef-ål-og'-raf-ē) *n* radiographic examination of cerebral ventricles after injection of air by means of a lumbar or cisternal puncture—**pneumoencephalogram** *n*.

pneumogastric (nū-mō-gas'-trik) *adj* pertaining to the lungs and stomach. → vagus.

pneumolysis (nū-mol'-is-is) *n* separation of the two pleural layers, or the outer pleural layer from the chest wall, to collapse the lung.

pneumomycosis (nū-mō-mī-kō'-sis) *n* fungus infection of the lung such as aspergillosis, actinomycosis, candidiasis—**pneumomycotic** *adj*.

pneumonectomy (nū-mon-ek'-to-mē) *n* excision of a lung.

pneumonia (nū-mō′-nē-à) *n* traditionally used for inflammation of the lung; that which is due to physical agents is pneumonitis, the word "pneumonia" being generally reserved for invasion by microorganisms.

pneumonitis (nū-mon-ī′-tis) *n* inflammation of lung tissue.

pneumoperitoneum (nū′-mō-pėr-it-on-ē′-um) *n* air or gas in the peritoneal cavity. Can be introduced for diagnostic or therapeutic purposes.

pneumothorax (nū-mō-thōr′-aks) *n* air or gas in the pleural cavity separating the visceral from the parietal pleura, so that lung tissue is compressed. Can be secondary to asthma, carcinoma of bronchus, chronic bronchitis, congenital cysts, emphysema, intermittent positive pressure ventilation, pneumonia, trauma or tuberculosis. *artificial pneumothorax* induced, in treatment of pulmonary tuberculosis. *spontaneous pneumothorax* occurs when an overdilated pulmonary air sac ruptures, permitting communication of respiratory passages and pleural cavity. *tension pneumothorax* occurs where a valvelike wound allows air to enter pleural cavity at each inspiration but not to escape on expiration, thus progressively increasing intrathoracic pressure and constituting an acute medical emergency—**pneumothoraces** *pl*.

podalic version (pō-dal′-ik) → version.

podiatry (pō-dī′-à-trē) *n* diagnosis and treatment of problems of the feet.

podophyllum (pō-dof′-il-um) *n* powerful purgative; a suspension in liquid paraffin is used to remove condylomata.

podopompholyx (pō-dō-pom′-fō-liks) *n* pompholyx* on the feet.

polioencephalitis (pō-lē-ō-en-sef′-à-lī′-tis) *n* inflammation of cerebral gray matter; may or may not include central nuclei—**polioencephalitic** *adj*.

poliomyelitis (pō-lē-ō-mī-el-ī′-tis) *n* (*syn* infantile paralysis) epidemic virus infection which attacks motor neurons of the anterior horns in the brain stem (*bulbar poliomyelitis*) and spinal cord. An attack may or may not lead to paralysis of the lower motor neuron type, with loss of muscular power and flaccidity. Vaccination is desirable. → Sabin vaccine, Salk vaccine.

polioviruses (pō-lē-ō-vī′-rus-ez) *npl* cause poliomyelitis.* → virus.

Politzer's bag (pol′-it-zėrs) rubber bag for inflation of the eustachian tube.

pollenosis (pol-en-ōs′-is) *n* allergic condition arising from sensitization to pollen.

pollicization (pol-is-īz-ā′-shun) *n* surgical procedure: index finger is rotated and shortened to produce apposition as a thumb.

polyarteritis (pol-ē-à-tėr-ī′-tis) *n* inflammation of many arteries. In *polyarteritis* nodosa (*syn* periarteritis nodosa) aneurysmal swellings and thrombosis occur in affected vessels. Further damage may lead to hemorrhage; clinical picture depends upon site affected. → collagen.

polyarthritis (pol-ē-ár-thrī'-tis) *n* inflammation of several joints at the same time. → Still's disease.

Polycillin™ ampicillin.*

polycystic (pol-ē-sis'-tik) *adj* composed of many cysts. Polycystic kidney disease comprises a number of separate conditions which may be rapidly or slowly fatal and are often associated with cysts of the liver.

polycythemia (pol-ē-sī-thē'-mē-á) *n* increase in number of circulating red blood cells, resulting from dehydration or as compensatory phenomenon to increase oxygen carrying capacity, as in congenital heart disease. *polycythemia vera* (*syn* erythremia) idiopathic condition in which red cell count is very high; patient complains of headache and lassitude. There is danger of thrombosis and hemorrhage.

polydactyly, polydactylism (pol-ē-dak'-til-ē, pol-ē-dak'-til-izm) *n* having more than the normal number of fingers or toes.

polydipsia (pol-ē-dip'-sē-á) *n* excessive thirst.

polyhydramnios (pol-ē-hī-dram'-nē-os) *n* excessive amount of amniotic fluid.

polymorphonuclear (pol-ē-mōr-fō-nū'klē-ar) *adj* having a many-shaped or lobulated nucleus, usually applied to phagocytic neutrophil leukocytes (granulocytes) which constitute 70% of white blood cells.

polymyalgia rheumatica (pol-ē-mī-al'-já roo-mat'-ik-á) syndrome occurring in the elderly: a sometimes crippling ache in shoulders, pelvic girdle muscles and spine, with pronounced morning stiffness and a raised ESR. Associated with temporal arteritis. Clinically distinct from rheumatoid arthritis. → arthritis.

polymyositis (pol-ē-mī-ō-sī'-tis) *n* manifests as muscle weakness, most commonly in middle age. Microscopic examination of muscle reveals inflammatory changes; they respond to corticosteroid drugs. → dermatomyositis.

polymyxin B (pol-ē-miks'-in bē) antibiotic occasionally used in Gram-negative infections, particularly those due to *Pseudomonas aeruginosa*. Usually given by slow intravenous infusion, as it causes pain when given intramuscularly. There are topical preparations for ear and eye infections. (Aerosporin.)

polyneuritis (pol-ē-nū-rī'-tis) *n* multiple neuritis—**polyneuritic** *adj*.

polyoma (pol-ē-ōm'-á) *n* one of the tumor-producing viruses.

polyopia (pol-ē-ō'-pē-á) *n* seeing many images of a single object.

polyp, polypus (pol'-ip[-us]) *n* a pedunculated tumor arising from any mucous surface, e.g., cervical, uterine, nasal, etc. Usually benign but may become malignant—**polypi** *pl*, **polypous** *adj*.

polypectomy (pol-ip-ek'-to-mē) *n* surgical removal of a polyp.

polypeptides (pol-ē-pep'-tīds) *npl* proteins which on hydrolysis yield more than two amino acids.

polypharmacy (pol-ē-får'-må -sē) *n* administration of several drugs at the same time.

polyploidy (pol'-ē-ployd-ē) *n* having a multiple of the haploid number of chromosomes.

polypoid (pol'-ip-oyd) *adj* resembling a polyp(us).

polyposis (pol-ē-pō'-sis) *n* numerous polypi in an organ. *polyposis coli* dominantly-inheritable condition; polypi occur throughout the large bowel. Often leads to carcinoma of the colon. Prevention is by removal of polyps.

polysaccharide (pol-ē-sak'-à-rīd) *n* carbohydrates ($C_6H_{10}O_5$) containing a large number of monosaccharide groups. Starch, inulin, glycogen, dextrin and cellulose are examples.

polyserositis (pol-ē-sėr-o-sī'-tis) *n* inflammation of several serous membranes. A genetic type is familial Mediterranean fever. → amyloidosis.

polythiazide (pol-ē-thī'-à-zīd) *n* saluretic diuretic. (Renese.)

polyuria (pol-ē-ūr'-ē-à) *n* excretion of an excessive amount of urine—**polyuric** *adj*.

pompholyx (pom'-fol-iks) *n* vesicular skin eruption associated with itching or burning. → cheiropompholyx.

POMR *abbr* problem-oriented medical record.

Pondimin™ fenfluramine.*

pons (ponz) *n* a bridge; a process of tissue joining two sections of an organ. *pons varolii* white convex mass of nerve tissue at the base of the brain which connects various lobes of the brain (→ Figure 1)—**pontine** *adj*.

Ponstel™ mefenamic* acid.

Pontiac fever (pon'-tē-ak) flulike illness with little or no pulmonary involvement and no mortality, caused by *Legionella* *pneumophilia*.

Pontocaine™ tetracaine.*

popliteal (pop-li-tē'-àl) *adj* pertaining to the popliteus. *popliteal artery* → Figure 9. *popliteal space* diamond-shaped depression at back of the knee joint, bounded by the muscles and containing the popliteal nerve and vessels. *popliteal vein* → Figure 10.

popliteus (pop-li-tē'-us) *n* muscle in the popliteal space which flexes the leg.

poradenitis (pōr-ad-en-ī'-tis) *n* painful mass of iliac glands, characterized by abscess formation. Occurs in lymphogranuloma* inguinale.

pore *n* a minute surface opening. Mouth of a duct (leading from the sweat glands) on the skin surface; controlled by fine papillary muscles, contracting and closing in the cold and dilating in the presence of heat.

porphyria (pōr-fir′-rē-à) *n* inborn error in porphyrin metabolism, usually hereditary, causing pathological changes in nervous and muscular tissue in some varieties and photosensitivity in others, depending on the level of metabolic block involved. Excess porphyrins or precursors are found in urine or stools or both. In some cases attacks are precipitated by certain drugs.

porphyrins (pōr′-fir-ins) *npl* light-sensitive organic compounds which form the basis of respiratory pigments, including hemoglobin. Naturally occurring porphyrins are uroporphyrin and coproporphyrin.* → porphyria.

porphyrinuria (pōr-fir-in-ū′-rē-à) *n* excretion of porphyrins in urine; produced as result of an inborn error of metabolism.

porta (pōr′-tà) *n* the depression (hilum) of an organ at which the vessels enter and leave. *porta hepatis* transverse fissure through which portal vein, hepatic artery and bile ducts pass on the under surface of the liver—**portal** *adj*.

portacaval (pōr-tà-kā′-vàl) *adj* pertaining to the portal vein and inferior vena cava. *portacaval anastomosis* a fistula made between the portal vein and inferior vena cava to reduce pressure within the portal vein in cirrhosis of the liver.

portahepatitis (pōr-tà-hep-à-tī′-tis) *n* inflammation around transverse fissure of the liver.

portal circulation that of venous blood (collected from intestines, pancreas, spleen and stomach) conveyed to the liver before return to the heart.

portal hypertension increased pressure in the portal vein. Usually caused by cirrhosis of the liver; results in splenomegaly, with hypersplenism and alimentary bleeding. → esophageal varices.

portal vein that conveying blood into the liver; about 75 mm long, formed by the union of superior mesenteric and splenic veins.

portwine stain purplish-red birthmark.

positive pressure ventilation positive pressure inflation of lungs to produce inspiration. Exhaled air, hand bellows or more sophisticated apparatus can be used. Expiration results from elastic recoil of the lung. *intermittent positive pressure ventilation* mechanically applied ventilation of the lungs for controlled ventilation during muscular paralysis as part of general anesthesia or intensive care.

postanal (pōst-ān′-àl) *adj* behind the anus.

postconcussional syndrome (pōst-kon-kush′-un-àl) headaches, giddiness and a feeling of faintness, which may persist for a considerable time after head injury.

postdiphtheritic (pōst-dif-thêr-it′-ik) *adj* following an attack of diphtheria. Refers esp. to paralysis of limbs and palate.

postencephalitic (pōst-en-sef-àl-it′-ik) *adj* following encephalitis lethargica. Commonly describes the syndrome of parkinsonism, which so often results from an attack of this encephalitis.

postepileptic (pōst-ep-il-ep′-tik) *adj* following on an epileptic seizure. *postepileptic automatism* is a fugue state, following a fit, when patient behavior, even involving violence, is not remembered (amnesia).

posterior (pos-tē′-rē-or) *adj* situated at the back. → anterior *opp. posterior chamber of the eye* space between anterior surface of the lens and posterior surface of the iris. → aqueous.

postganglionic (pōst-gang-lē-on′-ik) *adj* situated after a collection of nerve cells (ganglion), as a postganglionic nerve fiber.

postgastrectomy syndrome (pōst-gas-trek′-to-mē) after gastrectomy* symptoms of hypoglycemia when patient is hungry, and of vasovagal attack immediately after a meal.

posthepatic (pōst-hep-at′-ik) *adj* behind the liver.

postherpetic (pōst-hėr-pet′-ik) *adj* after shingles.*

posthitis (pōs-thī′-tis) *n* inflammation of the prepuce.*

postmature (pōst-mȧ-tūr′) *adj* past expected date of delivery; when birth is delayed beyond the usual 40 weeks—**postmaturity** *n*.

postmenopausal (pōst-men-ō-pawz′-ȧl) *adj* occurring after the menopause* has been established.

postmortem (pōst-mōr′-tem) *adj* after death, usually implying dissection of the body. → antemortem *opp,* autopsy. *postmortem wart* → verruca.

postmyocardial infarction syndrome pyrexia and chest pain associated with inflammation of the pleura, lung or pericardium. Due to sensitivity to released products from dead muscle.

postnasal (pōst-nā′-zȧl) *adj* situated behind the nose and in the nasopharynx.

postnatal (pōst-nā′-tȧl) *adj* after delivery. → antenatal *opp. postnatal depression* a low mood experienced by some mothers for a few days following birth of a baby; sometimes called "baby blues." Less severe than puerperal* psychosis. *postnatal examination* routine examination 6 weeks after delivery.

postpartum (pōst-pȧr′-tum) *adj* after a birth (parturition).

postperfusion syndrome result of transfusion with blood containing cytomegalovirus (CMV); with fever of several weeks duration, hepatic inflammation and often involvement of other body systems (renal, pulmonary, GI tract).

postprandial (pōst-pran′-dē-ȧl) *adj* following a meal.

postural (pos′-tū-rȧl) *adj* pertaining to posture. *postural albuminuria* orthostatic* albuminuria. *postural drainage* usually implies drainage from respiratory tract, by elevation of the foot of the bed or by using a special frame.

postvaccinal (pōst-vak′-sin-ȧl) *adj* after vaccination.

postvagotomy diarrhea (pōst-vā-got′-o-mē) three types: (a) transient diarrhea shortly after operation, lasting from a few hours to a day or two; episodes disappear in 3–6 months; (b) continued recurrence with longer attacks (recurrent episodic diarrhea); (c) an increased daily bowel frequency; may be of disabling severity, but often acceptable in contrast to preoperative constipation.

Potaba-6™ potassium para-aminobenzoate.*

potassium chlorate mild antiseptic used in mouthwashes and gargles. Distinguished from potassium chloride.

potassium chloride used in potassium replacement solutions, and as a supplement in thiazide diuretic therapy.

potassium citrate alkalinizes urine; still used in cystitis and during sulfonamide therapy to prevent renal complications.

potassium deficiency disturbed electrolyte balance; can occur after excessive vomiting and/or diarrhea; after prolonged use of diuretics, steroids, etc. Signs and symptoms are variable, but nausea and muscle weakness are often present. Heart failure can quickly supervene.

potassium hydroxide caustic potash; occasionally used for warts.

potassium iodide expectorant used in bronchitis and asthma; also used in prophylaxis of simple goiter, and preoperatively in toxic goiter.

potassium para-aminobenzoate (pa-rà-à-mē-nō-ben′-zō-āt) used in scleroderma and Peyronie's disease. Has an antifibrotic effect. 3 g capsules perorally four times daily with meals for several months. (Potaba-6.)

potassium permanganate (pér-mang′-àn-āt) purple crystals with powerful disinfectant and deodorizing properties. Used as lotion 1 in 1000; 1 in 5000 to 10,000 for baths.

Pott's disease spondylitis; spinal caries; spinal tuberculosis. Resultant necrosis of vertebrae causes kyphosis.

pouch *n* a pocket or recess. *pouch of Douglas* the rectouterine pouch.

povidone iodine (pov′-i-dōn ī′-ō-dīn) liquid from which iodine is slowly liberated when in contact with the skin and mucous membranes. Useful for preoperative skin preparation and as a douche. (Betadine.)

PPD *abbr* purified protein derivative. → Mantoux reaction.

PPLO *abbr* pleuropneumonia-like organism, similar to the agent that causes contagious pleuropneumonia in cattle. → Mycoplasma.

Prader-Willi syndrome (prā′-dér-wil′-ē) metabolic condition characterized by congenital hypotonia, hyperphagia, obesity, and mental retardation. Diabetes mellitus develops in later life.

prazosin (praz′-ō-sin) *n* antihypertensive agent; acts peripherally by direct vasodilation. (Minipress.)

precancerous *adj* occurring before cancer, with special reference to nonmalignant pathological changes which are believed to lead to cancer.

precipitin (prē-sip'-it-in) *n* antibody which is capable of forming an immune complex with an antigen and becoming insoluble—a precipitate. Basis of many delicate diagnostic serological tests for identification of antigens in serum and other fluids. → immunoglobulins.

precordial (prē-kōr'-dē-ȧl) *adj* pertaining to the area of the chest immediately over the heart.

prediabetes (prē-dī-ab-ē'-tēz) *n* potential predisposition to diabetes* mellitus. Preventive mass urine testing can detect the condition. Early treatment prevents ketoacidosis and may help to prevent the more serious complications such as retinopathy and neuropathy—**prediabetic** *adj, n.*

predigestion (prē-dī-jes'-chun) *n* artificial digestion of protein (e.g., in peptonized foods) or amylolysis (e.g., in malt extracts or dextrinized cereals) before digestion takes place in the body.

prednisolone (pred-nis'-o-lōn) *n* a synthetic hormone with properties similar to those of cortisone* but side-effects, such as salt and water retention, are markedly reduced. Widely prescribed for connective tissue diseases, conditions involving immune reaction including autoimmune disorders. (Delta-Cortef, Hydeltrasol.)

prednisone (pred'-ni-sōn) *n* converted into prednisolone* in the liver, therefore prescribed for the same conditions as prednisolone.

preeclampsia (prē-ē-klamp'-sē-ȧ) *n* condition characterized by albuminuria, hypertension and edema, arising usually in the latter part of pregnancy—**preeclamptic** *adj.*

prefrontal (prē-front'-ȧl) *adj* situated in the anterior portion of the frontal lobe of the cerebrum. → leukotomy.

preganglionic (prē-gang-lē-on'-ik) *adj* preceding or in front of a collection of nerve cells (ganglion), as a preganglionic nerve fiber.

pregnancy *n* being with child, i.e., gestation from last menstrual period to parturition, normally 40 weeks or 280 days. → ectopic pregnancy, phantom pregnancy. *pregnancy-associated hypertension* solely a disease of pregnancy, most commonly, of the primigravida.* Blood pressure returns to normal and protein and urea, if present in the blood, resolve quickly after delivery in nearly all instances.

pregnanediol (preg-nan-e-dī'-ol) *n* a urinary excretion product from progesterone.*

Pregnyl™ preparation of human* chorionic gonadotropin; useful for undescended and ectopic testes.

Preludin™ phenmetrazine.*

Premarin™ preparation of conjugated estrogens. Can be given orally. Useful for menopausal symptoms.

premature *adj* occurring before the proper time. *premature baby* where birth weight is less than 2.5 kg (5½ lb) and implying need for special treatment. Not all low birthweight babies are premature, but are included in category "small for dates." → placental insufficiency. *premature beat* → extrasystole.

premedication *n* drugs given before administration of another drug, e.g., those given before an anesthetic. The latter are of several types: (a) sedative or anxiolytic, e.g., morphine, meperidine, which also have sedative properties; (b) drugs which inhibit secretion of saliva and of mucus from the upper respiratory tract and cause tachycardia.

premenstrual (prē-men'-stroo-ål) *adj* preceding menstruation. *premenstrual* (cyclical) syndrome (PMS) a group of physical and mental changes which begin any time between 2 and 14 days before menstruation and which are relieved almost immediately once flow starts. Recent research reveals a deficiency of essential fatty acids.

premolars (prē-mōl'-arz) *npl* the teeth, also called bicuspids, situated fourth and fifth from the midline of the jaws, used with the molars for gripping and grinding food.

prenatal (prē-nā'-tål) *adj* pertaining to the period between the last menstrual period and birth of the child, normally 40 weeks or 280 days.

preparalytic (prē-pār-å-lit'-ik) *adj* before onset of paralysis, usually referring to the early stage of poliomyelitis.

prepatellar (prē-på-tel'-år) *adj* in front of the kneecap, as applied to a large bursa. → bursitis.

prepubertal (prē-pū'-bėr-tål) *adj* before puberty.

prepuce (prē'-poos) *n* foreskin of the penis (→ Figure 16).

prerenal (prē-rē'-nål) *adj* literally, before or in front of the kidney, but used to denote states in which, for instance, renal failure has arisen not within the nephrons but in the vascular fluid compartment, as in severe dehydration.

presbycusis (prez-bē-ku'-sis) *n* hearing loss that occurs in the normal course of aging.

presbyopia (prez-bē-ō'-pē-å) *n* long-sightedness, due to failure of accommodation in those of 45 years and older—**presbyopic** *adj*, **presbyope** *n*.

prescription *n* a written formula, signed by a physician, directing a pharmacist to supply required drugs.

presenile dementia (prē-sēn'-īl dē-men'-shå) → dementia.

presenility (prē-sē-nil'-i-tē) *n* condition occurring before senility is established. → dementia—**presenile** *adj*.

presentation *n* part of the fetus which first enters the pelvic brim and will be felt by the examining finger through the cervix in labor. May be vertex, face, brow, shoulder or breech.

pressor (pres'-or) *n* substance which raises blood pressure.

pressure areas bony prominences of the body, over which the flesh of bedridden patients is denuded of its blood supply as it is compressed between bone and surfaces of bed, splint, chair, etc.

pressure point a place at which an artery passes over a bone, against which it can be compressed, to stop bleeding.

pressure sore (*syn* bedsore, decubitus ulcer) classified as superficial or deep: *superficial pressure sores* involve destruction of epidermis with exposure to microorganisms that penetrate the tissue, which is moist with lymph. *deep pressure sores* are caused by damage to microcirculation in deeper tissues, usually resulting from shearing force. Inflammatory and necrotic residue then tracks out to the skin surface destroying the dermis and epidermis. Deep sores are usually infected, discharging an exudate which results in protein and fluid loss from the body. Deep sores can take many weeks or months to heal and quite often require surgical closure to prevent further debility.

presystole (prē-sis'-to-lē) *n* period preceding the systole or contraction of the heart muscle—**presystolic** *adj*.

prevesical (prē-ves'-i-kál) *adj* anterior to the bladder.

priapism (prī'-áp-izm) *n* prolonged penile erection in the absence of sexual stimulation.

prickly heat → miliaria.

primaquine (prī'-má-qwin) *n* antimalarial; useful for eradication of *Plasmodium vivax* from the liver.

primary complex (*syn* Ghon focus) the initial tuberculous infection, manifest as a small focus of infection in lung tissue and enlarged caseous, hilar glands. Usually heals spontaneously.

primidone (prim'-i-dōn) *n* anticonvulsant used mainly in major epilepsy, but sometimes effective in minor epilepsy. (Mysoline.)

primigravida (prīm-i-grav'-i-dá) *n* a woman who is pregnant for the first time—**primigravidae** *pl*.

primipara (prī-mip'-ar-á) *n* a woman who has given birth to a child for the first time—**primiparous** *adj*.

Priscoline™ tolazoline.*

proband (prō'-band) *n* in genetically-inherited diseases, the first family member to present for investigation.

Pro-Banthine™ propantheline.*

probenecid (prō-ben'-e-sid) *n* drug which inhibits renal excretion of certain compounds, notably penicillin* and para-aminosalicylic* acid; used to increase blood level of such drugs. Also hinders reabsorption of urates by the renal tubules, so increasing excretion of uric acid, hence used in treatment of gout. (Benemid.)

procainamide (prō-kān'-à-mīd) *n* derivative of procaine* used in cardiac arrhythmias such as paroxysmal tachycardia. Also helps to relax voluntary muscle and thus overcome myotonia. Given orally or by slow intravenous injection. (Pronestyl.)

procaine (prō'-kān) *n* once widely-used local anesthetic of high potency and low toxicity. Used mainly for infiltration and anesthesia as a 0.5–2% solution. Now replaced by lidocaine. (Novocain.)

procarbazine (prō-kàr'-bà-zēn) *n* drug of the nitrogen* mustard group useful in Hodgkin's disease. (Matulane.)

process *n* prominence or outgrowth of any part.

prochlorperazine (prō-klōr-pér'-à-zēn) *n* a phenothiazine. Has sedative and anti-emetic properties. Useful for vertigo, migraine, Ménière's disease, severe nausea and vomiting, schizophrenia. (Compazine.)

procidentia (pro-si-den'-shà) *n* complete prolapse of the uterus, so that it lies within the vaginal sac but outside the contour of the body.

proctalgia (prok-tal'-jà) *n* pain in the rectal region.

proctitis (prok-tī'-tis) *n* inflammation of the rectum.* *granular proctitis* acute proctitis, so called because of granular appearance of the inflamed mucous membrane.

proctoclysis (prok-tō-klī'-sis) *n* → enterolysis.

proctocolectomy (prok-tō-kōl-lek'-to-mē) *n* surgical excision of the rectum and colon.

proctocolitis (prok-tō-kō-lī'-tis) *n* inflammation of rectum and colon; usually a type of ulcerative colitis.*

proctoscope (prok'-tō-skōp) *n* instrument for examining the rectum. → endoscope—**proctoscopic** *adj*, **proctoscopy** *n*.

proctosigmoiditis (prok'-tō-sig-moyd-īt'-is) *n* inflammation of rectum and sigmoid colon.

procyclidine (prō-sī'-kli-dēn) *n* spasmolytic drug similar in action to benzhexol*; used in treatment of parkinsonism. Reduces rigidity but has little action on tremor. (Kemadrin.)

prodromal (prō-drō'-màl) *adj* preceding, as transitory rash before the true rash of an infectious disease.

pro-drug *n* compound with reduced intrinsic activity, but which, after absorption, is metabolized to release active components. Avoids side-effects in gastrointestinal tract.

Progestasert™ flexible T-shaped unit, like an IUCD; contains the hormone progesterone,* released at a continuous rate of 65 mg daily.

progestational (prō-jes-tā'-shun-al) *adj* before pregnancy. Favoring pregnancy—**progestation** *n*.

progesterone (prō-jes'-tėr-ōn) *n* hormone of the corpus luteum.* Used in treatment of functional uterine hemorrhage, and in threatened abortion. Given by intramuscular injection.

progestogen (prō-jes'-tō-jen) *n* any natural or synthetic progestational hormone progesterone.*

proglottis (prō-glot'-is) *n* a sexually mature segment of tapeworm—**proglottides** *pl*.

prognosis (prog-nō'-sis) *n* a forecast of probable course and termination of a disease—**prognostic** *adj*.

prolactin (prō-lak'-tin) *n* a hormone secreted by the anterior pituitary, concerned with lactation and reproduction. Increased levels found in some pituitary tumors (prolactinomas); result in amenorrhea and infertility.

prolapse (prō'-laps) *n* descent; the falling of a structure. *prolapse of an intervertebral disk (PID)* protrusion of disk nucleus into the spinal canal. Most common in the lumbar region, where it causes low back pain and/or sciatica. *prolapse of the iris* iridocele.* *prolapse of the rectum* lower portion of the intestinal tract descends outside the external anal sphincter. *prolapse of the uterus* uterus descends into the vagina and may be visible at vaginal orifice. → procidentia.

Prolixin™ fluphenazine.*

promazine (prom'-à-zēn) *n* tranquilizing drug similar to but less hepatotoxic than chlorpromazine.* Also useful in obstetrics, treatment of alcoholism, senile agitation and for shivering attacks. (Sparine.)

promethazine (prō-meth'-à-zēn) *n* antihistamine of high potency and low toxicity. Hypnotic side-effect useful in psychiatry and obstetrics. Also useful for travel sickness. Given 2 hours before a journey its effect will last for 6–12 h. (Phenergan.)

pronate (prō'-nāt) *vt* to place ventral surface downward, e.g., on the face; to turn (palm of the hand) downwards. → supinate *opp*—**pronation** *n*.

pronator (prō'-nā-tor) *n* that which pronates, usually applied to a muscle. → supinator *opp*. *pronator teres* → Figure 4.

prone *adj* 1 lying on the anterior surface of the body with face turned to one side. 2 of the hand, with the palm downwards. → supine *opp*.

Pronestyl™ procainamide.*

propantheline (prō-pan'-thel-ēn) *n* synthetic compound with atropine*-like action. Used for its antispasmodic effects in pylorospasm, peptic ulcer, etc. Dryness of mouth may occur in some patients. (Pro-Banthine.)

prophylaxis (prō-fil-aks'-is) *n* (attempted) prevention—**prophylactic** *adj*.

propranolol (prō-pran'-ol-ol) *n* effective drug in prevention or correction of cardiac arrhythmias and dysrhythmias. Reduces frequency of anginal attacks by blocking effects of beta-receptor activation in the heart. Bronchoconstriction may occur as a side-effect in some patients. Prepared as eye drops for glaucoma. (Inderal.)

proptosis (prop-tō'-sis) *n* forward protrusion, esp. of the eyeball.

propylthiouracil (prō-pil-thī-ūr'-à-sil) *n* inhibits thyroid activity; used occasionally in thyrotoxicosis.

prostacyclin (pros-tà-sī'-klin) *n* naturally occurring substance formed by endothelial cells of blood vessel walls; inhibits platelet aggregation.

prostaglandins (pros-tà-glan'-dins) *npl* share some of the properties of hormones, vitamins, enzymes and catalysts. All body tissues probably contain some prostaglandins. Used pharmaceutically to terminate early pregnancy, and for asthma and gastric hyperacidity.

prostate (pros'-tāt) *n* small conical gland at the base of the male bladder and surrounding the first part of the urethra. (→ Figure 16)— **prostatic** *adj*.

prostatectomy (pros-tà-tek'-to-mē) *n* surgical removal of the prostate* gland. *retropubic prostatectomy* the prostate is reached through a lower abdominal (suprapubic) incision, the bladder being retracted upwards to expose the prostate behind the pubis. *transurethral prostatectomy* chippings of prostatic tissue are cut from within the urethra using either a cold knife or electric cautery; usually restricted to small fibrous glands or to cases of prostatic carcinoma. → resectoscope. *transvesical prostatectomy* prostate is approached through the bladder, using a lower abdominal (suprapubic) incision.

prostatic acid phosphatase (prost-at'ik as'-id fos'-fà-tās) enzyme in seminal fluid secreted by the prostate gland. *prostatic acid phosphatase test* (PAP test) an increase in this enzyme in blood is indicative of carcinoma of the prostate gland.

prostatism (pros'-tàt-ism) *n* general condition produced by hypertrophy or chronic disease of the prostate gland, characterized by the obstructive symptoms of hesitancy, a poor stream and post-micturition dribbling.

prostatitis (pros-tà-tī'-tis) *n* inflammation of the prostate* gland.

prostatocystitis (pros-tà-tō-sis-tī'-tis) *n* inflammation of prostate gland and male urinary bladder.

prosthesis (pros-thē'-sis) *n* artificial substitute for a missing part—**prostheses** *pl*, **prosthetic** *adj*.

prosthetics (pros-thet'-iks) *n* branch of surgery which deals with prostheses.

prosthokeratoplasty (pros-thō-kėr'-ȧt-ō-plas'-tē) *n* keratoplasty in which corneal implant is of some material other than human or animal tissue.

Prostigmin™ neostigmine.*

Prostin™ pessaries containing prostaglandin E_2; given to induce labor.

protamine sulfate (prō'-tȧ-mēn) a protein of simple structure used as an antidote to heparin*; 1 ml of 1% solution will neutralize effects of about 1000 units of heparin.

protamine zinc insulin an insoluble form of insulin,* formed by combination with protamine (a simple protein) and a trace of zinc. Action lasts over 24 h, and with initial doses of soluble insulin permits a wide degree of control.

protease (prō'-tē-ās) *n* any enzyme which digests protein: a proteolytic enzyme.

protein calorie malnutrition (PCM) (protein energy malnutrition—PEM) depleted body fat and protein resulting from an inadequate diet.

proteins (prō'-tēnz) *npl* complex nitrogenous compounds found in all animal and vegetable tissues. Built up of amino* acids; essential for growth and repair of the body. Those from animal sources are of high biological value since they contain the essential amino acids. Those from vegetable sources contain not all, but some essential amino acids. Proteins are hydrolyzed in the body to produce amino acids, which are then used to make new body proteins.

proteinuria (prō-tēn-ūr'-ē-ȧ) *n* albuminuria.*

proteolysis (prō-tē-ol'-is-is) *n* hydrolysis of peptide bonds of proteins, with formation of smaller polypeptides—**proteolytic** *adj*.

proteolytic enzymes (prō-tē-ō-li'-tik) enzymes that promote proteolysis*; of limited use in liquefying slough and necrotic tissue, and as debriding agents.

proteose (prō'-tē-ōs) *n* mixture of cleavage products from breakdown of proteins, intermediate between protein and peptone.

Proteus (prō'-tē-us) *n* bacterial genus. Gram-negative motile rods which swarm in culture. Found in damp surroundings. Sometimes a commensal of the intestinal tract. May be pathogenic, esp. in wound and urinary tract infections as a secondary invader.

prothrombin (prō-throm'-bin) *n* a precursor of thrombin formed in the liver. *prothrombin time,* a measure of its production and concentration in blood, is the time taken for plasma to clot after addition of thrombokinase. Inversely proportional to the amount of prothrombin present. Prothrombin time is lengthened in certain hemorrhagic combinations and patients on anticoagulant drugs. → thrombin. *prothrombin test* indirectly reveals amount of prothrombin in blood:

to a sample of oxalated blood are added all the factors needed to bring about clotting, except prothrombin. Time taken for clot to form is therefore dependent on amount of prothrombin present. Normal time is 10–12 s.

protoplasm (prō′-tō-plazm) *n* → cytoplasm—**protoplasmic** *adj*.

protozoa (prō-tō-zō′-à) *npl* the smallest type of animal life; unicellular organisms. Phylum includes the genera *Plasmodium* (malarial parasites) and *Entamoeba*. Commonest protozoan infestation is *Trichomonas vaginalis,* classed with the intestinal flagellates—**protozoon** *sing,* **protozoal** *adj*.

protriptyline (prō-trip′-tl-in) *n* antidepressant similar to imipramine,* but response to treatment is more rapid. Has no sedative effect. (Vivactil.)

proud flesh excessive granulation tissue.

Provera™ medroxyprogesterone.*

provitamin (prō-vīt′-à-min) *n* a vitamin precursor, e.g., carotene is converted into vitamin A.

proximal (proks′-i-màl) *adj* nearest to the head or source.

Prozac™ fluoxetine.*

prune belly syndrome condition found in male infants, with obstructive uropathy and atrophy of abdominal musculature.

prurigo (proo-rī′-gō) *n* chronic, itching disease occurring most frequently in children. *prurigo estivale* hydroa* estivale. *Besnier's prurigo* → Besnier's.

pruritus (proo-rī′-tis) *n* itching. Generalized pruritus may be a symptom of systemic disease, as in diabetes, icterus, Hodgkin's disease, carcinoma—**pruritic** *adj*.

prussic acid (prus′-ik) → hydrocyanic acid.

pseudoangina (soo-dō-an-jī′-nà) *n* false angina. Sometimes referred to as "left mammary pain," it occurs in anxious individuals. Usually no cardiac disease present; may be part of effort* syndrome.

pseudoarthrosis (soo-dō-àr-thrō′-sis) *n* a false joint, e.g., due to ununited fracture; also congenital malformation.

pseudobulbar paralysis (soo-dō-bul′-bàr) gross disturbance in control of tongue, bilateral hemiplegia and mental changes following on a succession of "strokes."

pseudocholinesterase (soo-dō-kō-lin-es′-tèr-āz) enzyme present in plasma and tissues (other than nerve tissue); synthesized in the liver.

pseudocoxalgia (soo-dō-koks-al′-jà) *n* → Perthes' disease.

pseudocrisis (soo-dō-krī′-sis) *n* rapid reduction of body temperature resembling a crisis, followed by further fever.

pseudocyesis (soo-dō-sī-ē′-sis) *n* usual signs of pregnancy without conception. Also phantom pregnancy.

pseudoephedrine (soo-dō-e-fed′-rin) *n* isomer of ephedrine; a nasal deconges-tant. May cause hallucinations in some young children.

pseudohermaphrodite (soo-dō-hėr-maf′-rō-dīt) *n* person in whom gonads of one sex are present, while external genitalia comprise those of the opposite sex.

Pseudomonas (soo-dō-mō′-nas) *n* bacterial genus. Gram-negative motile rods. Found in water and decomposing vegetable matter. Some are pathogenic to plants and animals; *P. aeruginosa (pyocanea)* can cause disease in man. Found commonly as a secondary invader in urinary tract infections and wound infec-tions. Produces a blue pigment (pyocyanin) which colors the exudate or pus.

pseudomucin (soo-dō-mū′-sin) *n* gelatinous substance (not mucin) found in some ovarian cysts.

pseudoparalysis (soo-dō-pȧr-ál′-is-is) *n* a loss of muscular power not due to a lesion of the nervous system. *pseudoparalysis of Parrot* inability to move one or more of the extremities because of syphlitic osteochondritis: occurs in neo-natal congenital syphilis.

pseudoparkinsonism (soo-dō-pȧr′-kin-son-izm) *n* signs and symptoms of par-kinsonism when they are not postencephalitic.

pseudopodia (soo-dō-pō′-dē-ȧ) *npl* literally false legs; cytoplasmic projections of an amoeba or other motile cell which help it to move. Not to be confused with cilia or microvilli, which are nonretractile projections from the cell surface—**pseudopodium** *sing*.

pseudopolyposis (soo-dō-pol-i-pōs′-is) *n* widely scattered polypi, usually result of previous inflammation—sometimes ulcerative colitis.

psittacosis (sit-ȧ-kō′-sis) *n* disease of parrots, pigeons and other birds which is occasionally responsible for a form of pneumonia in man. Caused by *Chla-mydia psittaci*. It behaves as a bacterium though multiplying intracellularly. Sensitive to sulfonamides and antibiotics.

psoas (sō′-as) *n* muscles of the loin. *psoas abscess* a cold abscess* in the psoas muscle, resulting from tuberculosis of lower dorsal or lumbar vertebrae. Pres-sure in the abscess causes pus to track along the tough ligaments so that the abscess appears as a firm smooth swelling which does not show signs of inflammation—hence the adjective "cold."

psoralen (sōr′-ȧ-len) *n* naturally occurring photosensitive compound which on exposure to ultraviolet increases melanin* in the skin. Pharmaceutical psoralen has been used in psoriasis and vitiligo.

psoriasis (sōr-ī′-ȧ-sis) *n* genetically-determined chronic skin disease in which erythematous areas are covered with adherent scales. May occur on any part of the body, but characteristic sites are extensor surfaces, esp. over the knees and elbows. A common cause of erythroderma—**psoriatic** *adj*.

psoriatic arthritis (sōr-ī-at'-ik) articular symptoms similar to those of rheumatoid arthritis; occurs in 3–5% of patients with psoriasis.

psychiatry (sī-kī'-at-rē) *n* branch of medical study devoted to diagnosis and treatment of mental illness—**psychiatric** *adj*.

psychochemotherapy (sī-kō-kē-mō-thėr'-à-pē) *n* use of drugs to improve or cure pathological changes in the emotional state—**psychochemotherapeutic** *adj*.

psychodynamics (sī-kō-dī-nam'-iks) *n* science of the mental processes, esp. of causative factors in mental activity.

psychogenesis (sī-kō-jen'-es-is) *n* the development of the mind.

psychogenic (sī-kō-jen'-ik) *adj* arising from the psyche or mind. *psychogenic symptom* originates in the mind rather than in the body.

psychogeriatric (sī-kō-jėr-ē-at'-rik) *adj* pertaining to psychology as applied to the elderly. *psychogeriatric dependency rating scales* are based on three aspects—psychological deterioration, physical infirmity and psychological agitation.

psychology (sī-kol'-o-jē) *n* study of the behavior of an organism in its environment. Medically, the study of human behavior.

psychometry (sī-kom'-e-trē) *n* science of mental testing.

psychomotor (sī-kō-mō'-tor) *adj* pertaining to the motor effect of psychic or cerebral activity.

psychoneuroimmunology (PNI) (sī-kō-noo-rō-im-ūn-ol'-o-jē) *n* study of white blood cell counts and their correlation with stressful conditions and illness.

psychoneurosis (sī-kō-noo-rō'-sis) *n* → neurosis.

psychopathic personality (sī-kō-path'-ik) persistent condition of mind which results in abnormally aggressive or seriously irresponsible conduct, deviant from social norms. Antisocial personality—**psychopath** *n*.

psychopathology (sī-kō-pa-thol'-o-jē) *n* pathology of abnormal mental processes—**psychopathological** *adj*.

psychopathy (sī-kop'-à-thē) *n* any disease of the mind—**psychopathic** *adj*.

psychopharmacology (sī-kō-fàr-mà-kol'-o-jē) *n* use of drugs which influence the affective and emotional state.

psychoprophylactic (sī-kō-prō-fil-ak'-tik) *adj* that which aims at preventing mental disease.

psychosis (sī-kō'-sis) *n* a major mental disorder of organic or emotional origin in which ability to think, respond emotionally, remember, communicate, interpret reality and behave appropriately is impaired. Insight is usually absent—**psychoses** *pl*, **psychotic** *adj*.

psychosomatic (sī-kō-som-at′-ik) *n* mind-body illness; illness in which emotional factors produce physical symptoms. These arise mainly from overactivity of the autonomic nervous system, which is influenced by emotional state.

psychotherapy (sī-kō-thĕr′-a-pē) *n* treatment of mental disorder by psychological means using discussion, explanation and reassurance—**psychotherapeutic** *adj*.

psychotropic (sī-kō-trō′-pik) *adj* that which exerts its specific effect upon brain cells.

psyllium (sil′-ē-um) *n* seed of an African plant that contains mucilage, which swells on contact with water; useful as a bulk-forming laxative. (Metamucil).

pteroylglutamic acid (tēr′-ō-il-gloo-tam′-ik) → folic acid.

pterygium (te-rij′-ē-um) *n* wing-shaped degenerative condition of the conjunctiva which encroaches on the cornea—**pterygial** *adj*.

ptomaine (tō′-mān) *n* one of a group of poisonous substances formed in the decay of protein by bacterial action.

ptosis (tō′-sis) *n* a drooping, particularly that of the eyelid. → visceroptosis—**ptotic** *adj*.

ptyalin (tī′-à-lin) *n* salivary amylase,* a slightly acid medium (pH 6.8) which converts starch into dextrin* and maltose.*

ptyalism (tī′-à-lizm) *n* excessive salivation.

ptyalolith (tī′-al-ō-lith) *n* a salivary calculus.

pubertas praecox (pū′-ber-tas prā′-coks) premature (precocious) sexual development.

puberty (pū′-bĕr-tē) *n* age at which reproductive organs become functionally active; accompanied by secondary characteristics—**pubertal** *adj*.

pubes (pū′-bēz) *n* hairy region covering the pubic bone.

pubiotomy (pū-bē-ot′-o-mē) *n* cutting the pubic bone to facilitate delivery of a live child.

pubis (pū′-bis) *n* the pubic bone, or os pubis, forming the center bone of the front of the pelvis—**pubic** *adj*.

PUBS *abbr* percutaneous umbilical blood sampling; samples of fetal blood taken from the umbilical cord through the abdomen of the mother.

pudendal block (pū-den′-dàl) rendering the pudendum insensitive by injection of local anesthetic. Used mainly for episiotomy and forceps delivery. → transvaginal.

pudendum (pū-den′-dum) *n* external reproductive organs, esp. of the female—**pudenda** *pl*, **pudendal** *adj*.

Pudenz-Hayer valve (pū′-denz–hāy′-er) one-way valve implanted at operation for relief of hydrocephalus.

puerperal (pū-ėr'-pe-rǎl) *adj* pertaining to childbirth. *puerperal psychosis* a mental illness (psychosis) occurring in the puerperium.* *puerperal sepsis* infection of genital tract occurring within 21 days of abortion or childbirth.

puerperium (pū-ėr-pėr'-ē-um) *n* period immediately following childbirth to complete involution, usually 6–8 weeks—**puerperia** *pl*.

pulmoflator (pul'-mō-flā-tor) *n* apparatus for inflation of lungs.

pulmonary (pul'-mon-ār-ē) *adj* pertaining to the lungs. *pulmonary artery* → Figures 7, 9. *pulmonary circulation* deoxygenated blood leaves the right ventricle, flows through the lungs, where it becomes oxygenated, and returns to left atrium of the heart. *pulmonary emphysema* stretching of the alveolar membrane, rendering it less efficient in the diffusion of gases. Can be generalized, as may result from chronic bronchitis; or can be localized, either distal to partial obstruction of a bronchiole or bronchus (obstructive emphysema), or in alveoli adjacent to a segment of collapsed lung (compensatory emphysema). *pulmonary hypertension* raised blood pressure within blood vessels supplying the lungs, due to increased resistance within the pulmonary circulation; associated with increased pressure in the right cardiac ventricle. May be due to disease of the left side of the heart or in the lung. In primary pulmonary hypertension the cause is not known. Usually leads to death from congestive heart failure in 2–10 years. *pulmonary edema* form of "waterlogging" of the lungs because of left ventricular failure or mitral stenosis. *pulmonary vein* → Figures 7, 10.

pulp *n* the soft, interior part of some organs and structures. *dental pulp* found in the pulp cavity and root canals of teeth; carries blood, nerve and lymph vessels. *digital pulp* tissue pad of the fingertip; infection referred to as "pulp space infection."

pulsatile (pul'-sǎ-tīl) *adj* beating, throbbing.

pulse *n* impulse transmitted to arteries by contraction of the left ventricle, and customarily palpated in radial artery at the wrist. *pulse rate* number of beats or impulses per minute; about 130 in newborns, 70–80 in adults and 60–70 in old age. *pulse rhythm* regularity—can be regular or irregular. *pulse volume* amplitude of expansion of arterial wall during passage of the wave. *pulse force* (or tension) strength, estimated by force needed to obliterate it by pressure of the finger. *pulse deficit* difference in rate of the heart (counted by stethoscope) and pulse (counted at the wrist); occurs when some ventricular contractions are too weak to open the aortic valve and hence produce a beat at the heart but not at the wrist; occurs commonly in atrial fibrillation. *pulse pressure* difference between systolic and diastolic pressures. → beat.

"pulseless" disease progressive obliterative arteritis of vessels arising from the aortic arch, resulting in diminished or absent pulse in neck and arms. Thromboendarterectomy or a bypass procedure may prevent blindness by improving carotid blood flow at its commencement in the aortic arch.

pulsus alternans (pul'-sus awl'-tĕr-nans) regular pulse with alternate beats of weak and strong amplitude; a sign of left ventricular disease.

pulsus bigeminus (pul'-sus bī-jem'-in-us) double pulse wave produced by interpolation of extrasystoles. A heart rhythm of paired beats, each pair followed by a prolonged pause. The second, weaker beat of each pair may not be strong enough to open the aortic valve, in which case it does not produce a pulse beat. Often due to excessive digitalis administration.

pulvis (pul'-vis) *n* a powder.

punctate (pungk'-tāt) *adj* dotted or spotted, e.g., punctate basophilia describes the immature red cell in whose cytoplasm are droplets of blue-staining material—**punctum** *n*, **puncta** *pl*.

puncture *n* a stab; a wound made with a sharp pointed hollow instrument for withdrawal or injection of fluid or other substance. *cisternal puncture* insertion of a special hollow needle with stylet through the atlanto-occipital ligament between occiput and atlas into the cisterna magna. One method of obtaining cerebrospinal fluid. *lumbar puncture* insertion of a special hollow needle with stylet either through the space between third and fourth lumbar vertebrae or, lower, into the subarachnoid space to obtain cerebrospinal fluid.

PUO *abbr* pyrexia* of unknown origin.

pupil *n* opening in the center of the iris of the eye to allow passage of light (→ Figure 15)—**pupillary** *adj*.

pupillary reflex constriction of the pupil when exposed to light.

purgative (pur'-gà-tiv) *n* drug causing evacuation of fluid feces. *drastic purgative* even more severe in action, when the fluid feces may be passed involuntarily.

purines (pū'-rēnz) *npl* constituents of nucleoproteins from which uric acid is derived. Gout is thought to be associated with the disturbed metabolism and excretion of uric acid, and foods of high purine content are excluded in its treatment.

Purinethol™ mercaptopurine.*

Purkinje's fibers (poor-kin'-jēz) muscle cell fibers found beneath the endocardium of the heart; make up the impulse-conducting network of the heart.

Purodigin™ digitoxin.*

purpura (pur'-pur-à) *n* disorder characterized by extravasation of blood from capillaries into the skin, or into or from the mucous membranes. Manifest either by small red spots (petechiae) or large bruises (ecchymoses) or by oozing from minor wounds, the latter, in the absence of trauma, being confined to mucous membranes. May arise through impaired integrity of capillary walls or defective quality or quantity of blood platelets. Purpura can be caused by many conditions, e.g., infective, toxic, allergic, nutritional. → Henoch-Schönlein purpura. *anaphylactoid purpura* excessive reaction between antigen and IgG (antibody). Antigen often unknown, but may be derived from beta-hemolytic streptococci, or drugs such as sulfonamides, which may interact chemically with body proteins. *purpura hemorrhagica* (thrombocytopenic purpura) characterized by greatly diminished platelet count. Clotting time is normal but bleeding time is prolonged; patient is usually well, but intracranial hemorrhage can occur.

purulent (pū'-rū-lent) *adj* pertaining to or resembling pus.

pus *n* a liquid, usually yellowish in color, formed in certain infections and composed of tissue fluid containing bacteria and leukocytes. Various bacteria are associated with pus having distinctive features, e.g., fecal smell of pus due to *Escherichia coli;* green color of pus due to *Pseudomonas aeruginosa.*

pustule (pus'-tūl) *n* small inflammatory swelling containing pus. *malignant pustule* → anthrax—**pustular** *adj.*

putrefaction (pū-tre-fak'-shun) *n* the process of rotting; destruction of organic material by bacteria—**putrefactive** *adj.*

PUVA *abbr* psoralen* with long wavelength ultraviolet light.

pyelitis (pī-el-ī'-tis) *n* mild form of pyelonephritis* with pyuria but minimal involvement of renal tissue. Pyelitis on the right side is a common complication of pregnancy.

pyelography (pī-el-og'-ra-fē) *n* → urography—**pyelographic** *adj,* **pyelogram** *n.*

pyelolithotomy (pī-el-ō-lith-ot'-o-mē) *n* operation for removal of a stone from the renal pelvis.

pyelonephritis (pī-el-ō-nef-rī'-tis) *n* form of renal infection that spreads outwards from the pelvis to the cortex of the kidney. Origin of infection is usually from the ureter and below, or from the blood stream—**pyelonephritic** *adj.*

pyelonephrosis (pī-el-ō-nef-rō'-sis) *n* any disease of the kidney pelvis.

pyeloplasty (pī'-el-ō-plas'-tē) *n* a plastic operation on the kidney pelvis. → hydronephrosis.

pyelostomy (pī-el-os'-to-mē) *n* surgical formation of an opening into the kidney pelvis.

pyemia (pī-ēm'-ē-à) *n* grave form of septicemia in which blood-borne bacteria lodge and grow in distant organs, e.g., brain, kidneys, lungs and heart, to form multiple abscesses—**pyemic** *adj.*

pyknolepsy (pik'-nō-lep-sē) *n* frequently recurring form of minor epilepsy seen in children. Attacks may number a hundred or more in a day.

pylephlebitis (pī-lē-fleb-ī'-tis) *n* inflammation of veins of the portal system secondary to intraabdominal sepsis.

pylethrombosis (pī-lē-throm-bō'-sis) *n* intravascular blood clot in the portal vein or any of its branches.

pyloroduodenal (pī-lōr-ō-dū-od'-en-ȧl) *adj* pertaining to pyloric sphincter and duodenum.

pyloromyotomy (pī-lōr-ō-mī-ot'-o-mē) *n* (*syn* Ramstedt's operation) incision of the pyloric sphincter muscle, as in pyloroplasty.

pyloroplasty (pī-lōr'-ō-plas'-tē) *n* a plastic operation on the pylorus designed to widen the passage.

pylorospasm (pī-lōr'-ō-spazm) *n* spasm of the pylorus usually due to presence of a duodenal ulcer.

pylorus (pī-lōr'-us) *n* opening of the stomach into the duodenum, encircled by a sphincter muscle—**pyloric** *adj*.

pyocolpos (pī-ō-kol'-pos) *n* pus in the vagina.

pyodermia, pyoderma (pī-ō-dėr'-mē-ȧ) *n* chronic cellulitis of the skin, manifesting in granulation tissue, ulceration, colliquative necrosis or vegetative lesions—**pyodermic** *adj*.

pyogenic (pī-ō-jen'-ik) *adj* pertaining to the formation of pus.

pyometra (pī-ō-mē'-trȧ) *n* pus retained in the uterus and unable to escape through the cervix, due to malignancy or atresia—**pyometric** *adj*.

pyonephrosis (pī-ō-nef-rō'-sis) *n* distension of the renal pelvis with pus—**pyonephrotic** *adj*.

Pyopen™ carbenicillin.*

pyopericarditis (pī-ō-per-ē-kȧr-dī'-tis) *n* pericarditis* with purulent effusion.

pyopneumothorax (pī-ō-nū-mō-thōr'-aks) *n* pus and gas or air within the pleural sac.

pyorrhea (pī-ō-rē'-ȧ) *n* a flow of pus, usually referring to that caused by periodontal* disease, *pyorrhea alveolaris*.

pyosalpinx (pī-ō-sal'-pinks) *n* a fallopian tube containing pus.

pyothorax (pī-ō-thōr'-aks) *n* pus in the pleural cavity.

pyramid of the kidney → Figure 20.

pyramidal (pir-am'-id-ȧl) *adj* applied to some conical eminences in the body. *pyramidal cells* nerve cells in the pre-Rolandic area of the cerebral cortex, from which originate impulses to voluntary muscles. *pyramidal tracts* in the brain and spinal cord transmit fibers arising from the pyramidal cells to voluntary muscles.

pyrantel pamoate (pir-an'-tel) antthelmintic used for treating roundworm and pinworm. (Antiminth.)

pyrazinamide (pir-à-zin'-à-mīd) *n* oral antituberculosis drug. Hepatotoxicity guarded against by SGOT* tests twice weekly. Can produce gastrointestinal side-effects. (Tebrazid.)

pyrexia (pī-reks'-ē-à) *n* → fever—**pyrexial** *adj.*

Pyridium™ phenazopyridine.*

pyridostigmine (pī-ri-dō-stig'-mēn) *n* drug which inhibits breakdown of acetylcholine at neuromuscular junctions. Used in myasthenia gravis. Less toxic and potent, and has more prolonged action than neostigmine. (Mestinon.)

pyridoxine (pī-ri-doks'-ēn) *n* vitamin* B_6; deficiency may lead to dermatitis and neuritic pains. Used in nausea of pregnancy and radiation sickness, muscular dystrophy, pellagra, premenstrual syndrome.

pyrimethamine (pī-ri-meth'-à-mēn) *n* powerful antimalarial widely used in prophylaxis. Suitable for administration to children. (Daraprim.)

pyrogen (pī'-rō-jen) *n* substance capable of producing fever—**pyrogenic** *adj.*

pyrosis (pī-rō'-sis) *n* (*syn* heartburn) eructation of acid gastric contents into the mouth, accompanied by a burning sensation felt behind the sternum.

pyrotherapy (pī-rō-ther'-à-pē) *n* production of fever by artificial means. → hyperthermia.

pyrvinium pamoate (per-vin'-ē-um pam'-ō-āt) anthelmintic effective against threadworm; turns stools red.

pyuria (pī-ū'-rē-à) *n* pus in the urine (more than three leukocytes per highpower field)—**pyuric** *adj.*

PZI *abbr* protamine zinc insulin.

Q

Q fever febrile disease caused by *Coxiella burnetti*. Human infection transmitted from sheep and cattle in which the organism does not produce symptoms. Pasteurization of milk kills *C. burnetti*.

quadriceps (kwod'-ri-seps) *n* the quadriceps extensor femoris muscle of the thigh, which possesses four heads and is composed of four parts (→ Figure 4).

quadriplegia (kwod-ri-plē'-jà) *n* → tetraplegia—**quadriplegic** *adj*.

quadruple vaccine vaccine for immunization against diphtheria, pertussis, poliomyelitis and tetanus.

quarantine *n* a period of isolation* of infected or suspected people with the object of preventing spread to others. Usually the same period as the longest incubation period for the specific disease.

quartan (kwar'-tan) *adj* applies to intermittent fever with paroxysms occurring every 72 h (fourth day).

Queckenstedt's test (kwek'-en-stets) performed during lumbar puncture. Compression on the internal jugular vein produces a rise in CSF pressure if there is no obstruction to circulation of fluid in the spinal region.

quelling reaction swelling of the capsule of a bacterium when exposed to specific antisera. Test identifies the genera, species or subspecies of bacteria causing a disease.

Questran™ lemon-flavored cholestyramine.*

quickening *n* first perceptible fetal movements felt by the mother, usually at 16–18 weeks gestation.

quiescent (kwē-es'-ent) *adj* becoming quiet. Used esp. of a skin disease which is settling under treatment.

quinacrine (kwin'-à-krēn) *n* synthetic antimalarial substance, more effective than quinine, and better tolerated. (Atabrine.)

quinestrol (kwin-es'-trol) *n* synthetic female sex hormone which suppresses lactation. (Estrovis.)

quinethazone (kwin-eth'-à-zōn) *n* a thiazide diuretic. (Hydromox.)

Quinidex™ quinidine.*

quinidine (kwin'-i-dēn) *n* alkaloid similar to quinine,* but with specific effect on atrial muscle of the heart. Sometimes used in early atrial fibrillation, but only about 50% of patients respond. Therapy should not be continued for more than 10 days unless adequate response has been obtained. (Cardioquin, Quinidex.)

quinine (kwī′-nīn) *n* chief alkaloid of cinchona; once the standard treatment for malaria. For routine use and prophylaxis, synthetic antimalarials are now preferred, but with increasing risk of drug-resistant malaria, quinine is coming back into use in some areas. Drug also has some oxytocic action and has been employed as a uterine stimulant in labor. Main use is in management of "night cramps," given as 300–600 mg of bisulfate.

quininism (kwīn′-in-izm) *n* headache, noises in the ears and partial deafness, disturbed vision and nausea arising from idiosyncratic reaction to or long-continued use of quinine.

quinsy (kwin′-zē) *n* → peritonsillar* abscess.

quotient *n* a number obtained by division. *respiratory quotient* ratio between inspired oxygen and expired carbon dioxide during a specified time.

R

RA latex test for rheumatoid arthritis; detects presence in the blood of rheumatoid factor.

rabies (rā´-bēz) *n* (*syn* hydrophobia) a fatal viral infection in man; infection follows the bite of a rabid animal, e.g., dog, cat, fox, vampire bat. Of worldwide distribution; vaccines are available—**rabid** *adj.*

rabbit fever tularemia.*

racemose (ras´-i-mōs) *adj* resembling a bunch of grapes.

radial artery → Figure 9.

radial vein → Figure 10.

radiation sickness transient nausea, vomiting, malaise sometimes following therapeutic irradiation. Loosely refers, as well, to acute effects of massive radiation dose, leading to cerebral inflammation, mucosal atophy in GI tract and failure of hematopoiesis; fatal.

radiculography (rad-i-kū-log´-rå-fē) *n* X-ray of spinal nerve roots after rendering them radiopaque to locate site and size of a prolapsed intervertebral disk—**radiculogram** *n.*

radiobiology (rā-dē-ō-bī-ol´-o-jē) *n* study of effects of radiation on living tissue—**radiobiological** *adj.*

radiograph (rā´-dē-ō-graf) *n* photographic image formed by exposure to X-rays; the correct term for an "X-ray"—**radiographic** *adj.*

radiography (rā-dē-og´-raf-ē) *n* use of X-radiation (a) to create images of the body from which medical diagnosis can be made (diagnostic radiography); or (b) treatment of (malignant) disease, according to a medically prescribed regime (therapeutic radiography)—**radiographer** *n.*

radioiodinated human serum albumin (RIHSA) (rā´-dē-ō-ī´-ō-din-āt-ed) used for detection and localization of brain lesions, determination of blood and plasma volumes, circulation time and cardiac output.

radioisotope (rā´-dē-ō-īs´-ō-tōp) *n* (*syn* radionuclide) forms of an element having the same atomic number but different mass numbers, exhibiting property of spontaneous nuclear disintegration. When taken orally or by injection, can be traced by a Geiger counter. *radioisotope scan* pictorial representation of amount and distribution of radioactive isotope present in a particular organ.

radiology (rā-dē-ol'-o-jē) *n* study of the diagnosis of disease by using X-rays and other allied imaging techniques—**radiological** *adj*, **radiologist** *n*.

radiomimetic (rā'-dē-ō-mim-et'-ik) *adj* produces effects similar to those of radiotherapy.

radiopaque (rā-dē-ō-pāk') *adj* having the property of significantly absorbing X-rays, thus becoming visible on a radiograph. Barium and iodine compounds are used, as contrast media, to produce artificial radiopacity—**radiopacity** *n*.

radiosensitive *adj* affected by X-rays. Applied to tumors treatable by X-rays.

radiotherapy (rā-dē-ō-thėr'-à-pē) *n* treatment of proliferative disease, esp. cancer, by X-rays and other forms of radiation—**radiotherapist** *n*.

radius (rā'-dē-us) *n* → Figures 2, 3.

radon seeds (rā'-don) capsules containing radon—a radioactive gas produced by the breaking up of radium atoms. Used in radiotherapy.

rale (ral) *n* abnormal sound heard on auscultation of lungs when fluid is present in bronchi.

Ramsay Hunt syndrome herpes zoster of the ear lobe with facial paralysis and loss of taste.

ramus (rā'-mus) *n* a branch, as of a blood vessel or nerve—**rami** *pl.*

ranitidine (ra-ni'-ti-dīn) *n* antiulcer drug; a histamine H_2 receptor antagonist which decreases gastric acid secretion. (Zantac.)

ranula (ran'-ū-là) *n* cystic swelling beneath the tongue due to blockage of a duct—**ranular** *adj*.

raphe (raf'-ē) *n* a seam, suture, ridge or crease; the median furrow on dorsal surface of the tongue.

rarefaction (rār-e-fak'-shun) *n* becoming less dense, as applied to diseased bone—**rarefied** *adj*.

rash *n* skin eruption. *nettle rash* → urticaria.

Rashkind's septostomy (rash'-kīnds sep-tos'-to-mē) when the pulmonary and systemic circulations do not communicate, an artificial atrial septal communication is produced by passing an inflatable balloon catheter through the foramen ovale, filling the balloon with contrast media and pulling it back into the right atrium.

RAST *abbr* radioallergosorbent test; an allergen specific IgE measurement.

rat-bite fever a relapsing fever caused by *Spirillum minus* or by *Streptobacillus moniliformis*. Blood Wassermann* test is positive in the spirillary infection.

rauwolfia (raw-wol'-fē-à) *n* dried root contains several alkaloids including reserpine*; once prescribed as a tranquilizer, now occasionally used as antihypertensive.

Rauzide™ bendroflumethazide.*

Raynaud's disease (rā′-nōz) idiopathic trophoneurosis. Paroxysmal spasm of digital arteries producing pallor or cyanosis of fingers or toes, and occasionally resulting in gangrene. Disease of young women.

Raynaud's phenomenon (rā′-nōz) → vibration syndrome.

RBC *abbr* red blood cell or corpuscle. → blood.

RDS *abbr* respiratory* distress syndrome.

reagin (rē′-à-jin) *n* IgE antibody.

rebore *n* → disobliteration.

recannulation (rē-kan-ū-lā′-shun) *n* re-establishment of patency of a vessel.

receptaculum (rē-sep-tak′-ū-lum) *n* receptacle, often acting as a reservoir. *receptaculum chyli* pear-shaped commencement of the thoracic duct in front of the first lumbar vertebra. Receives digested fat from the intestine.

receptive sensory aphasia type of aphasia* with inability to associate meaning with words, though other forms of communication, such as miming, drawing and writing, may be understood.

receptor *n* sensory afferent nerve ending capable of receiving and transmitting stimuli.

recessive *adj* receding; having a tendency to disappear. *recessive trait* a genetically controlled trait that is expressed only when the specifying allele* is present at both paired chromosomal loci (i.e., "in double dose"). When specifying allele is present at only one locus, the trait is not manifest, as its presence is negated by a dominant allele at the partner locus. The exception is for X-linked genes in males, in which a single recessive allele on the X-chromosome will express itself, so that its specific trait is manifest.

Recklinghausen's disease (rek′-ling-howz-enz) name given to two conditions: (a) osteitis fibrosa cystica, the result of overactivity of the parathyroid glands (hyperparathyroidism) resulting in decalcification of bones and formation of cysts; (b) multiple neurofibromatosis,* with tumors that can be felt beneath the skin along the course of nerves. There may be pigmented spots (café au lait) on the skin, and pheochromocytoma.

recliner's reflux syndrome severe disturbance of the antireflux mechanism, which allows stomach contents to leak at any time, regardless of posture, although most likely to happen in reclining positions.

recombinant DNA (rē-kom′-bi-nant) altered DNA, produced by piecing together (recombining chemically) the genic DNA of two different organisms. Used to study structure and function of both normal and abnormal genes and so, for example, the molecular basis of human genetic disorders. Practical applications are in diagnosis (including prenatal diagnosis) and in manufacture of special gene products used in treatment, such as insulin.

Recombivax-HB™ hepatitis* B vaccine produced from yeast cultures.

recrudescence (rē-kroo-des′-ens) *n* return of symptoms.

rectal bladder term for ureters transplanted into the rectum, which is closed, with the establishment of a proximal colostomy; only in severe disease of urinary bladder.

rectal varices (var′-i-sēz) hemorrhoids.*

rectocele (rek′-tō-sēl) *n* prolapse* of the rectum, so that it lies outside the anus. Usually reserved for herniation of anterior rectal wall into posterior vaginal wall caused by injury to the levator muscles at childbirth. Repaired by a posterior colporrhaphy. → procidentia.

rectoscope (rek′-tō-skōp) *n* instrument for examining the rectum. → endoscope—**rectoscopic** *adj*.

rectosigmoid (rek-tō-sig′-moyd) *adj* pertaining to the rectum and sigmoid portion of colon.

rectosigmoidectomy (rek-tō-sig-moyd-ek′-to-mē) *n* surgical removal of the rectum and sigmoid colon.

rectouterine (rek-tō-ū′-ter-in) *adj* pertaining to rectum and uterus.

rectovaginal (rek-tō-vaj′-in-ȧl) *adj* pertaining to rectum and vagina.

rectovesical (rek-tō-ves′-ik-ȧl) *adj* pertaining to rectum and bladder.

rectum (rek′-tum) *n* lower part of the large intestine between the sigmoid* flexure and anal canal (→ Figure 18)—**rectal** *adj*.

rectus abdominis (rek′-tus ab-dom′-in-is) → Figure 4.

rectus femoris (rek′-tus fem-ōr′-is) → Figure 4.

Reed-Sternberg cells multinucleated histiocytes (a macrophage type) found in Hodgkin's disease; diagnostic.

referred pain pain occurring at a distance from its source, e.g., pain felt in upper limbs from angina pectoris; that from the gallbladder felt in the scapular region.

reflex **1** *adj* literally, reflected or thrown back; involuntary, not able to be controlled by the will. *reflex action* involuntary motor or secretory response by tissue to a sensory stimulus, e.g., sneezing, blinking, coughing. Testing various reflexes facilitates diagnosis of diseases involving the nervous system. *reflex zone therapy* treatment of the feet for disorders in other parts of the body whether or not these disorders have resulted in signs and symptoms. **2** *n* a reflex action. *accommodation reflex* constriction of the pupils and convergence of the eyes for near vision. *conditioned reflex* reaction acquired by repetition or practice. *corneal reflex* reaction of blinking when the cornea is touched (often absent in hysterical conditions).

reflux (rē′-fluks) *n* backward flow.

refractory (rē-frak'-tōr-ē) *adj* resistant to treatment; stubborn, unmanageable; rebellious.

regeneration *n* renewal of tissue.

regional ileitis (il-ē-ī'-tis) (*syn* Crohn's disease) nonspecific chronic recurrent granulomatous disease of the ileum affecting mainly young adults and characterized by a necrotizing, ulcerating inflammatory process, usually with an abrupt demarcation between it and healthy bowel. Healthy bowel ("skip" area) may intervene between two diseased segments. Colon, rectum and anus may also be involved.

Regitine™ phentolamine.*

Reglan™ metoclopramide.*

Regroton™ reserpine.*

Reiter protein complement fixation (RPCF) test test for syphilis; uses an extract prepared from cultivatable treponemata.

Reiter's syndrome (ri'-terz) condition in which arthritis occurs together with conjunctivitis and urethritis (or cervicitis in women). Commonly, but not always, a sexually transmitted infection and should be considered as a cause of knee effusion in young men when trauma has not occurred.

rejection *n* process which leads to destruction of grafted tissues.

relapsing fever louse-borne or tick-borne infection caused by spirochetes of genus *Borrelia*. Prevalent in many parts of the world. Characterized by a febrile period of a week or so, with apparent recovery, followed by a further bout of fever.

relaxant *n* that which reduces tension. → muscle.

relaxin (rē-laks'-in) *n* polypeptide secreted by ovaries to soften the cervix and loosen the ligaments in preparation for birth.

REM sleep *abbr* → paradoxical sleep.

remission *n* the period of abatement of a fever or other disease.

remittent *adj* increasing and decreasing at periodic intervals.

renal (rē'-nål) *adj* pertaining to the kidney. *renal adenocarcinoma* cancer of the kidney. *renal artery* → Figures 9, 19, 20. *renal asthma* hyperventilation of lungs occurring in uremia as a result of acidosis. *renal calculus** stone in the kidney. *renal capsule* → Figure 20. *renal erythropoietic factor* an enzyme released in response to renal (and therefore systemic) hypoxia. Once secreted into blood, it reacts with a plasma globulin to produce erythropoietin. *renal failure* can only be described within context, whether acute or chronic. Acute renal failure (ARF) occurs when previously healthy kidneys suddenly fail (as through toxic, inflamed or ischemic state); condition is potentially reversible. Chronic renal failure (CRF) occurs when irreversible and progressive pathological destruction of the kidney leads to terminal or end stage renal disease (ESRD). Process usually takes several years but once ESRD is reached, death will follow unless patient is treated with some type of dialysis or renal transplant. → crush syndrome, tubular necrosis, uremia, *renal function tests* → kidney function tests. *renal glycosuria* occurs in patients with normal blood sugar and a lowered renal threshold for sugar. *renal edema* inefficient kidney filtration disturbing electrolyte balance and resulting in edema.* *renal rickets* → rickets. *renal transplant* kidney* transplant. *renal uremia* uremia* following kidney disease itself, in contrast to uremia from failure of blood circulation (extrarenal uremia). *renal vein* → Figures 19, 20.

Renese™ polythiazide.*

renin (ren'-in) *n* enzyme released into blood from the kidney cortex in response to sodium loss. Reacts with angiotensinogen (a plasma protein fraction) to produce angiotensin I, which in turn is converted into angiotensin II by an enzyme in the lungs. Excessive production of renin results in hypertensive kidney disease.

renogram (rē'-nō-gram) *n* X-ray of renal shadow following injection of opaque medium, demonstrated in aortograph series—**renographic** *adj*.

reovirus (rē'-ō-vī-rus) *n* previously called respiratory enteric orphan virus,* one of a group of RNA-containing viruses that can infect respiratory and intestinal tracts without causing serious disease.

reproductive system organs and tissues necessary for reproduction. In the male, includes the testes, vas deferens, prostate gland, seminal vesicles, urethra and penis (→ Figure 16). In the female,

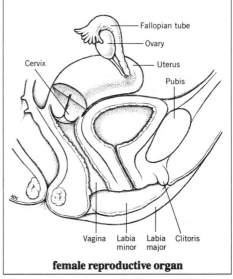

Fallopian tube
Ovary
Cervix
Uterus
Pubis
Vagina
Labia minor
Labia major
Clitoris

female reproductive organ

includes the ovaries, fallopian tubes, uterus, vagina and vulva (→ Figure 17).

RES *abbr* reticuloendothelial* system.

resection *n* surgical excision. *submucous resection (of nasal septum)* incision of nasal mucosa, removal of deflected nasal septum, replacement of mucosa.

resectoscope (rē-sek'-to-skōp) *n* instrument passed along the urethra; permits resection of tissue from base of the bladder and prostate under direct vision. → prostatectomy.

reserpine (rē-ser'-pēn) *n* chief alkaloid of rauwolfia.* Used mainly in hypertension, sometimes with other drugs. Severe depression has occurred after full and prolonged therapy. Interferes with transmission in sympathetic adrenergic nerves, esp. sympathetically mediated vascular reflexes and thus can lead to postural and exercise hypotension. (Regroton, Serpalan.)

residual *adj* remaining. *residual air* air remaining in the lung after forced expiration. *residual urine* urine remaining in the bladder after micturition.

resolution *n* subsidence of inflammation; earliest indications of a return to normal, as when, in lobar pneumonia, consolidation begins to liquefy.

resonance *n* the musical quality elicited on percussing a cavity which contains air. *vocal resonance* reverberating note heard through the stethoscope when patient is asked to say "one, one, one" or "99".

resorcinol (rē-sōr'-sin-ol) *n* drug which acts as a skin abrasive. Useful in a cream for acne and in a lotion for dandruff.

resorption (rē-sōrp'-shun) *n* act of absorbing again, e.g., absorption of (a) callus following bone fracture, (b) roots of the deciduous teeth, (c) blood from a hematoma.

respiration *n* process of gaseous exchange between a cell and its environment. *external respiration* absorption of oxygen from air in the alveoli into lung capillaries, and excretion of carbon dioxide from the blood in lung capillaries into the air in the lungs. *internal* or *tissue respiration* is the reverse process—blood vessels supplying the cells carry oxygen which passes from blood into tissue cells, and carbon dioxide from cells passes into the blood in vessels draining the cells. *paradoxical respiration* occurs when ribs on one side are fractured in two places. During inspiration air is drawn into the unaffected lung via the normal route but also from the lung on the affected side. During expiration air is forced from the lung on the unaffected side, some of which enters the lung on the affected side, resulting in inadequate oxygenation of blood. → abdominal breathing, anaerobic respiration. Cheyne Stokes respiration, resuscitation— **respiratory** *adj*.

respirator *n* **1** apparatus worn over nose and mouth and designed to purify the air breathed through it. **2** apparatus that mechanically and rhythmically inflates and deflates the lungs when natural nervous or muscular control of respiration is impaired, as in anterior poliomyelitis. Apparatus works by creating low pressure around the thorax (tank respirators).

respiratory distress syndrome (RDS) *neonatal respiratory distress syndrome (NRDS)* dyspnea in the newly born. Due to failure of secretion of protein-lipid complex (pulmonary surfactant) by type II pneumocytes in tiny air spaces of the lung on first entry of air. Causes atelectasis. Formerly called hyaline membrane disease. Environmental temperature of 32–34° C (90–94° F), oxygen and infusion of sodium bicarbonate are used in treatment. Clinical features include severe retraction of chest wall with every breath, cyanosis, an increased respiratory rate and an expiratory grunt. → lecithin-sphingomyelin ratio. *adult respiratory distress syndrome* (ARDS) acute respiratory failure due to noncardiogenic pulmonary edema.

respiratory failure failure of the lungs to oxygenate blood adequately. *acute respiratory failure* respiratory insufficiency secondary to an acute insult to the lung; hypoxemia develops, frequently terminating in bronchopneumonia. *acute on chronic respiratory failure* hypoxemia resulting from chronic obstructive airways disease such as chronic bronchitis and emphysema.

respiratory function tests numerous tests available for assessing respiratory function, including measurements of vital capacity (VC), forced* vital capacity (FVC), forced expiratory volume (FEV, the volume of air that can be expired in 1 s) and maximal breathing capacity (MBC, quantity of air that can be shifted in 1 min).

respiratory quotient → quotient.

respiratory syncytial virus (RSV) (sin-sish′-ål) causes severe respiratory infection with occasional fatality in very young children. Infections are less severe in older children.

respiratory system deals with gaseous exchange. Comprises nose, nasopharynx, larynx, trachea, bronchi and lungs. → Figures 6, 7.

restless leg syndrome restless legs characterized by paresthesias, like creeping, crawling, itching and prickling.

resuscitation *n* restoration to life of one who is apparently dead (collapsed or shocked). External massage is carried out for cardiac arrest by placing patient on his back on a firm surface. Lower portion of the sternum is depressed 35–50 mm each second. To carry out artificial respiration, the exhaled breath of the operator inflates patient's lungs via one of three routes (a) mouth-to-mouth, (b) mouth-to-nose, (c) mouth to nose and mouth—**resuscitative** *adj.*

retardation *n* **1** slowing of a process which has already been carried out at a quicker rate or higher level. **2** arrested growth or function from any cause.

rete (rē′-tē) *n* a netlike process or structure, esp. of veins or arteries.

retention *n* **1** retaining of facts in the mind. **2** accumulation of that which is normally excreted. *retention cyst* a cyst* caused by the blocking of a duct. → ranula. *retention of urine* accumulation of urine within the bladder due to interference of nerve supply, obstruction or psychological factors.

reticular (re-tik′-ū-lår) *adj* resembling a net.

reticulocyte (re-tik'-ū-lō-sīt) *n* a young circulating red blood cell which still contains traces of the nucleus that was present in the cell when developing in the bone marrow.

reticulocytoma (re-tik-ū-lō-sī-tō'-mȧ) *n* → Ewing's tumor.

reticulocytosis (re-tik'-ū-lō-sī-tō'-sis) *n* increase in number of reticulocytes in blood, indicating active red blood cell formation in the marrow.

reticuloendothelial system (RES) (re-tik'-ū-lō-en-dō-thē'-lē-ȧl) widely scattered system of cells, of common ancestry and fulfilling many vital functions, e.g., defense against infection, antibody, blood cell and bile pigment formation and disposal of cell breakdown products. Main sites of reticuloendothelial cells are bone marrow, spleen, liver and lymphoid tissue.

reticuloendotheliosis (re-tik'-ū-lō-en-dō-thē-lē-ōs'-is) *n* term loosely used for conditions in which there is a reaction of reticuloendothelial cells.

retina (ret'-in-ȧ) *n* the light-sensitive internal coat of the eyeball, consisting of eight superimposed layers, seven of which are nervous and one pigmented (→ Figure 15). It is fragile, translucent and of a pinkish color—**retinal** *adj*.

retinitis (ret-in-ī'-tis) *n* inflammation of the retina. *retinitis pigmentosa* noninflammatory familial, degenerative condition which progresses to blindness, for which the term pigmentary retinopathy is becoming more widely used.

retinoblastoma (ret'-in-ō-blas-tō'-mȧ) *n* malignant tumor of the neuroglial element of the retina, occurring exclusively in children.

retinopathy (ret-in-op'-ȧ-thē) *n* any noninflammatory disease of the retina. → retinitis.

retinoscope (ret'-in-ō-skōp) *n* instrument for detection of refractive errors by illumination of retina using a mirror.

retinotoxic (ret-in-ō-toks'-ik) *adj* toxic to the retina.

retractile (rē-trak'-tīl) *adj* capable of being drawn back, i.e., retracted.

retractor (re-trak'-tor) *n* surgical instrument for holding apart the edges of a wound to reveal underlying structures.

retrobulbar (ret-rō-bul'-bȧr) *adj* pertaining to the back of the eyeball. *retrobulbar* neuritis inflammation of that portion of the optic nerve behind the eyeball.

retrocecal (ret-rō-sē'-kȧl) *adj* behind the cecum, e.g., a retrocecal appendix.

retroflexion (ret-rō-flek'-shun) *n* state of being bent backwards. → anteflexion *opp*.

retrograde (ret'-rō-grād) *adj* going backward. *retrograde pyelography* → pyelography.

retrolental fibroplasia (ret-rō-len'-tȧl fī-brō-plā'-zē-ȧ) → fibroplasia.

retroperitoneal (ret'-rō-pėr-it-on-ē'-ȧl) *adj* behind the peritoneum.

retropharyngeal (ret'-rō-far-in-jē'-ȧl) *adj* behind the pharynx.

retroplacental (ret'-rō-plá-sent'-ál) *adj* behind the placenta.

retropubic (ret-rō-pu'-bik) *adj* behind the pubis.

retrosternal (ret-rō-stern'-ál) *adj* behind the breastbone.

retroversion (ret-rō-ver'-zhun) *n* turning backward. → anteversion *opp. retroversion of the uterus* tilting of the whole of the uterus backward with the cervix pointing forward—**retroverted** *adj.*

revascularization (rē-vas'-kū-lár-ī-zā'-shun) *n* regrowth of blood vessel into a tissue or organ after deprivation of its normal blood supply.

Reye's syndrome (rīz) "wet brain and fatty liver," as described in 1963. Cerebral edema without cellular infiltration, and diffuse fatty infiltration of liver and other organs, including the kidney. The age range of recorded cases is 2 months–15 years. Presents with vomiting, hypoglycemia and disturbed consciousness, jaundice being conspicuous. There is an association with salicylate administration and chicken pox.

Rh *abbr* Rhesus factor. → blood groups.

rhabdomyolisis (rab-dō-mī-ol'-is-is) *n* sporadic myoglobinurea; group of disorders characterized by muscle injury leading to degenerative changes. *nontraumatic rhabdomyolisis* → crush syndrome.

rhagades (rag'-a-dēz) *npl* superficial elongated scars radiating from the nostrils or angles of the mouth and which are found in congenital syphilis. → stigmata.

Rheomacrodex™ low molecular weight dextran.* Antithrombotic. Used to prevent clots in grafted vein.

Rhesus factor (rē'-sus) → blood groups.

Rhesus incompatability, isoimmunization problem arising when a Rhesus negative mother carries a Rhesus positive fetus. During birth there is mixing of fetal and maternal bloods. The mother's body then develops antibodies against rhesus positive blood. If a subsequent fetus is also Rhesus positive, then the mother's antibodies will attack fetal blood supply causing severe hemolysis.

rheumatic fever → rheumatism.

rheumatism (roo'-má-tizm) *n* nonspecific term embracing a diverse group of diseases and syndromes which have in common disorder or diseases of connective tissue and hence usually present with pain, or stiffness, or swelling of muscles and joints. Main groups are rheumatic fever, rheumatoid arthritis, ankylosing spondylitis, nonarticular rheumatism, osteoarthritis and gout. *acute rheumatism* (*syn* rheumatic fever), a disorder, tending to recur but initially commonest in childhood, classically presenting as fleeting polyarthritis of the larger joints, pyrexia and carditis within three weeks following a streptococcal throat infection. Atypically, but not infrequently, symptoms are trivial and ignored, but carditis may be severe and result in permanent cardiac damage. *nonarticular rheumatism* involves soft tissues and includes fibromyositis, lumbago, bursitis, etc.—**rheumatic** *adj*.

rheumatoid (roo′-mȧ-toyd) *adj* resembling rheumatism. *rheumatoid arthritis* a disease of unknown etiology but probably autoimmune, characterized by chronic polyarthritis mainly affecting smaller peripheral joints, accompanied by general ill health and resulting eventually in varying degrees of crippling joint deformity and associated muscle wasting. Not just joints but every system may be involved in some way. Many rheumatologists therefore prefer the term "rheumatoid disease." *rheumatoid factors* macro gammaglobulins found in most people with severe rheumatoid arthritis. It is not yet known whether they are the cause of, or the result of, arthritis. → pneumoconiosis, Still's disease.

rheumatology (roo-mȧ-tol′-o-jē) *n* science or the study of the rheumatic diseases.

rhinitis (rī-nī′-tis) *n* inflammation of nasal mucous membrane.

rhinology (rī-nol′-o-jē) *n* study of diseases affecting the nose—**rhinologist** *n*.

rhinophyma (rī-nō-fī′-mȧ) *n* nodular enlargement of the skin of the nose.

rhinoplasty (rī′-nō-plas′-tē) *n* plastic surgery of the nasal framework.

rhinorrhea (rī-nōr-rē′-ȧ) *n* nasal discharge.

rhinoscopy (rī-nos′-ko-pē) *n* inspection of the nose using a nasal speculum or other instrument—**rhinoscopic** *adj*.

rhinosporidosis (rī′-nō-spōr-i-dō′-sis) *n* fungal condition affecting mucosa of nose, eyes, ears, larynx and occasionally the genitalia.

Rhinosporidium (rī′-nō-spōr-id′-ē-um) *n* genus of fungi parasitic to man.

rhinovirus (rī′-nō-vī′-rus) *n* a cause of the common cold; over a 100 varieties.

rhizotomy (rī-zot′-o-mē) *n* surgical division of a root; usually posterior root of a spinal nerve. *chemical rhizotomy* accomplished by injection of a chemical, often phenol.*

rhodopsin (rō-dop′-sin) *n* the visual purple contained in retinal rods. Its color is preserved in darkness; bleached by daylight. Formation dependent on vitamin A.

RhoGam (rō′-gam) → anti-Rhesus* (Rh) serum.

rhonchus (rong′-kus) *n* adventitious sound heard on auscultation of the lung. Passage of air through bronchi obstructed by edema or exudate produces a musical note.

rhythm *n* **1** a measured or regular period of time or movement. **2** means of birth control consisting of calculating intermenstrual periods of fertility in the female and avoiding coitus during that time.

riboflavin (rī′-bō-flā-vin) *n* constituent of the vitamin* B group. Given in Menière's disease, angular stomatitis and a variety of other conditions.

ribonuclease (rī-bō-nū′-klē-āz) *n* enzyme that catalyzes depolymerization of ribonucleic acid. Can be made synthetically.

ribonucleic acid (RNA) (rī-bō-noo-klē′-ik) nucleic acids found in all living cells. On hydrolysis they yield adenine, guanine, cytosine, uracil, ribose and phosphoric acid. They play an important part in protein synthesis.

ribosomes (rī′-bō-sōmz) *npl* submicroscopic protein-making agents inside all cells.

ribs *npl* the twelve pairs of bones which articulate with the twelve dorsal vertebrae posteriorly and form the walls of the thorax (→ Figure 6). Upper seven pairs are *true ribs* and are attached to the sternum anteriorly by costal cartilage. Remaining five pairs are the *false ribs;* first three pairs have no attachment to the sternum but are bound to each other by costal cartilage. Lowest two pairs are the *floating ribs,* which have no anterior articulation. *cervical ribs* are formed by an extension of the transverse process of the 7th cervical vertebra in the form of bone or a fibrous tissue band; this causes an upward displacement of the subclavian artery. A congenital abnormality.

rice-water stool the stool of cholera.* The "rice grains" are small pieces of desquamated epithelium from the intestine.

rickets *n* disorder of calcium and phosphorus metabolism associated with a deficiency of vitamin D, and beginning most often in infancy and early childhood between the age of 6 months and 2 years. With proliferation and deficient ossification of the growing epiphyses of bones, producing "bossing," softening and bending of long weight-bearing bones, muscular hypotonia, head sweating and, if the blood calcium falls sufficiently, tetany. *fetal rickets* achondroplasia.* *renal rickets* condition of decalcification (osteoporosis) of bones associated with chronic kidney disease and clinically simulating rickets; occurs in later age groups and is characterized by excessive urinary calcium loss. *vitamin D resistant rickets* due to disease of lower extremities, producing short legs. Genetic illness; no deficiency of vitamin D; serum levels of phosphorus low; no associated renal disease. Thought to be due to a defect in the tubular reabsorption of phosphorus and a lowered calcium absorption from the gut, causing secondary hyperthyroidism and a vitamin D abnormality.

Rickettsia (rik-et′-sē-à) *n* small pleomorphic parasitic microorganisms naturally inhabiting cells of the gut of arthropods. Some are pathogenic to mammals and man, in whom they cause the typhus group of fevers. Smaller in size than bacteria and larger than the viruses. Physiologically similar to bacteria but, like the viruses, they are obligate intracellular parasites.

Riedel's thyroiditis (re′-delz thī-royd-ī′-tis) a chronic fibrosis of the thyroid gland; ligneous goiter.

Rifadin™ rifampin.*

rifampin (rif-am'-pin) *n* antibiotic. Main indication is in treating tuberculosis, in association with other antitubercular drugs; also useful in leprosy; colors urine, sputum and tears red, which confirms maintenance of treatment dosage. (Rifadin, Rimactane.)

Rift valley fever one of the mosquito-transmitted hemorrhagic fevers.

rigor *n* a sudden chill, accompanied by severe shivering. Body temperature rises rapidly and remains high until perspiration ensues and causes it to fall gradually. *rigor mortis* stiffening of the body after death.

Rimactane™ rifampin.*

Ringer's lactate Hartmann's solution.

ringworm *n* (*syn* tinea) generic term for contagious infection of skin by a fungus; common manifestations are circular (circinate) scaly patches. → dermatophytes.

Rinne's test (rin'-nēz) testing of air conduction and bone conduction hearing, by tuning fork.

risus sardonicus (ris'-us sàr-don'-i-kus) the spastic grin of tetanus.*

Ritalin™ methylphenidate.*

river blindness form of onchocerciasis.*

RN *abbr* registered nurse.

RNA *abbr* ribonucleic* acid.

Robaxin™ methocarbamol.*

Robinul™ glycopyrrolate.*

Rocephin™ ceftriaxone.*

Rocky Mountain spotted fever a tick-borne typhus fever caused by the parasite *Rickettsia* rickettsii.

rodent ulcer a basal cell carcinoma on the face or scalp which, although locally invasive, does not give rise to metastases.

ROM *abbr* range of motion.

Romberg's sign (rom'-bergz) a sign of ataxia.* Inability to stand erect (without swaying) when eyes are closed and feet together. Also called "Rombergism."

rosacea (rō-zā'-shà) *n* skin disease which shows on flush areas of the face. In areas affected there is chronic dilation of superficial capillaries and hypertrophy of sebaceous follicles, often complicated by a papulopustular eruption.

roseola (rō-zē-ōl'-à) *n* a faint, pink spot, widespread in distribution except for the skin of hands and face.

rotaviruses (rō-tà-vī'-rus-es) *npl* viruses associated with gastroenteritis in children and infants. Related to, but easily distinguished from, reoviruses.*

rotator *n* a muscle having the action of turning a part.

Roth spots (roth) round white spots in the retina in some cases of bacterial endocarditis, thought to be of embolic origin.

roughage *n* → dietary fiber, bran.

rouleau (roo′-lō) *n* a row of red blood cells, resembling a roll of coins.

round ligament of the uterus → Figure 17.

roundworm *n* (*Ascaris lumbricoides*) look like earth worms. Worldwide distribution; parasitic to man. Eggs passed in stools; ingested, hatch in bowel, migrate through tissues, lungs and bronchi before returning to the bowel as mature worms. During migration worms can be coughed up—which is unpleasant and frightening. Heavy infections can produce pneumonia. A tangled mass can cause intestinal obstruction or appendicitis. Best drug for treatment is piperazine. Roundworm of the cat and dog is called *Toxocara*.

Rous sarcoma virus (RSV) (rous) a virus of chickens that can cause tumors (sarcomas). A typical member of the RNA tumor virus group; despite much research no viruses belonging to this group have as yet been isolated from human tumors.

Rovsing's sign (rov′-singz) pressure in the left iliac fossa causes pain in the right iliac fossa in appendicitis.

RPCF *abbr* Reiter protein complement fixation.

RSV *abbr* 1 respiratory* syncytial virus. 2 Rous* sarcoma virus.

rubefacients (rū-be-fāsh′-ents) *npl* substances which, when applied to the skin, cause redness (hyperemia).

rubella (rū-bel′-à) *n* (*syn* German measles) acute, infectious, eruptive fever (exanthema) caused by a virus and spread by droplet infection. With mild fever, a scaly, pink macular rash and enlarged occipital and posterior cervical glands. Complications are rare, except when contracted in early months of pregnancy, when it may produce fetal deformities. Occasionally followed by a painful arthritis.

Rubenstein-Taybi syndrome a constellation of abnormal findings first described in 1963; includes mental and motor retardation, broad thumbs and toes, growth retardation, susceptibility to infection in the early years and characteristic facial features.

rubor (rū′-bor) *n* redness; usually in context of the four classical signs of inflammation—the others being calor,* dolor,* tumor.*

RU 486™ mifepristone.*

S

Sabin vaccine (sa'-bin) live attenuated polio virus which can be given orally. Produces active immunity against poliomyelitis.

sac *n* small pouch or cystlike cavity—**saccular, sacculated** *adj*.

saccharides (sak'-à-rīdz) *npl* one of the three main classes of carbohydrates (i.e., sugars).

sacculation (sak-ū-lā'-shun) *n* appearance of several saccules.

saccule (sak'-ūl) *n* a minute sac—**saccular, sacculated** *adj*.

sacral (sā'-kràl) *adj* pertaining to the sacrum. *sacral nerve* → Figure 11.

sacroanterior (sā-krō-an-tēr'-ē-or) *adj* describes a breech presentation in obstetrics; fetal sacrum is directed to one or other acetabulum of the mother.

sacrococcygeal (sā-krō-kok-sij'-ē'-àl) *adj* pertaining to sacrum* and coccyx.*

sacroiliac (sak-rō-il'-ē-ak) *adj* pertaining to sacrum* and ilium.*

sacroiliitis (sak-rō-il-ē-ī'-tis) *n* inflammation of a sacroiliac joint. Involvement of both joints characterizes such conditions as ankylosing spondylitis, Reiter's syndrome and psoriatic arthritis.

sacrolumbar (sāk-rō-lum'-bàr) *adj* pertaining to sacrum* and loins.*

sacroposterior (sak-rō-pos-tēr'-ē-or) *adj* describes a breech presentation in obstetrics; fetal sacrum is directed to one or other sacroiliac joint of the mother.

sacrospinalis muscle (sāk-rō-spin-al'-is) → Figure 5.

sacrum (sāk'-rum) *n* triangular bone lying between the fifth lumbar vertebra and the coccyx (→ Figures 2, 3). Consists of five vertebræ fused together, and it articulates on each side with the innominate bones of the pelvis, forming the sacroiliac joints—**sacral** *adj*.

saddle nose one with a flattened bridge, often a sign of congenital syphilis.*

sagittal (saj'-it-àl) *adj* resembling an arrow. In the anteroposterior plane of the body. *sagittal suture* immovable joint formed by the union of the two parietal bones.

salicylamide (sal-i-sil'-à-mīd) *n* mild analgesic similar in action to the salicylates, but less likely to cause gastric disturbance.

salicylic acid (sal-i-sil'-ik) has fungicidal and bacteriostatic properties; used in a variety of skin conditions. A constituent of Whitfield's ointment.

saline (sā'-lēn) *n* solution of salt and water. Normal or physiological saline is a 0.9% solution with the same osmotic pressure as that of blood. → hypertonic, isotonic.

saliva (så-lī'-vå) *n* secretion of the salivary glands (spittle); contains water, mucus and ptyalin*—**salivary** *adj*.

salivary (sal'-i-vār-ē) *adj* pertaining to saliva. *salivary calculus* a stone formed in the salivary ducts. *salivary glands* the glands which secrete saliva, i.e., the parotid, submaxillary and sublingual glands.

salivation (sal-iv-ā'-shun) *n* increased secretion of saliva.

Salk vaccine (solk) preparation of killed poliomyelitis virus used as antigen to produce active artificial immunity to poliomyelitis; given by injection.

Salmonella (sal-mon-el'-å) *n* genus of bacteria. Gram-negative rods. Parasitic in many animals and man, in whom they are often pathogenic. Some species, such as *S. typhi*, are host-specific, infecting only man, in whom they cause typhoid fever. Others, such as *S. typhimurium*, may infect a wide range of host species, usually through contaminated foods. *S. enteritidis* a motile Gram-negative rod, widely distributed in domestic and wild animals, particularly rodents, and sporadic in man as a cause of food poisoning.

salpingectomy (sal-pin-jek'-to-mē) *n* excision of a fallopian tube.

salpingitis (sal-pin-jī'-tis) *n* acute or chronic inflammation of the fallopian tubes. → hydrosalpinx, pyosalpinx.

salpingogram (sal-ping'-ō-gram) *n* radiological examination of tubal patency by retrograde introduction of opaque medium into the uterus and along the tubes—**salpingographic** *adj*, **salpingography** *n*.

salpingo-oophorectomy (sal-ping-ō-ō-o-fōr-ek'-to-mē) *n* excision of a fallopian tube and ovary.

salpingostomy (sal-ping-gos'-to-mē) *n* operation to restore tubal patency.

salpinx (sal'-pingks) *n* a tube, esp. the fallopian tube or the eustachian tube.

salsalate (sal'-så-lāt) *n* nonsteroidal anti-inflammatory drug; an ester of salicylic* acid, which is insoluble in gastric juice and therefore less likely than aspirin* to cause gastric irritation and erosion. (Disalcid.)

salve (sav) *n* an ointment.

sal volatile (sal vol'-å-til) aromatic solution of ammonia. A household analeptic.

Sandimmune™ cyclosporin.*

sanguineous (sang-gwin'-ē-us) *adj* pertaining to or containing blood.

Sanorex™ mazindol.*

Sansert™ methysergide.*

saphenous (sà-fē′-nus) *adj* apparent; manifest. Name given to the two main veins in the leg, the internal and the external (→ Figure 10), and to the nerves (→ Figure 11) accompanying them.

sapremia (sa-prē′-mē-à) *n* a general bodily reaction to circulating toxins and breakdown products of saprophytic (nonpathogenic) organisms, derived from one or more foci in the body.

saprophyte (sap′-rō-fīt) *n* free-living microorganisms obtaining food from dead and decaying animal or plant tissue—**saprophytic** *adj*.

sarcoid (sàr′-koyd) *adj* term applied to a group of lesions in skin, lungs or other organs, which resemble tuberculous foci in structure, but the true nature of which is still uncertain.

sarcoidosis (sàr-koyd-ōs′-is) *n* a granulomatous disease of unknown etiology in which histological appearances resemble tuberculosis. May affect any organ of the body, but most commonly presents as a condition of the skin, lymphatic glands or bones of the hand.

sarcolemma (sàr-kō-lem′-mà) *n* delicate outer membranous covering of muscle fibrils.

sarcoma (sàr-kō′-mà) *n* malignant growth of mesodermal tissue (e.g., connective tissue, muscle, bone)—**sarcomata** *pl*, **sarcomatous** *adj*.

sarcomatosis (sàr-kō-mà-tō′-sis) *n* sarcomata widely spread throughout the body.

Sarcoptes (sàr-kop′-tēz) *n* genus of mites. *S. scabiei* is the itch mite which causes scabies.*

sartorius (sàr-tō′-rē-us) *n* the "tailor's muscle" of the thigh, since it flexes one leg over the other (→ Figures 4, 5).

scab *n* dried crust forming over an open wound.

scabies (skā′-bēz) *n* parasitic skin disease caused by itch mites. Highly contagious.

scalenus syndrome (ska-lē′-nus) pain in arm and fingers often with wasting, because of compression of lower trunk of the brachial plexus behind scalenus anterior muscle at the thoracic outlet.

scalpel (skal′-pl) *n* a surgeon's knife, which may or may not have detachable blades.

scanning speech form of dysarthria occurring in disseminated sclerosis; speech is jumpy, staccato or slow.

scaphoid (skaf′-oyd) *n* boat-shaped, as a bone of the tarsus and carpus. *scaphoid abdomen* concavity of the anterior abdominal wall, often associated with emaciation.

scapula (skap′-ū-là) *n* shoulder blade (→ Figures 2, 3)—**scapular** *adj*.

scar *n* (*syn* cicatrix) dense, avascular white fibrous tissue; end result of healing, esp. in the skin.

scarification (skår-if-i-kā'-shun) *n* making a series of small, superficial incisions or punctures in the skin.

scarlatina (skår-lå-tē'-nå) *n* (*syn* scarlet fever) infection by Group A β-hemolytic streptococcus. Occurs mainly in children. Begins commonly with throat infection, leading to fever and outbreak of a punctuate erythematous rash on skin of the trunk. Characteristically the area around the mouth escapes (circumoral pallor)—**scarlatinal** *adj*.

scarlet fever → scarlatina.

SCAT *abbr* sheep cell agglutination test. Rheumatoid factor in blood is detected by the sheep cell agglutination titer.

Scheuermann's disease (shoy'-er-manz) osteochondritis* of the spine affecting the ring epiphyses of the vertebral bodies. Occurs in adolescents.

Schick test (shik) test used to determine susceptibility or immunity to diphtheria; injection of 2 or 3 minims of freshly prepared toxin beneath the skin of the left arm. A similar test is made in the right arm, but with serum in which toxin has been destroyed by heat, leaving only associated protein. Positive reaction consists in appearance of a round red area on the left arm within 24–48 h, reaching maximum intensity on the fourth day, then gradually fading. Indicates susceptibility or absence of immunity. No reaction indicates immunity to diphtheria. Occasionally a pseudoreaction occurs, caused by associated protein, in which case redness appears on both arms.

Schilder's disease (shil'-dèrz) genetically determined degenerative disease associated with mental subnormality.

Schilling test (shil'-ing) estimation of absorption of radioactive vitamin B_{12} for confirmation of pernicious anemia.

Schistosoma (skis-tō-sō'-mà) *n* (*syn Bilharzia*) genus of blood flukes that require fresh water snails as an intermediate host before infesting humans. *S. haematobium* found mainly in Africa and the Middle East; *S. japonicum* in Japan, the Philippines and eastern Asia. *S. mansoni* is indigenous to Africa, the Middle East, Caribbean and South America.

schistosomiasis (skis-tō-sō-mī'-à-sis) *n* (*syn* bilharziasis) infestation by *Schistosoma*, which enter via the skin or mucous membrane. A single fluke can live in one part of the body, depositing eggs frequently for many years. Prevention is by chlorination of drinking water, proper disposal of human waste and eradication of fresh water snails. Schistosomiasis is a serious problem in the tropics and the Orient. The eggs are irritating to mucous membranes, which thicken and bleed causing anemia, together with pain and dysfunction of the afflicted organ; fibrosis of mucous membranes can cause obstruction.

schistosomicide (skis-tō-sō'-mi-sīd) *n* any agent lethal to *Schistosoma*—**schistosomicidal** *adj*.

schizophrenia (skiz-ō-frē'-nē-à) *n* group of psychotic mental illnesses characterized by disorganization of personality. Course can be at times chronic, at times marked by intermittent attacks. A complete return to the pre-morbid personality is unlikely. Three elements are common to all cases: shallowness of emotional life; inappropriateness of emotion; unrealistic thinking. *catatonic schizophrenia* characterized by episodes of immobility with muscular rigidity or stupor, interspersed with periods of acute excitability. *simple schizophrenia* least disorganized form, with apathy and withdrawal. Onset is usually at an early age, but hallucinations and delusions are absent—**schizophrenic** *adj*.

Schlatter's disease (shlat'-ėrz) (*syn* Osgood-Schlatter's disease) osteochondritis* of the tibial tubercle.

Schlemm's canal (shlemz) lymphaticovenous canal in the inner part of the sclera, close to its junction with the cornea, which it encircles.

Scholz's disease (shōlz) genetically determined degenerative disease associated with mental subnormality.

Schönlein's disease (shān'-līnz) Henoch*-Schönlein purpura.

Schultz-Charlton test (shultz–chȧrl'-ton) blanching produced in skin of a patient showing scarlatinal rash, around an injection of serum from a convalescent case, indicating neutralization of toxin by antitoxin.

Schwan cells cells forming an enveloping sheath around nerve fibers, including the myelin* sheath around larger fibers, which is both protective and electrically insulating.

sciatica (sī-at'-i-kȧ) *n* pain in the line of distribution of the sciatic nerve (buttock, back of thigh, calf and foot).

scirrhus (skir'-us) *n* a carcinoma which provokes a considerable growth of hard, connective tissue; a hard carcinoma of the breast—**scirrhous** *adj*.

scissor leg deformity the legs are crossed in walking—following double hip-joint disease, or as manifestation of Little's disease (spastic cerebral diplegia).

scissors gait → gait.

sclera (skle'-rà) *n* the "white" of the eye (→ Figure 15); the opaque bluish-white fibrous outer coat of the eyeball covering the posterior five-sixths; it merges into the cornea at the front—**sclerae** *pl*, **scleral** *adj*.

sclerema (skler-ē'-mà) *n* rare disease in which hardening of skin results from deposition of mucinous material.

scleritis (skler-ī'-tis) *n* inflammation of the sclera.*

sclerocorneal (skler-ō-kōr'-nē-al) *adj* pertaining to sclera* and cornea,* as the circular junction of these two structures.

scleroderma (skler-ō-der′-mà) *n* disease in which localized edema of the skin is followed by hardening, atrophy, deformity and ulceration. Occasionally becomes generalized, producing immobility of the face, contraction of the fingers; diffuse fibrosis of myocardium, kidneys, digestive tract and lungs. When confined to the skin it is termed morphea. → collagen, dermatomyositis.

sclerosis (skler-ōs′-is) *n* abnormal hardening or fibrosis of a tissue. → multiple sclerosis, tuberous sclerosis—**sclerotic** *adj*.

sclerotherapy (skler-ō-thėr′-a-pē) *n* injection of a sclerosing agent for treatment of varicose veins. When, after the injection, rubber pads are bandaged over the site to increase localized compression, the term *compression sclerotherapy* is used. Sclerotherapy for esophageal varices involves use of an esophagoscope, either rigid or flexible—**sclerotherapeutic** *adj*.

sclerotomy (skler-ot′-o-mē) *n* incision of sclera for relief of acute glaucoma, prior to a decompression operation.

scolex (skō′-leks) *n* head of the tapeworm, by which it attaches itself to the intestinal wall, and from which segments (proglottides) develop.

scoliosis (skō-lē-ōs′-is) *n* lateral curvature of the spine, congenital or acquired, due to abnormality of vertebrae, muscles and nerves. *idiopathic scoliosis* is characterized by a lateral curvature together with rotation and associated rib hump or flank recession. Treatment is by spinal brace, traction or internal fixation with accompanying spinal fusion—**scoliotic** *adj*.

scopolamine (skō-pol′-à-mēn) *n* (*syn* hyoscine) hypnotic alkaloid obtained from belladonna and hyoscyamus. (Tramsderm-Scop.)

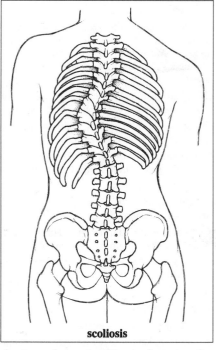

scoliosis

scorbutic (skōr-bū′-tik) *adj* pertaining to scorbutus, the old name for scurvy.*

scotoma (skō-tō′-mà) *n* a blind spot in the field of vision. May be normal or abnormal. *scotopic vision* ability to see well in poor light—**scotomata** *pl*.

scrapie (skrā′-pē) *n* a virus disease of sheep and goats.

Scriver test (skrī′-vėr) remarkably efficient in detecting, by a single procedure, 22 aminoacidopathies.

scrofula (skrof′-ū-là) *n* tuberculosis of bone or lymph gland—**scrofulous** *adj*.

scrotum (skrō′-tum) *n* pouch in the male which contains the testes (→ Figure 16)—**scrotal** *adj*.

scurvy (skur′-vē) *n* deficiency disease caused by lack of vitamin* C (ascorbic acid). Clinical features include fatigue and hemorrhage, which may take the form of oozing at the gums or large ecchymoses. Tiny bleeding spots on the skin around hair follicles are characteristic. In children painful subperiosteal hemorrhage (rather than other types of bleeding) is pathognomonic.

scybala (sib′-à-là) *npl* rounded, hard, fecal lumps—**scybalum** *sing*.

Sea Legs™ meclizine.*

sebaceous (se-bā′-shus) *adj* literally, pertaining to fat; usually refers to sebum.* *sebaceous cyst* (*syn* wen) a retention cyst in a sebaceous (oil-secreting) gland in the skin. Most commonly found on scalp, scrotum and vulva. *sebaceous glands* cutaneous glands which secrete an oily substance called "sebum;" ducts are short and straight, and open into the hair follicles (→ Figure 12).

seborrhea (seb-ōr-ē′-à) *n* greasy condition of scalp, face, sternal region and elsewhere due to overactivity of sebaceous* glands.

sebum (sē′-bum) *n* normal secretion of the sebaceous* glands; contains fatty acids, cholesterol and dead cells.

secobarbital (sek-ō-bȧrb′-i-tol) *n* short-acting barbiturate with general properties of the group, used in mild insomnia and anxiety conditions. (Seconal.)

Seconal™ secobarbital.

secretin (se-krē′-tin) *n* hormone produced in duodenal mucosa; causes copious secretion of pancreatic juice.

secretion (se-krē′-shun) *n* a fluid or substance formed or concentrated in a gland and passed into the alimentary tract, the blood, or to the exterior.

secretory (sē′-krē-tōr-ē) *adj* involved in the process of secretion; describes a gland which secretes.

Sectral™ acebutolol.*

sedation *n* production of a state of lessened functional activity.

sedative *n* agent which lessens functional activity.

sedimentation rate → erythrocyte sedimentation rate.

segregation *n* in genetics, separation from one another of two alleles, each carried on one of a pair of chromosomes; this happens at meiosis* when the haploid, mature germ cells (egg and sperm) are made.

selenomethionine (sel-en-ō-meth-ī′-o-nēn) *n* injection in which the sulfur atom present in the amino acid methionine is replaced by radioactive selenium. Taken up selectively by the pancreas; valuable in diagnosis of pancreatic disease.

self-monitoring of blood glucose (SMBG) blood from a finger prick is applied to a reagent strip to read hemoglobin A_{1c} ($H6A_{1c}$) level, which reflects blood glucose level.

sella turcica (sel′-là tur′-si-kà) pituitary* fossa.

semen (sē′-men) *n* secretion from the testicles and accessory male organs, e.g., prostate; contains spermatozoa.*

semicircular canals three membranous semicircular tubes contained within the bony labyrinth of the internal ear (→ Figure 13). Concerned with appreciation of the body's position in space.

semicomatose (sem-ē-kō′-mà-tōs) *adj* describes a condition bordering on the unconscious.

semilunar (sem-ē-lū′-nàr) *adj* shaped like a crescent or half moon. *semilunar* cartilages crescentic interarticular cartilages of the knee joint (menisci).

semimembranosus muscle (sem-ē-mem-brăn-ōs′-us) → Figure 5.

seminal (sem′-i-nàl) *adj* pertaining to semen. *seminal vesicle* → Figure 16.

seminiferous (sem-in-if′-ėr-us) *adj* carrying or producing semen.

seminoma (sem-in-ō′-mà) *n* malignant tumor of the testis—**seminomata** *pl*, **seminomatous** *adj*.

semispinalis muscle (sem-ē-spin-àl′-is) → Figure 5.

semitendinosus muscle (sem-ē-ten-din-ōs′-us) → Figure 5.

senescence (sē-nes′-ens) *n* normal changes of mind and body in increasing age—**senescent** *adj*.

Sengstaken tube (sengz′-tā-ken) incorporates a balloon which, after being positioned in the lower esophagus, is inflated to apply pressure to bleeding esophageal varices.

senile (sē′-nīl) *adj* suffering from senescence* complicated by morbid processes commonly called degeneration—**senility** *n*.

senna (sen′-nà) *n* leaves and pods of a purgative plant from Egypt and India. Once used extensively as "black draught" or compound senna mixture. (Senokot.)

Senokot™ standardized senna.*

sensitization (sen-si-tī-zā′-shun) *n* rendering sensitive. Persons may become sensitive to a variety of substances, such as food, bacteria, plants, chemical substances, drugs, sera, etc. Tendency is much greater in some persons than others. → allergy, anaphylaxis.

sensorineural (sen-sor-i-nūr'-ȧl) *adj* pertaining to sensory neurons. *sen-sorineural deafness* a discriminating term for nerve deafness.*

sensory *adj* pertaining to sensation. *sensory nerves* those which convey impulses to the brain and spinal cord (→ Figure 1).

sepsis (sep'-sis) *n* state of being infected with pus-producing organisms—**septic** *adj*.

septicemia (sep-ti-sēm'-ē-ȧ) *n* persistence and mutliplication of living bacteria in the blood stream—**septicemic** *adj*.

Septra™ cotrimoxazole.*

septum (sep'-tum) *n* partition between two cavities, as between the nasal cavities. *septal defect* congenital malformation, with opening(s) in tissue separating ventricular or atrial chambers of the heart; surgery is generally required—**septa** *pl*, **septal, septate** *adj*.

sequela (sē-kwē'-lȧ) *n* pathological consequences of a disease, as pockmarks of smallpox—**sequelae** *pl*.

sequestrectomy (sē-kwes-trek'-to-mē) *n* excision of a sequestrum.*

sequestrum (sē-kwes'-trum) *n* piece of dead bone which separates from healthy bone but remains within the tissues—**sequestra** *pl*.

Serax™ oxazepam.*

serology (sē-rol'-o-jē) *n* study of sera—**serological** *adj*.

seropurulent (sē-rō-pūr'-e-lent) *adj* containing serum* and pus.*

serosa (sē-rōz'-ȧ) *n* a serous membrane,* as the peritoneal covering of the abdominal viscera—**serosal** *adj*.

serositis (sē-rō-sī'-tis) *n* inflammation of a serous membrane.*

serotonin (sē-rō-tōn'-in) *n* a product of tryptophan metabolism. Liberated by blood platelets after injury and found in high concentrations in many body tissues including the CNS. A vasoconstrictor, inhibits gastric secretion, stimulates smooth muscle. Serves as a central neurotransmitter and is a precursor of melatonin. Together with histamine it may be concerned in allergic reactions. Called also 5-hydroxytryptamine and 5-HT.

serous (sē'-rus) *adj* pertaining to serum.* *serous membrane* → membrane.

Serpalan™ reserpine.*

serpiginous (sėr-pij'-in-us) *adj* snakelike, coiled, irregular; used to describe the margins of skin lesions, esp. ulcers and ringworm.

Serratia (sėr-ā'-shȧ) *n* genus of Gram-negative bacilli capable of causing infection in humans; an endemic hospital resident. → infection.

serration (sėr-ā'-shun) *n* a sawlike notch—**serrated** *adj*.

serratus muscles (sėr'-ȧ-tus) → Figures 4, 5.

serum (sē'-rum) *n* supernatant fluid which forms when blood clots. *serum sickness* → anaphylaxis—**sera** *pl*.

serum gonadotropin (gō-nad-ō-trō'-pin) ovarian stimulating hormone obtained from blood serum of pregnant mares; used in amenorrhea, often in association with estrogens.

sex-linked refers to genes which are located on the sex chromosomes or, more esp., on the X chromosome. To avoid confusion it is now customary to refer to the latter genes (and the characters determined by them) as X-linked.

sexually transmitted disease previously called venereal disease.

SGA *abbr* small for gestational age.

SGOT *abbr* obsolete for aspartate* transaminase.

SGPT *abbr* obsolete for alanine* transaminase.

shelf operation an operation to deepen the acetabulum in congenital dislocation of the hip joint, involving use of a bone graft. Performed at 7–8 years, after failure of conservative treatment.

Shigella (shi-gel'-lȧ) *n* genus of bacteria containing some of the organisms causing dysentery. *S. flexneri* a pathogenic, Gram-negative rod; most common cause of bacillary dysentery epidemics, and sometimes infantile gastroenteritis. Found in the feces of cases of dysentery and carriers, whence it may pollute food and water supplies.

shin bone the tibia, the medial bone of the foreleg.

shingles *n* condition arising when the infecting agent (herpes zoster virus) attacks sensory nerves, causing severe pain and appearance of vesicles along the nerve's distribution (usually unilateral). → herpes zoster virus.

Shirodkar's operation (shir-od'-kȧrs) placing of a purse-string suture around an incompetent cervix during pregnancy; removed when labor starts.

shock *n* circulatory disturbance produced by severe injury or illness and due in large part to reduction in blood volume; features includes a fall in blood pressure, rapid pulse, pallor, restlessness, thirst and a cold clammy skin.

short-circuit operation anastomosis* to bypass an obstruction in a conducting channel, e.g., gastrojejunostomy.

shortsightedness *n* → myopia.

shoulder girdle formed by the clavicle and scapula on either side.

shoulder lift → Australian lift.

"show" *n* popular term for the blood-stained vaginal discharge at commencement of labor.

shunt *n* passage of blood through other than the usual channel.

sialagogue (sī-al'-ȧ-gog) *n* agent which increases flow of saliva.

sialogram (sī-al′-ō-gram) *n* radiographic image of salivary glands and ducts, after injection of an opaque medium—**sialography** *n*, **sialographic** *adj*.

sialolith (sī-al′-ō-lith) *n* a stone in a salivary gland or duct.

sickle-cell anemia → anemia.

side-effect any physiological change other than that desired from drug administration, e.g., the antispasmodic drug propantheline may cause dry mouth. Term also covers undesirable drug reactions. Some are predictable, the result of a known metabolic action of the drug, as yellowing of skin and eyes with mepacrine; thinning of skin and bone and formation of striae with corticosteroids; loss of hair with cyclophosphamide. Unpredictable reactions can be: (a) immediate: anaphylactic shock, angioneurotic edema; (b) erythematous: all forms of erythema, including nodosum and multiforme and purpuric rashes; (c) cellular eczematous rashes and contact dermatitis; (d) specific, as light-sensitive eruptions with ledermycin and griseofulvin.

sideroblast (sid′-er-ō-blast) *n* a nucleated precursor cell to the red blood cell (erythrocyte)—**sideroblastic** *adj*.

siderosis (sid-ér-ōs′-is) *n* excess of iron in blood or tissues. Inhalation of iron oxide can cause one form of pneumoconiosis.*

SIDS *abbr* sudden infant death syndrome → crib death.

sigmoid (sig′-moyd) *adj* shaped like the letter S. *sigmoid colon* → Figure 18. *sigmoid flexure* → flexure.

sigmoidoscope (sig-moyd′-o-skōp) *n* instrument for visualizing the rectum and sigmoid flexure of the colon. → endoscope—**sigmoidoscopic** *adj*, **sigmoidoscopy** *n*.

sigmoidostomy (sig-moyd-os′-to-mē) *n* the formation of a colostomy in the sigmoid* colon.

sign *n* any objective evidence of disease.

silicone (sil′-i-kōn) *n* organic compound that is water-repellant. *silicone foam dressing* a soft durable substance that fits exactly the contours of an open granulating wound in which it encourages healing.

silicosis (sil-i-kō′-sis) *n* form of pneumoconiosis* or "industrial dust disease" found in metal grinders, stone workers, etc.

Silvadene™ silver* sulfadiazine.

silver nitrate in the form of small sticks, used as a caustic for warts. Occasionally used as antiseptic eye drops (1%), and as an application to ulcers. Now being used in 0.5% solution for burns to control bacterial infection in postburn period. Causes sodium and chloride loss from wound surface. Sodium chloride given orally or intravenously. Urine tested for chlorides.

silver sulfadiazine silver derivative of sulfadiazine. Topical bacteriostatic agent, esp. in burns. A burn area cannot be sterilized, but silver sulfadiazine greatly limits bacterial activity and penetration. (Silvadene.)

Silverman score method of rating respiratory distress by assessing movement of accessory muscles and degree of expiratory grunt.

simian crease (sim′-ē-àn) fused crease on the palm of the hand associated with congenital abnormalities including Down syndrome.

Simmond's disease (sim′-onds) patient becomes emaciated, suffers from early senility, face wrinkles, hair becomes gray and sparse, blood pressure lowers, pulse slows, bones become frail. Previously called hypopituitary cachexia.

Sim's position (simz) an exaggerated left lateral position with the right knee well flexed and left arm drawn back over edge of the bed.

sinciput (sin′-si-put) *n* upper half of the skull, including the forehead.

Sinemet™ levodopa* combined with carbidopa* in 10:1 ratio.

Sinequan™ doxepin.*

sinew *n* a ligament or tendon.

sinoatrial node (sī-nō-ā′-trē-àl) → node.

sinus (sī′-nus) *n* **1** a hollow or cavity, esp. the nasal sinuses (→ Figure 14). **2** a channel containing blood, esp. venous blood, as the sinuses of the brain. **3** a recess or cavity within a bone. **4** any suppurating tract or channel. *sinus arrhythmia* increase of the pulse rate on inspiration, decrease on expiration. Appears to be normal in some children. → cavernous, pilonidal.

sinusitis (sī-nus-ī′-tis) *n* inflammation of a sinus, used exclusively for the para-nasal sinuses.

sinusoid (sī′-nus-oyd) *n* a dilated channel into which arterioles or veins open in some organs and which take the place of the usual capillaries.

sitz-bath (sits–bath) a hip bath.

Sjögren-Larsson syndrome (shō′-gren–làr′-son) genetically determined con-genital ectodermosis. Associated with mental subnormality.

Sjögren syndrome (shō′-gren) deficient secretion from lacrimal, salivary and other glands, mostly in postmenopausal women; with keratoconjunctivitis, dry tongue and hoarse voice. Thought due to an autoimmune process. Also called keratoconjunctivitis sicca.

skeleton *n* bony framework of the body, supporting and protecting the soft tis-sues and organs (→ Figures 2, 3). *appendicular skeleton* bones forming the upper and lower extremities. *axial skeleton* bones forming the head and trunk—**skeletal** *adj*.

Skene's glands (skēnz) two small glands at the entrance to the female urethra; the paraurethral glands.

skin *n* tissue which forms the outer covering of the body; two main layers: (a) the epidermis, or cuticle, forming the outer coat (b) the dermis, or cutis vera, the inner or true skin, lying beneath the epidermis. → Figure 12.

skull *n* bony framework of the head (→ Figure 2). → cranium.

sleep *n* a naturally altered state of consciousness occurring in humans in a 24 h biological rhythm. A *sleep cycle* consists of orthodox* sleep and paradoxical* sleep; each cycle lasts approximately 60–90 min, and needs to be completed for the person to gain benefit. *sleep apnea* →

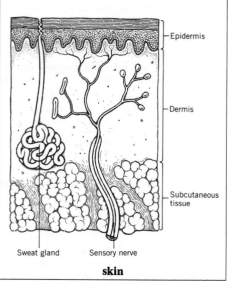

Epidermis

Dermis

Subcutaneous tissue

Sweat gland   Sensory nerve

skin

apnea. *sleep deprivation* cumulative condition arising from continued disturbance of established rhythm of paradoxical* sleep. Can result in slurred, rambling speech; irritability; disorientation; slowed reaction time; malaise, progressing to illusions; delusions; paranoia and hyperactivity.

sleeping sickness disease endemic in Africa, characterized by increasing somnolence, caused by infection of the brain by trypanosomes. → trypanosomiasis.

sleep-walking → somnambulism.

slipped disk *n* prolapsed intervertebral disk. → prolapse.

slipped epiphysis (e-pif′-i-sis) displacement of an epiphysis, esp. the upper femoral one. → epiphysis.

slough (sluf) *n* septic tissue which becomes necrosed and separates from healthy tissue.

Slow K™ slow-release potassium chloride product.

slow release drugs drug formulations which do not dissolve in the stomach but in the small intestine where the drug is slowly released and absorbed. Some drugs are now incorporated into a skin patch, which after application permits slow release.

slow virus an infective agent which only produces disease after a long latent period; many cases may never develop overt symptoms but may still be a link in the chain of infectivity. → Creutzfeldt-Jakob disease.

small-for-dates → low birthweight.

smallpox *n* (*syn* variola) caused by a virus eradicated following WHO world-wide campaign. Prophylaxis is by vaccination. → vaccinia.

smear *n* film of material spread out on a glass slide for microscopic examination. *cervical smear* microscopic examination of cells scraped from the cervix to detect carcinoma-in-situ. → carcinoma.

smegma (smeg'-mà) *n* sebaceous secretion which accumulates beneath the pre-puce and clitoris.

smelling salts mixture of compounds usually containing some form of ammonia, which acts as a stimulant when inhaled.

smokers' blindness (*syn* tobacco amblyopia) absorption of cyanide in smoke. Sight worsens, color vision goes, the victim can go blind. Cyanide prevents absorption of vitamin B_{12}. Injection of hydroxycobalamin is therapeutic.

snare *n* surgical instrument with a wire loop at the end; used for removal of polyps.

Snellen's test types (snel'-enz) a chart for testing visual acuity.

snow *n* solid carbon dioxide. Used for local freezing of tissues in minor surgery.

snuffles *n* snorting inspiration due to congestion of nasal mucous membrane. A sign of early congenital (prenatal) syphilis, when the nasal discharge may be purulent or blood-stained.

S.O.A.P. notes method of recording nursing notes using subjective and objective data, assessment and plan.

SOB *abbr* shortness of breath.

sodium bicarbonate (sō-dē-um bī-kàr'-bon-āt) a domestic antacid, given for heartburn, etc. For prolonged therapy alkalis that cause less rebound acidity are preferred.

sodium chloride (klōr'-īd) salt, present in body tissues. Used extensively in shock and dehydration as intravenous normal saline, or as dextrosesaline in patients unable to take fluids by mouth. Used orally as replacement therapy in Addison's disease, in which salt loss is high. When salt is lost from the body, there is compensating production of renin.

sodium citrate (sī'-trāt) alkaline diuretic very similar to potassium citrate. Used also as an anticoagulant for stored blood, and as an addition to milk feeds to reduce curdling.

sodium fluoride (flōr'-īd) white powder used in drinking water and solutions for preventing dental caries.

sodium iodide (ī'-ō-dīd) used occasionally as an expectorant, and as a contrast agent in retrograde pyelography.

sodium perborate (pėr'-bōr-āt) aqueous solutions having antiseptic properties similar to hydrogen peroxide, used as mouth-washes, etc.

sodium peroxide (pėr-oks'-īd) used for bleaching.

sodium propionate (prō'-pē-on-āt) used as an antimycotic in fungal infections as gel, ointment, lotion and pessaries.

sodium salicylate (sal-is'-il-āt) has analgesic action of salicylates in general, and formerly used in rheumatic fever. Large doses are essential. Chronic rheumatoid conditions do not respond well.

sodium sulfate (sul'-fāt) popular domestic purgative. A 25% solution is used as a wound dressing. Given intravenously as a 4.3% solution in anuria.

sodium tetradecyl sulfate (tet'-rȧ-dek'-l sul'-fāt) sclerosant liquid for injection into veins to obliterate them and shrink varicosities.

soft palate → Figure 14.

soft sore primary ulcer of the genitalia occurring in chancroid.*

solar plexus (sō'-lȧr pleks'-us) large network of sympathetic (autonomic) nerve ganglia and fibers, extending from one adrenal gland to the other; supplies abdominal organs.

soleus muscle (sō'-lē-us) → Figures 4, 5.

Solu-Cortef™ hydrocortisone sodium succinate, used for severe asthma.

somatic (som-at'-ik) *adj* pertaining to the body. *somatic cells* body cells, as distinct from germ cells.* *somatic nerves* nerves controlling activity of striated, skeletal muscle.

somatostatin (som-at'-ō-sta'-tin) *n* growth hormone-release inhibiting hormone (GH-RIH).

somatotropin (som-at-ō-trō'-pin) *n* → growth hormone.

Sombulex™ hexobarbital.*

somnambulism (som-nam'-bū-lizm) *n* (*syn* sleepwalking) a state of dissociated consciousness in which sleeping and waking states are combined. Considered normal in children but as an illness having a hysterical basis in adults.

Somophyllin™ aminophylline.*

Sonne dysentery (son'-nē dis'-en-tėr-ē) bacillary dysentery caused by infection with *Shigella sonnei* (Sonne bacillus). The organism is excreted by cases and carriers in feces, and contaminates hands, food and water, from which new hosts are infected.

sonograph (son'-ō-graf) *n* graphic record of sound waves—**sonogram** *n*.

soporific (sop-ōr-if'-ik) *adj, n* describes an agent which induces profound sleep.

Sorbitol™ liquid for parenteral feeding.

sordes (sōr'-dēz) *npl* dried, brown crusts that form in the mouth, esp. on the lips and teeth, in illness.

sotalol (sot'-à-lol) *n* antihypertensive of the beta-adrenoceptor blocking type exemplified by propanolol.

souffle (soo'-fl) *n* puffing or blowing sound. *funic souffle* auscultatory murmur of pregnancy. Synchronizes with fetal heartbeat and is caused by pressure on the umbilical cord. *uterine souffle* soft, blowing murmur which can be auscultated over the uterus after fourth month of pregnancy.

sound *n* instrument to be introduced into a hollow organ or duct to detect a stone or to dilate a stricture.

spansules (span'-sūls) *n* chemically prepared formulation for drugs designed to obtain controlled release via oral route.

Sparine™ promazine.*

spasm *n* convulsive, involuntary muscular contraction.

spasmodic colon megacolon.*

spasmodic dysmenorrhea (dis'-men-ōr-ē'-a) → dysmenorrhea.

spasmolytic (spaz-mō-lit'-ik) *adj, n* an antispasmodic drug—**spasmolysis** *n*.

spastic (spas'-tik) *adj* of a condition of muscular rigidity or spasm, as spastic diplegia (Little's disease). *spastic dystonic syndrome* abnormality of gait and foot posture usually due to brain damage at birth. Difficult to treat because imbalance in various opposing muscles has developed over a long period. *spastic gait* → gait. *spastic paralysis* results mainly from upper motor neuron lesions; with exaggerated tendon reflexes—**spasticity** *n*.

spatula (spat'-ū-là) *n* flat flexible knife with blunt edges for making poultices and spreading ointment. *tongue spatula* a rigid, blade-shaped instrument for depressing the tongue.

spectinomycin (spek-tin'-ō-mī'-sin) *n* antibiotic useful for resistant microorganisms; drug of choice in treatment of gonorrhea. (Trobicin.)

speculum (spek'-ū-lum) *n* instrument used to hold the walls of a cavity apart, so that interior of the cavity can be examined—**specula** *pl*.

sperm *n, npl* abbreviated form of the word spermatozoon* or spermatozoa. *sperm count* an infertility test: less than 60 million sperm in an ejaculation of semen implies sterility; between 300 and 500 million is normal.

spermatic (sper-mat'-ik) *adj* pertaining to or conveying semen. *spermatic cord* suspends the testicle in the scrotum and contains the spermatic artery and vein and the vas deferens. → Figure 16.

spermaticidal (sper-mat-is-ī'-dal) *adj* lethal to spermatozoa.*

spermatogenesis (sper-mat-ō-jen'-es-is) *n* formation and development of spermatozoa—**spermatogenetic** *adj*.

spermatorrhea (sper-mat-ōr-ē'-á) *n* involuntary discharge of semen without orgasm.

spermatozoon (sper-mat-ō-zō'-on) *n* a mature, male reproductive cell—**spermatozoa** *pl*.

spermicide, spermatocide (sperm'-i-sīd) *n* agent that kills spermatozoa—**spermicidal** *adj*.

sphenoid (sfē'-nóyd) *n* wedge-shaped; of a bone at the base of the skull containing a cavity, the sphenoidal sinus—**sphenoidal** *adj*.

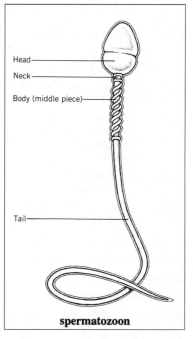

Head

Neck

Body (middle piece)

Tail

spermatozoon

spherocyte (sfēr'-ō-sīt) *n* round red blood cell, as opposed to biconcave—**spherocytic** *adj*.

spherocytosis (sfēr-ō-sī-tō'-sis) *n* (*syn* acholuric jaundice) hereditary genetic disorder transmitted as a dominant gene, i.e., with a one in two chance of transmission. Exists from birth but can remain in abeyance throughout life; sometimes discovered by "accidental" examination of the blood. → jaundice.

sphincter (sfink'-tér) *n* a circular muscle, contraction of which serves to close an orifice (→ Figure 19).

sphincterotomy (sfink-tér-ot'-o-mē) *n* surgical division of a muscular sphincter.

sphingomyelinase (sfing-gō-mī'-el-in-āz) *n* an essential enzyme in lipid metabolism and storage.

sphygmocardiograph (sfig-mō-kár'-dē-ō-graf) *n* apparatus for simultaneous graphic recording of radial pulse and heartbeats—**sphygmocardiographic** *adj*.

sphygmograph (sfig'-mō-graf) *n* apparatus attached to the wrist, over the radial artery, which records the movements of the pulse beat—**sphygmographic** *adj*.

sphygmomanometer (sfig-mō-man-om'-e-tėr) *n* instrument used for measuring blood pressure.

spica (spī'-kȧ) *n* a bandage applied in a figure-of-eight pattern.

spicule (spī'-kūl) *n* small, spikelike fragment, esp. of bone.

spigot (spig'-ot) *n* glass, wooden or plastic peg used to close a tube.

spina bifida (spī'-nȧ bif'-id-ȧ) congenital defect with incomplete closure of the neural canal, usually in the lumbo-sacral region. *spina bifida occulta* defect does not affect spinal cord or meninges; often marked externally by pigmentation, a hemangioma, a tuft of hair or lipoma which may extend into the spinal canal. *spina bifida cystica* an externally protruding spinal lesion; varies in severity from meningocele to myelomeningocele. Condition can be detected in utero in mid-pregnancy by an increased concentration of alphafetoprotein in amniotic fluid or by ultrasonography.

spinal *n* pertaining to the spine. *spinal anesthetic* local anesthetic solution injected into the subarachnoid space, rendering the area supplied by selected spinal nerves insensitive. *spinal canal* → vertebral canal. *spinal caries* disease of the vertebral bones. *spinal column* → vertebral column. *spinal cord* the continuation of nervous tissue of the brain down the spinal canal to the level of the first or second lumbar vertebra (→ Figures 1, 11). *spinal fluid* cerebrospinal* fluid. *spinal nerves* 31 pairs leave the spinal cord and pass out of the spinal canal to supply the periphery. *spinal tap* needle puncture of lumbar subarachnoid space to inject contrast medium or drugs, or to aspirate sample of cerebrospinal fluid (CSF) for diagnostic purposes. Site is usually between third and fourth or fouth and fifth lumbar vertebrae (→ lumbar* puncture).

spine *n* **1** vertebral* column. **2** a sharp process of bone—**spinous, spinal** *adj*.

spinnbarkheit (spin'-bȧr-kīt) *n* viscosity of cervical mucus, useful in estimating time of ovulation.

Spirillum (spī-ril'-um) *n* bacterial genus. Cells are rigid screwlike shapes. Common in water and organic matter. *S. minus* is found in rodents and may infect man, in whom it causes one form of rat-bite* fever—**spirilla** *pl*, **spirillary** *adj*.

spirochete (spī'-rō-kēt) *n* bacterium having a spiral shape—**spirochetal** *adj*.

spirochetemia (spī-rō-kēt-ēm'-ē-ȧ) *n* spirochetes in the blood stream; occurs in secondary stage of syphilis and in the syphilitic fetus—**spirochetemic** *adj*.

spirograph (spī'-rō-graf) *n* apparatus which records lung movements—**spirographic** *adj*, **spirography** *n*.

spirometer (spī-rom'-ėt-ėr) *n* instrument for measuring lung capacity— **spirometric** *adj*, **spirometry** *n*.

spironolactone (spī-ron-o-lak'-tōn) *n* potassium-sparing antialdosterone preparation; acts on complex biochemical processes involved in edematous accumulation and causes renal excretion of sodium and water. (Aldactone.)

splanchnic (splangk'-nik) *adj* pertaining to or supplying the viscera.

splanchnicectomy (splangk-ni-sek'-to-mē) *n* surgical removal of the splanchnic nerves, whereby the viscera are deprived of sympathetic impulses; occasionally performed in the treatment of hypertension or for the relief of certain kinds of visceral pain.

splanchnology (splangk-nol'-o-jē) *n* study of structure and function of the viscera.

spleen *n* a lymphoid, vascular organ immediately below the diaphragm, at the tail of the pancreas, behind the stomach. Enlarged in reactive and neoplastic conditions affecting the reticuloendothelial system.

splenectomy (splen-ek'-to-mē) *n* surgical removal of the spleen.

splenic anemia (splen'-ik a-nē'-mē-à) *n* → anemia.

splenitis (splen-ī'-tis) *n* inflammation of the spleen.*

splenius capitis muscle (splen'-ē-us kap'-i-tus) → Figure 5.

splenocaval (splen-ō-kā'-vàl) *adj* pertaining to the spleen and inferior vena cava, usually referring to anastomosis of the splenic vein to the latter.

splenogram (splen'-ō-gram) *n* radiographic picture of the spleen after injection of radio-opaque medium—**splenograph, splenography** *n,* **splenographical** *adj*.

splenomegaly (splen-ō-meg'-à-lē) *n* enlargement of the spleen.

splenoportal (splen-ō-pōr'-tàl) *adj* pertaining to the spleen and portal vein.

splenoportogram (splen-ō-port'-ō-gram) *n* radiographic demonstration of the spleen and portal vein after injection of radio-opaque medium—**splenoportographical** *adj*, **splenoportograph, splenoportography** *n*.

splenorenal (splen-ō-rē'-nàl) *adj* pertaining to the spleen and kidney, as anastomosis of the splenic vein to the renal vein; a procedure carried out in some cases of portal hypertension.

splint *n* device for immobilizing a joint.

spondyl(e) (spon'-dil) *n* a vertebra.*

spondylitis (spon-dil-ī'-tis) *n* inflammation of one or more vertebrae. *ankylosing spondylitis* a condition characterized by ossificiation of spinal ligaments and ankylosis of sacroiliac joints; occurs chiefly in young men—**spondylitic** *adj*.

spondylography (spon-dil-og'-raf-ē) *n* method of measuring degree of kyphosis by directly tracing the line of the back.

spondylolisthesis (spon-dil-ō-lis-thē'-sis) *n* forward displacement of lumbar vertebra(e)—**spondylolisthetic** *adj*.

spondylosis deformans (spon-dil-ōs'-is dē-fōr'-manz) degeneration of the whole intervertebral disk, with new bone formation at periphery of the disk. Commonly called "osteoarthritis of spine."

spongioblastoma multiforme (spon-jē-ō-blas-tō'-mȧ mul'-ti-form) highly malignant rapidly growing brain tumor.

spore *n* a phase in the life cycle of a limited number of bacterial genera: the vegetative cell becomes encapsulated and metabolism almost ceases. Spores are highly resistant to heat and desiccation. Only thorough sterilization ensures spore destruction of such ubiquitous species as *Clostridium tetani* and *Clostridium botulinum* .

sporicidal (spōr-i-sīd'-ȧl) *adj* lethal to spores—**sporicide** *n*.

sporotrichosis (spōr-ō-tri-kōs'-is) *n* infection of a wound by a fungus (*Sporotrichum schenkii*), with a primary sore, lymphangitis and subcutaneous painless granulomata. Occurs among agricultural workers.

sporulation (spōr-ū-lā'-shun) *n* formation of spores by bacteria.

spotted fever 1 cerebrospinal fever. Organism responsible is *Neisseria meningitides,* transferred by droplet infection. Occurs in epidemics. → meningitis. 2 Rocky Mountain spotted fever is a tick borne typhus* fever.

sprain *n* injury to soft tissues surrounding a joint, resulting in discoloration, swelling and pain.

Sprengel's shoulder deformity (spreng'-elz) congenital high scapula, a permanent elevation of the shoulder, often associated with other congenital deformities, as the presence of a cervical rib or the absence of vertebrae.

sprue (sprͻͻ) *n* chronic malabsorption disorder associated with glossitis, indigestion, weakness, anemia and steatorrhea.

spurious diarrhea (spū'-rē-us dī'-ȧ-rē'-ȧ) leakage of fluid feces past a solid impacted mass of feces. More likely to occur in children and the elderly.

sputum (spū'-tum) *n* spittle.

squamous (skwā'-mus) *adj* scaly. *squamous epithelium* nonglandular epithelial covering of skin and mucous membrane. *squamous carcinoma* carcinoma arising in squamous epithelium; epithelioma.

squills (skwilz) *npl* dried bulbs of Mediterranean plant, used in Gee's linctus and other cough preparations as an expectorant.

squint *n* (*syn* strabismus) incoordinated action of muscles of the eyeball, such that visual axes of the two eyes fail to meet at the objective point. *convergent* *squint* eyes turned towards the medial line. *divergent squint* eyes turned outwards.

SSE *abbr* soap suds enema.

staccato speech (stȧ-kȧ'-tō) with interruptions between words or syllables. The scanning speech of disseminated sclerosis and cerebellar disease.

stagnant loop syndrome stagnation of contents of any surgically created "loop" of intestine with consequent increase in bacterial population and interference with absorption of food.

St Anthony's fire disease characterized by either (a) a burning sensation and later gangrene of the extremities, or (b) convulsions. Due to a mixture of mycotoxins.*

stapedectomy (stā-pe-dek'-to-mē) *n* surgical removal of stapes for otosclerosis. After stapedectomy, stapes can be replaced by a prosthesis. Normal hearing is restored in 90% of patients.

stapedial mobilization, stapediolysis (stā-ped-ē'-ȧl) release of a stapes rendered immobile by otosclerosis.

stapes (stā'-pēz) *n* stirrup-shaped medial bone of the middle ear. *mobilization of stapes* forcible pressure on stapes to restore its mobility. Gain in hearing is not permanent, but a stapedectomy can be done later—**stapedial** *adj*.

Staphcillin™ methicillin.*

Staphylococcus (staf-il-ō-kok'-us) *n* genus of bacteria. Gram-positive cocci occurring in clusters. May be saprophytes or parasites. Common commensals of man; responsible for much minor pyogenic infection, and a lesser amount of more serious infection. Produce several exotoxins, including leukocidins, which kill white blood cells, and hemolysins, which destroy red blood cells. A common cause of hospital cross infection. *S. epidermis* one of the most common microorganisms causing bacteremia in patients who have had bone marrow transplant. In addition to an overall 8% fatality rate, protracted illness, extensive soft tissue infections, endocarditis, pneumonia and infected emboli have occurred. Organism is frequently resistant to all antimicrobials except vancomycin—**staphylococcal** *adj*.

staphyloma (staf-il-ōm'-ȧ) *n* protrusion of the cornea or sclera of the eye—**staphylomata** *pl*.

stasis (stā'-sis) *n* stagnation; cessation of motion. *intestinal stasis* sluggish bowel contractions resulting in constipation.

status (stat'-us) *n* state; condition. *status asthmaticus* repeated attacks of asthma* without any period of freedom between spasms. *status epilepticus* epileptic attacks following each other almost continuously. *status lymphaticus* a condition found postmortem in patients who have died without apparent cause;

thymus may be found hypertrophied with increase in lymphatic tissue elsewhere.

STD *abbr* sexually* transmitted diseases.

steapsin (stē-ap'-sin) *n* the lipase* of the pancreatic juice which splits fat into fatty acids and glycerine.

steathorrea (stē-at-ō-rē'-à) *n* passage of pale, bulky, greasy, foul-smelling stools.

steatosis (stē-a-tō'-sis) *n* (*syn.* fatty liver) fat-saturated liver seen in alcoholics; degenerative changes are present in some areas.

Stein-Leventhal syndrome (stīn–lev'en-thal) secondary amenorrhea, infertility, bilateral polycystic ovaries and hirsutism occurring in the second or third decades of life. Sometimes treated by wedge resection of ovary.

Stelazine™ trifluoperazine.*

stellate (stel'-āt) *adj* star-shaped. *stellate ganglion* large collection of nerve cells (ganglion) on the sympathetic chain in the root of the neck. *stellate ganglionectomy* surgical removal of the stellate ganglion; sometimes performed for Meniere's disease when attacks of vertigo are crippling and are unrelieved by conventional treatment.

Stellwag's sign (stel'-wags) occurs in exophthalmic goiter (thyrotoxicosis). Patient does not blink as often as usual and eyelids close only imperfectly.

stem cell any primitive, precursor cell that produces a line of differentiated cells as it divides; esp. the precursor to blood cells.

stenosis (ste-nō'-sis) *n* a narrowing. **1** *pyloric stenosis* narrowing of pylorus due to scar tissue formed during healing of a duodenal ulcer. **2** *congenital hypertrophic pyloric stenosis* due to thickened pyloric sphincter muscle—**stenoses** *pl*, **stenotic** *adj*.

stercobilin (stėr-kō-bī'-lin) *n* the brown pigment of feces; derived from the bile pigments.

stercobilinogen (stėr-kō-bil-in'-ō-jen) *n* → urobilinogen.

stercoraceous (stėr-kōr-ash'-ē-us) *adj* pertaining to or resembling feces—**stercoral** *adj*.

stereotactic surgery (stē-rē-ō-tak'-tik) electrodes and cannulae are passed to a predetermined point in the brain for physiological observation or destruction of tissue in diseases such as paralysis agitans, multiple sclerosis and epilepsy. Intractible pain can be relieved by this method—**stereotaxy** *n*.

sterilization (stėr-il-ī-zā'-shun) *n* **1** treatment that achieves the killing or removal of all types of microorganisms including spores; utilizes heat, radiation, chemicals or filtration. **2** rendering incapable of reproduction—**sterile** *adj*, **sterility** *n*.

sternal puncture insertion of a special guarded hollow needle with a stylet into the body of the sternum for aspiration of a bone marrow sample.

sternoclavicular (stèr-nō-cla-vik′-ū-lår) *adj* pertaining to sternum* and clavicle.*

sternocleidomastoid muscle (stèr-nō-klī-dō-mas′-toyd) straplike neck muscle arising from the sternum and clavicle, and inserting into the mastoid process of temporal bone. → torticollis.

sternocostal (stèr-nō-kos′-tal) *adj* pertaining to sternum* and ribs.

sternotomy (stèr-not′-o-mē) *n* surgical division of the sternum.*

sternum (stèr′-num) *n* the breastbone—**sternal** *adj*.

steroids (stèr′-oyds) *npl* naturally occurring group of chemicals allied to cholesterol and including sex hormones, adrenal cortical hormones, bile acids, etc. By custom, implies esp. the natural adrenal glucocorticoids, hydrocortisone and cortisone, or synthetic analogues such as prednisolone and prednisone.

sterol (ster′-ol) *n* a solid alcohol. Cholesterol and many hormones secreted by the adrenal cortex and gonads are examples. All have the same basic ring structure.

stertor (stèr′-tor) *n* loud snoring; sonorous breathing—**stertorous** *adj*.

stethoscope (steth′-ō-skōp) *n* instrument used for listening to various body sounds, esp. those of the heart and chest. **stethoscopic** *adj*.

Stevens-Johnson syndrome severe variant of the allergic response—erythema multiforme. Acute hypersensitivity state, which can follow infection or administration of drugs—such as long-acting sulfonamides, some anticonvulsants and antibiotics. Occasionally no cause is evident. Lung complications during acute phase can be fatal. Mostly a benign condition, with complete recovery.

stigmata (stig-må′-tà) *npl* marks of disease, or congenital abnormalities, as facies of congenital syphilis—**stigma** *sing*.

stilette (stil-et′) *n* wire or metal rod for maintaining patency of hollow instruments.

stillborn *n* born dead.

Still's disease form of rheumatoid polyarthritis, involving enlargement of spleen, lymphatic nodes and glands, occurring in infants and young children. Sufferers are often retarded. Also called "arthritis deformans juvenilis."

stimulant *n* agent which excites or increases function.

stimulus (stim′-ū-lus) *n* anything which excites functional activity in an organ or part.

stitch *n* 1 a sudden, sharp, darting pain. 2 a suture.

Stockholm technique (stok′-hōlm) method of treating carcinoma of the cervix by radium on three successive occasions at weekly intervals.

Stokes-Adams syndrome a fainting (syncopal) attack, commonly transient, which occurs in patients with heart block. If severe, may take the form of a convulsion, or patient may become unconscious.

stoma (stō'-mà) *n* the mouth; any opening—**stomata** *pl,* **stomal** *adj.*

stomach (stum'-ak) *n* the most dilated part of the digestive tube, situated between the esophagus (cardiac orifice) and the beginning of the small intestine (pyloric orifice); it lies in the epigastric, umbilical and left hypochrondriac regions of the abdomen. The wall is composed of four coats: serous, muscular, submucous and mucous. *stomach pH electrode* an apparatus used to measure gastric contents in situ.

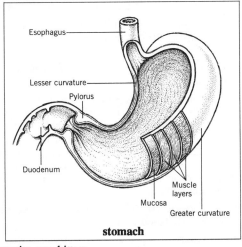

Esophagus

Lesser curvature

Pylorus

Duodenum

Muscle layers

Mucosa

Greater curvature

stomach

stomachics (stum-ak'-iks) *npl* agents which increase appetite, esp. bitters.

stomatitis (stō-mà-tī'-tis) *n* inflammation of the mouth. *angular stomatitis* fissuring in the corners of the mouth consequent upon riboflavin deficiency. Sometimes misapplied to: (a) the superficial maceration and fissuring at the labial commisures in perleche* and (b) chronic fissuring at the site in elderly persons with sagging lower lip or malapposition of artificial dentures. *aphthous stomatitis* recurring crops of small ulcers in the mouth. Relationship to herpes simplex suspected, but not proven. → aphthae. *gangrenous stomatitis* → cancrum oris.

stone *n* calculus; a hardened mass of mineral matter.

stool *n* the feces. An evacuation of the bowels.

strabismus (stà-biz'-mus) *n* → squint.

strain *n* damage, usually muscular, that results from excessive physical effort.

stramonium (strà-mō'-nē-um) *n* plant resembling belladonna* in its properties, used as an antispasmodic in bronchitis and parkinsonism.

strangulated hernia → hernia.

strangulation *n* constriction that impedes circulation—**strangulated** *adj.*

strangury (strang'-gū-rē) *n* painful urge to micturate with slow voiding of small amounts of urine.

stratified (strat'-i-fīd) *adj* arranged in layers.

stratum (stra'-tum) *n* layer or lamina, as the various layers of the epithelium of skin: stratum granulosum, stratum lucidum—**strata** *pl*.

strawberry tongue tongue thickly furred with projecting red papillae. As the fur disappears the tongue is vividly red, like an overripe strawberry. Characteristic of scarlet* fever.

Streptobacillus (strep-tō-ba-sil'-us) *n* pleomorphic bacterium which may be Gram-positive in young cultures.

Streptococcus (strep-tō-kok'-us) *n* genus of bacteria. Gram-positive cocci, often arrayed as chains. Require enriched media for growth and colonies are small. Saprophytic and parasitic species. Pathogenic species produce powerful exotoxins; including leukocidins, which kill white blood cells, and hemolysins, which kill red blood cells. Streptococci cause numerous infections, such as scarlatina, tonsillitis, erysipelas, endocarditis and wound infections in hospital, with rheumatic fever and glomerulonephritis as possible sequelae—**streptococcal** *adj*.

streptodornase (strep-tō-dōr'-nāz) *n* enzyme used with streptokinase* in liquefying pus and blood clots.

streptokinase (strep-tō-kī'-nāz) *n* enzyme derived from cultures of certain hemolytic streptococci. Plasminogen activator. Used with streptodornase.* Its fibrinolytic effect has been used as thrombolytic therapy to speed removal of intravascular fibrin.

streptolysins (strep-tō-lī'-sins) *npl* exotoxins produced by streptococci. Antibody produced in the tissues against streptolysin may be measured and taken as an indicator of recent streptococcal infection.

streptomycin (strep-tō-mī'-sin) *n* antibiotic effective against many organisms, but used mainly in tuberculosis. Treatment must be combined with other drugs to reduce drug resistance. Not absorbed when given orally, hence used in some intestinal infections.

Streptothrix (strep'-to-thriks) *n* a filamentous bacterium which shows true branching. → Streptobacillus.

stress test evaluates heart function through controlled exercise, as on a treadmill.

striae (strī'-ē) *npl* streaks; stripes; narrow bands. *striae gravidarum* lines which appear, esp. on the abdomen, as a result of skin stretching pregnancy, due to rupture of lower layers of the dermis. Red at first and then become silvery-white—**stria** *sing*, **striated** *adj*.

stricture (strik'-tūr) *n* a narrowing, esp. of a tube or canal, due to scar tissue or tumor.

stridor (strī'-dor) *n* a harsh sound in breathing, caused by air passing through constricted air passages—**stridulous** *adj*.

stroke *n* popular term for apoplexy resulting from a vascular accident in the brain, which can result in hemiplegia. → cerebrovascular accident.

stroma (strō'-må) *n* interstitial or foundation substance of a structure.

Strongyloides (stron-ji-loy'-dēz) *n* genus of intestinal worms that can infest man.

strongyloidiasis (threadworm) (stron-ji-loy-dī'-à-sis) *n* infestation with *Strongyloides stercoralis*, usually acquired through the skin from contaminated soil, but can be through mucous membrane. At the site of larval penetration there may be an itchy rash. As the larvae migrate through the lungs, pulmonary symptoms may develop, with larvae in sputum. Abdominal symptoms may also arise. Because of autoinfective life cycle, treatment aims at complete elimination of the parasite. Thiabendazole 25 mg per kg twice daily for 2 days; given either as a suspension or tablets which should be chewed.

strophanthus (strō-fan'-thus) *n* African plant with cardiac properties similar to digitalis, but of more rapid action. The active principle, strophanthin, is sometimes given by intravenous injection.

STS *abbr* serological test for syphilis.

student's elbow olecranon bursitis.*

stupe (stūp) *n* a medical fomentation.* Opium may be added to relieve pain. Turpentine may be added to produce counterirritation.

stupor *n* state of marked impairment of, but not complete loss of consciousness; gross lack of responsiveness, usually reacting only to noxious stimuli. Psychiatry defines three main varieties of stupor: depressive, schizophrenic and hysterical—**stuporous** *adj*.

St Vitus' dance (sānt vi'-tus) → chorea.

sty *n* (*syn* hordeolum) abscess in the follicle of an eyelash.

styloid (stī'-loyd) *adj* long and pointed; resembling a pen or stylus.

styptic (stip'-tik) *n* astringent applied to stop bleeding. A hemostatic.

subacute *adj* moderately severe. Often the stage between acute and chronic phases of disease. *subacute bacterial endocarditis* septicemia due to bacterial infection of a heart valve. Petechiae of the skin and embolic phenomena are characteristic. The term infective endocarditis is now preferred, since other microorganisms may be involved. *subacute combined degeneration of the spinal cord* a complication of untreated pernicious anemia (PA); affects the posterior and lateral columns. *subacute sclerosing panencephalitis (SSPE)* a slow* virus infection caused by the measles virus; characterized by diffuse inflammation of brain tissue.

subarachnoid hemorrhage bleeding, usually from a ruptured berry aneurysm, into the subarachnoid space, accompanied by headache and a stiff neck. Blood is present in the CSF. Cerebral angiography reveals the site of bleeding and treatment depends on this.

subarachnoid space (sub-à-rak'-noyd) space beneath the arachnoid membrane, between it and the pia mater; contains cerebrospinal fluid.

subcarinal (sub-ka-rī'-nal) *adj* below a carina,* usually referring to the carina tracheae.

subclavian (sub-klā'-vē-an) *adj* beneath the clavicle. *subclavian artery* → Figure 9. *subclavian vein* → Figure 10.

subclinical *adj* insufficient to cause the classical identifiable disease.

subconjunctival (sub-kon-jungk-tī'-vàl) *adj* below the conjunctiva.

subconscious *adj, n* that portion of the mind outside the range of clear consciousness, but capable of affecting conscious mental or physical reactions.

subcostal (sub-kos'-tàl) *adj* beneath the rib.

subcutaneous (sub-kū-tā'-nē-us) *adj* beneath the skin. subcutaneous edema demonstrable by the "pitting" produced by pressure of the finger. *subcutaneous tissue* → Figure 12.

subcuticular (sub-kū-tik'-ū-làr) *adj* beneath the cuticle, as a subcuticular abscess.

subdural (sub-dūr'-àl) *adj* beneath the dura mater; between the dura and arachnoid membranes. *subdural hematoma* result of bleeding from a small vein or veins lying between the dura and brain; develops slowly and may present as a space-occupying lesion with vomiting, papilledema, fluctuating level of consciousness, weakness, usually a hemiplegia on the opposite side to the clot. Finally there is a rise in blood pressure and a fall in pulse rate.

subendocardial (sub-en-dō-kàr'-dē-àl) *adj* immediately beneath the endocardium.

subhepatic (sub-he-pat'-ik) *adj* beneath the liver.

subinvolution (sub-in-vol-ū'-shun) *n* failure of the gravid uterus to return to normal size within a normal time after childbirth. → involution.

subjective *adj* internal; personal; arising from the senses and not perceptible to others. → objective *opp.*

sublimate (sub'-li-māt) **1** *n* a solid deposit resulting from the condensation of a vapor. **2** *vt* in psychiatry, to redirect a primitive desire into some more socially acceptable channel—**sublimation** *n*.

Sublimaze™ fentanyl.*

subliminal (sub-lim′-in-ål) *adj* inadequate for perceptible response. Below the threshold of consciousness. → liminal.

sublingual (sub-ling′-gwål) *adj* beneath the tongue.

subluxation (sub-luks-ā′-shun) *n* incomplete dislocation of a joint.

submandibular (sub-man-dib′-ū-lår) *adj* below the mandible.

submaxillary (sub-maks′-il-ār-ē) *adj* beneath the lower jaw.

submucosa (sub-mū-kō′-så) *n* layer of connective tissue beneath a mucous membrane—**submucous, submucosal** *adj*.

submucous (sub-mū′-kus) *adj* beneath a mucous membrane. *submucous resection* removal of a deflected nasal septum.

subnormality *n* state of arrested or incomplete development of mind (not amounting to severe subnormality) which includes subnormality of intelligence and is of a nature or degree that requires or is susceptible to medical treatment or other special care or training of the patient. *severe subnormality* degree that includes subnormality of intelligence so that patient is incapable of living an independent life.

suboccipital (sub-ok-sip′-it-ål) *adj* beneath the occiput; in the nape of the neck.

subperiosteal (sub-per-ē-os′-tē-ål) *adj* beneath the periosteum of bone.

subphrenic (sub-fren′-ik) *adj* beneath the diaphragm.

subscapularis muscle (sub-skap-ū-lār′-is) → Figure 4.

subsultus (sub-sul′-tus) *adj* muscular tremor. *subsultus tendinum* twitching of tendons and muscles particularly around the wrist in severe fever, such as typhoid.

succinylcholine (sucks-in-il-kōl′-ēn) *n* short-acting muscle relaxant.

succus (suk′-us) *n* a juice, esp. that secreted by the intestinal glands and called *succus entericus.*

succussion (su-kush′-un) *n* splashing sound produced by fluid in a hollow cavity on shaking the patient, as liquid content of dilated stomach in pyloric stenosis. *hippocratic succussion* splashing sound, on shaking, when fluid accompanies a pneumothorax.

sucrose (sū′-krōs) *n* a disaccharide obtained from sugar cane, sugar beet and maple syrup; normally hydrolyzed into dextrose and fructose in the body.

sucrosuria (sū-krōs-ū′-rē-å) *n* presence of sucrose in urine.

suction abortion abortion performed by an instrument that sucks contents from the uterus.

sudamina (sū-dam′-in-å) *n* sweat rash.

sudden infant death syndrome → crib death.

sudor (sū′-dor) *n* sweat—**sudoriferous** *adj*.

sudorific (sū-dor-if'-ik) *adj*, *n* (*syn* diaphoretic) describes an agent which induces sweating.

sulcus (sul'-kus) *n* a furrow or groove, particularly those separating the gyri or convolutions of the cortex of the brain—**sulci** *pl*.

sulfacetamide (sul-fà-sēt'-à-mīd) *n* a sulfonamide* used mainly as eye drops, and systemically for urinary tract infections. (Cetamide, Sulfamide.)

sulfadiazine (sul-fà-dī'-à-zīn) *n* powerful sulfonamide* compound for systemic use in many infections. Often the drug of choice in meningococcal infections, as its penetration into cerebrospinal fluid is greater than other sulfonamides. Less effective against staphylococcal infections.

sulfamethoxazole (sul-fà-meth-oks'-à-zōl) *n* sulfonamide that has a pattern of absorption and excretion very similar to trimethoprim, and so used in mixed products. (Gantanol.)

Sulfamide™ sulfacetamide.*

sulfasalazine (sul-fà-sal'-à-zēn) *n* sulfonamide compound which, after ingestion, is distributed largely in connective tissue. Used in treatment of ulcerative colitis. (Azulfidine.)

sulfhemoglobin (sulf-hē-mō-glo'-bin) *n* a sulfide oxidation product of hemoglobin,* produced in vivo by certain drugs; cannot transport oxygen or carbon dioxide and, not being reversible in the body, is an indirect poison. A variant compound is sulfmethemoglobin.

sulfhemoglobinemia (sulf-hē-mō-glō'-bin-ēm'-ē-à) *n* a condition of circulating sulfhemoglobin* in blood.

sulfinpyrazone (sulf-in-pī'-rà-zōn) *n* uricosuric* agent. (Anturane.)

sulfonamides (sul-fon'-à-mīds) *npl* group of bacteriostatic agents, effective orally. They are antimetabolites, obstructing bacterial formation of essential folic acid.

sulfonamidopyrimidines (sul-fon-à-mīd'-ō-pi-rim'-i-dēnz) *npl* oral blood-sugar lowering agents.

sulfones (sul'-fōnz) *npl* group of synthetic drugs, represented by dapsone,* useful for leprosy.

sulfonylureas (sul-fon-il-ū'-rē-az) *npl* sulfonamide* derivatives; oral hypoglycemic agents. They increase insulin output from a functioning pancreas so that injections of insulin may be unnecessary. Of chief value in "middle-age onset" diabetes.

sunstroke *n* → heat stroke.

supercilium (sū-per-sil'-ē-um) *n* the eyebrow—**superciliary** *adj*.

Superinone™ tyloxapol.*

superior *adj* in anatomy, pertaining to the upper of two parts.

supernumerary (sū-per-nū'-mer-ār-ē) *adj* in excess of the normal number; additional.

supinate (sū'-pin-āt) *vt* turn or lay face or palm upward. → pronate *opp*.

supinator (sū'-pin-āt-or) *n* that which suppinates, usually applied to a muscle. → pronator *opp*.

supine (sū'-pīn) *adj* 1 lying on the back with face upwards. 2 of the hand, with the palm upwards. → prone *opp*.

suppository (su-poz'-i-tōr-ē) *n* medicament in a base that melts at body temperature. Inserted into the rectum.

suppression *n* 1 cessation of a secretion (e.g., urine) or a normal process (e.g., menstruation). 2 in psychology, the voluntary forcing out of mind of painful thoughts; may result in the precipitation of a neurosis.

suppuration (sup-er-ā'-shun) *n* the formation of pus—**suppurative** *adj*, **suppurate** *vi*.

supraclavicular (sū-prȧ-klȧ-vik'-ū-lȧr) *adj* above the collar bone (clavicle).

supracondylar (sū-prȧ-kon'-dil-ȧr) *adj* above a condyle.*

supraorbital (sū-prȧ-ōr'-bit-ȧl) *adj* above the orbits. *supraorbital ridge* the ridge covered by the eyebrows.

suprapubic (sū-prȧ-pū'-bik) *adj* above the pubis.

suprarenal (sū-prȧ-rē'-nȧl) *adj* above the kidney. → adrenal.

supraspinatus muscle (sū-prȧ-spin-ā'-tus) → Figure 5.

suprasternal (sū-prȧ-ster'-nȧl) *adj* above the breastbone (sternum).

surface muscles → Figures 4, 5.

surfactant (sur-fak'-tant) *n* mixture of phospholipids, chiefly lecithin* and sphingomyelin, secreted into the pulmonary alveoli; reduces surface tension of pulmonary fluids, contributing to the elastic properties of pulmonary tissues. Can be instilled via a tracheal catheter for respiratory distress syndrome. → pneumocytes, zinc.

surgery *n* that branch of medicine which treats diseases, deformities and injuries, wholly or in part, by manual or operative procedures.

surgical emphysema air in the subcutaneous tissue-planes following trauma of surgery or injury.

Surmontil™ trimipramine.*

suspensory bandage applied so that it supports and suspends the scrotum.*

suspensory ligaments → Figure 15.

suture (sū'-tūr) *n* 1 the junction of cranial bones. 2 in surgery, a ligature.*

swab *n* small piece of cotton wool or gauze, sometimes on the end of a shaft of wire or wood, usually enclosed in a protecting tube; used to collect material for bacteriological examination.

sweat *n* secretion from the sudoriferous glands. *sweat gland* → Figure 12.

sweat test petri dish prepared with agar, silver nitrate and potassium chromate. With palm of hand pressed to this, excessive chorides in sweat leaves distinctive white print, as in cystic fibrosis.

swimmer's ear otitis externa, caused by water remaining in the ear canal after swimming.

sycosis barbae (sī-kō'-sis bàr'-bē) (*syn* barber's itch) pustular folliculitis of the beard area in men. Now rare due to antibiotics and improved hygiene.

sycosis nuchae (sī-kō'-sis nook'-ē) a folliculitis at the nape of the neck which leads to keloid thickening (acne keloid).

Sydenham's chorea (sīd'-en-hamz kōr-ē'-à) St. Vitus Dance. → chorea.

symbiosis (sim-bī-ō'-sis) *n* relationship between two or more organisms in which the participants are of mutual aid and benefit to one another. → antibiosis *opp*—**symbiotic** *adj*.

symblepharon (sim-blef'-à-ron) *n* adhesion of the lid to the eyeball.

Symmetrel™ amantadine.*

sympathectomy (sim-pà-thek'-tō-mē) *n* surgical excision of part of the sympathetic nervous system.

sympathetic nervous system a portion of the autonomic nervous system; composed of a chain of ganglia on either side of the vertebral column in the thoracolumbar region, sending fibers to all plain muscle tissue.

sympatholytic (sim-pàth-ō-lit'-ik) *n* drug which opposes the effects of the sympathetic nervous system.

sympathomimetic (sim-pàth-ō-mim-et'-ik) *adj* capable of producing changes similar to those produced by stimulation of the sympathetic nerves.

symphysis (sim'-fis-is) *n* a fibrocartilaginous union of bones—**symphyseal** *adj*.

symptom (sim'-tum) *n* a subjective phenomenon or manifestation of disease. *symptom complex* a group of symptoms which, occurring together, typify a particular disease or syndrome—**symptomatic** *adj*.

symptomatology (sim-tum-à-tol'-o-jē) *n* 1 branch of medicine concerned with symptoms. 2 the combined symptoms typical of a particular disease.

Synalar™ fluocinolone.*

synapse, synapsis (sin'-aps, sin-ap'-sis) *n* point of communication between two adjacent neurons.

synchysis (sin'-kis-is) *n* degenerative condition of the vitreous humor of the eye, rendering it fluid. *synchysis scintillans* fine opacities in the vitreous.

syncope (sin'-ko-pē) *n* (*syn* faint) literally, sudden loss of strength. Caused by reduced cerebral circulation often following a fright, when vasodilation is responsible. May be symptomatic of cardiac arrhythmia, e.g., heart block.

syncytium (sin-si'-shum) *n* a mass of protoplasm that is multinucleated.

syndactyly, syndactylism, syndactylia (sin-dak'-til-ē) *n* webbed fingers or toes—**syndactylous** *adj*.

syndrome (sin'-drōm) *n* group of symptoms and/or signs which, occurring together, produce a pattern or symptom complex, typical of a particular disease.

synechia (sin-ek'-ē-à) *n* abnormal union of parts, esp. adhesion of the iris to the cornea in front, or the lens capsule behind—**synechiae** *pl*.

Synkavite™ menadiol.*

synkinesis (sin-kin-ē'-sis) *n* ability to carry out precision movements.

synovectomy (sin-ō-vek'-to-mē) *n* excision of synovial membrane.

synovial fluid (sin-ō'-vē-al) fluid secreted by the membrane lining a joint cavity.

synovial membrane (sin-ō'-vē-àl) → membrane.

synovioma (sin-ō-vē-ōm'-à) *n* tumor of synovial membrane—benign or malignant.

synovitis (sī-nō-vī'-tis) *n* inflammation of a synovial membrane.

synthesis (sin'-the-sis) *n* process of building complex substances from simpler substances by chemical reactions—**synthetic** *adj*.

Synthroid™ levothyroxine.*

Syntocinon™ synthetic oxytocin.*

syphilide (sif'-il-īd) *n* a syphilitic skin lesion.

syphilis (sif'-il-is) *n* venereal disease caused by *Treponema pallidum*. Infection is acquired or may be congenital—when it is prenatal. *acquired syphilis* manifests in: (a) primary stage, commences 4–5 weeks (or later) after infection when a primary chancre associated with swelling of local lymph glands appears; (b) secondary stage, in which skin eruption (syphilide) appears; (c) third (tertiary) stage, occurs 15–30 years after initial infection. Gummata appear, or neurosyphilis* and cardiovascular syphilis supervene. Commonest types of nervous system involvement are general paralysis of the insane and tabes dorsalis (locomotor ataxia). Cardiovascular involvement produces aortic aneurysm and impairment or destruction of the aortic valve. *congenital syphilis* is acquired by the fetus from the infected mother—**syphilitic** *adj*.

syringe (si-rinj') *n* device for injecting, instilling or withdrawing fluids; principal components are a cylindrical barrel, to one end of which a hollow needle is attached, and a close-fitting plunger.

syringomyelia (si-ring'-gō-mī-ēl'-ē-à) *n* uncommon, progressive disease of the nervous system of unknown cause, beginning mainly in early adult life. Cavitation and surrounding fibrous tissue reaction, in the upper spinal cord and brain stem, interfere with sensation of pain and temperature, and sometimes with motor pathways. Characteristic symptom is painless injury, particularly of the exposed hands. Touch sensation is intact. → Charcot's joint.

systemic circulation oxygenated blood leaves the left ventricle and after flowing throughout the body returns deoxygenated to the right atrium.

systole (sis'-tol-ē) *n* contraction phase of the cardiac cycle, as opposed to diastole*—**systolic** *adj*.

systolic murmur (sis-tol'-ik) cardiac murmur occurring between the first and second heart sounds due to valvular disease, e.g., mitral systolic murmur.

T

T cells group of lymphocytes that play a major role in immunity*; subsets of various types act in ways not yet fully elucidated, but in general are divided into T-helper (CD4) and T-killer (CD8) classes. T-helpers promote several immune responses, secreting cytokines* that stimulate production of immunoglobulins (by B* cells) and growth of lymphocyte population, and activate macrophages.* T-killers (cytotoxic) attack antigens directly. Some members of both subsets act to suppress (T-suppressor) immune activity when antigenic challenge is removed.

TAB *abbr* vaccine containing killed *Salmonella typhi, Salmonella paratyphi A* and *S. paratyphi B;* used to produce active artificial immunity against typhoid* and paratyphoid* fever.

tabes (tā'-bēz) *n* wasting away. *tabes dorsalis* variety of neurosyphilis: posterior (sensory) columns of the spinal cord and sensory nerve roots are diseased. → Charcot's joint, locomotor ataxia. *tabes mesenterica* tuberculous enlargement of peritoneal glands found in children—**tabetic** *adj*.

taboparesis (tā-bō-par-ēs'-is) *n* condition of general paralysis of the insane in which spinal cord shows the same lesions as in tabes* dorsalis.

TACE™ chlorotrianisene.*

tachycardia (tak-ē-kàr'-dē-à) *n* excessively rapid action of the heart. *paroxys-* mal tachycardia temporary but sudden marked increase in frequency of heart-beats, because conducting stimulus is originating in an abnormal focus.

tachyphasia (tak-ē-fā'-zhà) *n* extreme rapidity of flow of speech occurring in some mental disorders.

tachypnea (tak'-ip-nē-à) *n* abnormal frequency of respiration—**tachypneic** *adj*.

Taenia (tē'-nē-à) *n* genus of flat, parasitic worms; cestodes or tapeworms. *T.* echinococcus adult worm lives in dog's intestine (the definitive host), and man (the intermediate host) is infested by swallowing eggs from dog's excrement. These become embryos in the human small intestine, pass via the blood stream to organs, particularly the liver, and develop into hydatid cysts. *T. saginata* larvae present in infested, undercooked beef. In human intestinal lumen they develop into adult tapeworm, attaching itself to the gut wall by four suckers. *T. solium* resembles *T. saginata,* but has hooklets as well as suckers. Commonest species in Eastern Europe. Larvae are ingested in infested, undercooked pork;

man can also be the intermediate host for this worm by ingesting eggs which, developing into larvae in the stomach, pass via the bowel wall to reach organs, and there develop into cysts. In the brain these may give rise to epilepsy.

taenia (tē'-nē-à) *n* a flat band. *taenia coli* three flat bands running the length of the large intestine and consisting of the longitudinal muscle fibers.

taeniacide (tē'-nē-à-sīd) *n* agent that destroys tapeworms—**taeniacidal** *adj*.

taeniafuge (tē'-nē-à-fūj) *n* agent that expels tapeworms.

Tagamet™ cimetidine.

talipes (tal'-i-pēz) *n* any of a number of deformities of foot and ankle.

talus (tāl'-us) *n* the astragalus; situated between the tibia proximally and the calcaneus* distally, thus directly bearing the weight of the body. Second largest bone of the ankle.

Talwin™ pentazocine.*

Tambocor™ flecainide.*

tamoxifen (ta-moks'-i-fen) *n* synthetic anti-estrogenic compound. Drug of choice for postmenopausal metastatic breast cancer. (Nolvadex.)

tamponade (tam-pon-ād') *n* insertion of a tampon. → cardiac.

Tandearil™ oxyphenbutazone.*

tannic acid brown powder obtained from oak galls; has astringent properties, and is used as suppositories for hemorrhoids.

tapeworm *n* → taenia.

Taractan™ chlorprothixene.*

tarsalgia (tàr-sal'-jà) *n* pain in the foot.

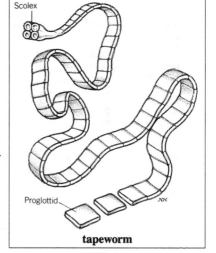

tapeworm

tarsometatarsal (tàr-sō-met-à-tàr'-sàl) *adj* pertaining to the tarsal and metatarsal region.

tarsoplasty (tàr'-sō-plas-tē) *n* any plastic operation to the eyelid.

tarsorrhaphy (tàr-sōr'-rà-fē) *n* suturing of the lids together to protect the cornea when it is anesthetic, or to allow healing.

tarsus (tàr'-sus) *n* **1** the seven small bones of the foot (→ Figure 2). **2** the thin elongated plates of dense connective tissue found in each eyelid, contributing to its form and support—**tarsal** *adj*.

tartar *n* the deposit, calculus, which forms on the teeth. *tartar emetic* → antimony and potassium tartrate.

Taxol™ paclitaxel.*

Tay-Sachs' disease (tā'-saks) *(syn* gangliosidosis) recessive inherited deficiency of the enzyme hexosaminidase, which leads to massive accumulation of a specific lipid substance called GM_2, or Tay-Sachs ganglioside.

Tay's choroiditis (tāz kōr-oyd-ī'-tis) → choroiditis.

tears *npl* secretion formed by the lacrimal gland; contain the enzyme lysozyme,* which acts as an antiseptic.

Tebrazid™ pyrazinamide.*

teeth *npl* structures used for mastication. The deciduous, milk or primary set, 20 in number, is shed by 7 years, and is normally replaced by permanent or secondary teeth. The permanent set, 32 in number, is usually complete in the late teens. *bicuspid teeth* → bicuspid. *canine or eye teeth* have sharp fanglike edge for tearing. *Hutchinson's teeth* have a notched edge and are characteristic of congenital syphilis. *incisor teeth* have knifelike edge for biting. *premolar and molar teeth* have a square termination for chewing and grinding. *wisdom teeth* the last molar teeth, one at either side of each jaw—**tooth** *sing*.

Tegopen™ cloxacillin.*

Tegretol™ carbamazepine.*

telangiectasis (tel-an-jē-ek'-tå-sis) *n* dilatation of the capillaries on a body surface.

Telepaque™ iopanoic* acid.

Temaril™ trimeprazine.*

temazepam (te-maz'-e-pam) *n* short-acting benzodiazepine.*

Temovate™ clobetasol* proprionate.

temporal (tem'-por-ål) *adj* of the temple. *temporal bones* one on each side of the head below the parietal bone, containing the middle ear.

temporomandibular (tem'-por-ō-man-dib'-ū-lár) *adj* pertaining to the temporal region or bone, and the lower jaw.

temporomandibular joint syndrome (TMJ) pain in the region of temporomandibular joint frequently caused by malocclusion of the teeth, resulting in malposition of the condylar heads in the joint and abnormal muscle activity, and by bruxism.*

tenaculum (te-nak'-ū-lum) *n* instrument with a hook on the end for holding parts, as in an operation.

tendinitis (ten-din-ī'-tis) *n* inflammation of a tendon.

tendon *n* firm, white, fibrous inelastic cord which attaches muscle to bone—**tendinous** *adj*.

tenesmus (ten-ez'-mus) *n* painful, ineffectual straining to empty the bowel or bladder.

tennis elbow → epicondylitis.

tenoplasty (ten'-ō-plas-tē) *n* reconstructive operation on a tendon—**tenoplastic** *adj*.

Tenormin™ atenolol.*

tenorrhaphy (ten-ōr'-rȧ-fē) *n* suturing of a tendon.

tenosynovitis (ten-ō-sī-nō-vī'-tis) *n* inflammation of thin synovial lining of a tendon sheath, as distinct from its outer fibrous sheath. May be caused by mechanical irritation or by bacterial infection.

tenotomy (ten-ot'-o-mē) *n* division of a tendon.

Tenuate™ diethylpropion.*

teratogen (tėr-at'-ō-jen) *n* anything capable of disrupting fetal growth and producing malformation: drugs, poisons, radiation, physical agents such (as ECT), infections (as rubella), and rhesus and thyroid antibodies. → dysmorphogenic—**teratogenic, teratogenetic** *adj*, **teratogenicity, teratogenesis** *n*.

teratology (ter-ȧ-tol'-o-jē) *n* scientific study of teratogens and their mode of action—**teratological** *adj*, **teratologist** *n*.

teratoma (ter-ȧ-tō'-mȧ) *n* tumor of embryonic origin and composed of various structures, including both epithelial and connective tissues; most commonly found in ovaries and testes, the majority being malignant—**teratomata** *pl*, **teratomatous** *adj*.

terbutaline (ter-bū'-tȧ-lēn) *n* bronchodilator useful in acute exacerbations of asthma. (Bricanyl.)

teres muscles (tē'-rēz) → Figure 5.

Terramycin™ oxytetracycline.*

testicle (tes'-tik-l) *n* → testis—**testicular** *adj*.

testis (tes'-tis) *n* one of two glandular bodies contained in the scrotum (→ Figure 16); they form spermatozoa and the male sex hormones. *undescended testis* organ remains within the bony pelvis or inguinal canal. → cryptorchism—**testes** *pl*.

testosterone (tes-tos'-ter-ōn) *n* hormone derived from the testes and responsible for development of secondary male characteristics. Used in carcinoma of the breast, to control uterine bleeding and in male underdevelopment.

tetanus (tet'-ȧ-nus) *n* (*syn* lockjaw) disease caused by *Clostridium tetani*, an anaerobe commonly found in ruminants and manure. Causes severe tonic muscle spasms. Tetanus toxoid injections produce active immunity. ATS injection produces passive immunity—**tetanic** *adj*.

tetany (tet′-à-nē) *n* condition of muscular hyperexcitability in which mild stimuli produce cramps and spasms. Found in parathyroid deficiency and alkalosis. Associated in infants with gastrointestinal upset and rickets.

tetracaine (tet′-rà-kān) *n* ophthalmic anesthetic. (Pontocaine.)

tetrachloroethylene (tet-rà-klōr-ō-eth′-il-ēn) *n* anthelmintic given in hookworm; single dose.

tetracoccus (tet-rà-kok′-us) *n* coccal bacteria arranged in cubical packets of four.

tetracycline (tet-rà-sī′-klin) *n* broad-spectrum antibiotic related to both chlortetracycline* and oxytetracycline* and used for similar purposes. As a rule, it causes less gastrointestinal disturbance, with less absorption of oral tetracycline when the stomach is full, or contains aluminium, calcium or magnesium. Causes fluorescence in body cells, which is retained by cancerous cells for 24–30 h after dosage ceases. (Achromycin.)

tetradacytlous (tet-rà-dak′-til-us) *adj* having four digits on each limb.

tetralogy of Fallot (fal-lō′) form of congenital heart defect which comprises cyanosis, septal defect between the ventricles, hypertrophy of the right ventricle, with narrowing of the outlet, and displacement of the aorta to the right. Amenable to corrective surgery.

tetraplegia (tet-rà-plē′-jē-à) *n* (*syn* quadriplegia) paralysis of all four limbs— **tetraplegic** *adj*.

thalamotomy (thal-à-mot′-o-mē) *n* usually operative (stereotaxic) destruction of a portion of thalamus. Can be done for intractable pain.

thalamus (thal′-à-mus) *n* body of grey matter at the base of the cerebrum (→ Figure 1). Sensory impulses from the whole body pass through on the way to the cerebral cortex—**thalami** *pl*, **thalamic** *adj*.

thalassemia (thal-à-sēm′-ē-à) *n* a hemolytic anemia which is inherited in an autosomal recessive pattern. Three classifications: (a) *minor*, denotes the carrier, who is asymptomatic; (b) *intermediate*, mild form which may require an occasional blood transfusion; (c) *major*, severe form in which affected bone marrow produces fetal-type hemoglobin. Breakdown of hemoglobin and recurrent blood transfusion leads to iron overload, treated with chelating agents such as desferrioxamine.

THAM™ tromethamine.*

thanatology (than-à-tol′-o-jē) *n* scientific study of death, including its etiology and diagnosis.

theca (thē′-kà) *n* an enveloping sheath, esp. of a tendon. *theca vertebralis* membranes enclosing the spinal cord—**thecal** *adj*.

thenar (thē′-nàr) *adj* pertaining to palm of the hand and sole of the foot. *thenar* eminence palmar eminence below the thumb.

theobromine (thē-ō-brō'-mēn) *n* drug allied to caffeine,* but with a less stimulating and more powerful diuretic action.

theophylline (thē-of'-il-in) *n* diuretic related to caffeine* but more powerful. Used mainly in its derivative aminophylline* in treatment of congestive heart failure, dyspnea and asthma.

therapeutic embolization deliberate infarction of a tumor to reduce its size and vascularity before removal by surgery.

therapeutics *n* branch of medical science dealing with treatment of disease— **therapeutic** *adj*.

thermogenesis (thér-mō-jen'-es-is) *n* production of heat—**thermogenetic** *adj*.

thermolabile (thér-mō-lā'-bīl) *adj* capable of being easily altered or decomposed by heat.

thermolysis (thér-mol'-is-is) *n* heat-induced chemical dissociation. Dissipation of body heat—**thermolytic** *adj*.

thermophil (thér'-mō-fil) *n* microorganism accustomed to growing at a high temperature—**thermophilic** *adj*.

thermostable (thér-mō-stā'-bl) *adj* unaffected by heat. Remaining unaltered at a high temperature, which is usually specified—**thermostability** *n*.

thermotherapy (thér-mō-thér'-à-pē) *n* heat treatment. → hyperthermia.

thiabendazole (thī-à-ben'-dà-zōl) *n* best available treatment for *Strongyloides* infestation. No starvation or purgation necessary. Stated to clear infection in about 50% of patients with trichuriasis. Effective orally for larva migrans caused by some species of *Ancylostoma*.(Mintezol.)

thiamine (thī'-à-min) *n* (*syn* vitamin B_1) concerned in carbohydrate metabolism; indicated therapeutically in thiamine deficiency disorders, such as beriberi, and some forms of neuritis; also as adjunct to oral antibiotic therapy; deficiency may cause mental confusion or cardiomyopathy.

thiazides (thī'-à-zīdz) *npl* saluretic diuretic group of drugs. → diuretics.

Thiersch skin graft (tērsh) thin sheet of split skin graft applied to a raw surface.

thiethylperazine (thī-eth-il-pér'-à-zēn) *n* a phenothiazine* tranquilizer useful for nausea, vomiting and vertigo. (Torecan.)

thioguanine (thī-ō-gwan'-ēn) *n* an antimetabolite. Interferes with synthesis of nucleoprotein, thus useful in acute leukemia.

thiopental (thī-ō-pen'-tàl) *n* barbiturate given intravenously as a short-acting basal anesthetic. Effect can be extended by additional doses, and in combination with curare compounds, adequate relaxation for major surgery can be achieved. (Pentothal.) → barbiturates.

thioridazine (thī-ō-rid'-a-zēn) *n* sedative, tranquilizer. Closely resembles chlorpromazine.* (Mellaril.)

thiothixene (thī-ō-thiks'-ēn) *n* antipsychotic used in schizophrenia. (Navane.)

thoracentesis (thōr-å-sen-tē'-sis) *n* aspiration of the pleural cavity.

thoracic (thōr-as'-ik) *adj* pertaining to the thorax. *thoracic aorta* → Figure 9. *thoracic nerve* → Figure 11. *thoracic duct* a channel conveying lymph (chyle) from the receptaculum chyli in the abdomen to the left subclavian vein. *thoracic inlet syndrome* → cervical rib.

thoracoplasty (thōr'-å-kō-plas'-tē) *n* operation on the thorax: ribs are resected to allow chest wall to collapse and the lung to rest; used in treatment of tuberculosis. Rarely necessary since advent of antituberculous drugs.

thoracoscope (thōr'-å-kō-skōp) *n* instrument that can be inserted into pleural cavity through a small incision in the chest wall, to permit inspection of pleural surfaces and division of adhesions by electric diathermy—**thoracoscopic** *adj*, **thoracospy** *n*.

thoracotomy (thōr-å-kot'-o-mē) *n* surgical exposure of the thoracic cavity.

thorax (thōr'-aks) *n* the chest cavity—**thoracic** *adj*.

Thorazine™ chlorpromazine.*

threadworm *n* strongyloidiasis.*

threonine (thrē'-o-nēn) *n* an essential amino* acid.

thrill *n* vibration as perceived by the sense of touch.

thrombectomy (throm-bek'-to-mē) *n* surgical removal of a thrombus from within a blood vessel.

thrombin (throm'-bin) *n* not normally present in circulating blood; enzyme generated from prothrombin (Factor II), activates factor VIII and itself combines with fibrinogens to form a stable clot. Extrinsic and intrinsic pathways lead to production of thrombin: extrinsic pathway is tested by the prothrombin time (PT); intrinsic pathway involves principally factors VIII and IX. Partial thromboplastin time (PTT) or a modification called the partial thromboplastin time with kaolin detects abnormalities in this pathway. → blood, Christmas disease, hemophilia.

thromboangiitis (throm-bō-an-jē-īt'-is) *n* clot formation within an inflamed vessel. *thromboangiitis obliterans* → Buerger's disease.

thromboarteritis (throm-bō-år-ter-īt'-is) *n* inflammation of an artery with clot formation.

thrombocyte (throm'-bō-sīt) *n* (*syn* platelet) plays a part in the clotting of blood. → blood.

thrombocythemia (throm-bō-sī-thē'-mē-å) *n* condition with an increase in circulating blood platelets, which can encourage clotting within blood vessels. → thrombocytosis.

thrombocytopenia (throm-bō-sī-tō-pē'-nē-à) *n* reduction in number of platelets in blood, which can result in spontaneous bruising and prolonged bleeding after injury—**thrombocytopenic** *adj*.

thrombocytopenic purpura (throm-bō-sī-tō-pē'-nik pur'-pur-à) syndrome characterized by low blood platelet count, intermittent mucosal bleeding and purpura. Can be symptomatic, i.e., secondary to known disease or to certain drugs; or idiopathic, a rare condition of unknown cause (purpura hemor-rhagica) occurring principally in children and young adults. In both forms the bleeding time is prolonged.

thrombocytosis (throm-bō-sī-tō'-sis) *n* increase in number of platelets in blood; can arise in course of chronic infections and cancers. Likely to cause throm-bosis.

thromboembolic (throm-bō-em'-bol-ik) *adj* describes phenomenon in which a thrombus, or clot, detaches itself and is carried in the bloodstream to block a blood vessel in another part of the body.

thromboendarterectomy (throm-bō-en-dàr-ter-ek'-to-mē) *n* removal of a thrombus and atheromatous plaques from an artery.

thromboendarteritis (throm-bō-en-dàr-ter-īt'-is) *n* inflammation of inner lin-ing of an artery with clot formation.

thrombogen (throm'-bō-jen) *n* a precursor of thrombin.

thrombogenic (throm-bō-jen'-ik) *adj* capable of clotting blood—**thrombo-genesis, thrombogenicity** *n*.

thrombokinase (throm-bō-kī'-nāz) *n* → thromboplastin.

thrombolytic (throm-bō-lit'-ik) *adj* pertaining to disintegration of a blood clot. *thrombolytic therapy* attempted removal of preformed intravascular fibrin occlusions using fibrinolytic agents—**thrombolysis** *n*.

thrombophlebitis (throm-bō-fle-bī'-tis) *n* inflammation of the wall of a vein with secondary thrombosis within involved segment. *thrombophlebitis migrans* recurrent episodes of thrombophlebitis affecting short lengths of superficial veins; deep vein thrombosis is uncommon and pulmonary embolism rare—**thrombophlebitic** *adj*.

thromboplastin (throm'-bō-plas-tin) *n* (*syn* thrombokinase) enzyme that con-verts prothrombin into thrombin. *intrinsic thromboplastin* produced by inter-action of several factors during clotting of blood. Much more active than tissue thromboplastin.

thrombosis (throm-bō'-sis) *n* intravascular formation of a blood clot—**throm-boses** *pl*, **thrombotic** *adj*.

thrombus (throm'-bus) *n* an intravascular blood clot—**thrombi** *pl*.

thrush *n* → candidiasis.

thymectomy (thī-mek'-to-mē) *n* surgical excision of the thymus.

thymocytes (thī'-mō-sīts) *npl* cells found in dense lymphoid tissue in the lobular cortex of the thymus gland—**thymocytic** *adj*.

thymoma (thī-mō'-mȧ) *n* tumor arising in the thymus—**thymomata** *pl*.

thymosin (thī-mō'-sin) *n* hormone secreted by epithelial cells of the thymus gland. Provides stimulus for lymphocyte production within the thymus; confers on lymphocytes elsewhere in the body the capacity to respond to antigenic stimulation.

thymus (thī'-mus) *n* gland lying behind the breastbone and extending upward as far as the thyroid gland. Well developed in infancy and attains its greatest size towards puberty; then the lymphatic tissue is replaced by fatty tissue. It has an immunological role.

thyrocalcitonin (thī-rō-kal-si-tō'-nin) *n* → calcitonin.

thyroglossal (thī-rō-glos'-ȧl) *adj* pertaining to thyroid gland and tongue. *thyro-glossal cyst* retention* cyst caused by blockage of thyroglossal duct; appears on side of the neck. *thyroglossal duct* fetal passage from thyroid gland to back of the tongue, where its vestigial end remains as the foramen cecum. In this area thyroglossal cyst or fistula can occur.

thyroid (thī'-royd) *n* ductless gland found on both sides of the trachea. Secretes thyroxine,* which controls basal metabolic rate. *thyroid cartilage* → Figure 6. *thyroid antibody test* presence and severity of autoimmune thyroid disease is diagnosed by levels of thyroid antibody in blood. *thyrotropin-releasing hormone (TRH)* secreted by hypothalamus, influences amount of TSH secretion. *thyroid-stimulating hormone (TSH), thyrotropin* secreted by the pituitary gland to control levels of thyroid hormone (T_3 and T_4) produced by the thryoid gland. Radioimmunoassay of TSH level is useful in diagnosing mild hypothyroidism. *thyroid storm* life-threatening crisis, with fever, weakness, confusion, shock and potential systemic collapse, due to great excess of thyroid hormone.

thyroidectomy (thī-royd-ek'-to-mē) *n* surgical removal of the thyroid gland.

thyroiditis (thī-royd-īt'-is) *n* inflammation of thyroid gland. *Autoimmune thyroiditis* or Hashimoto's disease, a firm goiter ultimately resulting in hypothyroidism. *Riedel's thyroiditis* → Riedel's.

thyrotoxicosis (thī-rō-toks-i-kōs'-is) *n* an autoimmune thyroid disease; due to excessive production of the thyroid gland hormone (thyroxine*), and resulting classically in anxiety, tachycardia, sweating, increased appetite with weight loss, fine tremor of the out-stretched hands, and prominence of the eyes (Graves' disease). More common in women than in men. In older patients cardiac irregularities may be a prominent feature. Thyrotoxicosis may also be due to increased thyroxine production by a single thyroid nodule or a multinodular goiter—**thyrotoxic** *adj*.

thyrotoxic crisis sudden worsening of symptoms in thyrotoxicosis; may occur immediately after thyroidectomy.

thyrotropic (thī-rō-trō'-pik) *adj* of a substance which stimulates the thyroid gland, as thyrotropin (thyroid-stimulating hormone, TSH) secreted by the anterior pituitary gland.

thyroxine (T4) (thī-roks'-ēn) *n* principal hormone of the thyroid gland; raises basal metabolic rate. Used in treatment of hypothyroidism. (Eltroxin.)

TIA *abbr* transient* ischemic attack.

tibia (tib'-ē-à) *n* shinbone; larger of the two bones in lower part of the leg; it articulates with the femur,* fibula* and talus*—**tibial** *adj.*

tibial artery → Figure 9.

tibial vein → Figure 10.

tibiofibular (tib-ē-ō-fib'-ū-làr) *adj* pertaining to the tibia and the fibula.

tic douloureux (tik doo-loo-re) (trigeminal neuralgia) spasms of excruciating pain in the distribution of the trigeminal nerve.

tidal air volume of air which passes in and out of the lungs in normal breathing.

Tietze syndrome (tēt'-sē) costochondritis which is self-limiting and of unknown etiology. No specific treatment.

timolol maleate (tim'-o-lol mal'-ē-āt) hypotensive beta-blocking agent. (Blocadren.)

tincture (tink'-tūr) *n* solution of a drug in alcohol.

tine test multiple puncture test using disposable equipment. Plastic holder has four small tines coated with undiluted tuberculin; reaction is read in 48–72 h.

tinea (tin'-ē-à) *n* → ringworm. *tinea barbae* sycosis* barbae. *tinea capitis* ringworm of the head. *tinea corporis* (*syn* circinata) ringworm of the body. *tinea cruris* ringworm of the crotch area. *tinea incognita* unrecognized ringworm to which topical corticosteroids have been inappropriately applied, obscuring usual signs of ringworm. *tinea pedis* ringworm of the foot.

Tinel's sign after injury to a peripheral nerve, a sharp tapping at site of injury may elicit tingling further along distribution of the nerve; an indication of regenerating nerve tissue.

tinnitus (tin-ī'-tus) *n* buzzing, thumping or ringing sound in the ears.

tissue *n* collection of cells or fibers of similar function, forming a structure. *tissue respiration* → respiration.

titer (tī'-ter) *n* a standard of concentration per volume, as determined by titration.

titration (tī-trā'-shun) *n* volumetric analysis by aid of standard solutions.

TMJ *abbr* temporomandibular* joint syndrome.

TNM system method of staging extent of the malignant process. Initial letters indicate Tumor, Nodes (lymph) and Metastases (distant). Each category has four main divisions—T1–4, N and M 0–3. Combined score permits allocation to Stages 1–4.

tobacco amblyopia (am-blē-ōp'-ē-à) → smokers' blindness.

tobramycin (tō-brà-mī'-sin) *n* antibiotic similar to gentamicin.* (Nebcin.)

tocography (to-kog'-raf-ē) *n* process of recording uterine contractions using a tocograph or a parturiometer.

tocopherol (to-kof'-èr-ol) *n* synthetic vitamin E, similar to that found in wheatgerm oil.

Tofranil™ imipramine.*

tolazamide (tol-az'-à-mīd) *n* a sulfonylurea.* (Tolinase.)

tolazoline (tol-az'-o-lēn) *n* peripheral vasodilator, used in circulatory disorders such as Raynaud's disease and related conditions. Has also been used in ophthalmic conditions such as keratitis. (Priscoline.)

tolbutamide (tol-bū'-tà-mīd) *n* sulfonamide* derivative which stimulates functioning islets of Langerhans to pour out more insulin. Some success in oral treatment of diabetes, so that insulin injections may be reduced or withdrawn. Of no value in juvenile diabetes. (Orinase.) *tolbutamide test* after blood is withdrawn for estimation of its fasting sugar content, intravenous injection of tolbutamide is given. Blood is taken for glucose levels 20 and 30 min later. Differentiates diabetes that can be controlled by oral antidiabetic drugs (noninsulin dependent) from diabetes which cannot (insulin dependent).

tolerance *n* ability to endure application or administration of a substance, usually a drug. Dosage may have to increase as tolerance develops. *exercise tolerance* exercise accomplished without pain or marked breathlessness. American Heart Association's classification of functional capacity: Class I—no symptoms on ordinary effort; Class II—slight disability on ordinary effort; Class III—marked disability on ordinary effort which prevents any attempt at housework; Class IV—symptoms at rest or heart failure.

Tolinase™ tolazamide.*

tolnaftate (tol-naf'-tāt) *n* antifungal agent, useful for athlete's foot. (Tinactin.)

tomography (to-mog'-raf-ē) *n* technique of using X-rays to create image of a specific, thin layer through the body (rather than the whole body)—**tomographic** *adj,* **tomogram, tomograph** *n.*

tongue *n* mobile muscular organ contained in the mouth; concerned with speech, mastication, swallowing and taste. → strawberry tongue.

tonic *adj* of a state of continuous muscular contraction, as opposed to intermittent contraction.

tonography (ton-og'-raf-ē) *n* continuous measurement of blood or intraocular pressure. *carotid compression tonography* occlusion of one common carotid artery causes an ipsilateral fall of intraocular pressure. Used as a screening test for carotid insufficiency.

tonometer (ton-om'-ėt-ėr) *n* instrument for measuring intraocular pressure.

tonsillectomy (ton-sil-lek'-to-mē) *n* removal of the tonsils. *tonsillectomy position* three-quarters prone position to prevent inhalation (aspiration) pneumonia and asphyxiation.

tonsillitis (ton-sil-lī'-tis) *n* inflammation of the tonsils.

tonsilloliths (ton-sil'-lō-liths) *npl* concretions arising in the body of the tonsil.

tonsillopharyngeal (ton-sil-lō-far-in-jē'-ėl) *adj* pertaining to tonsils* and pharynx.*

tonsillotome (ton-sil'-lō-tōm) *n* instrument for excision of tonsils.

tonsils *npl* small bodies, one on each side, covered by mucous membrane, embedded in the fauces between the palatine arch; composed of about 10–18 lymph follicles—**tonsillar** *adj*.

tooth *n* → Figure 14.

topectomy (top-ek'-to-mē) *n* modified frontal lobotomy. Small incisions made in thalamofrontal tracts.

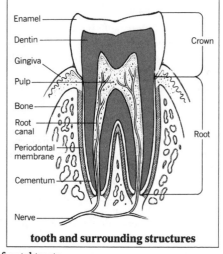

Enamel
Dentin
Gingiva
Pulp
Bone
Root canal
Periodontal membrane
Cementum
Nerve

Crown
Root

tooth and surrounding structures

tophus (tō'-fus) *n* small, hard concretion forming on the ear lobe, on the joints of the phalanges, etc., in gout—**tophi** *pl*.

topical *adj* describes local application of anesthetics, drugs, powders and ointments to skin and mucous membrane.

TOPV *abbr* trivalent oral polio vaccine.

TORCH infections infectious diseases which may be transmitted to the fetus through the placenta. Includes toxoplasmosis, rubella, cytomegalovirus and herpes simplex.

Torecan™ thiethylperazine.*

torsion *n* twisting.

torticollis (tōr-ti-kol′-is) *n* (*syn* wryneck) painless contraction of one sternoclei-domastoid* muscle; head is slightly flexed and drawn towards contracted side, with the face rotated over the other shoulder.

torulosis *n* crptococcosis.*

total colonic lavage (*syn* whole gut irrigation) preoperative procedure before extensive bowel surgery. A large amount of fluid, e.g., 1 l per half hour, is introduced into the stomach via a nasogastric tube while patient sits on a pad-ded commode. Infusion is continued until effluent is clear, usually 4–6 h. Has been used for fecal impaction.

total parenteral nutrition (TPN) solutions containing all essential nutrients administered by a central venous line; only liquids and low density solutions are administered. → parenteral feeding.

Tourette's syndrome inherited neurologic disorder; with involuntary move-ment, tics, often including vocal tics that may manifest in scatalogical outbursts (coprolalia). Condition can be socially, as well as physically, disabling.

tourniquet (turn′-i-ket) *n* apparatus for compression of the blood vessels of a limb. Designed for compression of a main artery to control bleeding; also used to obstruct venous return from a limb and so facilitate withdrawal of blood from a vein. Tourniquets vary from a simple rubber band to a pneumatic cuff.

toxemia (toks-ē′-mē-à) *n* generalized poisoning of the body by products of bac-teria or damaged tissue—**toxemic** *adj*.

toxic *adj* poisonous, caused by a poison. *toxic epidermal necrolysis (TEN)* syn-drome with semblance of scalded skin; may occur in response to a drug, staphylococcal infection, systemic illness, or can be idiopathic. *toxic shock syndrome* (*syn* tampon shock syndrome) cluster of signs and symptoms which occur in some women who use tampons, with high temperature, vomiting and diarrhea. *Staphylococcus aureus,* present in vagina of about 5% of women, is causative agent.

toxicity (toks-is′-i-tē) *n* quality or degree of being poisonous.

toxicology (toks-i-kol′-o-jē) *n* science dealing with poisons, their mechanisms of action and antidotes to them—**toxicological** *adj*.

toxin (toks′-in) *n* product of bacteria that damages or kills cells.

Toxocara (toks-ō-kar′-à) *n* genus of roundworm of the cat and dog. Man can be infested (toxocariasis) by eating with hands soiled from these pets. The worms cannot become adult in man (incorrect host), so larval worms wander through the body, attacking mainly the liver and the eye. Treatment is unsatisfactory, but condition usually clears after several months.

toxoid (toks′-oyd) *adj* toxin altered in such a way that it has lost its poisonous properties but retained its antigenic properties. *toxoid antitoxin* mixture of toxoid and homologous antitoxin in floccule form, used as a vaccine, e.g., in immunization against diphtheria.

Toxoplasma (toks-ō-plaz'-mà) *n* protozoon whose natural host in the US is the domestic cat.

toxoplasmosis (toks-ō-plaz-mō'-sis) *n Toxoplasma* parasites which, commonly occurring in mammals and birds, may infect man. Intrauterine fetal and infant infections are often severe, producing encephalitis, convulsions, hydrocephalus and eye diseases, resulting in death or, in those who recover, mental retardation and impaired sight. Infection in older children and adults may result in pneumonia, nephritis or skin rashes. Skull X-ray reveals flecks of cerebral calcification. Skin and antibody tests confirm the diagnosis.

TPI test *Treponema pallidum* immobilization test; modern, highly specific test for syphilis in which syphilitic serum immobilizes and kills spirochetes grown in pure culture.

TPN *abbr* total* parenteral nutrition.

trabeculae (trà-bek'-ū-lē) *npl* fibrous bands or septa projecting into the interior of an organ, e.g., the spleen; they are extensions from the capsule surrounding the organ—**trabecula** *sing*, **trabecular** *adj*.

trabeculotomy (trà-bek-ū-lot'-o-mē) *n* operation for glaucoma: a channel is created through the trabecular meshwork from the canal of Schlemm to the angle of the anterior chamber.

trace elements metals and other elements regularly present in small amounts in tissues and known to be essential for normal metabolism (e.g., copper, cobalt, manganese, fluorine, etc.).

tracer *n* substance or instrument used to gain information. Radioactive tracers have extended knowledge in physiology; some are used in diagnosis.

trachea (trā'-kē-à) *n* (*syn* windpipe) fibrocartilaginous tube lined with mucous membrane passing from the larynx* to the bronchi* (→ Figure 6); about 115 mm long and about 25 mm wide—**tracheal** *adj*.

tracheitis (trā-kē-ī'-tis) *n* inflammation of the trachea; most commonly result of viral infection such as the common cold.

trachelorrhaphy (trā-kel-ōr'-rà-fē) *n* operative repair of a uterine cervical laceration.

tracheobronchial (trā-kē-ō-brong'-kē-àl) *adj* pertaining to the trachea* and the bronchi.*

tracheobronchitis (trā'-kē-ō-brong-kī'-tis) *n* inflammation of the trachea and bronchi → acute bronchitis.

tracheoesophageal (trā'-kē-ō-ē-sof-à-jē'-àl) *adj* pertaining to the trachea* and the esophagus.* *tracheoesophageal fistula* usually occurs in conjunction with esophageal atresia; generally connects distal esophagus to the trachea.

tracheostomy (trā-kē-os'-to-mē) *n* fenestration in the anterior wall of the trachea by removal of a circular piece of cartilage from the third and fourth rings, for establishment of a safe airway and reduction of "dead space."

tracheotomy (trā-kē-ot'-o-mē) *n* vertical slit in anterior wall of the trachea at the level of the third and fourth cartilaginous rings.

trachoma (trȧ-kō'-mȧ) *n* contagious inflammation affecting conjunctiva, cornea and eyelids; due to *Chlamydia trachomatis* which is sensitive to sulfonamides and antibiotics. Leads to blindness if untreated.

Tracrium™ atracurium.*

traction *n* drawing or pulling on the body to overcome muscle spasm and to reduce or prevent deformity. A steady pulling exerted on some part (limb or head) by means of weights and pulleys.

tractotomy (trak-tot'-o-mē) *n* incision of a nerve tract. Surgical relief of intractable pain. Using stereotactic measures, operation performed for some forms of mental illness.

tragus (trā'-gus) *n* projection in front of the external auditory meatus—**tragi** *pl*.

Trandate™ labetalol.*

tranquilizers (tran'-kwi-lī-zerz) *npl* drugs used to relieve tension or combat psychotic symptoms without significant sedation. Do not affect a basic disease, but reduce symptoms. Greatly exaggerate the effects of alcohol.

transabdominal (tranz-ab-dom'-in-ȧl) *adj* through the abdomen, as transabdominal approach for nephrectomy.

transamniotic (tranz-am-nē-ot'-ik) *adj* through the amniotic membrane and fluid, as a transamniotic transfusion of the fetus for hemolytic disease.

transcutaneous (tranz-kū-tā'-nē-us) *adj* through the skin, as for absorption of applied drugs. *transcutaneous electrical nerve supply* four pads are placed on either side of the spine from a battery-operated apparatus, controlled by the patient, for relief of pain.

transection (tran-sek'-shun) *n* cutting across or mechanical severance of a structure.

transfrontal (tranz-front'-ȧl) *adj* through the frontal bone; an approach used for hypophysectomy.

transfusion *n* introduction of fluid into tissue or into a blood vessel. *blood transfusion* intravenous replacement of lost or destroyed blood by compatible citrated human blood. Also used for severe anemia with deficient blood production. Fresh blood from a donor or stored blood from a blood bank may be used. Can be given "whole," or with some plasma removed ("packed-cell" transfusion). If incompatible blood is given severe reaction follows. → blood groups. *intrauterine transfusion* of a fetus endangered by Rhesus incompatibility. Red cells are transfused directly into the abdominal cavity of the fetus, on one or more occasions, thus enabling labor to be postponed until a time more favorable to fetal welfare.

TransdermNitro™ preparation of glyceryl trinitrate (nitroglycerine) that facilitates controlled absorption via the skin so that a constant blood level can be maintained.

Transderm-Scop™ scopolamine*; derivative of hyoscine (hyoscine-N-butyl bromide), antispasmodic which relaxes smooth muscle in peptic ulcer, colic and related conditions; most effective by injection.

transient ischemic attacks (TIA) → drop attacks, vertebrobasilar insufficiency.

transillumination *n* transmission of light through the sinuses for diagnostic purposes.

transirrigation *n* diagnostic puncture and lavage, as performed in maxillary sinusitis.

translocation *n* transfer of a segment of a chromosome to a different site on the same chromosome (shift) or to a different one. Can be a direct or indirect cause of congenital abnormality.

translumbar (tranz-lum′-bår) *adj* through the lumbar region. Route used for injecting aorta prior to aortography.

transmethylation (tranz-meth-il-ā′-shun) *n* process in metabolism of amino acids in which a methyl group is transferred from one compound to another.

transmigration *n* transit of a cell across a membrane from one side of a vessel to the other.

transmural *adj* through the wall, e.g., of a cyst, organ or vessel.

transnasal *adj* through the nose.

transonic *adj* allowing passage of ultrasound.

transperitoneal *adj* (tranz-pėr-i-ton-ē′-ål) across or through the peritoneal cavity. → dialysis.

transplacental (tranz-pla-sen′-tål) *adj* through the placenta.

transplant *n* customarily refers to surgical grafting of an organ into its proper anatomical bed, *orthotopic transplant* (e.g., liver and heart), or into another site, *heterotopic transplant*—**transplantation** *n*, **transplant** *vt*.

transplantation *n* commonly refers to transplantation of healthy bone marrow to treat inborn errors including immune deficiency, deficiency anemias such as thalassemia and aplastic anemia, and mucopolysaccharidoses, a group of diseases in which the enzyme that breaks down body mucus is absent.

transrectal (tranz-rek′-tål) *adj* through the rectum, as a transrectal injection into a tumor.

transsphenoidal (tran-sfen-oyd'-ål) *adj* through the sphenoid bone; an approach used for hypophysectomy.

transthoracic (tranz-thōr-as'-ik) *adj* across or through the chest, as in transthoracic needle biopsy of a lung mass.

transudate (tranz'-ū-dāt) *n* fluid that has passed out of the cells either into a body cavity (e.g., ascitic fluid in the peritoneal cavity) or to the exterior (e.g., serum from the surface of a burn).

transurethral (tranz-ū-rēth'-rål) *adj* by way of the urethra.

transvaginal (tranz-vaj'-in-ål) *adj* through the vagina, as an incision to drain the uterorectal pouch, transvaginal injection into a tumor, pudendal block or culdoscopy.

transverse colon → Figure 18.

transvesical (tranz-ves'-ik-ål) *adj* through the bladder, by custom, referring to the urinary bladder.

tranylcypromine (tra-nl-sī'-prō-mēn) *n* a monoamine* oxidase inhibitor. (Parnate.)

trapezius muscles (trå-pē'-zē-us) → Figures 4, 5.

Trasicor™ oxprenolol.*

trauma *n* 1 bodily injury. 2 emotional shock—**traumatic** *adj*.

Trecator™ ethionamide.*

Trematoda (trem-å-tō'-då) *n* class of parasitic worms which include many pathogens of man such as the *Schistosoma* of schistosomiasis.

tremor *n* involuntary trembling. *intention tremor* involuntary tremor which only occurs on attempting voluntary movement; a characteristic of multiple sclerosis.

trench fever louse-borne disease rickettsial caused by *Rochalimaea quintana;* with fever, weakness, severe pain in back and legs. Name refers to widespread infection of trench-bound soldiers in World War I.

trench foot (*syn* immersion foot) occurs in frostbite* or other conditions of exposure where there is "deprivation" of local blood supply and secondary bacterial infection.

trench mouth infection of tonsils by Vincent's bacillus.

Trendelenburg's sign test of the stability of the hip, and esp. the ability of hip abductors (gluteus medius and minimus) to steady the pelvis upon the femur: normally, when one leg is raised, the pelvis tilts upwards on that side, through the hip abductors of the standing limb. If the abductors are inefficient (e.g., in poliomyelitis, severe coxa vara and congenital dislocation of the hip), they are unable to sustain the pelvis against body weight and it tilts downwards instead of rising.

Treponema (trep-o-nēm′-à) *n* genus of slender spiral-shaped bacteria which are actively motile. Best visualized with dark-ground illumination. Cultivated in the laboratory with great difficulty. *T. pallidum* causative organism of syphilis; *T. pertenue* spirochete that causes yaws. *T. carateum;* spirochete that causes pinta.

treponematosis (trep-o-nēm-à-tōs′-is) *n* term applied to the treponemal diseases.

treponemicide (trep-o-nēm′-i-sīd) *n* substance lethal to *Treponema*—**treponemicidal** *adj*.

triage (trē-azh) *n* system of priority classification of patients in any emergency situation.

triamcinolone (trī-am-sin′-o-lōn) *n* steroid with good anti-inflammatory effect and little electrolyte-retaining activity. Because of stimulation of protein breakdown, can cause muscle wasting. (Aristocort, Kenalog.)

triamterene (trī-am′-ter-ēn) *n* diuretic that increases excretion of sodium chloride but lessens potassium loss at distal kidney tubule. (Dyrenium.)

TRIC *abbr* trachoma inclusion conjunctivitis. Agent responsible for infections of eye, genital tract and urethritis. → conjunctivitis.

triceps (trī′-seps) *n* three-headed muscle on the back of the upper arm. → Figures 4, 5.

trichiasis (tri-kī′-à-sis) *n* abnormal ingrowing eyelashes causing irritation from friction on the eyeball.

trichinosis (trik-i-nō′-sis) *n* disease caused by eating undercooked pig meat infected with *Trichinella spiralis* (the trichina worm). Female worms living in the small bowel produce larvae that invade the body and, in particular, form cysts in skeletal muscles; usual symptoms are diarrhea, nausea, colic, fever, facial edema, muscular pains and stiffness.

trichloracetic acid (trī-klōr-à-sē′-tik) powerful caustic and astringent. Used as a crystal for application to warts and ulcers.

trichomonacide (trik-ō-mōn′-à-sīd) *n* substance lethal to protozoa belonging to genus *Trichomonas.*

Trichomonas (trik-ō-mōn′-às) *n* protozoan parasite of man. *T. vaginalis* produces infection of urethra and vagina often associated with profuse discharge (leukorrhea). Organism is best recognized by microscopic examination of the discharge. → amoeba, protozoa.

trichomoniasis (trik-ō-mō-nī′-à-sis) *n* inflammation of the vagina (urethra in males) caused by *Trichomonas vaginalis.*

trichophytosis (trik-ō-fī-tō′-sis) *n* infection with a species of the fungus *Trichophyton,* e.g., ringworm* of the hair or skin.

trichuriasis (tri-kū-rī'-à-sis) *n* infestation with *Trichuris trichiura*.

Trichuris (tri-kū'-ris) *n* genus of nematodes. *T. trichiura* whipworm.

triclofos (trī'-klō-fōs) *n* derivative of chloral* hydrate causing less gastric irriation. (Triclos.)

Triclos™ triclofos.*

tricuspid (trī'-kus'-pid) *adj* having three cusps. *tricuspid regurgitation* incomplete closure of tricuspid valve, resulting in backflow of some blood into right atrium with each ventricular contraction. *tricuspid valve* that between the right atrium and ventricle of the heart.

trifluoperazine (trī-flū-ō-pèr'-à-zēn) *n* tranquilizer and antiemetic. More potent and less sedative than chlorpromazine.* (Stelazine.)

trigeminal (trī-jem'-in-àl) *adj* triple; separating into three sections, e.g., trigeminal nerve, the fifth cranial nerve, which has three branches, supplying skin of the face, the tongue and teeth. *trigeminal neuralgia* → tic douloureux.

trigger finger condition in which the finger can be actively bent but cannot be straightened without help; usually due to a thickening on the tendon which prevents free gliding.

trigone (trī'-gōn) *n* a triangular area, esp. applied to the bladder base, bounded by the ureteral openings at the back and the urethral opening at the front— **trigonal** *adj*.

trihexyphenidyl (trī-heks-ē-fen'-i-dl) *n* antispasmodic used mainly for rigidity of parkinsonism. Side-effects include dryness of mouth, nausea and vertigo. (Artane.)

triiodothyronine (T3) (trī-ī-ō-dō-thī'-rō-nēn) *n* a thyroid hormone that plays a part in maintaining the body's metabolic process.

Trilafon™ perphenazine.*

trimeprazine (trī-mep'-rà-zēn) *n* antihistamine with sedative action. A phenothiazine* derivative. Used in treatment of pruritis, urticaria and preoperatively for children. (Temaril.)

trimethaphan (trī-meth'-à-fan) *n* brief-acting blocking agent used by intravenous injection to produce a fall in blood pressure during bloodless field surgery. (Arfonad.)

trimethoprim (trī-meth'-ō-prim) *n* antibacterial agent. Has selective inhibiting action on the enzyme that converts folic acid into folinic acid, needed by many bacteria. When used with sulfonamides* the ensuing action is bactericidal. The sulfonamide must have a similar pattern of absorption and excretion. → cotrimoxazole.

trimipramine (trī-mip'-rà-mēn) *n* antidepressant similar to imipramine.* (Surmontil.)

tripelennamine (trī-pel-en′-à-mēn) *n* an antihistamine, useful in the treatment of allergies. (PBZ.)

triple antigen (*syn* DPT) contains diphtheria, whooping cough and tetanus antigens.

triple test a Dreiling tube is passed through the mouth into the duodenum and pancreatic function tests are carried out. The enzymes secretin and pancreozymin are given to stimulate the pancreas, and its juice is aspirated as it flows into the duodenum. Presence of a pancreatic tumor may be recognized at once by the volume and chemistry of the juice. Some of the juice is then examined, using Papanicolaou's method, to detect cancer cells and thirdly, a radiological hypotonic duodenogram is obtained, which reliably demonstrates tumors of the pancreas or ampulla. The test takes 2 h to complete.

triple vaccine → vaccines.

triploid (trip′-loyd) *adj* possessing three chromosomal sets. → genome, haploid.

trismus (triz′-mus) *n* spasm in the muscles of mastication.

trisomy (trī′-sō-mē) *n* the presence in triplicate of a chromosome that should normally be present only in duplicate. Increases the chromosome number by one (single trisomy), e.g., to 47 in man. *trisomy 18* → Edward syndrome. *trisomy 21* → Down syndrome.

Trobicin™ spectinomycin.*

trocar (trō′-kàr) *n* a pointed rod which fits inside a cannula.*

trochanters (trō-kan′-ters) *npl* two processes, the larger one (*trochanters major*) on the outer, the other (*trichanters minor*) on the inner side of the femur between the shaft and neck; they serve for the attachment of muscles— **trochanteric** *adj*.

trochlea (trō′-klē-à) *n* any part which is like a pulley in structure or function— **trochlear** *adj*.

tromethamine (trō-meth′-à-mēn) *n* an alkali used to treat acidosis. (THAM.)

trophoblastic tissue (trof-ō-blas′-tik) cells, covering the embedding ovum and concerned with nutrition of the ovum.

tropicamide (tro-pik′-à-mīd) *n* synthetic drug with mydriatic and cyclophegic actions. (Mydracil.)

Trouseau's sign (troo-sōz′) → carpopedal spasm.

Trypanosoma (trip-an-ō-sō′-mà) *n* genus of parasitic protozoa. Life cycle alternates between blood-sucking arthropods and vertebrate hosts, and in the latter they appear frequently in the blood stream as fusiform, actively motile structures some 10–40 μm in length. A limited number of species are pathogenic to man.

trypanosomiasis (trip-an-ō-sō-mī'-à-sis) *n* disease produced by infestation with *Trypanosoma*. In man this may be with *T. rhodesiense* in East Africa or *T. gambiense* in West Africa, both transmitted by the tsetse fly, and with *T. cruzii*, transmitted by bugs, in South Africa. In West Africa infection of the brain commonly produces the symptomatology of "sleeping sickness."

tryparsamide (trī-pàr'-sà-mīd) *n* organic arsenic compound of value in treatment of trypanosomiasis; usually given by intravenous injection.

trypsin (trip'-sin) *n* proteolytic enzyme present in pancreatic juice. Given in digestive disorders. Specially purified forms are used to liquefy clotted blood and other secretions, and in ophthalmology, to facilitate removal of cataracts.

tryptophan (trip'-tō-fan) *n* an essential amino* acid, necessary for growth; a precursor of serotonin.* Adequate levels of tryptophan may compensate deficiencies of niacin and thus mitigate pellagra.

tubal (tū'-bàl) *adj* pertaining to a tube. *tubal abortion* → abortion. *tubal ligation* tying of both fallopian tubes as a means of sterilization. *tubal pregnancy* → ectopic pregnancy.

Tubarine™ tubocurarine.*

tubercle (tū'-bėr-kl) *n* **1** small rounded prominence, usually on bone. **2** the specific lesion produced by *Mycobacterium tuberculosis*.

tuberculide, tuberculid (tū-ber'-kū-līd) *n* a small lump. Metastatic manifestation of tuberculosis,* producing a skin lesion, e.g., papulonecrotic tuberculide, rosacealike tuberculide.

tuberculin (tū-bėr'-kū-lin) *n* sterile extract of either the crude (old tuberculin) or refined (PPD) complex protein constituents of the tubercle bacillus. Its commonest use is in determining whether a person has or has not previously been infected with the tubercle bacillus. → Mantoux reaction.

tuberculoid (tū-bėr'-kū-loyd) *adj* resembling tuberculosis.* Describes one of the two types of leprosy.

tuberculoma (tū-bėr-kū-lō'-mà) *n* a caseous tubercle, usually large, its size suggesting a tumor.

tuberculosis (tū-bėr-kū-lō'-sis) *n* specific infective disease caused by *Myco-bacterium tuberculosis* (Koch's tubercle bacillus). *avian tuberculosis* endemic in birds and rarely seen in man. *bovine tuberculosis* endemic in cattle and transmitted to man via infected cow's milk. → bovine. *human tuberculosis* endemic in man and the usual cause of pulmonary and other forms of tuberculosis. *miliary tuberculosis* a generalized acute form in which, as a result of blood stream dissemination, minute, multiple tuberculous foci are scattered throughout many organs of the body—**tubercular, tuberculous** *adj*.

tuberculostatic (tū-bėr-kū-lō-stat'-ik) *adj* inhibiting growth of *Myobacterium tuberculosis*.

tuberous sclerosis (tū'-bėr-us skler-ōs'is) (*syn* epiloia) inherited sclerosis of brain tissue resulting in mental defect; may be associated with epilepsy.

tuberosity (tū-bėr-os'-i-tē) *n* a bony prominence.

tubocurarine (tū-bō-kūr-ár'-ēn) *n* muscle-relaxing drug derived from the South American arrow poison curare. Action reversed by neostigmine given intravenously together with atropine,* which depresses vagus nerve and so quickens heart beat. Causes hypertension and histamine release and is now often replaced by pancuronium,* alcuronium* or vecuronium.* (Tubarine.)

tuboovarian (tū-bō-ō-vėr'-ē-an) *adj* pertaining to or involving both tube and ovary, e.g., tubo-ovarian abscess.

tubular necrosis acute necrosis of renal tubules which may follow crush syndrome, severe burns, hypotension, intrauterine hemorrhage and dehydration. Urine flow is greatly reduced and acute renal* failure develops.

tubule (tū'-būl) *n* a small tube. *collecting tubule* straight tube in the kidney medulla conveying urine to the kidney pelvis. *convoluted tubule* coiled tube in the kidney cortex. *seminiferous tubule* coiled tube in the testis. *uriniferous tubule* nephron.*

Tuinal™ mixture of amobarbital* and secobarbital.*

tularemia (tū-là-rē'-mē-à) *n* (*syn* deer-fly fever, rabbit fever, tick fever) endemic disease of rodents, caused by *Pasteurella tularensis;* transmitted by biting insects and acquired by man either in handling infected animal carcasses or by the bite of an infected insect. Suppuration at the inoculation site is followed by inflammation of the draining lymph glands and by severe constitutional upset—**tularemic** *adj.*

tumescence (tū-mes'-ens) *n* a state of swelling; turgidity.

tumor *n* a swelling. A mass of abnormal tissue which resembles normal tissues in structure, but which fulfills no useful function and which grows at the expense of the body. Benign, simple or innocent tumors are encapsulated, do not infiltrate adjacent tissue or cause metastases and are unlikely to recur if removed. *malignant tumor* not encapsulated, infiltrates adjacent tissue and causes metastases. → cancer—**tumorous** *adj.*

tunica (too'-ni-ka) *n* a lining membrane; a coat. *tunica adventitia* outer coat of an artery. *tunica intima* lining of an artery. *tunica media* middle, muscular coat of an artery.

tunnel reimplantation operation surgical procedure used to reimplant the ureter.

turbinate (tur'-bin-āt) *adj* shaped like a top or inverted cone. *turbinate bone* three on either side forming the lateral nasal walls.

turbinated *adj* scroll-shaped, as the three turbinate processes which project from the lateral nasal walls.

turbinectomy (tur-bin-ek′-to-mē) *n* removal of turbinate bones.

turgid *adj* swollen; firmly distended, as with blood by congestion—**turgescence, turgidity** *n*.

Turner syndrome condition of multiple congenital abnormalities in females, with infantile genital development, webbed neck, cubitus valgus and, often, aortic coarctation. Ovaries are almost completely devoid of germ cells and there is failure of pubertal development. Most subjects with Turner syndrome have a single sex chromosome, the X, and thus only 45 chromosomes in their body cells.

tussis (tus′-sis) *n* a cough.

Tylenol™ acetaminophen.*

tylosis (tī-lō′-sis) *n* → keratosis.

tyloxapol (tī-loks′-à-pol) *n* drug which increases volume and decreases viscosity of bronchial mucus. (Superinone.)

tympanic (tim-pan′-ik) *adj* pertaining to the tympanum.* *tympanic membrane* → membrane.

tympanites (tim-pan-i′-tēz) *n* (*syn* meteorism) abdominal distension due to accumulation of gas in the intestine.

tympanitis (tim-pan-ī′-tis) *n* inflammation of the tympanum.

tympanoplasty (tim′-pan-ō-plas′-tē) *n* any reconstructive operation on the middle ear to improve hearing. Normally carried out in ears damaged by chronic suppurative otitis media with associated conductive deafness—**tympanoplastic** *adj*.

tympanum (tim′-pan-um) *n* cavity of the middle ear.

typhoid fever infectious fever usually spread by contamination of food, milk or water supplies with *Salmonella typhi*, either directly by sewage, indirectly by flies or by faulty personal hygiene. Symptomless carriers harboring agent in the gallbladder and excreting it in stools are the main source of outbreaks of disease in this country. Average incubation period is 10–14 days. A progressive febrile illness marks onset, which develops, as the microbe invades lymphoid tissue, including that of the small intestine (Peyer's patches), to profuse diarrheal (pea soup) stools which may become frankly hemorrhagic; recovery usually begins by end of the third week. A rose-colored rash may appear on the upper abdomen and back at the end of the first week. → TAB.

typhus (tī′-fus) *n* acute infectious rickettsial disease characterized by high fever, skin eruption and severe headache. A disease of war, famine or catastrophe, being spread by lice, ticks or fleas. Infecting organism in epidemic typhus is *Rickettsia prowazekii*, sensitive to sulfonamides and antibiotics. Other species are responsible for murine typhus, scrub typhus (tsutsugamushi), trench fever, Q fever, rickettsialpox.

tyramine (tī'-rà-mēn) *n* amine present in several foodstuffs, esp. cheese. Has an effect in the body similar to epinephrine,* consequently patients taking drugs in the monoamine oxidase inhibitor (MAOI) group should not eat cheese, as a dangerously high blood pressure may result.

tyrosine (tī'-rō-sēn) *n* an amino acid essential for growth. Combines with iodine to form thyroxine.

tyrosinosis (tī-rō-sin-ō'-sis) *n* due to abnormal metabolism of tyrosine; excess parahydroxyphenylpyruvic acid is excreted in urine.

tyrothricin (tī-roth'-ri-sin) *n* mixture of gramicidin* and other antibiotics; too toxic for systemic therapy, but is valuable in a number of infected skin conditions.

U

ulcer (ul'-sėr) *n* destruction of mucous membrane or skin from whatever cause, producing a crater or indentation. An inflammatory reaction occurs and if it penetrates a blood vessel bleeding ensues. An ulcer in the lining of a hollow organ can perforate the wall.

ulcerative (ul'-sėr-à-tiv) *adj* pertaining to or of the nature of an ulcer. → colitis.

ulcerogenic (ul-sėr-ō-jen'-ik) *adj* capable of producing an ulcer.

Ullrich syndrome (ul'-rik) → Noonan syndrome.

ulna (ul'-nà) *n* inner bone of the forearm. → Figures 2, 3.

ulnar artery (ul'-når) → Figure 9.

ultrasonography (ul-trà-son-og'-raf-ē) *n* production of a visible image using ultrasound. A controlled beam is directed into the body; reflected echoes are used to build up an electronic image of various structures of the body. *realtime ultrasonography* ultrasound imaging technique involving rapid pulsing to enable continuous viewing of movement, rather than stationary images—**ultrasonograph** *n*.

ultrasound *n* sound waves of frequency over 20 kHz and inaudible to human ear.

umbilical cord (um-bil'-i-kàl) the navel string attaching fetus to placenta.

umbilicated (um-bil'-i-kāt-ed) *adj* having a central depression, e.g., a smallpox vesicle.

umbilicus (um-bil'-i-kus) *n* (*syn* navel) abdominal scar left by separation of the umbilical cord after birth—**umbilical** *adj*.

uncinate (un'-sin-āt) *adj* hook-shaped, unciform.

"underarm, pill" six small capsules containing levonorgestrel* inserted under the skin of a woman's forearm; the implants release small amounts of the drug. Effect is achieved in 24 h and lasts for 5 years.

undine (un'-dēn) *n* small, thin glass flask used for irrigating the eyes.

undulant fever (un'-dū-lant) brucellosis*.

unguentum (un-gwen'-tum) *n* ointment.

unilateral (ū-ni-lat'-ėr-àl) *adj* relating to or on one side only.

uniocular (ū-nē-ok'-ū-làr) *adj* pertaining to, or affecting one eye.

uniovular (ū-nē-ō′-vū-lar) *adj* (*syn* monovular) pertaining to one ovum, as uniovular twins (identical). → binovular *opp*.

unipara (ū-nip′-à-rà) *n* woman who has borne only one child. → primipara— **uniparous** *adj*.

Unipen™ nafcillin.*

upper respiratory infection (URI) upper respiratory tract is commonest site of infection in all age groups. Infections include rhinitis—usually viral— sinusitis, tonsillitis, adenoiditis, pharyngitis, otitis media and croup (laryngitis), often involving tonsils and posterior cervical lymph glands. Such infections seldom require hospital treatment, but epiglottitis can be rapidly fatal.

urachus (ū′-rak-us) *n* stemlike structure connecting the bladder with the umbilicus in the fetus; in postnatal life it is represented by a fibrous cord situated between the apex of the bladder and the umbilicus, known as the median umbilical ligament—**urachal** *adj*.

urate (ū′-rāt) *n* any salt of uric acid; such compounds are present in blood, urine and tophi, or calcareous concretions.

urea (ū-rē′-à) *n* chief nitrogenous end product of protein metabolism; excreted in urine, of which it is the main nitrogenous constituent. Can be given as an osmotic diuretic by intravenous infusion to reduce intracranial and intraocular pressure and topically to moisturize and soften dry, rough skin. *urea clearance test, urea concentration test* urine is collected after administration of oral dose of urea; speed and concentration at which urea appears in urine is a measure of the level at which kidneys are functioning.

Ureaphil™ urea preparation used to produce dehydration in cerebral edema, raised intraocular pressure, and as a diuretic in resistant cases. Has a low potential for sodium retention, thus increases urinary output.

Urecholine™ bethanechol.*

uremia (ūr-ēm′-ē-à) *n* clinical syndrome due to renal failure resulting from either disease of the kidneys themselves, or from disorder or disease elsewhere in the body which induces kidney dysfunction and which results in gross biochemical disturbance, including retention of urea and other nitrogenous substances in blood (azotemia). Depending on cause, it may or may not be reversible. Fully developed syndrome is characterized by nausea, vomiting, headache, hiccough, weakness, dimness of vision, convulsions and coma. → renal—**uremic** *adj*.

uremic snow → uridrosis.

ureter (ūr′-ē-tèr) *n* tube passing from each kidney to the bladder for conveyance of urine (→ Figures 19, 20); length from 25–30 cm—**ureteric, ureteral** *adj*.

ureterectomy (ū-rēt-èr-ek′-to-mē) *n* excision of a ureter.

ureteritis (ū-rēt-èr-ī′-tis) *n* inflammation of a ureter.

ureterocele (ū-rēt'-ėr-ō-sēl) *n* intrusion of lower end of ureter into the bladder; result of ureter expansion from cystic restriction of output.

ureterocolic (ū-rēt'-ėr-ō-kol-ik) *adj* pertaining to the ureter* and colon,* usually indicating anastomosis of the two structures.

ureterocolostomy (ū-rēt'-ėr-ō-kol-os'-to-mē) *n* (*syn* utero-colic anastomosis) surgical transplantation of ureters from bladder to colon so that urine is passed by the bowel; sometimes carried out to relieve strangury in tuberculosis of the bladder, or prior to cystectomy for bladder tumors.

ureteroileal (ū-rēt'-ėr-ō-il'-ē-ȧl) *adj* pertaining to ureters* and ileum,* as the anastomosis necessary in ureteroileostomy (ileal conduit).

ureteroileostomy (ū'-rēt'-ėr-ō-il-ē-os'-to-mē) *n* → ileoureterostomy.

ureterolith (ū-rē'-tėr-ō-lith) *n* a calculus* in the ureter.

ureterolithotomy (ū-rēt'-ėr-ō-lith-ot'-o-mē) *n* surgical removal of a stone from a ureter.

ureterosigmoidostomy (ū-rēt'-ėr-ō-sig-moyd-os'-to-mē) *n* ureterocolostomy.*

ureterostomy (ū-rēt-ėr-os'-to-mē) *n* formation of a permanent fistula through which ureter discharges urine. → cutaneous, ileoureterostomy, rectal bladder.

ureterovaginal (ū-rēt-ėr-ō-vaj'-in-ȧl) *adj* pertaining to the ureter* and vagina.*

ureterovesical (ū-ēt-ėr-ō-ves'-i-kȧl) *adj* pertaining to ureter* and urinary bladder.*

urethra (ū-rēth'-rȧ) *n* passage from the bladder through which urine is excreted (→ Figure 19); in the female it measures 25–40 mm; in the male, 250 cm—**urethral** *adj*.

urethritis (ū-rēth-rī'-tis) *n* inflammation of the urethra. *nonspecific urethritis* → nongonococcal urethritis.

urethrocele (ū-rēth'-rō-sēl) *n* prolapse of the urethra, usually into anterior vaginal wall.

urethrography (ū-rēth-rog'-raf-ē) *n* radiological examination of urethra—**urethrographic** *adj*, **urethrogram** *n*, **urethrograph** *n*.

urethrometry (ū-rēth-rom'-ėt-rē) *n* measurement of urethral lumen using a urethrometer—**urethrometric** *adj*.

urethroplasty (ū-rēth'-rō-plas-tē) *n* any plastic operation on the urethra—**urethroplastic** *adj*.

urethroscope (ū-rēth'-rō-skōp) *n* instrument designed to allow visualization of interior of the urethra—**urethroscopic** *adj*, **urethroscopy** *n*.

urethrostenosis (ū-rēth-rō-sten-ōs'-is) *n* urethral stricture.*

urethrotomy (ū-rēth-rot'-o-mē) *n* incision into the urethra; usually part of an operation for stricture.

urethrotrigonitis (ū-rēth-rō-trig-on-ī'-tis) *n* inflammation of the urinary bladder. → trigone.

URI *abbr* upper respiratory infection.

uric acid acid formed in breakdown of nucleoproteins in tissues, the end product of purine metabolism, and excreted in urine. Relatively insoluble and excessive amounts may give rise to stones. Present in excess in blood in gout and a goutlike syndrome occurring in male infants, manifesting as early as 4 months, with self-destructive behavior, cerebral palsy and mental retardation.

uricosuric (ū-ri-kō-sū'-rik) *adj* enhances renal excretion of uric acid due to impairment of tubular reabsorption. Such substances are used in chronic gout.

uridrosis (ūr-id-rō'-sis) *n* (*syn* uremic snow) excess of urea in sweat; may be deposited on skin as fine white crystals.

urinalysis (ūr-in-ȧl'-is-is) *n* examination of urine.

urinary (ūr'-in-ār-ē) *adj* pertaining to urine. *urinary bladder* a muscular distensible bag situated in the pelvis (→ Figures 16, 19); receives urine from the kidneys via two ureters and stores it until the volume causes reflex evacuation through the urethra. *urinary system* comprises two kidneys, two ureters, one urinary bladder and one urethra. The kidneys filter urine from the blood; ureters convey it to the bladder, where it is stored until conveyed to the exterior by the urethra. → Figures 19, 20. *urinary tract infection* second most prevalent infection in hospitals, but the most common hospital-acquired infection. Occurs most frequently in use of indwelling catheter; most common infecting agent is *Escherichia coli,* suggesting autogenous infection via periurethral route.

urination *n* → micturition.

urine *n* amber-colored fluid excreted from kidneys at the rate of about 1500 ml every 24 h in the adult; slightly acid, with specific gravity of 1.005–1.030.

uriniferous (ūr-in-if'-ér-us) *adj* conveying urine.*

urinogenital (ūr-in-ō-jen'-i-tȧl) *n* → urogenital.

urinometer (ūr-in-om'-ét-ér) *n* instrument for estimating specific gravity of urine.

Urispas™ flavoxate.*

urobilin (ūr-ō-bil'-in) *n* brownish pigment formed by oxidation of urobilinogen and excreted in feces and sometimes found in urine left standing in contact with air.

urobilinogen (ūr-ō-bil-in'-ō-jen) *n* (*syn* stercobilinogen) pigment formed from bilirubin* in the intestine by bacterial action. May be reabsorbed into the circulation and converted back to bilirubin in the liver and re-excreted in bile or urine.

urobilinuria (ūr-ō-bil-in-ūr′-ē-à) *n* presence of increased amounts of urobilin in urine. Evidence of increased production of bilirubin in the liver, as after hemolysis.

urochrome (ūr′-ō-krōm) *n* yellow pigment that gives urine its normal color.

urodynamics (ūr-ō-dī-nam′-iks) *n* use of sophisticated equipment to measure bladder function. Particularly useful in diagnosing cause of urinary incontinence.

Urografin™ contrast medium suitable for urography.

urography (ū-rog′-raf-ē) *n* (*syn* pyelography) radiographic visualization of renal pelvis and ureter by injection of radiopaque liquid, which may be injected into the blood stream, whence excreted by the kidney (intravenous urography), or injected directly into renal pelvis or ureter by way of a fine catheter introduced through a cystoscope (retrograde or ascending urography). *intravenous urography (IVU)* demonstration of urinary tract following intravenous injection of opaque medium—**urographic** *adj*, **urogram** *n*.

urokinase (ūr-ō-kīn′āz) *n* enzyme which dissolves fibrin clot. Used for traumatic and postoperative hyphema.

urology (ūr-ol′-o-jē) *n* science which deals with disorders of female urinary tract and male genitourinary tract—**urological** *adj*, **urologist** *n*.

uropathy (ūr-op′-à-thē) *n* disease in any part of urinary system.

URI *abbr* upper* respiratory infection.

urticaria (ur-ti-kār′-ē-à) *n* (*syn* nettlerash, hives) allergic skin eruption characterized by multiple, circumscribed, smooth, raised, pinkish, itchy weals, developing very suddenly, usually lasting a few days and leaving no visible trace. Common provocative agents in susceptible subjects are ingested foods such as shellfish, injected sera and contact with, or injection of, antibiotics such as penicillin and streptomycin. → angioedema. *factitial urticaria* → dermographia.

uterine tubes (ū′-tèr-in) fallopian tubes.* → Figure 17.

uteroplacental (ū-tèr-ō-pla-sen′-tàl) *adj* pertaining to the uterus* and placenta.*

uterorectal (ū-tèr-ō-rek′-tàl) *adj* pertaining to uterus* and rectum.*

uterosacral (ū-tèr-ō-sā′-kràl) *adj* pertaining to uterus* and sacrum.*

uterosalpingography (ū-tèr-ō-sal-ping-og′-raf-ē) *n* (*syn* hysterosalpingography) radiological examination of uterus and uterine tubes involving retrograde introduction of an opaque medium during fluoroscopy. Used to investigate patency of fallopian tubes.

uterovaginal (ū-tèr-ō-vaj′-in-àl) *adj* pertaining to uterus* and vagina.*

uterovesical (ū-tèr-ō-ves′-ik-àl) *adj* pertaining to uterus* and urinary bladder.*

uterus (ū'-tėr-us) *n* the womb (→ Figure 17); a hollow muscular organ into which the ovum is received through the fallopian tubes and where it is retained during development, and from which the fetus is expelled through the vagina. → bicornuate—**uteri** *pl,* **uterine** *adj.*

utricle (ū'-tri-kl) *n* a little sac or pocket (→ Figure 13).

uvea (ū'-vē-á) *n* pigmented part of the eye, including iris, ciliary body and choroid—**uveal** *adj.*

uveitis (ū-vē-ī'-tis) *n* inflammation of the uvea.*

uvula (ū'-vū-lá) *n* central, taglike structure hanging down from the free edge of the soft palate (→ Figure 14).

uvulectomy (ū-vū-lek'-to-mē) *n* excision of the uvula.

uvulitis (ū-vū-lī'-tis) *n* inflammation of the uvula.

V

vaccination *n* originally described inoculation with discharge from cowpox for protection from smallpox. Now applied to inoculation of any antigenic material to produce active artificial immunity.

vaccines *npl* suspensions or products of infectious agents, used chiefly for producing active immunity. *triple vaccine* protects against diphtheria, tetanus and whooping cough. In addition to these, *quadruple vaccine* protects against poliomyelitis. → Sabin, Salk, TOPV, BCG.

vaccinia (vak-sin′-ē-à) *n* virus used to confer immunity against smallpox. Origins are obscure but it is probably a cowpox-smallpox hybrid—**vaccinial** *adj*.

vacuum extractor **1** instrument used to assist delivery of the fetus. **2** instrument used as a method of abortion.

vagal (vā′-gàl) *adj* pertaining to the vagus* nerve.

vagina (va-jī′-nà) *n* literally, a sheath; the musculomembranous passage extending from the cervix uteri to the vulva (→ Figure 17); measures 75 mm along the anterior wall and 90 mm along the posterior wall—**vaginal** *adj*.

vaginismus (vaj-in-iz′-mus) *n* painful muscular spasm of vaginal walls resulting in dyspareunia or painful coitis.

vaginitis (vaj-in-ī′-tis) *n* inflammation of the vagina. *senile vaginitis* can cause adhesions which may obliterate the vaginal canal. *Trichomonas vaginitis* characterized by an intensely irritating discharge; due to a ciliated protozoon that normally inhabits the bowel. → Trichomonas.

vagolytic (vā-gō-lit′-ik) *adj* that which neutralizes the effect of a stimulated vagus nerve.

vagotomy (vā-got′-o-mē) *n* surgical division of the vagus nerves; done in conjunction with gastroenterostomy in treatment of peptic ulcer or pyloroplasty.

vagus nerve (vā′-gus) the parasympathetic pneumogastric nerve; the 10th cranial nerve, composed of both motor and sensory fibers, with a wide distribution in neck, thorax and abdomen, sending important branches to heart, lungs, stomach—**vagi** *pl*, **vagal** *adj*.

valgus, valga, valgum (val′-gus) *adj* exhibiting angulation away from the midline of the body, e.g., hallux valgus.

valine (vā′-lēn) *n* an essential amino* acid, α-aminoisovalerianic acid.

Valium™ diazepam.*

Valley fever coccidioidomycosis.*

Valsalva maneuver (val-sal'-vă) the maximum intrathoracic pressure achieved by forced expiration against a closed glottis; occurs in such activities as lifting heavy objects or straining at stool; glottis narrows simultaneously with contraction of abdominal muscles.

valve *n* fold of membrane in a passage or tube permitting flow of contents in one direction only—**valvular** *adj*.

valvoplasty (val'-vō-plas-tē) *n* plastic operation on a valve, usually reserved for the heart; to be distinguished from valve replacement or valvotomy—**valvoplastic** *adj*.

valvotomy, valvulotomy (val-vot'-o-mē) *n* incision of a stenotic valve, by custom, referring to the heart, to restore normal function.

valvulitis (val-vū-lī'-tis) *n* inflammation of a valve, particularly in the heart.

Vanceril™ beclomethasone.

Vancocin™ vancomycin.*

vancomycin (van-kō-mī'-sin) *n* antibiotic for overwhelming staphylococcal infections. Natural resistance to vancomycin is rare. Has to be given intravenously. (Vancocin.)

Van den Bergh's test (van'den bergz) estimation of serum bilirubin.* Direct positive reaction (conjugated) occurs in obstructive and hepatic jaundice. Indirect positive reaction (unconjugated) occurs in hemolytic jaundice.

vanillylmandelic acid (van-il'-l-man-del'-ik) *n* metabolite of epinephrine* excreted in urine.

varicella (var-i-sel'-ă) *n* → chickenpox—**varicelliform** *adj*.

varicella zoster hyperimmune globulin (VZIG) blood product which when injected produces immunity to varicella and zoster.

varices (var'-i-sēz) *npl* dilated, tortuous (or varicose) veins. → varicose veins—**varix** *sing*.

varicocele (var'-i-kō-sēl) *n* varicosity of the veins of the spermatic cord.

varicose ulcer (var'-i-kōs) (*syn* gravitational ulcer) indolent type of ulcer* that occurs in the lower third of a leg afflicted with varicose* veins.

varicose veins dilated veins, the valves of which become incompetent so that blood flow may be reversed. Most commonly found in lower limbs, where they can result in a gravitational ulcer; in the rectum, as "rectal varices" (hemorrhoids); and in the lower esophagus, when they are called esophageal varices.

variola (var-ē-ō'-lă) *n* → smallpox.

varioloid (var'-ē-ō-loyd) *n* attack of smallpox modified by previous vaccination.

varix (var'-iks) *n* → varices.

varus, vara, varum (vār′-us) *adj* displaying displacement or angulation towards the midline of the body, e.g., coxa vara.

vas (vas) *n* a vessel. *vas deferens* excretory duct of the testis. *vasa vasorum* minute nutrient vessels of the artery and vein wall—**vasa** *pl*.

vascular (vas′-kū-lår) *adj* supplied with vessels, esp. referring to blood vessels.

vascularization (vas′-kū-lår-īz-ā′-shun) *n* the acquisition of a blood supply; process of becoming vascular.

vasculitis (vas-kū-lī′-tis) *n* (*syn* angiitis) inflammation of a blood vessel.

vasculotoxic (vas′-kū-lō-toks′-ik) *adj* any substance which brings about harmful changes in blood vessels.

vasectomy (va-sek′-to-mē) *n* surgical excision of part of the vas deferens, usually for sterilization.

vasoconstrictor (vaz-ō-kon-strik′-tor) *n* any agent which causes a narrowing of the lumen of blood vessels.

Vasodilan™ isoxuprine.*

vasodilator (vaz-ō-dī′-lā-tor) *n* any agent which causes a widening of the lumen of blood vessels.

vasoepididymostomy (vaz′-ō-ep-i-did-ē-mos′-to-mē) *n* anastomosis of vas deferens to the epididymis.

vasomotor nerves (vaz-ō-mō′-tor) nerves which cause changes in the caliber of the blood vessels, usually constriction.

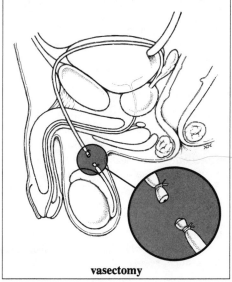

vasectomy

vasopressin (vaz-ō-pres′-in) *n* formed in the hypothalamus. Passes down nerves in the pituitary stalk to be stored in posterior lobe of the pituitary gland; the antidiuretic hormone (ADH). A synthetic preparation is available—pitressin, which can be given intranasally or by injection in diabetes insipidus.

vasopressor (vaz-ō-pres′-or) *n* a drug that increases blood pressure usually, but not always, by vasoconstriction of arterioles.

vasospasm (vaz′-ō-spazm) *n* constructing spasm vessel walls—**vasospastic** *adj*.

vasovagal attack (vaz-ō-vā'-gȧl) faintness, pallor, sweating, feeling of fullness in epigastrium. When part of the postgastrectomy* syndrome it occurs a few minutes after a meal.

Vasoxyl™ methoxamine.*

vastus muscles (vas'-tus) → Figure 4.

V-Cillin™ penicillin* V.

vector *n* a carrier of disease.

vegetations *npl* growths or accretions composed of fibrin and platelets occurring on the edge of the cardiac valves in endocarditis.

vehicle *n* inert substance in which a drug is administered, e.g., water in mixtures.

vein *n* a vessel conveying blood from capillaries back to the heart; has same three coats as an artery, the inner one being fitted with valves—**venous** *adj*.

Velban™ vinblastine.*

Velosef™ cephradine.*

vena cava (vē'-nȧ kā'-vȧ) → Figure 8.

venepuncture (vē'-ne-pungk'-tūr) *n* insertion of a needle into a vein.

venereal (ven-ėr'-ē-ȧl) *adj* pertaining to or caused by sexual intercourse. *venereal disease* → sexually-transmitted disease.

venesection (vē'-nė-sek'-shun) *n* (*syn* phlebotomy) clinical procedure, formerly by opening the cubital vein with a scalpel (now usually by venepuncture), whereby blood volume is reduced in congestive heart failure.

venoclysis (vē-nō-klī'-sis) *n* introduction of nutrient or medicinal fluids into a vein.

venography (vē-nog'-raf-ē) *n* (*syn* phlebography) radiological examination of venous system involving injection of an opaque medium—**venographic** *adj*, **venogram** *n*, **venograph** *n*.

venom *n* poisonous fluid produced by some scorpions, snakes and spiders.

venotomy (vē-not'-o-mē) *n* incision of a vein. → venesection.

venous (vē'-nus) *adj* pertaining to the veins.

ventilators *npl* apparatuses for providing assisted ventilation. Controls provide range from intermittent positive pressure to intermittent mandatory ventilation or even to continuous positive airways pressure.

Ventolin™ albuterol.*

ventral (ven'-trȧl) *adj* pertaining to the abdomen or the anterior surface of the body.

ventricle (ven'-tri-kl) *n* a small bellylike cavity. *ventricle of the brain* four cavities filled with cerebrospinal fluid within the brain. *ventricle of the heart* the two lower muscular chambers of the heart (→ Figure 8)—**ventricular** *adj*.

ventricular puncture (ven-trik'-ū-lár) highly skilled method of puncturing a cerebral ventricle for a sample of cerebrospinal fluid.

ventriculocysternostomy (ven-trik'-ū-lō-sis-tèrn-os'-to-mē) *n* artificial communication between cerebral ventricles and subarachnoid space. One of the drainage operations for hydrocephalus.

ventriculoscope (ven-trik'-ū-lō-skōp) *n* instrument via which cerebral ventricles can be examined—**ventriculoscopic** *adj*.

ventriculostomy (ven-trik'-ū-los'-to-mē) *n* artificial opening into a ventricle. Usually refers to a drainage operation for hydrocephalus.

ventrosuspension *n* fixation of a displaced uterus to anterior abdominal wall.

venule (ven'-ūl) *n* **1** a small vein. **2** a syringelike apparatus for collecting blood from a vein.

verapamil (ver-áp-am'-il) *n* synthetic drug with quinidinelike action on the myocardium. Useful for angina of effort. (Calan, Isoptin.)

vermicide (vèr'-mi-sīd) *n* agent which kills intestinal worms—**vermicidal** *adj*.

vermiform (vèr'-mi-form) *adj* wormlike. *vermiform appendix* the vestigial, hollow, wormlike structure attached to the cecum.

vermifuge (vèr'-mi-fūj) *n* agent which expels intestinal worms.

Vermox™ mebendazole.*

vernix caseosa (vèr'-niks kās-ē-ōs'-à) fatty substance which covers skin of the fetus at birth and keeps it from becoming sodden by the liquor amnii.

verruca (vè-roo'-kà) *n* wart. → condyloma. *verruca necrogenica* (postmortem wart) develops as result of accidental inoculation with tuberculosis while carrying out a postmortem. *verruca plana* the common, multiple, flat, tiny warts often seen on children's hands, knees and face. *verruca plantaris* a flat wart on the sole of the foot. Highly contagious. *verruca seborrheica* (*syn* basal cell papilloma) brown, greasy wart seen in seborrheic subjects, commonly on chest or back, which increase with aging. *verruca vulgaris* common wart of the hands or feet, of brownish color and rough pitted surface, caused by the human papillomavirus—**verrucae** *pl*, **verrucous, verrucose** *adj*.

version *n* turning—applied to the maneuver to alter the position of the fetus *in utero*. *cephalic version* turning the child so that head presents. *external cephalic version (ECV)* conversion of a transverse into a head presentation to facilitate labor. Technique is safer with use of ultrasound and tachographic monitoring. *internal version* turning the child by one hand in the uterus, and the other on patient's abdomen. *podalic version* turning the child to a breech presentation; may be external or internal.

vertebra (vėr'-te-brȧ) *n* one of the irregular bones making up the spinal column—**vertebrae** *pl,* **vertebral** *adj.*

vertebral column (vėr'-te-brȧl) (*syn* spinal column) made up of 33 vertebrae, articulating with the skull above and the pelvic girdle below. Vertebrae are so shaped that they enclose a cavity (spinal* canal, neural canal) which houses the spinal* cord. There is more low back pain and sciatica in people who have a narrow spinal canal.

vertebrobasilar insufficiency(VBI) (vėr'-te-brō-bās'-i-lȧr) syndrome caused by lack of blood to the hindbrain. May be progressive, episodic or both. Clinical manifestations include giddiness and vertigo, nausea, ataxia, drop* attacks and signs of cerebellar disorder such as nystagmus.

vertex *n* the top of the head.

vertigo (vėr'-ti-gō) *n* giddiness, dizziness—**vertiginous** *adj.*

vesical (ves'-i-kȧl) *adj* pertaining to urinary bladder.

vesicant (ves'-i-kant) *n* a blistering substance.

vesicle (ves'-i-kl) *n* **1** a small bladder, cell or hollow structure. **2** a skin blister—**vesicular** *adj,* **vesiculation** *n.*

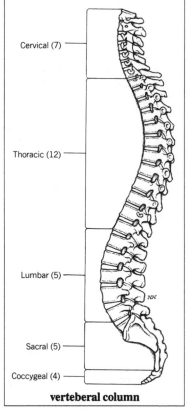

Cervical (7)

Thoracic (12)

Lumbar (5)

Sacral (5)

Coccygeal (4)

verteberal column

vesicostomy (ves-i-kos'-to-mē) *n* → cystostomy.

vesicoureteral (ves'-i-kō-ū-rē-tėr'-ȧl) *adj* pertaining to urinary bladder* and ureter.* Vesicoureteric reflux can cause pyelonephritis.

vesicovaginal (ves-i-kō-vaj'-i-nȧl) *adj* pertaining to urinary bladder* and vagina.*

vesiculitis (ves-ik'-ū-lī'-tis) *n* inflammation of a vesicle, particularly seminal vesicles.

vesiculopapular (ves-ik'-ū-lō-pap'-ū-lȧr) *adj* pertaining to or exhibiting both vesicles and papules.

vessel *n* a tube, duct or canal, holding or conveying fluid, esp. blood and lymph.

vestibule (ves'-ti-būl) *n* **1** middle part of the internal ear, lying between the semicircular canals and the cochlea (→ Figure 13). **2** triangular area between the labia minora—**vestibular** *adj*.

viable (vī'-à-bl) *adj* capable of living a separate existence—**viability** *n*.

Vibramycin™ doxycycline.*

vibration syndrome (*syn* Raynaud's phenomenon) impotency and paralysis of arms and hands in workers using vibrating machines.

Vibrio (vib'-rē-ō) *n* genus of curved, motile microorganisms. *V. cholerae*, or the comma vibrio, causes cholera.

Videx™ didanosine.*

villus (vil'-us) *n* microscopic fingerlike projection; found in mucous membrane of the small intestine or on the outside of the chorion of the embryonic sac—**villi** *pl*, **villous** *adj*.

vinblastine (vin-blas'-tēn) *n* alkaloid from periwinkle; antimitotic used mainly in Hodgkin's disease and choriocarcinoma resistant to other therapy. Given intravenously. (Velan.)

Vincent's angina (vin'-sents an-jī'-nà) infection of mouth or throat by spirochete and a bacillus in synergism. To be differentiated from Ludwig's angina.

vincristine (vin-kris'-tēn) *n* antileukemic drug. Derived from an extract of periwinkle plant. Given intravenously. (Oncovin.)

viral hemorrhagic fevers fevers that occur mainly in the tropics; often transmitted by mosquitoes or ticks. Usually with a petechial skin rash. Examples are Ebola, dengue, Lassa fever, Marburg disease, Rift valley fever and yellow fever.

viral hepatitis → hepatitis.

viremia (vī-rē'-mē-à) *n* presence of virus in blood *maternal viremia* can cause fetal damage—**viremic,** *adj*.

viricidal (vī-ri-sī'-dàl) *adj* lethal to a virus—**viricide** *n*.

virilism (vir'-il-ism) *n* appearance of secondary male characteristics in the female.

virology (vī-rol'-o-jē) *n* study of viruses and the diseases caused by them—**virological** *adj*.

virulence (vir'-ū-lens) *n* infectiousness; the disease-producing power of a microorganism; the power of a microorganism to overcome host resistance—**virulent** *adj*.

virus *n* small microorganism parasitic within living cells. Viruses differ from bacteria in having only one kind of nucleic acid, either DNA or RNA; in lacking apparatus necessary for energy production and protein synthesis; and by reproducing (replicating) by independent synthesis and assembly of their component parts. Cause many acute and chronic diseases in man. Some of the more important groups are: (a) *pox-viruses,* as smallpox, molluscum contagiosum, (b) *herpes viruses,* as herpes simplex virus, cytomegalovirus, varicella-zoster virus, Epstein-Barr virus, (c) *adenoviruses,* (d) *papillomaviruses,* as polyoma virus, which can cause tumors in laboratory animals, (e) *reoviruses,* as rotaviruses, (f) *toga-viruses,* as yellow fever virus, (g) *picornaviruses,* (h) *myxoviruses,* (i) *para-myxoviruses,* (j) *rhabdo-viruses,* as rabies virus, (k) *coronaviruses,* as some

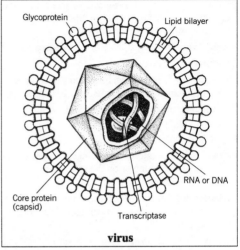

virus

common cold viruses, (l) *arenaviruses,* as Lassa fever virus. Groups a–d are DNA viruses, groups e–l are RNA viruses. Those viruses which are spread by arthropods—insects and ticks—are known as arboviruses, these include reoviruses, togaviruses and rhabdoviruses.

viscera (vis'-ėr-à) *npl* the internal organs—**viscus** *sing,* **visceral** *adj*.

visceroptosis (vis-ėr-op-tō'-sis) *n* downward displacement or falling of the abdominal organs.

viscid (vis'-id) *adj* sticky, glutinous, mainly used to describe sputum.

Vistaril™ hydroxyzine.*

visual *adj* pertaining to vision. *visual acuity* → acuity. *visual field* area within which objects can be seen. *visual purple* purple pigment in the retina of the eye, which is called rhodopsin.

vital capacity amount of air expelled from the lungs after a deep inspiration. → forced vital capacity.

vitalograph (vī-tal'-ō-graf) *n* apparatus for measuring the forced* vital capacity.

vitamin *n* essential food factor, chemical in nature, present in certain foodstuffs; some vitamins synthesized commercially. Absence causes deficiency diseases.

vitamin A (*syn* retinol) fat-soluble anti-infective substance present in all animal fats. In its provitamin form, β carotene, present in carrots, cabbage, lettuce, tomatoes and other fruits and vegetables; in the body converted into retinol. Essential for healthy skin and mucous membranes; aids night vision. Deficiency can result in stunted growth, night blindness and xerophthalmia, and is an important cause of blindness in certain parts of the world, e.g., India.

vitamin B refers to any one of a group of water-soluble vitamins—the vitamin B complex, all chemically related and often occurring in the same foods. → biotin, cyanocobalamin, folic acid, nicotinic acid, pantothenic acid, pyridoxine, riboflavine, thiamine.

vitamin B1 thiamine.*

vitamin B2 riboflavine.*

vitamin B6 pyridoxine.*

vitamin B12 cyanocobalamin.*

vitamin C ascorbic* acid.

vitamin D fat-soluble vitamin with two main forms: ergocalciferol (vitamin D_2, calciferol*) and cholecalciferol (vitamin D_3); production of both is dependent on UVR acting on two different sterols. Good sources are oily fish and dairy produce. *vitamin D resistant rickets* → rickets.

vitamin E group of chemically related compounds known as tocopherols.* Intracellular fat-soluble antioxidant, maintaining stability of polyunsaturated fatty acids and other fatlike substances. It is thought that deficiency results in muscle degeneration, hemolytic blood disease, and is associated with the aging process. *vitamin E deficiency syndrome* occurs in small infants, less than 2 kg and under 35 weeks gestation. Diagnosis at between 6 and 11 weeks reveals low hemoglobin and reticulocytosis; good response to vitamin E including a rise in hemoglobin and loss of edema. Condition is aggravated by giving iron. Deficiency in older children results in cerebellar* ataxia and is associated with abetalipoproteinemia.

vitamin K menadiol,* phytomenadione.* *vitamin K test* after injection of vitamin K, serum prothrombin rises in obstructive jaundice, but remains depressed in toxic jaundice.

vitiligo (vit-i-lī'-gō) *n* skin disease of probable autoimmune origin characterized by areas of complete loss of pigment.

vitrectomy (vit-rek'-to-mē) *n* surgical removal of vitreous humor from the vitreous chamber.

vitreous (vit'-rē-us) *adj* glassy. *vitreous chamber* cavity inside the eyeball and behind the lens. *vitreous humor* jellylike substance contained in the vitreous chamber. (→ Figure 15).

Vivactil™ protriptyline.*

vocal cords membranous folds stretched anteroposteriorly across the larynx. Sound is produced by their vibration as air from the lungs passes between them.

volition *n* the will to act—**volitional** *adj.*

Volkmann's ischemic contracture (vŏlk'-manz) flexion deformity of wrist and fingers from fixed contracture of flexor muscles in the forearm. Cause is ischemia of the muscles by injury or obstruction to brachial artery, near the elbow.

voluntary *adj* under control of the will; free and unrestricted; as opposed to reflex or involuntary.

volvulus (vol'-vū-lus) *n* twisting of a section of bowel, so as to occlude the lumen; a cause of intestinal obstruction.

vomit *n vt, vi* ejection of stomach contents through the mouth.

vomiting of pregnancy → hyperemesis.

vomitus (vom'-it-us) *n* vomited matter.

von Willebrand's disease (von vil'-e-brandz) inherited bleeding disease due to deficiencies relating to factor VIII proteins in plasma. Inheritance is autosomal dominant, affecting both sexes, and is essentially a disorder of the primary hemostatic mechanism with deranged platelet-endothelial cell interaction. In severe cases von Willebrand's disease results in a clotting defect resembling hemophilia.*

vulva (vul'-và) *n* external genitalia of the female—**vulval** *adj.*

vulvectomy (vul-vek'-to-mē) *n* excision of the vulva.

vulvitis (vul-vī'-tis) *n* inflammation of the vulva.

vulvovaginal (vul-vō-vaj'-in-àl) *adj* pertaining to the vulva* and the vagina.*

vulvovaginitis (vul-vō-vaj-in-ī'-tis) *n* inflammation of the vulva and vagina.

W

Waldeyer's ring (val'-dī-erz) a lymphatic circle surrounding the pharynx.

warfarin (wawr'-fār-in) *n* the oral anticoagulant of choice. Coumarin derivative. (Coumadin.)

wart *n* → verruca. *venereal warts, genital warts* moist pink or red growths, often in groups, caused by human papillomavirus (HPV). Preferred site is genital or anal area; often acquired in sexual contact. These warts are associated with subsequent dysplastic changes in tissue and development of cancer. Treatment and follow-up are necessary.

Wasserman test (wos'-êr-man) for diagnosis of syphilis; a complement-fixation test and not entirely specific. → TPI test.

Waterhouse-Friderichsen syndrome (wot'-er-hows–frid-er-ik'-sen) shock with widespread skin hemorrhages occurring in meningitis, esp. meningococcal. There is bleeding in the adrenal glands.

WBC *abbr* white blood cell or corpuscle. → blood.

weal (wēl) *n* a superficial swelling, characteristic of urticaria, nettle stings, etc.

Weber's test (web'-êrz) tuning fork test for diagnosis of deafness.

Wegener's granulomatosis inflammation of upper and lower respiratory tract, with progressive formation of granulomatous tissue and necrosis. Cause unknown; treatment with immunosuppressive drugs is successful if begun early.

Weil-Felix test (vīl–fē'-liks) agglutination reaction used in diagnosis of the typhus group of fevers. Patient's serum is titrated against a heterologous antigen.

Weil's disease (vīlz) spirochetosis icterohemorrhagica, type of jaundice with fever caused by a leptospire voided in urine of rats. A disease of miners, sewer workers, etc., who work in dirty water.

wen *n* → sebaceous.

Wharton's jelly (war'-tunz) jellylike substance contained in the umbilical cord.

whiplash *n* injury through rapid acceleration of the head, with hyperextension of muscles and ligaments supporting cervical spine. Site of damage usually at third and fourth cervical vertebrae; painful and slow to heal.

Whipple's disease uncommon but serious inflammatory disease affecting joints and organs but always causing great damage to intestinal mucosa; with anemia, skin pigmentation, joint pain and severe malabsorption. Fatal if untreated (with prolonged antibiotic regimen) and recovery is slow.

whipworm *n Trichuris trichiura,* roundworm which infests the intestine of man in the humid tropics. Eggs are excreted in stools. Worms do not normally produce symptoms, but heavy infestations of over 1000 worms cause bloody diarrhea, anemia and prolapse of the rectum. Treatment is unsatisfactory but thiabendazole has cleared infestation in about 50% of patients treated.

white fluids emulsions of tar acids and phenols in water, widely used for general disinfectant purposes.

white leg thrombophlebitis* occurring in women after childbirth.

White's tar paste zinc paste with the addition of about 6% coal tar. Valuable in infantile eczema.

whitlow (wit'-lō) *n* → paronychia.

WHO *abbr* World Health Organization.

whole gut irrigation → total colonic lavage.

whooping cough → pertussis.

Widal test (vē-dal') agglutination reaction for typhoid fever. Patient's serum is put in contact with *Salmonella typhi;* result is positive if agglutination occurs, proving presence of antibodies in serum.

Wilms' tumor (vilmz) commonest abdominal tumor of childhood, and one which usually affects the kidneys. Usually diagnosed during the preschool period. Prognosis is uncertain and depends on the stage of the tumor and child's age at onset of diagnosis and treatment.

Wilson's disease hepaticolenticular degeneration with choreic movements. Due to disturbance of copper metabolism. No urinary catecholamine excretion. Associated with mental subnormality. Can be treated with BAL and penicillamine. Asymptomatic relatives can be given prophylactic penicillamine.

window (oval and round) → Figure 13.

windpipe *n* → trachea.

wintergreen *n* → methylsalicylate.

womb *n* the uterus.*

Wood's light ultraviolet light used for detection of ringworm.

woolsorters' disease → anthrax.

worms *npl* → ascarides, taenia, *Trichuris.*

wound *n* most commonly used when referring to injury to skin or underlying tissues of organs by a blow, cut, missile or stab. Also includes injury to skin caused by chemicals, cold, friction, heat, pressure and rays; and manifestation in skin of internal conditions, e.g., pressure sores and ulcers.

wound drains most commonly used in abdominal wounds. May be inserted as a therapeutic measure, as to drain an abscess, or to prevent complications (prophylaxis). Drainage is active where the drain is attached to suction apparatus producing a "closed wound suction." A passive drain provides a path of least resistance to the skin and exudate seeps into a surgical dressing; this system provides a route for bacteria to enter the body. → healing.

wound dressings (*syn* surgical dressings) previously they absorbed exudate from the wound, which dried, so that when separated from the wound some newly formed tissue was removed. It has been demonstrated conclusively that wounds heal more quickly in a moist environment than in a dry one. Modern dressings aim to be permeable to water vapor and gases but not to bacteria or liquids; this retains serous exudate, which is actively bactericidal. They do not adhere to wound surface and on removal do not damage new tissue.

wrist *n* the carpus (→ Figure 3). *wrist drop* paralysis of the muscles which raise the wrist because of damage to the radial nerve.

wryneck *n* → torticollis.

Wycillin™ penicillin* G.

Wydase™ hyaluronidase.*

X

Xanax™ alprazolam.*

xanthelasma (zan-thel-az′-mà) *n* a variety of xanthoma. *xanthelasma* palpebrarum small yellowish plaques appear on the eyelids.

xanthine (zan′-thēn) *n* 2,6-dioxypurine found in liver, muscle, pancreas and urine. Some derivatives are diuretic. Present in some renal calculi and possesses stimulant properties to muscle tissue, esp. the heart.

xanthinuria (zan-then-ūr′-ē-à) *n* rare hereditary disorder in man in which xanthine oxidase enzyme is lacking, resulting in excessive urinary xanthine and hypoxanthine in place of uric acid.

xanthoma (zan-thō′-mà) *n* collection of cholesterol under the skin producing a yellow discoloration—**xanthomata** *pl*.

Xenopsylla (zen-op-sil′-à) *n* genus of fleas. *X. cheopis* is the rat flea that transmits bubonic plague.

xeroderma, xerodermia (zē-rō-dér′-mà) *n* dryness of the skin → ichthyosis. *xeroderma pigmentosum* (*syn* Kaposi's disease) a familial dermatosis probably caused by failure of normal skin repair following ultraviolet damage. Pathological freckle formation (ephelides*) may give rise to keratosis, neoplastic growth and a fatal termination.

xerophthalmia (zē-rōf-thal′-mē-à) *n* dryness and ulceration of the cornea which may lead to blindness. Associated with lack of vitamin A.

xerosis (zē-rō′-sis) *n* dryness. *xerosis conjunctivae* → Bitot's spots.

xerostomia (zē-rō-stō′-mē-à) *n* dry mouth.

xiphoid process (zī′-foyd) lower tip of the sternum.

X-linked *adj* → sex-linked.

X-rays *npl* short wavelength, penetrating rays of electromagnetic spectrum, produced by electrical equipment. Word is popularly used to mean radiographs.*

Xylocaine™ lidocaine.*

xylometazoline (zī-lō-me-taz′-ō-lēn) *n* nasal vasoconstrictor; gives quick relief but action is short; danger of rebound congestion after repeated use. (Neo-Synephrine.)

xylose (zī′-lōs) *n* wood sugar.

xylose test more convenient than fat balance and equally accurate. Xylose is given orally and its urinary excretion is measured. Normally 25% of loading dose is excreted. Less than this indicates malabsorption syndrome.

XXY syndrome Klinefelter* syndrome.

Y

yaws *n* tropical disease which resembles syphilis so closely that they may be one and the same disease but modified by differences of climate, social habit and hygiene. Pinta (S. America) and bejel (Transjordan) may be similar variants. All these diseases are caused by an identical spirochete and produce a positive Wassermann test in blood. Only syphilis is a sexually-transmitted disease. General term for the group is "treponematosis."

yellow fever acute febrile illness of tropical areas, caused by a group B arbovirus and spread by a mosquito (*Aedes aegypti*). Characteristic features are jaundice, black vomit and anuria. An attenuated virus variant known as 17D is prepared as vaccine for immunization.

Yersinia (yer-sin'-ē-à) *n* newly named genus of the family Enterobacteriaceae; comprises several species previously within the genus *Pasteurella*,* including *Y. pestis*, the plague bacillus.

Z

Zantac™ ranitidine.*

Zarontin™ ethosuximide.*

Zaroxolyn™ metolazone.*

Zinacef™ cefuroxime.*

zinc (zingk) *n* trace element; an essential part of many enzymes. Zinc absorption is reduced by alcohol and the contraceptive pill. Deficiency in zinc is associated with anemia, short stature, hypogonadism, impaired wound healing and geophagia.* Zinc salts have many topical applications (e.g., astringents, antiseptics and deodorants) but when absorbed are often poisonous, causing chronic symptoms resembling those produced by lead. *zinc oxide* widely used mild astringent, present in calamine lotion and cream. Lassar's paste, Unna's paste and many other dermatological applications. *zinc peroxide* white powder with antiseptic action similar to that of hydrogen* peroxide, but slower and prolonged in action. Used as ointment, lotion and mouthwash. *zinc stearate* mild astringent used as a dusting powder in eczematous conditions.

Zoladex™ goserelin.*

Zollinger-Ellison syndrome (zol'-in-ger—el'-i-son) presence of ulcerogenic tumor of the pancreatic islets of Langerhans, hypersecretion of gastric acid, fulminating ulceration of esophagus, stomach, duodenum and jejunum. Frequently accompanied by diarrhea. Diagnosed by gastric secretion and blood gastrin studies.

zona (zō'-nà) *n* a zone; a girdle; herpes zoster. *zona pellucida* vitelline membrane surrounding the ovum.

zonula ciliaris (zōn'-ū-là sil-ē-ār'-is) suspensory ligament attaching periphery of the lens of the eye to ciliary body.

zonule (zōn'-ūl) *n* small zone, belt or girdle. Zonula.

zonulolysis (zōn-ū-lol'is-is) *n* breaking down the zonula ciliaris, sometimes necessary before intracapsular extraction of the lens—**zonulolytic** *adj*.

zoonosis (zō-on-ōs'-is) *n* disease in man transmitted from animal. Farm workers are at risk—**zoonoses** *pl*.

Zovirax™ acyclovir.*

zygoma (zī-gō'-mà) *n* the cheekbone—**zygomatic** *adj*.

zygote (zī′-gōt) *n* the fertilized ovum. The diploid* cell derived from fusion after fertilization of two gametes, ova and sperm, each of which carries a haploid* chromosome complement.

Zyloprim™ allopurinal.*

zymogen (zī′-mō-jen) *n* inactive precursor of an active enzyme which is converted to active form by the action of acid, another enzyme or by other means.

Appendices

Appendices

Appendix 1
Illustrations of
Major Body Systems

Acknowledgments
Figures 1, 2, 3, 4, 5, 8, 11, 13, 14, 15, 18, 19, and 20 from the Royal Society of Medicine
Family Medical Guide, Longman

Figures 6, 7, 9, 10, 12, 16, and 17 from Wilson KJW: Ross & Wilson's Foundations of
Anatomy and Physiology, 5th ed Churchill Livingstone, Edinburgh, 1981.

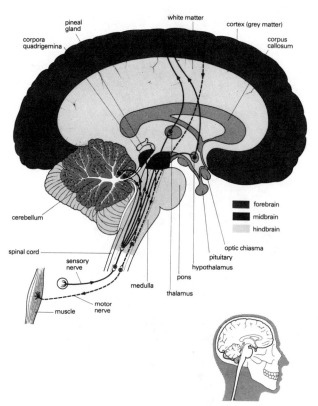

Figure 1 Brain – midline section

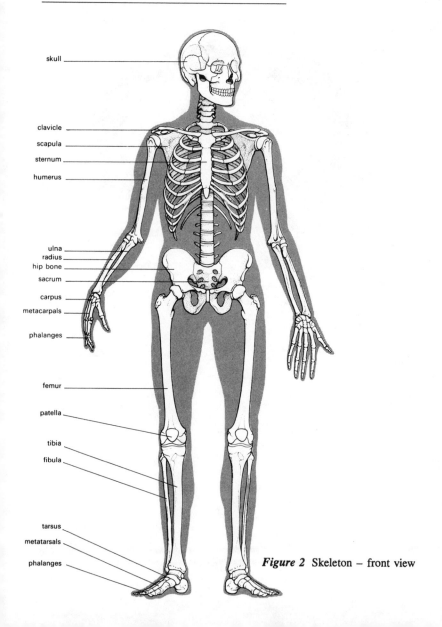

skull

clavicle
scapula
sternum
humerus

ulna
radius
hip bone
sacrum
carpus
metacarpals

phalanges

femur

patella

tibia
fibula

tarsus
metatarsals
phalanges

Figure 2 Skeleton – front view

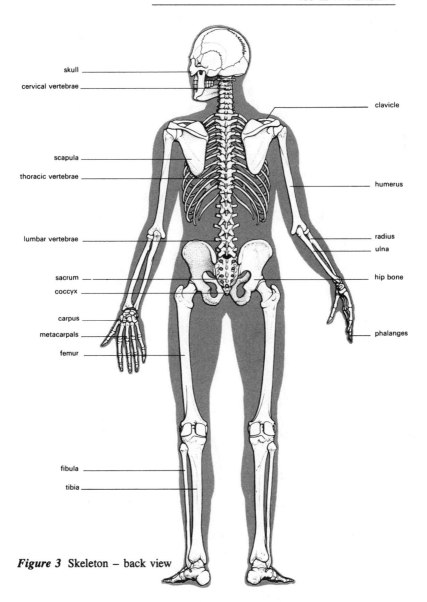

skull

cervical vertebrae

clavicle

scapula

thoracic vertebrae

humerus

lumbar vertebrae

radius

ulna

sacrum

hip bone

coccyx

carpus

metacarpals

phalanges

femur

fibula

tibia

Figure 3 Skeleton – back view

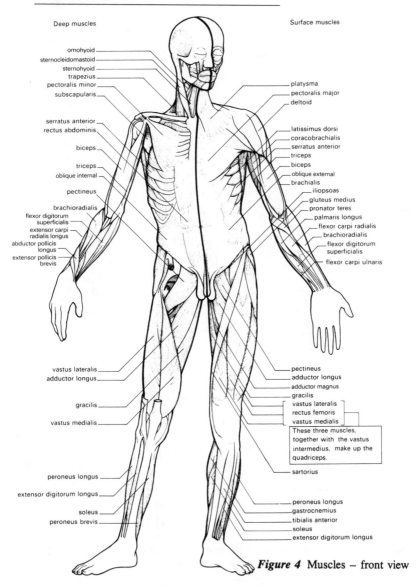

Deep muscles

Surface muscles

omohyoid
sternocleidomastoid
sternohyoid
trapezius
pectoralis minor
subscapularis

serratus anterior
rectus abdominis

biceps

triceps
oblique internal

pectineus

brachioradialis
flexor digitorum
superficialis
extensor carpi
radialis longus
abductor pollicis
longus
extensor pollicis
brevis

platysma
pectoralis major
deltoid

latissimus dorsi
coracobrachialis
serratus anterior
triceps
biceps
oblique external
brachialis
iliopsoas
gluteus medius
pronator teres
palmaris longus
flexor carpi radialis
brachioradialis
flexor digitorum
superficialis
flexor carpi ulnaris

vastus lateralis
adductor longus

gracilis

vastus medialis

pectineus
adductor longus
adductor magnus
gracilis
vastus lateralis
rectus femoris
vastus medialis

These three muscles,
together with the vastus
intermedius, make up the
quadriceps.

sartorius

peroneus longus

extensor digitorum longus

soleus
peroneus brevis

peroneus longus
gastrocnemius
tibialis anterior
soleus
extensor digitorum longus

Figure 4 Muscles – front view

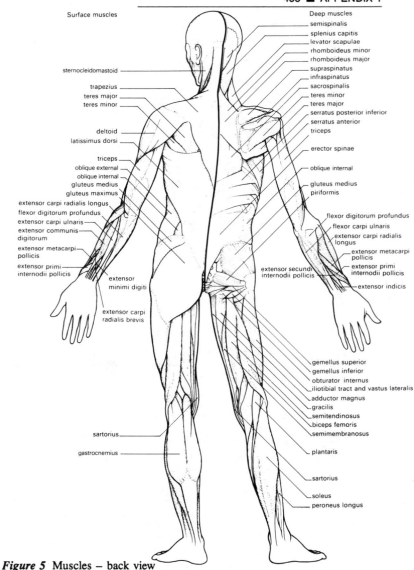

Figure 5 Muscles – back view

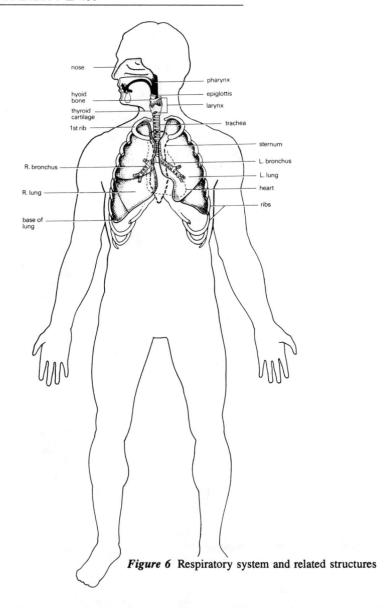

Figure 6 Respiratory system and related structures

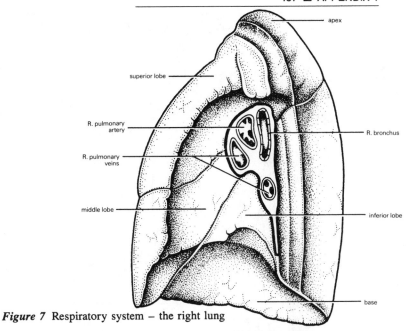

Figure 7 Respiratory system – the right lung

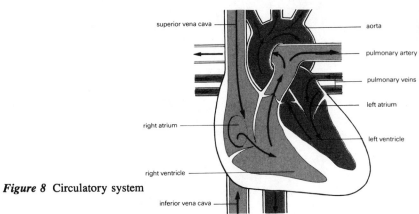

Figure 8 Circulatory system

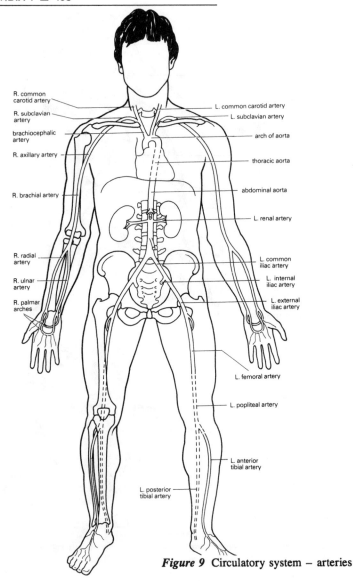

R. common carotid artery
R. subclavian artery
brachiocephalic artery
R. axillary artery
R. brachial artery
R. radial artery
R. ulnar artery
R. palmar arches

L. common carotid artery
L. subclavian artery
arch of aorta
thoracic aorta
abdominal aorta
L. renal artery
L. common iliac artery
L. internal iliac artery
L. external iliac artery
L. femoral artery
L. popliteal artery
L. anterior tibial artery
L. posterior tibial artery

Figure 9 Circulatory system – arteries

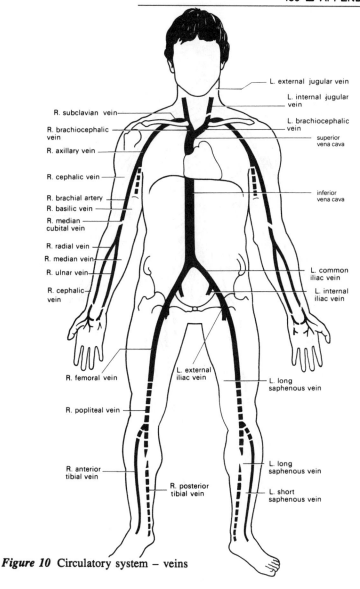

Figure 10 Circulatory system – veins

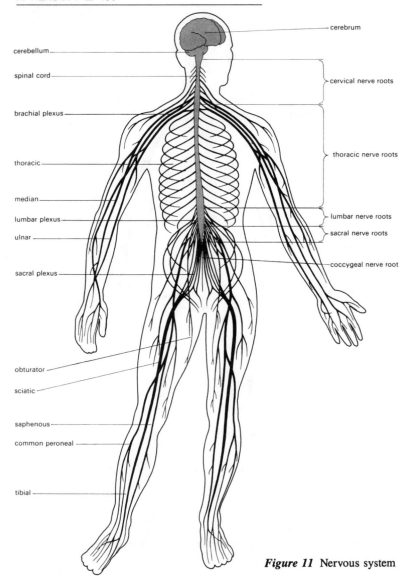

Figure 11 Nervous system

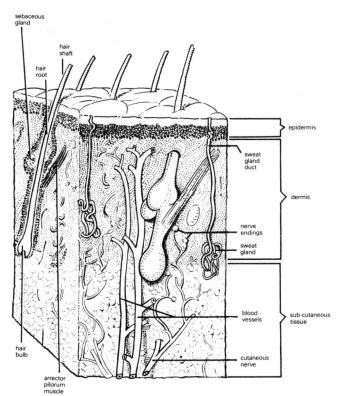

Figure 12 Skin

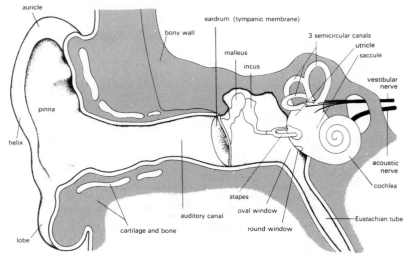

Figure 13 Ear

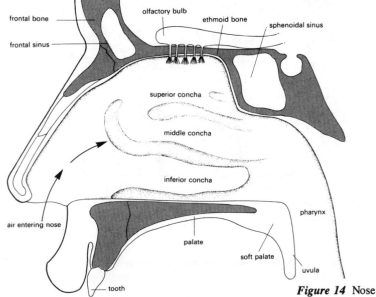

Figure 14 Nose

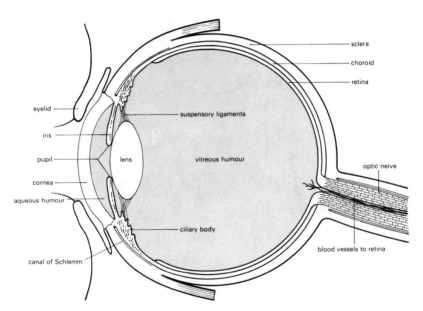

Figure 15 Eye

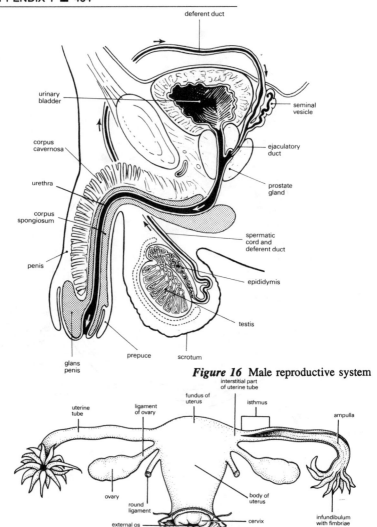

Figure 16 Male reproductive system

Figure 17 Female reproductive system

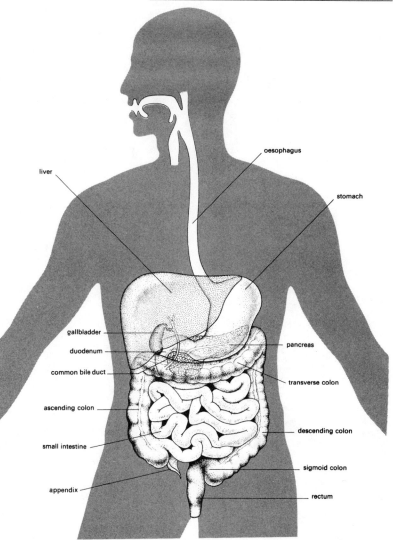

Figure 18 Digestive system

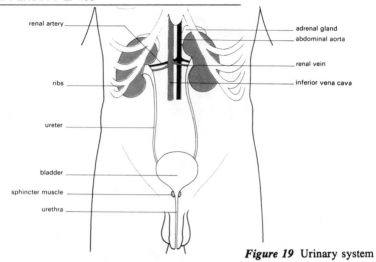

renal artery

adrenal gland
abdominal aorta

renal vein

ribs

inferior vena cava

ureter

bladder

sphincter muscle

urethra

Figure 19 Urinary system

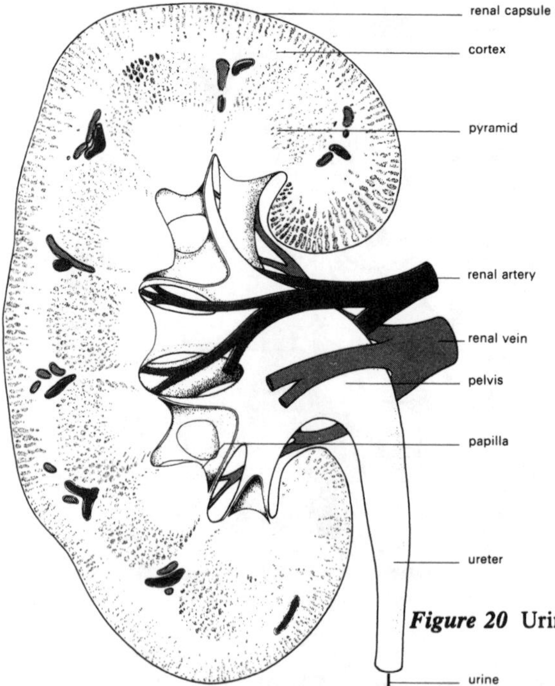

renal capsule

cortex

pyramid

renal artery

renal vein

pelvis

papilla

ureter

Figure 20 Urinary system – the kidney

urine

Appendix 2
SI Units and
the Metric System

Système International (SI) Units

At an international convention in 1960, the General Conference of Weights and Measures agreed to promulgate an International System of Units, frequently described as SI or Système International. This is merely the name for the current version of the metric system, first introduced in France at the end of the 18th century.

In any system of measurement, the magnitude of some physical quantities must be arbitrarily selected and declared to have unit value. These magnitudes form a set of standards and are called *basic units*. All other units are *derived units*.

Basic units
The SI has seven basic units.

Name of SI units	Symbol for SI unit	Quantity
meter	m	length
kilogram	kg	mass
second	s	time
mole	mol	amount of substance
ampere	A	electric current
kelvin	°K	thermodynamic temperature
candela	cd	luminous intensity

Derived units
Derived units are obtained by appropriate combinations of basic units:
– unit area results when unit length is multiplied by unit width
– unit density results when unit weight (mass) is divided by unit volume

Name of SI units	Symbol for SI unit	Quantity
joule	J	work, energy, quantity of heat
pascal	Pa	pressure
newton	N	force

Decimal multiples and submultiples

The metric system uses multiples of 10 to express number.

Multiples and submultiples of the basic unit are expressed as decimals and the following prefixes are used:

Multiples and sub-multiples of units

1 000 000 000 000	10^{12}	tera	T
1 000 000 000	10^{9}	giga	G
1 000 000	10^{6}	mega	M
1 000	10^{3}	kilo	k
100	10^{2}	hecto	h
10	10^{1}	deca	da
0.1	10^{-1}	deci	d
0.01	10^{-2}	centi	c
0.001	10^{-3}	milli	m
0.000 001	10^{-6}	micro	μ
0.000 000 001	10^{-9}	nano	n
0.000 000 000 001	10^{-12}	pico	p
0.000 000 000 000 001	10^{-15}	femto	f
0.000 000 000 000 000 001	10^{-18}	atto	a

Rules for using units

a.   The symbol for a unit is unaltered in the plural and should not be followed by a full stop except at the end of the sentence:

   5 cm *not* 5 cm. or 5 cms.

b.   The decimal sign between digits is indicated by a full stop in typing. No commas are used to divide large numbers into groups of three, but a half-space (whole space in typing) is left after every third digit. If the numerical value of the number is less than 1 unit, a zero should precede the decimal sign:

   0.123 456 *not* .123,456

c.   The SI symbol for "day" (i.e. 24 hours) is "d", but urine and fecal excretions of substances should preferably be expressed as "per 24 hours":

   g/24 h

d.   "Squared" and "cubed" are expressed as numerical powers and not by abbreviation: square centimeter is cm^2 *not* sq cm.

Commonly used measurements

a. Temperature is expressed as degrees Celsius (°C) and the standard thermometer is graded 32–42°C.

    1° Celsius = 1° Centigrade

b. The calorie is replaced by the joule:

    1 calorie = 4.2 J

    1 Calorie (dietetic use) = 4.2 kilojoules = 4.2 kJ

    The previous 1000 Calorie reducing diet is expressed (approximately) as a 4000 kJ diet.

1 g of fat provides	38 kJ
1 g of protein provides	17 kJ
1 g of carbohydrate provides	16 kJ

c. Equivalent concentration mEq/l is commonly used for reporting results of monovalent electrolyte measurements (sodium, potassium, chloride and bicarbonate). It is not part of the SI system and should be replaced by molar concentration—min these examples mmol/1. For these four measurements, the numerical value will not change.

d. The SI unit of pressure is the pascal (Pa). Blood gas measurements should be given in the SI unit kPa instead of mmHg.

    1 mmHg = 133.32 Pa

    1 kPa = 7.5006 mmHg

    Column measurement will be *retained* in clinical practice *as at present*.

    blood pressure (in mmHg)

    cerebrospinal fluid (in mmH_2O)

    central venous pressure (in cmH_2O)

Weights and measures

Metric   English

Linear measure

	1 millimeter	=	0.039	in	1 inch	=	25.4	mm
10 mm	= 1 centimeter	=	0.394	in	1 foot	=	0.305	m
10 cm	= 1 decimeter	=	3.94	in	1 yard	=	0.914	m
10 dm	= 1 meter	=	39.37	in	1 mile	=	1.61	km
1000 m	= 1 kilometer	=	0.6214	mile				

Square measure

	1 sq centimeter	=	0.155	sq in	1 square inch	=	6.452	cm^2
100 cm^2	= 1 sq meter	=	1.196	sq yd	1 square foot	=	9.29	dm^2
100 m^2	= 1 are	=	119.6	sq yd	1 square yard	=	0.836	m^2
100 ares	= 1 hectare	=	2.471	acres	1 acre	=	4047	m^2
100 ha	= 1 sq kilometer	=	0.386	sq miles	1 square mile	=	259	ha

Cubic measure

	1 cu centimeter	=	0.061	in^3	1 cubic inch	=	16.387	cm^3
1000 cm^3	= 1 cu decimeter	=	0.035	ft^3	1 cubic foot	=	0.0283	m^3
1000 dm^3	= 1 cu meter	=	1.308	yd^3	1 cubic yard	=	0.765	m^3

Capacity measure

	1 milliliter	=	0.002	pt	1 fluid ounce	=	29.6	cm^3
10 ml	= 1 centiliter	=	0.021	pint	1 pint	=	0.473	l
10 cl	= 1 deciliter	=	0.211	pt	1 quart	=	0.946	l
10 dl	= 1 liter	=	1.057	qt	1 gallon	=	3.785	l
1000 l	= 1 kiloliter	=	264.2	gal				

Weight

	1 milligram	=	0.015	grain	1 grain	=	64.8	mg
10 mg	= 1 centigram	=	0.154	grain	1 dram	=	1.772	g
10 cg	= 1 decigram	=	1.543	grain	1 ounce	=	28.35	g
10 dg	= 1 gram	=	15.43	grain	1 pound	=	0.4536	kg
		=	0.035	oz	1 stone	=	6.35	kg
1000 g	= 1 kilogram	=	2.205	lb	1 quarter	=	12.7	kg
1000 kg	= 1 tonne				1 hundred weight	=	50.8	kg
	(metric ton)	=	0.984	(long) ton	1 ton	=	1.016	tonnes
					1 short ton	=	0.907	tonnes

Temperature

$$°\text{Fahrenheit} = \left(\frac{9}{5} \times x°\text{C}\right) + 32$$

$$°\text{Centigrade} = \frac{5}{9} \times (x°\text{F} - 32)$$

where x is the temperature to be converted

Appendix 3
Normal Characteristics

Blood

Normal ranges vary between laboratories. These ranges should be taken as a guide only

Test	Measurement
Albumin *see* Protein	
Alkali reserve	55–70 ml
	CO_2/100 ml
	(23.8–34.6 mEq/l)
Amino acid nitrogen	2.5–4.0 mmol/l
Aminotransferases *see* Transaminases	
Ammonia	12–60 μmol/l
Amylase	90–300 iu/l
Antistreptolysin "O" titer	Up to 200 U/ml
Ascorbic acid	0.7–1.4 mg/100 ml
Bicarbonate	24–30 mmol/l
Bilirubin (total)	3–20 μmol/l
direct	Up to 6.8 μmol/l
Bleeding time	1–6 min
Blood volume	Approx $\frac{1}{12}$ or 8% body weight
Bromsulphthalein	Less than 15% after 25 min
Calcium	2.1–2.6 mmol/l
Carbon dioxide (whole blood)	4.5–6.0 kPa
Carbon monoxide (carboxyhemoglobin)	Less than 0.8 vol %

Test	Measurement
Ceruloplasmin (copper oxidase)	0.3–0.6 g/l
Chloride	95–105 mmol/l
Cholesterol	3.5–7.0 mmol/l
Cholinesterase	2–5 iu/l
Clotting time	4–10 min
factor V assay (AcG)	75–125%
factor VIII assay (AHG)	50–200%
factor IX assay (PTC, Christmas factor)	75–125%
factor X assay (Stuart factor)	75–125%
CO₂ combining power *see* Alkali reserve	
Copper	75–140 μg/100ml
Corticosteroids (cortisol)	0.3–0.7 μmol/l
Creatine	15–60 μmol/l
Creatine kinase	4–60 iu/l
Creatinine	60–120 μmol/l
Enzymes *see* individual enzymes	
Erythrocyte sedimentation rate (ESR)	
men	3–5 mm/1 h; 7–15 mm/2h (Westergren)
women	7–12 mm/1 h; 12–17/2h (Westergren)
Fasting blood sugar *see* Glucose	
Fatty acids (free)	0.3–0.6 mmol/l
Fibrinogen *see* Protein	
Flocculation tests *see under* individual tests	
Folic acid	greater than 3 ng/ml
Gammaglobulin *see* Protein	
Gamma-glutamyl-transpeptidase (GGT)	5–30 iu/l
Globulin *see* Protein	
Glucose (whole blood, fasting)	
venous	3.0–5.0 mmol/l
capillary (arterial)	3.3–5.3 mmol/l
Glucose tolerance	max. 180 mg/100 ml returns fasting 1½–2h
Glycerol *see* Triglyceride	
Haptoglobins	16–31 μmol/l
Hematocrit *see* PCV	

Test	*Measurement*
Hemoglobin	12–18g/dl
Iron	
men	13–32 μmol/l
women	Approx 3.25 μmol/l less
Iron-binding capacity (total)	45–70 μmol/l
Kahn	negative
Ketones	0.06–0.2 mmol/l
Lactate	0.75–2.0 mmol/l
Lactate dehydrogenase	
total	60–250 iu/l
"heart specific"	50–150 iu/l
Lead (whole blood)	0.5–1.7 μmol/l
LE cells	None
Lipase	18–280 iu/l
Lipids (total)	4.5–10 g/l
β-Lipoproteins	3.5–6.5 g/l
Liver function *see* individual tests	
Magnesium	0.7–1.0 mmol
5′-Nucleotidase	2.15 iu/l
Osmolality	275–295 mosmol/kg
Oxygen (whole blood)	11–15 kPa
Oxygen capacity	14.4–24.7 ml
pH	7.36–7.42
Phosphatase	
acid-total	3.5–20 iu/l
acid-prostatic	0–3.5 iu/l
alkaline-total	20–90 iu/l
Phosphate (inorganic)	0.8–1.4 mmol/l
Phospholipids	
(as fatty acids)	5.0–9.0 mmol/l
(as phosphorus)	1.9–3.2 mmol/l
Phosphorus *see* Phosphate, inorganic	
Platelets	$200–500 \times 10^9$/l
Potassium	3.8–5.0 mmol/l

Test	Measurement
Protein	
total	62–80 g/l
albumin	35–50 g/l
globulin (total)	18–32 g/l
gammaglobulin	7–15 g/l
fibrinogen	2–4 g/l
A–G ratio	1.5:1–2.5:1
Protein-bound iodine	0.3–0.6 μmol/l
Prothrombin time	11–18 s
Pseudocholinesterase *see also* Cholinesterase	60–90 Warburg units
Pyruvate (fasting)	0.05–0.08 mmol/l
Red cell count	
total	$4.0–6.0 \times 10^{12}/l$
reticulocytes	0.1–2.0/100 RBCs
packed cell volume (PCV)	
men	40–54%
women	36–47%
mean cell volume (MCV)	78–94 μm^3
mean corpuscular hemoglobin concentration (MCHC)	32–36%
mean corpuscular hemoglobin (MCH)	27–32 pg
mean cell diameter	6.7–7.7 μm
Red cell fragility	Hemolysis slight 0.44% NaCl Hemolysis complete 0.3% NaCl
Sodium	136–148 mmol/l
Sulfhemoglobin	None
Thyroxine	0.04–0.85 μmol/l
Transaminase	
alanine (ALT; at 30°C)	2–20 iu/l
aspartate (AST; at 30°C)	8–25 iu/l
Triglyceride	0.3–1.8 mmol/l
Urea	3.0–6.5 mmol/l
Uric acid	0.1–0.45 mmol/l

Test	Measurement
Vitamin A	1.0–3.0 μmol/l
Vitamin B$_{12}$	150–800 pg/ml
Vitamin C *see* Ascorbic acid	
White cell count	
total	4.0–10.0 × 10^9/l
differential	
neutrophils	2,500–7,500 × 10^6/l
eosinophils	200–400 × 10^6/l
basophils	0–50 × 10^6/l
lymphocytes	1,500 × 3,500 × 10^6/l
monocytes	400–800 × 10^6/l
Zinc sulfate reaction	2.8 units

Cerebrospinal fluid

Pressure (adult)	50 to 200 mm water
Cells	0 to 5 lymphocytes/mm^3
Glucose	3.3–4.4 mmol/l
Protein	100–400 mg/l

Feces

Normal fat content	
Daily output on normal diet	less than 7g
Fat (as stearic acid)	11–18 mmol/24h

Urine

Total quantity per 24 hours	1000 to 1500 ml
Specific gravity	1.012 to 1.030
Reaction	pH 4 to 8

Average amounts of inorganic and organic solids in urine each 24 hours

Calcium	2.5–7.5 mmol
Creatinine	9–17 mmol
5H1AA	15–75 μmol
HMMA*	10–35 μmol
Hydroxyproline	0.08–0.25 mmol
Magnesium	3.3–5.0 mmol

Phosphate	15–50 mmol
Urea	250–500 mmol
17-ketosteroids:	
men	8 to 22 mg/24 hours
women	5 to 12 mg/24 hours

*4-Hydroxy-3-methoxy mandelic acid.

Vitamins

Vitamin & daily intake	Sources	Function	Properties	Deficiencies
Fat-soluble				
A (retinol) 750–1200 μg (retinol equivalents)	Carrots, spinach, apricots, tomatoes, liver, kidney, oily fish, egg yolk, milk, butter, cheese	Normal development of bones and teeth. Antiinfective. Essential for healthy skin and mucous membranes. Aids night vision.	Synthesized in the body from carotene, present in vegetables. Can be stored in liver.	Poor growth. Rough dry skin and mucous membranes encouraging infection. Lessened ability to see in poor light. Xerophthalmia and eventual blindness.
D (calciferol)	Oily fish, egg yolk, butter, margarine. Ultra-violet rays of sunlight.	Anti-rachitic. Assists absorption and metabolism of calcium and phosphorus.	Produced in the body by action of sunlight on ergosterol in skin.	Rickets in children; osteomalacia and osteoporosis in adults.
E (tocopherol)	Wheat germ, egg yolk, milk, cereals, liver, green vegetables.	Not fully understood in human body, perhaps controls oxidation in body tissues.		
K	Green vegetables, especially cabbage, peas.	Antihemorrhagic. Essential for the production of prothrombin.	Only absorbed in the presence of bile.	Delayed clotting time. Liver damage.

Vitamin & daily intake	Sources	Function	Properties	Deficiencies
Water-soluble				
B-*complex*				
B1 aneurin (thiamin) 1–1.5 mg	Wholemeal flour and bread, brewers' yeast, cereals, milk, eggs, liver, fish, vegetables.	Anti-neuritic. Anti-beri-beri. Anti-pellagra. Health of nervous system.	Destroyed by excessive heat, e.g. toast and baking soda	Beri-beri. Neuritis. Poor growth in children.
B2 (riboflavin) 1.5–2.5 mg Nicotinic acid 15–18 mg		Steady and continuous release of energy from carbohydrates.	Can withstand normal cooking and food processing.	Fissures at corner of mouth and tongue. Inflammation. Corneal opacities. Pellagra: dermatitis diarrhea dementia.
B6 (pyridoxine)	As other B-complex foods	Protein metabolism.	Relieves post-radiotherapy nausea and vomiting.	Nervousness and insomnia.
B12 (cobalamin)	Liver, kidney, and other B-complex foods.	Essential for red blood cell formation.	Requires intrinsic factor secreted by gastric cells for absorption.	Pernicious anemia.
Cytamin	Prepared from growth of Streptomyces.	Maintenance therapy for patients with pernicious anemia.		
Folic acid	Liver and green vegetables	Assists production of red blood cells.	Some forms of macrocytic anemia. Premature babies and elderly people on poor diets.	

Vitamin & daily intake	*Sources*	*Function*	*Properties*	*Deficiencies*
C (ascorbic acid) 30–60 mg	Fresh fruit: oranges, lemons, grapefruit, black-currants; green leaf vegetables, potatoes, turnips, rose hip syrup	Formation of bones, connec-tive tissue, teeth and red blood cells.	Destroyed by cooking in the presence of air and by plant enzymes released when cutting and grating raw food. Lost by long storage.	Sore mouth and gums. Capillary bleeding. Scurvy. Delayed wound healing.

Appendix 4
Poisons

Acknowledgment
The information about poisons has been updated with the help of S.J. Hopkins PhD FPS,
Consultant Pharmacist, Addenbrooke's Hospital, Cambridge.

Basic principles of treatment

In all cases of poisoning, certain general principles should be followed. It is a
common misconception that for each poison there is a specific antidote. In practice, a true pharmacological antagonist is available in only 2.0% of poisonings.
In the great majority of instances, therefore, the treatment consists primarily in
the application of basic principles of supportive treatment. If the poison is a gas,
or the vapor of a volatile liquid, the patient must be removed at once to fresh air
and given oxygen and artificial respiration if needed. Subsequent treatment is
supportive to maintain vital functions. If the poison has been ingested in most
cases it is necessary to remove as much as possible of the unabsorbed substance
from the stomach. Outside of the hospital this is best achieved by pharyngeal
irritation using the finger or by administration of syrup of Ipecac as directed by
the local Poison Control Center. In the hospital, gastric aspiration and lavage
should be given provided the patient retains an adequate cough and gag reflex, or
is sufficiently unconscious to allow the introduction of a cuffed endotracheal
tube to protect the airway. These procedures should only be performed with the
patient lying on his side with the head dependent. An adequate size of tube must
be used, and 300 ml quantities of lukewarm water should be used for lavage until
the recovered fluid runs clear. As a general rule nothing should be left in the
stomach after lavage for fear of subsequent vomiting and pulmonary aspiration.
Emetic drugs have been enthusiastically recommended to avoid the use of gastric
aspiration and lavage. Apomorphine, common salt, mustard and copper sulfate
have been used as emetics, but are now regarded as dangerous, and should **not** be
used. Syrup of ipecac is quite widely used in a dose of 15 ml followed by 200 ml

of water, and provided its limitations are recognized is the treatment of choice in children. The onset of its emetic effect is usually delayed for about 18 min and occasionally it may produce undesirable toxic effects after absorption.

Common errors in treatment
1. Analeptic therapy
Bemegride is not a specific barbiturate antagonist and its use in poisonings due to hypnotic drugs is associated with frequent serious side-effects including cardiac arrhythmias, convulsions and even irreversible brain damage. The use of analeptics cannot be justified.

2. Bladder catheterization
This highly dangerous procedure is seldom necessary even in deeply unconscious patients. With adequate nursing care, there should be no undue risk of skin breakdown due to incontinence of urine. Bladder catheterization is justified in prolonged bladder distension and occasionally when forced diuresis therapy is being given.

3. Prophylactic antibiotics
With good nursing care, including frequent turning of the patient and careful attention to mouth hygiene prophylactic administration of antibiotics is unnecessary. These drugs should be given only when there is clear clinical or X-ray evidence of infection.

Guide to poisonous substances and treatment

Substance	Clinical features	Treatment
Acids Strong hydrochloric acid. Spirits of salts. Strong sulfuric acid (oil of vitriol). Strong nitric acid. (See Bleaches (b)) **Alkalis** Caustic soda (sodium hydroxide). Caustic potash (potassium hydroxide). Strong ammonia	Severe burning of mouth and throat, causing dyspnea due to edema of glottis. Severe abdominal pains, thirst, shock, dark and bloodstained vomit, gastroenteritis.	Plenty of water to dilute the poison. *Acids:* Neutralize with milk of magnesia or calcium hydroxide (56 ml to ½ liter of warm water). Carbonates, as chalk, sodium bicarbonate and washing soda also effective, but cause liberation of carbon dioxide. Soap can be used if no other alkali available. *Alkalis:* Neutralize with acetic acid (56 ml to ½ liter), or vinegar (112 ml to ½ liter): lemon juice also effective, if available in sufficient quantity. General measures include morphine for pain, and arachis or olive oil as demulcent.
Amphetamine and related substances	Alertness, tremor, confusion, delirium, hallucinations, panic attacks, lethargy, exhaustion, headache, sweating, cardiac arrhythmias, hypertension or hypotension, dryness of mouth, diarrhea and abdominal colic, ulcers of the lips in addicts, convulsions and deep unconsciousness.	Gastric aspiration and lavage. If markedly excited chlorpromazine i.m. is the most effective treatment. Intensive supportive therapy. Forced acid diuresis if essential. For severe hypertension, phentolamine 5–10 mg i.v.
Anticoagulants Phenindione Warfarin Rodenticides	Hematuria, hemoptysis, bruising and hematemesis; occasionally bleeding elsewhere. Orange yellow urine. Prolonged prothrombin time.	Gastric aspiration and lavage. Vit. K₁ 20 mg i.v. Blood transfusion if necessary.

Substance	Clinical features	Treatment
Antidepressants Amitriptyline Butriptyline Desipramine Doxepin Imipramine Nortriptyline Protriptyline Trimipramine	Dryness of the mouth, dilated pupils, tachycardia leading to bizarre cardiac arrhythmias, hypotension, cardiac failure or arrest, urinary retention, varying degrees of unconsciousness, pressure of speech, increased limb reflexes, convulsions, torticollis and ataxia. Respiratory failure. Cardiac complications are common and particularly dangerous in children.	Gastric aspiration and lavage. Intensive supportive therapy. In the majority of patients these measures are all that are necessary. The central nervous system effects and some of the cardiac abnormalities can be abolished by the slow i.v. injection of physostigmine salicylate 1–3 mg, which may be repeated once after 10 min. If ineffective, convulsions may be controlled by diazepam 10 mg i.v. or sodium phenobarbital 300 mg i.m. β-Adrenergic blocking drugs may correct difficult cardiac arrhythmias.
Antihistamines	In adults, toxic doses cause deep central depression. In children and infants, the effect is often stimulatory, and convulsion and convulsions may result. Hypotension, tachycardia and occasionally cardiac arrhythmias. Respiratory depression. Dryness of the mouth, nausea and constipation. Hyperpyrexia. Agranulocytosis and aplastic anemia may develop.	Intensive supportive therapy. Gastric aspiration and lavage. Sedation may be required in the form of diazepam or sodium phenobarbital i.m. Antibiotics, steroid drugs and blood transfusion may be necessary in severe blood dyscrasia.

Substance	Clinical features	Treatment
Atropine Belladonna Scopolamine Homatropine Propantheline and other anticholinergic drugs. Deadly Nightshade	Blurring of vision, taxia, mental confusion, hallucinations. Tachycardia, hypertension, cardiac arrhythmias. Dryness and burning of the mouth with marked thirst, nausea and vomiting. Urinary urgency and possible acute retention. Hyperpyrexia. Death usually results from respiratory failure.	Intensive supportive therapy. Gastric aspiration and lavage. Peripheral effects may be relieved by subcutaneous injection of neostigmine 0.25 mg. When central nervous stimulation is marked, sedation with a short-acting barbiturate or diazepam may be necessary. Physostigmine salicylate (1–4 mg) i.m. or i.v. will rapidly antagonize the central nervous complications, but repeat doses may be required every 1 to 2 hours.
Barbiturates *Long-acting* Barbital Phenobarbital *Medium-acting* Allobarbital Butobarbital Amylobarbital *Short-acting* Pentobarbital Cyclobarbital Quinalbarbital *Ultra-short-acting* Hexobarbital Thiopental	Impaired level of consciousness. Limb reflexes very variable. Withdrawal fits and delirium during the phase of recovery occur in patients habituated to the drug. Cardiovascular depression with hypotension and "shock". Respiratory depression. Hypothermia. Renal failure. Bullous lesions occur in 6% of patients with this condition.	Intensive supportive therapy. Gastric aspiration and lavage. Forced osmotic alkaline diuresis and/or hemodialysis are of value in patients severely poisoned with long-acting barbiturates but are less effective with the other types.

Substance	Clinical features	Treatment
Benzodiazepines Chlordiazepoxide Diazepam Flurazepam Lorazepam Oxazepam Temazepam	Physical dependence may occur when the drug has been taken for some time. Also an additive effect occurs when taken in combination with alcohol, barbiturate, phenothiazine, monoamine oxidase inhibitors and imipramine. Loss of consciousness, bradycardia and hypotension. Respiratory depression.	Intensive supportive therapy. Gastric aspiration and lavage.
Bleaches a. Containing sodium hypochlorite	If inhaled: Cough and pulmonary edema. If ingested: Irritation of the mouth and pharynx; edema of pharynx and larynx. Nausea and vomiting.	Gastric aspiration and lavage using 2.5% sodium thiosulfate (if not available milk or milk of magnesia). If severely ill sodium thiosulfate (1%) 250 ml i.v.
b. Containing oxalic acid	Irritation of the mouth and throat. Nausea and vomiting. Muscular twitchings and convulsions. Shock and cardiac arrest. Acute renal failure the onset of which may be delayed.	Intensive supportive therapy. Gastric aspiratin and lavage adding 10 g calcium lactate to the lavage fluid. Calcium gluconate 10% 10 ml i.v. and repeat as necessary. Provided the renal output is adequate at least 5 liters of fluid should be given for 3 days.
Carbamates Meprobamate	Impairment of consciousness, muscle weakness and incoordination, nystagmus. Respiratory depression. Hypotension. Hypothermia. Withdrawal fits may occur.	Intensive supportive therapy. Gastric aspiration and lavage. Forced osmotic alkaline diuresis in severely poisoned patients and, if ineffective, hemodialysis.

Substance	Clinical features	Treatment
Carbon monoxide and coal gas	Vertigo and ataxia; acute agitation and confusion; deep coma may develop. Papilledema, increased limb reflexes and possibly extensor plantar responses. Acute myocardial infarction, tachycardia, arrhythmias and hypotension. Respiratory stimulation, which may progress to respiratory failure. Nausea, vomiting, hematemesis and fecal incontinence are common. Bullous lesions may occur. Sequelae include Parkinsonism, hemiparesis and impairment of higher intellectual function.	Urgent. Remove from exposure. Intensive supportive therapy. Give a mixture of 95% O_2 and 5% CO_2 or by hyperbaric oxygen if available. In the presence of cerebral edema 500 ml of 20% mannitol i.v. over 15 min followed by 500 ml 5% dextrose over the next 4 hours.
Contraceptives, oral	Mild nausea or vomiting. Withdrawal bleeding in girls may occur.	Intensive supportive therapy. Gastric aspiration and lavage.
Cresol Phenol Lysol	Strong smell of carbolic acid in patient's breath or vomit. Corrosion of lips and buccal mucosa but little pain. Marked abdominal pain, nausea and vomiting. Hematemesis or gastric perforation. After absorption, initial excitement then impaired consciousness. Hypotension. Dark urine, oliguria and renal failure. Liver failure may occur. Respiratory failure is a common cause of death.	Intensive supportive therapy. Gastric aspiration and lavage with care. Wash ulcers with copious water or 50% alcohol. Medical measures for hepatic and renal failure. Hemodialysis may be required.

Substance	Clinical features	Treatment
Cyanide	Very toxic. *Mild poisoning* Headache, dyspnea, vomiting, ataxia and loss of consciousness occur gradually. *Severe poisoning* The above features develop very rapidly and the patient becomes deeply unconscious. The smell of bitter almonds is not necessarily present. The skin remains pink unless breathing has ceased. Rapid, thready pulse. Hypotension. Limb reflexes are often absent and the pupils are dilated.	Speed is essential. As long as the heart sounds are audible, recovery may be anticipated with appropriate treatment. Treatment includes: (1) If the poisoning is due to inhalation, remove from contaminated atmosphere. (2) Break an ampule of amyl nitrite under the patient's nose whilst applying artificial respiration where this is necessary. (3) Cobalt edetate (Kelocyanor), which is the treatment of choice. Dose 300–600 mg i.v. initially, but a second dose of 300 mg may be given if recovery does not occur within 1–2 minutes, followed by i.v. glucose 5%. (4) Alternatively, give sodium nitrite (3%) in a dose of 10 ml over 3 minutes i.v. (5) Slow i.v. infusion of 50 ml of 25% sodium thiosulfate. (6) If the poison has been ingested, gastric aspiration and lavage, with 300 ml 25% sodium thiosulfate left in the stomach. Hyperbaric oxygen may reduce the cellular anoxia. *Note:* Ketocyanor and the other antidotes should be kept in an emergency kit in all emergency depts. Ketocyanor may cause nausea and vomiting, but recovery is rapid.

Substance	Clinical features	Treatment
Cyanide (contd)		Remember that Ketocyanor is relatively toxic except in cyanide poisoning, so careful diagnosis is important. If given in error, treat cobalt toxicity with i.v. infusion of sodium calcium edetate.
Detergents	Nausea, vomiting and diarrhea. Most are not very toxic.	Supportive therapy
Digitalis and Digoxin	Nausea and vomiting, diarrhea. Bradycardia. Cardiac arrhythmias. Mental confusion.	Intensive supportive therapy. Gastric aspiration and lavage. In hypokalemic arrhythmia, potassium chloride 1.0 g orally every 20 min; if vomiting occurs 1 g in 200 ml 5% dextrose infused over 30 min. Lidocaine 500 mg in 500 ml saline/dextrose i.v. administered at a rate depending on the clinical response is the best treatment for ventricular ectopics. Atropine sulfate 0.6 mg i.m. repeated as necessary for bradycardia. Cardiac pacing may occasionally be required.
Glutethimide	Similar to barbiturate poisoning, but depth of coma may vary considerably. Sudden apnea may occur, probably due to sudden raised intracranial pressure. Pupils dilated and unresponsive to light. Hypotension may be severe. Myocardial infarction may occur.	Intensive supportive therapy. Gastric aspiration and lavage with a mixture of castor oil and water. Leave 50 ml of castor oil in stomach to reduce absorption. If there is any suspicion of raised intracranial pressure give 500 ml 20% mannitol i.v. over 20 min followed by 500 ml 5% dextrose over next 4 hours.

Substance	Clinical features	Treatment
Iron salts	*Stage 1.* Epigastric pain, nausea and vomiting. Hematemesis. Tachypnea and tachycardia followed by bloody diarrhea and collapse. *Stage 2.* An interval of hours or even several days may elapse during which there are no further signs and symptoms. Then severe headache, confusion, delirium, convulsions and loss of consciousness. Respiratory and circulatory failure. *Stage 3.* If patient survives, liver failure and renal failure may occur.	Intensive supportive therapy. Immediate i.m. injection of desferrioxamine 1–2 g, followed by gastric aspiration and lavage with desferrioxamine 2 g in 1 liter of water. Afterwards 10 g desferrioxamine should be left in the stomach. I.v. infusion of desferrioxamine 15 mg/kg per hour to a maximum dose of 80 mg/kg per 24 hours. Medical measures for hepatic and renal failure may be necessary.
Lead	Severe abdominal pain, vomiting, diarrhea, oliguria, collapse, coma, "Shock" and hepatic failure may occur. Acute hemolytic anemia.	Intensive supportive therapy. Gastric aspiration and lavage. When colic is severe calcium gluconate (10%) 10 ml i.v. Calcium sodium edetate up to 40 mg/kg twice daily for 5 days by i.v. infusion. Penicillamine orally in doses of 20–40 mg daily following initial therapy. Sodium bicarbonate (5%) or sodium lactate (M/6) by i.v. infusion for acidosis. Peritoneal or hemodialysis in severe poisoning.

Substance	Clinical features	Treatment
Methyl alcohol Methanol Wood alcohol	Headache, blurring of vision which may lead to blindness, dilatation of pupils and papilledema, loss of consciousness. Nausea and vomiting. Hyperventilation.	Intensive supportive therapy. Gastric aspiration and lavage. Ethylalcohol 50% 1 ml per kg stat, then 0.5 ml per kg every 2 hours. Treat acidosis with i.v. infusions of sodium bicarbonate 5% or sodium lactate (M/6), repeated if necessary for some hours.
Methaqualone	Hypertonia, myoclonia, extensor plantar responses, papilledema and impairment of level of consciousness. Tachycardia, acute myocardial infarction. Respiratory depression. Bleeding tendencies may occur.	Intensive supportive therapy. Gastric aspiration and lavage. Hemodialysis in severe poisoning.
Opium alkaloids Heroin Morphine Meperidene Codeine Dipipanone Pentazocine Propoxyphene	Impaired level of consciousness; pinpoint pupils. Convulsions may occur particularly in young children. Respiratory and circulatory depression. Methemoglobinemia may occur.	Intensive supportive therapy. Gastric aspiration and lavage. Naloxone (Narcan) 0.4 mg i.v. and repeated 3 min later is usually sufficient to re-establish normal respiration and conscious level.
Organophosphorous compounds	These insecticides are very toxic. Headache, restlessness, ataxia, muscle weakness, convulsions. Salivation, nausea, vomiting, colic and diarrhea. Bradycardia, hypotension, peripheral circulatory failure. Bronchospasm, cyanosis, acute pulmonary edema. Respiratory failure is the usual cause of death.	Intensive supportive therapy. Gastric aspiration and lavage if ingested. As soon as cyanosis is corrected, atropine sulfate 2 mg i.v. and repeated at 15-min intervals until fully atropinized. Pralidoxime 30 mg per kg i.v. slowly and repeat half-hourly as necessary. If sedation or control of convulsions is required, diazepam 10 mg may be used.

Substance	Clinical features	Treatment
Paracetamol	Pallor, nausea and sweating. Hypotension, tachycardia and other cardiac arrhythmias. Excitement and delirium progressing to CNS depression and stupor. Hypothermia, hypoglycemia and metabolic acidosis. Tachypnea. Hemolysis. Renal failure. Jaundice and hepatic failure, which is the commonest mode of death. Severity of poisoning best assessed on blood levels. If the plasma paracetamol level is above 2000 mmol per liter and especially if the plasma half-life is greater than 4 hours hepatic damage is likely.	Intensive supportive therapy. If the plasma paracetamol half-life is greater than 4 hours give acetylcysteine 150 mg/kg by i.v. infusion in glucose 5% over 15 minutes, followed by 50 mg/kg over 4 hours and 100 mg/kg over 16 hours may protect the liver against paracetamol damage. Methionine 2.5 g orally initially, repeated 4-hourly up to a total of 10 g is also of value. *Note* Acetylcysteine may increase liver damage unless given within 12 hours of poisoning. Intravenous infusions of sodium bicarbonate to correct acidemia, i.v. glucose for hypoglycemia, and if hemolysis is severe corticosteroids and blood transfusion may be necessary. Hemodialysis may be required for renal failure.
Paraquat	Burning sensation in mouth at time of ingestion followed by nausea, vomiting and diarrhea. After a few hours painful buccal ulceration develops. Several days after ingestion a progressive alveolitis and bronchiolitis is probable and is the usual cause of death. Severe renal and hepatic impairment may occur.	Careful gastric aspiration and lavage with 300 ml of Fuller's earth suspension 30% with 15 g of magnesium sulfate. Leave 300 ml of suspension in stomach. Give another 300 ml later to promote excretion of unabsorbed drug by purging. Intensive supportive therapy. Immediate forced diuresis is safe before renal damage occurs.

Substance	Clinical features	Treatment
Petroleum distillates	Nausea, vomiting and diarrhea. If inhaled or aspirated, intense pulmonary congestion and chemical pneumonitis. Depression of consciousness and respiration with occasional convulsions.	*No gastric aspiration or lavage.* 250 ml liquid paraffin orally. If pneumonitis, hydrocortisone 100 mg i.m. 6-hourly for 48 hours with antibiotics as indicated. Mechanical ventilation may be necessary.
Phenothiazines	Impaired level of consciousness, Parkinsonism, torticollis, oculogyric crises, restlessness and convulsions. Hypotension, tachycardia, cardiac arrhythmias. Hypothermia. Respiratory depression in severe poisoning.	Intensive supportive therapy. Gastric aspiration and lavage. Convulsions should be treated with diazepam 10 mg, or orphenadrine 20 mg or procyclidine 10 mg by injection. Cogentin (benztropine mesylate) 2 mg i.v. is effective for Parkinsonism.
Phenytoin	Stimulation and possibly euphoria, vertigo, headache, cerebellar ataxia, nystagmus, tremor, loss of consciousness. Nausea, and vomiting. Respiratory depression.	Intensive supportive therapy. Gastric aspiration and lavage.
Primidone	Similar to phenytoin but loss of consciousness tends to be more marked.	Intensive supportive therapy. Gastric aspiration and lavage. Forced alkaline osmotic diuresis or hemodialysis may be necessary in severe poisoning.
Quinine and quinidine	Tinnitus; blurred vision; headache and dizziness. Impaired consciousness; rapid, shallow breathing. Tachycardia, hypotension, cardiac arrhythmias and arrest may occur. Acute hemolysis and renal failure.	Intensive supportive therapy. Gastric aspiration and lavage. ECG monitoring is required and cardiac arrhythmias treated with appropriate drugs. In marked visual impairment stellate ganglion block may produce dramatic improvement. Forced acid diuresis may be of value in severe poisoning.

Substance	Clinical features	Treatment
Salicylates Aspirin (acetylsalicylic acid) Methyl salicylate Sodium salicylate	Alertness and restlessness, tinnitus, deafness. Hyperventilation. Hyperpyrexia and sweating. nausea and vomiting. Dehydration and oliguria. Unconsciousness may occur in severe poisoning; hypoprothrombinemia occurs in some patients. Hypokalemia may be severe. Metabolic acidemia and hypoglycemia are often marked in children.	Gastric aspiration and lavage in all patients. Forced alkaline diuresis if the plasma salicylate is above 500 mg/liter in adults or 300 mg/liter in children. In very severe poisoning hemodialysis. Intensive supportive therapy.
Snake bite pit vipers (Crotalidae)	Immediate symptoms: Swelling, some pain and redness. Later symptoms: Numbness of fingers, toes, metallic or rubbery taste in mouth, chills, weakness, rapid pulse; respiratory difficulty and shock may follow.	If within 30–40 min of a medical facility, keep site of bite immobile and below heart level and bring victim to facility. Treatment determined on basis of severity of signs and sensitivity to polyvalent antivenin (crotalid). Adrenaline should be available for serum reactions. If further than 40 min away from facility, a single incision, 1/4″ long and not more than 1/8″ deep is made, suction carried out for 30–60 min, wound cleansed and sterile dressing applied.
Thiazides	Polyuria, dehydration, hypokalemia, hyponatremia, hypochloremia and alkalemia. Acute renal failure may occur. Also acute hepatic failure is occasionally found and in susceptible patients an acute attack of gout may result.	Intensive supportive therapy. Gastric aspiration and lavage. Potassium chloride 2 g 3-hourly depending on the degree of hypokalemia. Intravenous fluids may be necessary to correct dehydration.

Further information may be obtained from various Poison Control Centers.

Appendix 5
Abbreviations Commonly Used in Medical and Nursing Records

a.a.	of each	BS	blood sugar
abd	abdomen	BSE	breast self exam
a.c.	before meals	BSP	bromosulfophthalein
Ac.	acid	BT	bleeding time
ACTH	adrenocorticotropin	BUN	blood urea nitrogen
ADL	activities of daily living	Bx	biopsy
ADP	adenosine diphosphate	C	centigrade
ad lib	as desired	c̄	with
adm	admission	Ca	calcium, cancer
alk.	alkaline	Cal	calorie
A.M.	morning	cap	capsule
a.m.a.	against medical advice	cath	catheter
amp	ampule	C.B.C.	complete blood count
amt	amount	C.B.R.	complete bed rest
ANS	autonomic nervous system	cc	cubic centimeter
ante	before	CC	chief complaint
AP	anteroposterior	C.C.U.	coronary care unit
AROM	artificial rupture of membranes	CF	cystic fibrosis
ASHD	arteriosclerotic heart disease	CHF	congestive heart failure
		CHO	carbohydrate
ASD	atrial septal defect	chol.	cholesterol
ATP	adenosine triphosphate	cm	centimeter
A-V	atrio-ventricular	CMV	cytomegalovirus
A&W	alive and well	CNS	central nervous system
		c/o	complains of
BCP	birth control pills	C.O.	cardiac output
B.E.	barium enema	contra	against
bene	well	CPD	cephalopelvic disproportion
b.i.d.	twice a day	C&S	culture and sensitivity
BM	bowel movement	CS	cesarean section
BMR	basal metabolic rate	CSF	cerebrospinal fluid
BP	blood pressure	CSS	central sterile supply
BRP	bathroom privileges	CST	convulsive shock therapy

CV	cardiovascular	F.B.S.	fasting blood sugar
CVA	cerebrovascular accident	Fe	iron
CVP	central venous pressure	FEV	forced expiratory volume
CVS	clean voided specimen	FH	family history
Cx	cervix	FHR	fetal heart rate
		fld	fluid
d.c.	discontinue	FSH	follicle stimulating hormone
D&C	dilation and curettage		
DD	differential diagnosis	G	gravida
dig.	digitalis	gal	gallon
dil.	dilute	GC	gonococcus
disch.	discharge	GH	growth hormone
DNA	deoxyribonucleic acid	GI	gastrointestinal
DOA	dead on arrival	Gm, g	gram
DOB	date of birth	gr	grain
DOE	dyspnea on exertion	gtt	drops
DPT	diphtheria, pertussis,	GTT	glucose tolerance test
	tetanus	GU	genitourinary
dr	dram		
Dr.	doctor	h(hr)	hour
D.R.	delivery room	Hb(Hgb)	hemoglobin
drsg.	dressing	HCL	hydrochloric
DSD	dry sterile dressing	Hct	hematocrit
DTs	delirium tremens	Hg	mercury
DTR	deep tendon reflex	HMD	hyaline membrane disease
D/W	dextrose and water	h/o	history of
Dx	diagnosis	HPI	history of present illness
		H.R.	heart rate
ECG, EKG	electrocardiogram	h.s.	hour of sleep
ECT	electroconvulsive therapy	ht	height
EDC	estimated date of	HT	hypertension
	confinement	Hx	history
EEG	electroencephalogram		
e.g.	for example	ICF	intracellular fluid
elix.	elixir	ICU	Intensive Care Unit
E.R.	emergency room	ID	intradermal
E.S.P.	extrasensory perception	I&D	incision and drainage
ESR	erythrocyte sedimentation	i.e.	that is
	rate	IM	intramuscular
et al.	and others	inj	injection
ext.	extract	I&O	intake and output
		IPPB	intermittent positive
f	frequency; female		pressure breathing
F	fahrenheit	IQ	intelligence quotient

IU	international unit	NSVD	normal spontaneous vaginal delivery
IUD	intrauterine device		
IV	intravenous	nullip	nullipara
IVP	intravenous pyelogram	N&V	nausea and vomiting
K	potassium	OA	occiput anterior
kg	kilogram	OB, Obs	obstetrics
		O.C.	oral contraceptive
L	left; liter	od	daily
lap	laparotomy	OD	right eye; overdose
lb	pound	OOB	out of bed
LE	lupus erythematosis	OP	occiput posterior
LGA	large for gestational age	OPD	outpatient department
LH	luteinizing hormone	O.R.	operating room
liq	liquid	Ortho	orthopedics
LLQ	left lower quadrant	os	opening
LMP	last menstrual period	OS	left eye
LOA	left occiput anterior	OT	occupational therapy
LOP	left occiput posterior	oz	ounce
LOT	left occiput transverse		
LP	lumbar puncture	p̄	after
LUQ	left upper quadrant	P	para; pulse
l&w	living and well	PA	physician's assistant
		Pap	Papanicolaou smear
m	meter	para	number of pregnancies
mEq	milliequivalent	path	pathology
mg	milligram	PBI	protein bound iodine
MI	myocardial infarction	p.c.	after meals
min	minute; minim	PE	physical examination
ml	milliliter	per	by; through
mm	millimeter	PERLA	pupils equal and reactive to light and accommodation
MS	multiple sclerosis		
MSU	midstream urine	P.H.	past history
multip	multipara	PI	present illness
		PID	pelvic inflammatory disease
NB	note carefully; newborn	PKU	phenylketonuria
neg	negative	p.m.	afternoon
neuro	neurology	P.O.R.	problem oriented record
N-G	nasogastric	pos	positive
nil	none	postop	postoperative
no.	number	preop	preoperative
noct	at night	prep	preparation
NPN	non protein nitrogen	p.r.	per rectum
NPO	nothing by mouth	p.r.n.	when needed
NS	normal saline		

pro time	prothrombin time	SIDS	sudden infant death syndrome
PSP	phenolsulfon phthalein		
pt	patient, pint	sig	label
PT	physical therapy	SOB	shortness of breath
PTA	prior to admission	s̄s̄	one half
PVC	premature ventricular contraction	SSE	soap suds enema
		stat	immediately
		Sx	symptoms
q.	every		
q.d.	every day	TB	tuberculosis
q.h.	every hour	Tbsp.; T.	tablespoon
q.h.s.	at bedtime	t.i.d.	three times a day
q.i.d.	4 times a day	TLC	tender loving care
q.o.d.	every other day	t.o.	telephone order
qt	quart	TPR	temperature, pulse, respiration
R, Rt	right	tsp	teaspoon
RBC	red blood cell	TUR	transurethral resection
RDS	respiratory distress syndrome	U	unit
REM	rapid eye movement	U/A	urinalysis
Rh	Rhesus factor	ung	ointment
RHD	rheumatic heart disease	URI	upper respiratory infection
RLQ	right lower quadrant	UTI	urinary tract infection
RNA	ribonucleic acid	vag	vaginal
R/O	rule out	VD	venereal disease
ROA	right occiput anterior	VDRL	venereal disease research laboratory
ROM	range of motion		
ROP	right occiput posterior	Vit	vitamin
ROT	right occiput transverse	v.o.	verbal order
RR	respiratory rate; recovery room	vol	volume
		VS	vital signs
RUQ	right upper quadrant		
Rx	therapy; treatment	WBC	white blood cell
		WC	wheelchair
s̄	without	WDWN	well developed, well nourished
sc	subcutaneous		
SD	standard deviation	WNL	within normal limits
sg	specific gravity	wt	weight
SGA	small for gestational age